Decision Making in
Reproductive Endocrinology

*We wish to dedicate this book
to our families whose support and concern was,
and is, so important to us*

Decision Making in Reproductive Endocrinology

EDITED BY

WILLIAM D. SCHLAFF

Chief, Section of Reproductive Endocrinology;
Associate Professor, Department of Obstetrics and Gynecology,
Division of Reproductive Endocrinology,
University of Colorado Health Sciences Center,
Denver, Colorado

JOHN A. ROCK

James Robert McCord Professor,
Chairman, Department of Gynecology and Obstetrics,
The Emory University School of Medicine,
Thomas K. Glenn Memorial Hospital,
Atlanta, Georgia

BOSTON
Blackwell Scientific Publications
OXFORD LONDON EDINBURGH MELBOURNE PARIS BERLIN VIENNA

© 1993 by
Blackwell Scientific Publications, Inc.
Editorial offices:
238 Main Street, Cambridge
  Massachusetts 02142, USA
Osney Mead, Oxford OX2 0EL, England
25 John Street, London WC1N 2BL
  England
23 Ainslie Place, Edinburgh EH3 6AJ
  Scotland
54 University Street, Carlton
  Victoria 3053, Australia

Other editorial offices:
Librairie Arnette SA
2, rue Casimir-Delavigne
75006 Paris
France

Blackwell Wissenschafts-Verlag
Meinekestrasse 4
D-1000 Berlin 15
Germany

Blackwell MZV
Feldgasse 13
A-1238 Wien
Austria

All rights reserved. No part of this book may be
reproduced in any form or by any electronic or
mechanical means, including information storage and
retrieval systems, without permission in writing from
the publisher, except by a reviewer who may quote brief
passages in a review.

First published 1993

Set by Setrite Typesetters Ltd, Hong Kong
Printed and bound in the United States of America by
Maple-Vail Book Manufacturing Group, Binghamton,
New York

93 94 95 96 5 4 3 2 1

DISTRIBUTORS

USA
  Blackwell Scientific Publications, Inc.
  238 Main Street, Cambridge
  Massachusetts, 02142
  (*Orders:* Tel: 800 759–6102
               617 876–7000)

Canada
  Times Mirror Professional Publishing
  130 Flaska Drive
  Markham, Ontario L6G 1B8
  (*Orders:* Tel: 800 268–4178
               416 470–6739)

Australia
  Blackwell Scientific Publications Pty Ltd
  54 University Street
  Carlton, Victoria 3053
  (*Orders:* Tel: 03 347–5552)

Outside North America and Australia
  Marston Book Services Ltd
  PO Box 87
  Oxford OX2 0DT
  (*Orders:* Tel: 0865 791155
               Fax: 0865 791927
               Telex: 837515)

Library of Congress Cataloging-in-Publication Data
Decision making in reproductive endocrinology/
  edited by William D. Schlaff, John A. Rock.
      p.   cm.
   Includes bibliographical references and index.
   ISBN 0–86542–214–1
   1. Endocrine gynecology — Decision making.
   2. Obstetrical endocrinology — Decision making.
   3. Infertility — Treatment — Decision making.
   I. Schlaff, William D.
   II. Rock, John A.
      [DNLM: 1. Decision Making.
   2. Endocrine Diseases — diagnosis.
   3. Endocrine Diseases — therapy.
   4. Genital Diseases, Female — diagnosis.
   5. Genital Diseases, Female — therapy.
   6. Infertility — diagnosis.
   7. Infertility — therapy.
   WP 140 D294]
   RG159.D43 1993
   618.1 — dc20
   DNLM/DLC

Contents

CONTENTS

CONTENTS

CONTENTS

Contributors

SEZER AKSEL MD
Director, Professor, Division of Reproductive Endocrinology, Department of Obstetrics and Gynecology, University of South Alabama College of Medicine, Mobile, Alabama

BRUCE H. ALBRECHT MD
Medical Director, Conceptions, Reproductive Technology Consultants; Assistant Clinical Professor, Department of Obstetrics and Gynecology, University of Colorado Health Sciences Center, Denver, Colorado

MARIA D. ALLO MD
Chairperson, Clinical Associate Professor, Department of Surgery, Santa Clara Valley Medical Center, San Jose, California

RICARDO H. ASCH MD
Director, Center for Reproductive Health; Professor, Department of Obstetrics and Gynecology; Assistant Dean, University of California at Irvine, Orange, California

SUZAN A. AYDINEL PhD
Director, Counseling and Psychological Research, Department of Obstetrics and Gynecology, Georgetown University Medical Center, Washington, DC

RICARDO AZZIZ MD
Associate Professor, Department of Obstetrics and Gynecology, University of Alabama School of Medicine, Birmingham, Alabama

THEODORE A. BARAMKI MD, FACOG
Head, Division of Reproductive Endocrinology, Greater Baltimore Medical Center; Associate Professor, Division of Reproductive Endocrinology, Department of Gynecology and Obstetrics, Johns Hopkins University School of Medicine, Baltimore, Maryland

GEORGE BETZ MD, PhD
Director, Department of Reproductive Endocrinology, Colorado Permanente Medical Group; Clinical Professor, University of Colorado, Denver, Colorado

RICHARD E. BLACKWELL PhD, MD
Director, Division of Reproductive Biology and Endocrinology; Professor of Obstetrics and Gynecology, University of Alabama School of Medicine, Birmingham, Alabama

KAREN D. BRADSHAW MD
Assistant Professor, Division of Reproductive Endocrinology, Department of Obstetrics and Gynecology, University of Texas Southwestern Medical Center, Dallas, Texas

ELY BRAND BS, MS, MD, FACOG, FACS
Director, Gynecologic Oncology, Assistant Professor, Department of Obstetrics and Gynecology, University of Colorado Health Sciences Center and Cancer Center, Denver, Colorado

EMMETT F. BRANIGAN MD
Assistant Professor, Department of Obstetrics and Gynecology, University of Washington Medical Center, Seattle, Washington

JAN M. BRUDER MD
Instructor, Division of Endocrinology, Department of Medicine, University of Colorado Health Sciences Center, Denver, Colorado

RONALD T. BURKMAN MD
C. Paul Hodgkinson, Chairman, Department of Obstetrics and Gynecology, Henry Ford Hospital, Detroit, Michigan

WILLIAM J. BUTLER MD
Medical Director, Center for Cancer Treatment and Research, Richland Memorial Hospital, Columbia, South Carolina

BRUCE R. CARR MD
Paul C. MacDonald Professor of Obstetrics and Gynecology, Division of Reproductive Endocrinology, Department of Obstetrics and Gynecology, University of Texas Southwestern Medical Center, Dallas, Texas

CONTRIBUTORS

SANDRA A. CARSON MD
Assistant Professor, Department of Obstetrics and Gynecology, University of Tennessee Health Science Center, Memphis, Tennessee

PETER R. CASSON MD
Assistant Professor, Department of Obstetrics and Gynecology, University of Tennessee Health Science Center, Memphis, Tennessee

MARCELLE I. CEDARS MD
Director, Center for Reproductive Health, Assistant Professor, Department of Obstetrics and Gynecology, University of Cincinnati Medical Center, Cincinnati, Ohio

GRACE M. CENTOLA PhD
Director, Andrology Laboratory and Rochester Regional Cryobank; Associate Professor, Department of Obstetrics and Gynecology, University of Rochester Medical Center, Rochester, New York

CHARLES C. CODDINGTON MD
Associate Professor, Department of Obstetrics and Gynecology, Eastern Virginia Medical School, Norfolk, Virginia

ANDREW S. COOK MD
Fertility Physicians of California, Fremont, California

DOUGLAS C. DALY MD
Director, Department of Reproductive Endocrinology, Blodgett Memorial Medical Center, Grand Rapids, Michigan; Clinical Associate Professor, Department of Obstetrics and Gynecology, Michigan State University

MARIAN D. DAMEWOOD MD
Associate Professor, Division of Reproductive Endocrinology, Department of Gynecology and Obstetrics, The Johns Hopkins University School of Medicine; Director, Women's Hospital Fertility Center, Baltimore, Maryland

RICHARD B. DAMEWOOD MD
Instructor in General Surgery, The Johns Hopkins School of Medicine; General Surgeon, Owing Mills, Maryland

M. YUSOFF DAWOOD MB, ChB, MMed, MD, FRCOG
Berel Held Professor, Director, Division of Reproductive Endocrinology, Department of Obstetrics, Gynecology, and Reproductive Sciences, University of Texas Medical School at Houston, Houston, Texas

MICHAEL P. DIAMOND MD
Associate Professor, Departments of Obstetrics and Gynecology and Surgery; Director, Division of Reproductive Endocrinology and Infertility, Vanderbilt University Medical Center, Nashville, Tennessee

RICHARD P. DICKEY MD, PhD
Clinical Professor and Director, Reproductive Endocrinology/ Infertility Service, Department of Obstetrics and Gynecology, Tulane University School of Medicine, New Orleans, Louisiana

JANETTE DURHAM MD
Assistant Professor, Department of Radiology, University of Colorado Health Sciences Center, Denver, Colorado

JILL T. FLOOD MD
Director, Beach Center for Infertility, Endocrinology and IVF, Virginia Beach, Virginia

GIRAUD V. FOSTER MD, PhD
Associate Professor, Department of Obstetrics and Gynecology, The Johns Hopkins University School of Medicine, Baltimore, Maryland

GARY FRISHMANN MD
Assistant Professor, Department of Obstetrics and Gynecology, Division of Reproductive Endocrinology Women's and Infants' Hospital, Providence, Rhode Island

RONALD S. GIBBS MD
Professor, Chairman, Department of Obstetrics and Gynecology, University of Colorado Health Sciences Center, Denver, Colorado

MARK GIBSON BS, MD
Professor, Chairman, Department of Obstetrics and Gynecology, West Virginia University, Morgantown, West Virginia

KENNETH A. GINSBURG MD
Assistant Director, Division of Reproductive Endocrinology and Infertility, Associate Professor, Department of Obstetrics and Gynecology, Hutzel Hospital/Wayne State University School of Medicine, Detroit, Michigan

DAVID S. GUZICK MD, PhD
Director, University of Pittsburgh School of Medicine, Magee-Women's Hospital, Pittsburgh, Pennsylvania

JOUKO K. HALME MD, PhD
Associate Professor, Division of Reproductive Endocrinology and Fertility, Department of Obstetrics and Gynecology, University of North Carolina School of Medicine, Chapel Hill, North Carolina

CHARLES B. HAMMOND MD
E.C. Hamblen Professor and Chairman, Department of Obstetrics and Gynecology, Duke University Medical Center, Durham, North Carolina

MARY G. HAMMOND MD
Associate Professor, Department of Obstetrics and Gynecology; Director, Division of Reproductive Endocrinology, University of North Carolina School of Medicine, Chapel Hill, North Carolina

RAY V. HANING JR MD
Director, Department of Reproductive Endocrinology, Brown University School of Medicine, Providence, Rhode Island

LISA J. HANSARD MD
Chief Resident, Department of Obstetrics and Gynecology, The University of Texas Health Sciences Center at San Antonio, San Antonio, Texas

JOHN HARRINGTON MD
Assistant Director, Department of Reproductive Endocrinology, Colorado Permanente Medical Group; Assistant Clinical Professor, University of Colorado, Denver, Colorado

JOHN S. HESLA MD
Assistant Professor, Director of Operative Endoscopy, Division of Reproductive Endocrinology, Department of Gynecology and Obstetrics, The Johns Hopkins University School of Medicine, Baltimore, Maryland

JOSEPH A. HILL MD
Associate Professor, Fearing Research Laboratory, Department of Obstetrics, Gynecology, and Reproductive Biology, Brigham and Women's Hospital, Harvard Medical School, Boston, Massachusetts

BRADLEY S. HURST MD
Assistant Professor, Division of Reproductive Endocrinology, Department of Obstetrics and Gynecology, University of Colorado Health Sciences Center, Denver, Colorado

GABOR B. HUSZAR MD
Director, Sperm Physiology Laboratory, Department of Obstetrics and Gynecology, Yale University School of Medicine, New Haven, Connecticut

JONATHAN P. JAROW MD, FACS
Associate Professor (Urology), Bowman Gray School of Medicine, Winston-Salem, North Carolina

JULIA V. JOHNSON MD
Assistant Professor, Division of Reproductive Endocrinology and Infertility, Department of Obstetrics and Gynecology, University of Vermont College of Medicine, Burlington, Vermont

OLIVER W. JONES, III MD
Assistant Professor, Department of Obstetrics and Gynecology, University of Colorado Health Sciences Center, Denver, Colorado

EUGENE KATZ MD
Division of Reproductive Endocrinology, Greater Baltimore Medical Center, Baltimore, Maryland

DAVID L. KEENAN MD
Assistant Professor, Department of Obstetrics and Gynecology, Emory University, Atlanta, Georgia

DANIEL KENIGSBERG MD
Clinical Associate Professor, State University of New York at Stony Brook; Long Island IVF, Port Jefferson, New York

WILLIAM R. KEYE JR MD
Director, Division of Reproductive Endocrinology and Infertility; Director, in vitro Fertilization Program, William Beaumont Hospital; Clinical Associate Professor, Department of Obstetrics and Gynecology, University of Michigan, Royal Oak, Michigan

SIMON KIPERSZTOK MD
Assistant Professor, Division of Reproductive Endocrinology and Fertility, Department of Obstetrics and Gynecology, University of Florida College of Medicine, Gainesville, Florida

NANCY A. KLEIN MD
Assistant Instructor, Division of Reproductive Endocrinology, Department of Obstetrics and Gynecology, University of Texas Health Sciences Center at San Antonio, San Antonio, Texas

OSCAR A. KLETZKY MD
Professor, Chief, Division of Reproductive Endocrinology, Department of Obstetrics and Gynecology, Harbor—UCLA Medical Center, Torrance, California

GEORGEANNA J. KLINGENSMITH MD
Associate Professor, Division of Pediatric Endocrinology, Children's Hospital, Denver, Colorado

GEORGE T. KOULIANOS MD
Assistant Professor, Division of Reproductive Endocrinology and Infertility, Department of Obstetrics and Gynecology, University of South Alabama, Mobile, Alabama

PETER A. LEE MD, PhD
Professor, Department of Pediatrics, University of Pittsburgh School of Medicine, Children's Hospital of Pittsburgh, Pittsburgh, Pennsylvania

BARBARA S. LEVY MD
Clinical Assistant Professor, Department of Obstetrics and Gynecology, University of Washington School of Medicine, Seattle, Washington

CONTRIBUTORS

ANTHONY A. LUCIANO MD
*Director of Reproductive Endocrinology and Infertility;
Associate Professor of Obstetrics and Gynecology, University
of Connecticut Health Center, Farmington, Connecticut*

HOWARD D. McCLAMROCK MD
*Assistant Professor, Division of Reproductive Endocrinology,
Department of Obstetrics and Gynecology, University of
Maryland School of Medicine, Baltimore, Maryland*

EDROY McMILLAN MD
*Department of Obstetrics and Gynecology, White Memorial
Medical Center, Los Angeles, California*

SANFORD M. MARKHAM MD
*Assistant Professor, Department of Obstetrics and
Gynecology, Georgetown University School of Medicine,
Washington, DC*

GEORGE B. MAROULIS MD
*Professor, Department of Obstetrics and Gynecology;
Director, Reproductive Endocrinology and Infertility,
University of South Florida College of Medicine, Tampa,
Florida*

DAN C. MARTIN MD
*Reproductive Surgeon, Clinical Associate Professor, Baptist
Memorial Hospital, University of Tennessee, Memphis,
Tennessee*

RANDALL B. MEACHAM MD
*Assistant Professor, Division of Urology, Department of
Surgery, University of Colorado Health Sciences Center,
Denver, Colorado*

DAVID R. MELDRUM MD
*Clinical Professor, Center for Advanced Reproductive Care,
UCLA School of Medicine, Redendo Beach, California*

AMIN A. MILKI MD
*Assistant Professor, Department of Gynecology and
Obstetrics, Stanford University Medical Center, Stanford,
California*

YOMNA T. MONLA MD
*Fellow, Division of Endocrinology, Department of Internal
Medicine, Baylor College of Medicine, Houston, Texas*

ARLENE J. MORALES MD
*Assistant Professor, Department of Reproductive Medicine,
University of California School of Medicine, San Diego, La
Jolla, California*

ANN MORRILL MD
*Fellow, Division of Endocrinology, Department of Medicine,
The Johns Hopkins University School of Medicine, Baltimore,
Maryland*

DEAN M. MOUTOS MD
*Assistant Professor, Department of Obstetrics and
Gynecology, University of Arkansas for Medical Science,
Little Rock, Arkansas*

ANA A. MURPHY MD
*Assistant Professor, Department of Reproductive Medicine,
University of California School of Medicine, San Diego, La
Jolla, California*

DENISE L. MURRAY MD
*Fellow, Division of Reproductive Endocrinology, Department
of Gynecology and Obstetrics, The Johns Hopkins University
School of Medicine, Baltimore, Maryland*

RONALD M. NELSON MD
*Chairman, Department of Obstetrics and Gynecology, White
Memorial Medical Center, Los Angeles, California*

MILES J. NOVY MD, FACOG
*Director, Division of Reproductive Endocrinology and
Infertility, Professor, Department of Obstetrics and
Gynecology, Oregon, Health Sciences University, Portland,
Oregon*

DAVID L. OLIVE MD
*Associate Professor, Director of Reproductive Endocrinology,
Department of Obstetrics and Gynecology, Yale University
School of Medicine, New Haven, Connecticut*

STEVEN J. ORY MD
*Associate Professor, Consultant Chairman, Section of
Reproductive Endocrinology and Fertility, Department of
Obstetrics and Gynecology, Mayo Clinic, Rochester,
Minnesota*

SANTIAGO L. PADILLA MD
Director, Fertility Center of Maryland, Towson, Maryland

PASQUALE PATRIZIO MD
*Research Fellow, Division of Reproductive Endocrinology,
Department of Obstetrics and Gynecology, University of
California at Irvine, Orange, California*

MICHELLE PETRI MD, MPH
*Associate Professor, Division of Molecular and Clinical
Rheumatology, The Johns Hopkins University School of
Medicine, Baltimore, Maryland*

CONTRIBUTORS

SUSAN POKORNY MD
Assistant Professor, Department of Obstetrics and Gynecology and Pediatrics, Baylor College of Medicine, Houston, Texas

MARY L. POLAN MD, PhD
Professor, Chairman, Department of Gynecology and Obstetrics, Stanford University Medical Center, Stanford, California

JOHN F. RANDOLPH, JR MD
Chief, Division of Reproductive Endocrinology; Associate Professor, Department of Obstetrics and Gynecology, University of Michigan Medical School, Ann Arbor, Michigan

JOHN T. REPKE MD
Associate Professor, Departments of Obstetrics and Gynecology and Reproductive Biology, Harvard Medical School; Medical Director, Labor and Delivery, Brigham and Women's Hospital, Boston, Massachusetts

ELI RESHEF MD
Assistant Professor, Department of Obstetrics and Gynecology, University of Oklahoma Health Sciences Center, Oklahoma City, Oklahoma

DANIEL RIDDICK MD
Professor and Chairman, Department of Obstetrics and Gynecology, University of Vermont School of Medicine, Burlington, Vermont

JOHN A. ROCK MD
James Robert McCord Professor, Chairman, Department of Gynecology and Obstetrics, The Emory University School of Medicine, Thomas K. Glenn Memorial Hospital, Atlanta, Georgia

GREGORY F. ROSEN MD, MS
Assistant Professor, Division of Reproductive Endocrinology and Infertility, Department of Obstetrics and Gynecology, University of California Medical School, Long Beach, California

GEORGE R. SAADE MD
Clinical Instructor, Department of Obstetrics and Gynecology, Baylor College of Medicine, Houston, Texas

WENDY J. SCHERZER MD
Assistant Professor, Division of Reproductive Endocrinology, Department of Obstetrics and Gynecology, University of Maryland School of Medicine, Baltimore, Maryland

WILLIAM D. SCHLAFF MD
Chief, Section of Reproductive Endocrinology; Associate Professor, Department of Obstetrics and Gynecology, Division of Reproductive Endocrinology, University of Colorado Health Sciences Center, Denver, Colorado

PETER N. SCHLEGEL MD
Assistant Professor, Division of Urology, Department of Surgery, New York Hospital–Cornell University Medical Center; Staff Scientist, Center for Biomedical Research, The Population Council, New York, New York

MINNA R. SELUB MD
Assistant Professor, Division of Reproductive Endocrinology and Infertility, Department of Obstetrics and Gynecology, Duke University Medical Center, Durham, North Carolina

FAYEK SHAMMA MD
Postdoctoral Associate, Division of Reproductive Endocrinology, Department of Obstetrics and Gynecology, Yale University School of Medicine, New Haven, Connecticut

ALVIN M. SIEGLER MD, DSc
Professor, Department of Obstetrics and Gynecology, Health Science Center at Brooklyn, State University of New York, Brooklyn, New York

KAYLEN M. SILVERBERG MD
Assistant Professor, Department of Obstetrics and Gynecology, University of Texas Health Sciences Center, San Antonio, Texas

JAMES A. SIMON MD
Chief, Division of Reproductive Endocrinology, Department of Obstetrics and Gynecology, Georgetown University Medical Center, Washington, DC

MICHAEL R. SOULES MD
Professor and Director, Division of Reproductive Endocrinology and Infertility, Department of Obstetrics and Gynecology, University of Washington Medical Center, Seattle, Washington

DANIEL I. SPRATT MD
Associate Professor, Division of Endocrinology, Department of Internal Medicine, Maine Medical Center and University of Vermont, Portland, Maine

KENNETH A. STEINGOLD MD
Director, Fertility Institute of Virginia, Richmond, Virginia

ROBERT J. STILLMAN MD
Director, Division of Reproductive Endocrinology and Fertility; Professor, Department of Obstetrics and Gynecology, George Washington University Medical Center, Washington, DC

CONTRIBUTORS

RONALD C. STRICKLER MD
Professor, Department of Obstetrics and Gynecology, Director, Division of Reproductive Endocrinology, Washington University School of Medicine; Chief, Department of Obstetrics and Gynecology, The Jewish Hospital of St Louis, St Louis, Missouri

LUTHER M. TALBERT MD
Professor, Department of Obstetrics and Gynecology, University of North Carolina School of Medicine, Chapel Hill, North Carolina

IAN H. THORNEYCROFT PhD, MD
Professor, Chairman, Section of Reproductive Endocrinology, Department of Obstetrics and Gynecology, University of South Alabama, Mobile, Alabama

AMY S. THURMOND MD
Assistant Professor, Department of Radiology, Obstetrics, and Gynecology; Director, Women's Imaging and Ultrasound, Oregon Health Sciences University, Portland, Oregon

BRUCE L. TJADEN DO
Chief, Department of Obstetrics and Gynecology, David Grant USAF Medical Center, Travis Air Force Base, California

MARIA D. URBAN MD
Associate Professor, Department of Pediatrics, Wright State University School of Medicine; Director of Pediatric Endocrinology, The Children's Medical Center, Dayton, Ohio

WULF H. UTIAN MB, BCh, PhD, FRCOG, FACOG, FICS
Arthur H. Bill Professor, Chairman, Department of Reproductive Biology, Case Western Reserve University, Cleveland, Ohio

RAFAEL F. VALLE MD
Associate Professor, Department of Obstetrics and Gynecology, Northwestern University Medical School, Chicago, Illinois

EDWARD E. WALLACH MD
Professor, Chairman, Department of Gynecology and Obstetrics, The Johns Hopkins University School of Medicine, Baltimore, Maryland

GARY S. WAND MD
Associate Professor, Division of Endocrinology, Department of Medicine, The Johns Hopkins University School of Medicine, Baltimore, Maryland

JOSEPH R. WAX MD
Attending Perinatologist, Department of Obstetrics and Gynecology, US Naval Hospital, Portsmouth, Virginia

ANNE COLSTON WENTZ MD
Head, Section of Reproductive Endocrinology and Infertility; Professor, Department of Obstetrics and Gynecology, Northwestern University Medical School, Chicago, Illinois

MARGUERITTE M. WHITE MD
Assistant Professor, Department of Obstetrics and Gynecology, University of Colorado Health Sciences Center, Denver, Colorado

MARGARET E. WIERMAN MD
Assistant Professor, Division of Reproductive Endocrinology, Department of Medicine, University of Colorado Health Sciences Center, Denver, Colorado

ROBERT A. WILD MD
Associate Professor, Section of Reproductive Endocrinology and Infertility; Research Coordinator and Director of Laboratories; Department of Obstetrics and Gynecology; Adjunct Associate Professor, Department of Medicine (Cardiology), University of Oklahoma Health Sciences Center, Oklahoma City, Oklahoma

CRAIG A. WINKEL MD
Associate Professor, Vice Chairman, Department of Obstetrics and Gynecology; Director, Division of Reproductive Endocrinology, Thomas Jefferson Medical College, Philadelphia, Pennsylvania

RICHARD J. WORLEY MD
Associate Clinical Professor, Department of Obstetrics and Gynecology, University of Colorado Health Sciences Center

HOWARD A. ZACUR MD, PhD
Associate Professor, Department of Gynecology and Obstetrics; Director, Division of Reproductive Endocrinology, The Johns Hopkins University School of Medicine, Baltimore, Maryland

BERNARD E. ZELIGMAN MD
Associate Professor, Department of Radiology, University of Colorado Health Sciences Center, Denver, Colorado

MICHAEL J. ZINAMAN MD
Associate Professor, Chief, Division of Reproductive Endocrinology and Infertility, Department of Obstetrics and Gynecology, Loyola University Medical Center, Maywood, Illinois

Preface

Problem solving in reproductive endocrinology is commonly encountered in the outpatient office. At times it is useful to have a ready reference that outlines the decision making process for a particular sign or symptom of a medical illness. In the busy office setting it is in some instances impossible to review detailed discussions of pathophysiology and management alternatives. The goal of this text is to provide a symptom or complaint-oriented series of brief chapters which provide a less detailed review of pathophysiology, but a more explicit and detailed approach to the diagnosis and management of reproductive disorders.

We wish to thank warmly the many contributors of this book who distilled a large body of information in each specific area into a brief discussion and focused plan of action. We wish also to acknowledge the editorial assistance of Ms Anne Terry and Peggy LeBrun and the efforts of Ms Lu Ann Lacey in coordinating the entire project.

Finally, the authors sincerely hope our colleagues, residents, and students find this text useful in the daily management and care of their patients.

William D. Schlaff
John A. Rock

Part I
Pediatric and adolescent abnormalities

1

Precocious puberty

PETER A. LEE

INTRODUCTION

The question of precocious puberty arises when a girl younger than age 8 years presents with one or more of the following findings: breast development, sexual hair, and menstruation [1].

The approach to each of these presentations is discussed below. If precocious puberty is present, complete early maturation should be evident by development of breasts, nipples, and areola (at least Tanner stage 2), pubic hair development (pigmented coarse hairs characteristic of sexual hair — at least Tanner stage 2), genital maturation with fullness of the labia, increased vaginal mucous membrane secretion, and estrogenization (pink versus red appearance) of the vaginal mucosa and accelerated linear growth and maturation evidenced by an accelerated growth rate, often with tall stature for age (>95% for height) and a significantly (20–24 months >chronologic age) advanced skeletal age. When clinical findings of complete puberty are present, the underlying etiology should be determined (Table 1.1) before treatment is considered. If true precocious puberty is present, hormone secretion is characterized by pubertal levels of luteinizing hormone (LH) and follicle stimulating hormone (FSH) secreted in response to endogenous gonadotropin-releasing hormone (GnRH) in an episodic, sleep-related fashion and by a robust response to exogenous GnRH stimulation [2,3].

It is important to realize that it is not immediately obvious whether or not puberty is actually beginning in most patients who present with the chief complaint of early development. The majority of patients do not have unequivocal findings of puberty and only a minority are found to have complete sexual precocity. The most common presenting finding of female pubertal development is breast development (Tanner stage 2) and the majority of these patients have premature thelarche. Therefore, when a child presents before age 8 years with breast development, it is necessary to ascertain if this represents the first evidence of precocious puberty or not.

BREAST MATURATION

When a girl presents before 8 years of age with breast development (Figs 1.1 and 1.2), this may be the first evidence of any of the forms of isosexual precocious puberty or only *premature thelarche*.

Premature thelarche is early breast maturation which is commonly an isolated finding but may be accompanied by other indications of mild estrogen stimulation (e.g., clear vaginal secretions) without clear evidence of other pubertal development or progression. It most commonly presents during the first 2 or 3 years of life as a mild progression of normal neonatal breast development. Breast growth is apparently stimulated by the estrogen secretion which occurs with the limited growth and maturation of ovarian follicles characteristic of the infant and, to a lesser extent, of the childhood ovary. In some instances of premature thelarche, an ovarian cyst can be demonstrated by ultrasonography. Regression of the cyst is often followed by receding breast development.

Ovarian cysts may occur not only in association with premature thelarche but also with true or pseudoprecocious puberty (Table 1.1) including the autonomous pubertal development which occurs in the McCune–Albright syndrome or as an incidental finding of normal childhood. Most cysts are self-limited; regression is spontaneous. Vaginal bleeding may occur after estrogen withdrawal accompanying cyst regression. Surgical intervention is indicated if large size or other characteristics suggest that rupture is probable. Treatment with medroxyprogesterone or testolactone may be used for recurrent estrogen-producing cysts [4].

Table 1.1 Precocious puberty in females

Complete

Central (true) — GnRH-stimulated gonadotropin secretion
  Idiopathic
  Associated with CNS abnormalities
    Congenital anomalies
    Consequence of radiation, chemotherapy, or surgery
    Hydrocephalus*
    Hypothalamic hamartomas
    Inflammatory or postinflammatory lesions
    Abscess
    Encephalitis
    Granulomas
    Meningitis
    Neurofibromatosis (with optic gliomas)
    Prader—Willi syndrome
    Septo-optic dysplasia
    Tay—Sachs
    Trauma
    Tuberous sclerosis
    Tumors or space-occupying lesions
    Arachnoid cysts
    Astrocytomas
    Craniopharyngiomas
    Ependymomas
    Gliomas
    Pituitary adenomas
    Suprasellar cysts

Pseudo (peripheral) non-GnRH-stimulated
  Adrenal adenomas or carcinomas (estrogen-secreting)
  Exogenous sex steroid or gonadotropin
  Nonhypothalamic GnRH-stimulated gonadotropin
    Chronic primary hypothyroidism*
    hCG-secreting tumors
  Gonadotropin-independent puberty
    Follicular cysts†
    McCune—Albright syndrome†
  Ovarian tumors
    Granulosa cell, granulosa-theca cell tumors
    Luteomas, luteinized cysts
    Ovarian carcinomas

Incomplete

Premature thelarche
Premature adrenarche

GnRH, Gonadotropin-releasing hormone; CNS, central nervous system; hCG, human chorionic gonadotropin.
hCG, human chorionic gonadotropin.
* Regression may follow treatment of primary problem.
† Spontaneous remissions may occur.

Evaluation of early breast development (<age 8 years) (Fig. 1.1)

History

1 Construction of a growth chart (Fig. 1.3) to ascertain height for age at current and previous available ages.
2 Construction of a growth velocity chart (Fig. 1.4) or calculation of annualized growth rate (≥7 cm/year is excessive for childhood after 3 years of age).
3 Neurologic abnormalities — hydrocephalus, seizures, congenital, infectious or neoplastic lesions, central nervous system (CNS) surgery, radiation, chemotherapy, or trauma.
4 Endocrinologic abnormalities — signs, symptoms, or previous diagnosis of gonadal, pituitary, or thyroid disease.
5 Possible exposure to exogenous gonadotropin or estrogens topically, orally, or parentally.

Physical examination

1 Height, weight, arm span, upper—lower segment ratios.
2 Tanner breast (Fig. 1.2) and pubic hair stages.
3 Genital maturation and appearance of vaginal mucosa.
4 Fundoscopic, visual field, and neurologic examination.
5 Inspection of skin for:
  (a) Temperature and texture (hypothyroidism).
  (b) Pigmentation (neurofibromatosis, McCune—Albright)
  (c) Acne (pubertal finding or androgen excess).

Diagnostic studies (Fig. 1.1)

The choice of diagnostic studies is based on findings of history and physical examination.

If it is clear that the breast development is accompanied by pubertal genital and pubic hair maturation, the child should be assessed for complete precocious puberty, as outlined below.

If breast development is an isolated finding on physical examination, but tall stature or an accelerated growth rate is evident, a full precocious puberty evaluation is warranted. However, if there is no evidence for progression of breast development or acceleration of growth rate and a normal height for age, a tentative diagnosis of premature thelarche can be made. At least one subsequent evaluation within 4—6 months should be done to substantiate that conclusion. However, if breast development

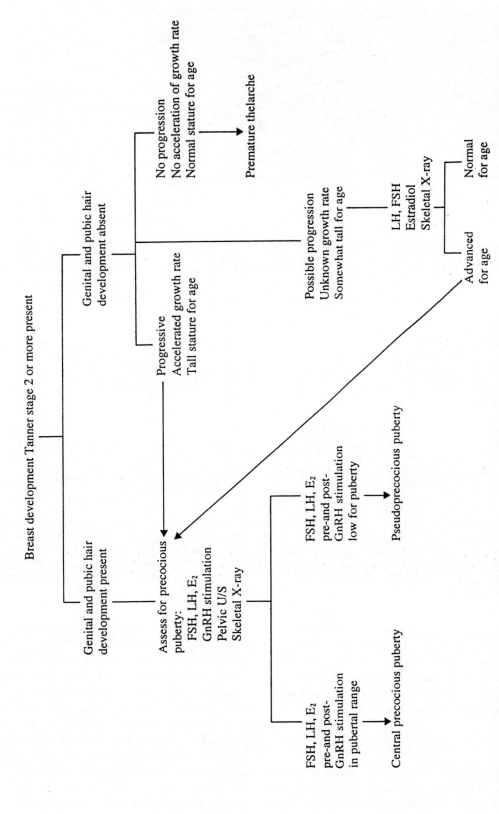

Fig. 1.1 Algorithm for assessment of pubertal development. E$_2$, estradiol; GnRH stim, GnRH stimulation test; U/S, ultrasound; skeletal X-ray, to determine bone age.

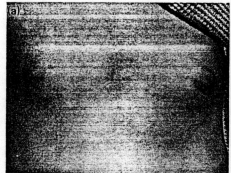
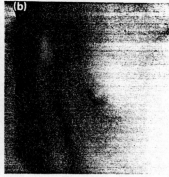

Fig. 1.2 Breast development (Tanner stage 3) of a 5 year old girl with idiopathic central sexual precocity (a), and (b) after regression to Tanner stage 2 at age 7 years after 2 years of GnRH analog therapy.

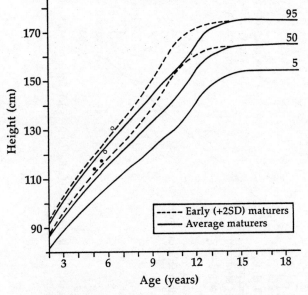
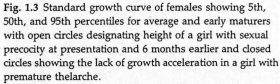

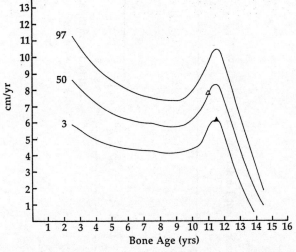

Fig. 1.3 Standard growth curve of females showing 5th, 50th, and 95th percentiles for average and early maturers with open circles designating height of a girl with sexual precocity at presentation and 6 months earlier and closed circles showing the lack of growth acceleration in a girl with premature thelarche.

Fig. 1.4 Female growth velocity chart showing velocity plotted for chronologic (open triangle) and bone age (closed triangle). While the velocity for the 11 year old is mean for age, the velocity for an 8 year old girl with sexual precocity while being mean for 8 years is only the 3rd percentile for her bone age of 11.75 years.

may have progressed, if growth rate cannot be documented, and particularly if the child is tall for age, basal hormone levels and bone age X-ray should be obtained. If hormone levels suggest that pubertal development or skeletal age is advanced, evaluation for sexual precocity should be pursued.

SEXUAL HAIR

Premature pubarche, the early growth of sexual (pubic or axillary) hair, may be the presenting finding of complete sexual precocity, disorders of androgen synthesis, but most commonly indicates premature adrenarche. *Premature adrenarche* is early onset of pubertal adrenal androgen secretion. Adrenarche is the gradual increase in the production of adrenal androgens, resulting in a progressive rise of circulating levels; sexual hair normally becomes apparent about 6 months after breast growth starts.

Evaluation of premature sexual hair is guided by concomitant findings: stature, growth acceleration, and other pubertal or virilizing effects. Early pubic hair resulting from adrenache may be an isolated finding or may be accompanied by other normal

6

pubertal androgen-mediated effects: acne, oily skin, body odor, and axillary hair. When the sexual hair is accompanied by no or minimal other findings, studies should include plasma dehydroepiandrosterone (DHEA) or DHEA sulfate (DHEAS) levels and skeletal age. If bone age is normal and DHEA or DHEAS levels are indicative of adrenarche, only reassessment of growth rate and pubertal development in 3–6 months is indicated. If there is excessive virilization, such as clitoromegaly, hirsutism, and severe acne, the differential diagnosis includes the congenital adrenal hyperplasias, adrenal and androgen-secreting ovarian tumors, and exogenous androgen. If premature sexual hair growth is accompanied by other findings associated with central sexual precocity, evaluation should be as indicated for that condition.

EARLY VAGINAL BLEEDING

Menarche in a child which is preceded by other early pubertal development should be assessed as precocious puberty. True precocious puberty can be expected to lead to premature menarche (<10 years of age), while withdrawal bleeding may occur in peripheral forms. Vaginal bleeding in a child without preceding pubertal development can be assumed not to be menstrual bleeding. While menstruation may be included as evidence for sexual precocity, vaginal bleeding occurring in the absence of other pubertal development is probably not hormonally caused. Causes include trauma with or without sexual abuse, foreign body, chronic irritation, infection, or sloughing of abnormal tissue. Rarely, endocrinopathies may be associated with such bleeding. The McCune Albright syndrome, chronic primary hyperthyroidism when it occurs in association with excessive prolactin, glycoprotein α-subunit and gonadotropin secretion, or ovarian cysts may cause enough estrogen stimulation to promote endometrial growth without breast development. Sudden cessation of this stimulation may be followed by vaginal discharge.

EVALUATION OF PRECOCIOUS PUBERTY

Pubertal development of breasts and pubic hair, accompanied by genital maturation and an accelerated growth rate, before 8 years of age constitutes *precocious puberty*.

If pubertal development is apparent, it is necessary to differentiate the underlying etiology and make a distinction between the following (Table 1.1):
— *Central* or *true precocious puberty* — normal physiologic pubertal hypothalamic–pituitary–ovarian (HPO) function occurring at an abnormally early age.
— *Pseudo-* or *peripheral precocious puberty* — sex steroid secretion or stimulation independent of hypothalamic GnRH–pituitary gonadotropin control.

Initial studies should document the degree of advanced maturity and differentiate central from peripheral causes:

1 *Plasma LH, FSH and estradiol* levels within the pubertal range suggest central puberty, although often pubertal patients will not have values from a single random sample above overlapping prepubertal–pubertal values. Inappropriately elevated estradiol levels for concomitantly obtained LH and FSH values suggest peripheral causes.

2 *Skeletal age X-ray*, an index of biologic age, serves as an index of maturity or advancement and as a baseline to document subsequent maturational rates.

3 *Pelvic ultrasound* will document ovarian and uterine size and symmetry, identify ovarian cysts and tumors, and, for central precocious puberty, should document symmetric increase in size of reproductive structures commensurate with pubertal development.

If all evidence suggests progressive normal but early puberty, *GnRH stimulation testing* and a head or magnetic resonance imaging (MRI) scan should be done. While episodic release of LH and FSH from nocturnal periodic sampling is indicative of central sexual precocity, this procedure is seldom needed to verify pubertal secretion.

1 GnRH testing with LH and FSH determinations before and periodically after an intravenous bolus of GnRH (100 mg of Factrel). The peak response of gonadotropins is generally within the first hour (Fig. 1.5). Appropriate sampling times are at 0, 20, 40, 60, and 90 min. In most gonadotropin assay systems, a greater FSH than LH response is typical of prepubertal girls while a robust response of LH is typical of puberty.

A mature gonadotropin response to GnRH stimulation confirms the diagnosis of central precocious puberty in a patient with premature onset and progression of physical pubertal characteristics including but not limited to breast and genital development, an accelerated growth rate, advanced bone age, and other hormone levels consistent with normal but early puberty.

2 *MRI scan* of the brain, with particular attention to the pituitary and hypothalamic area, should be done

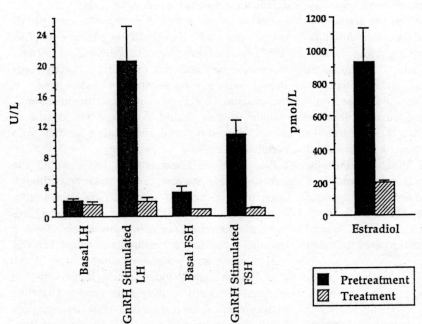

Fig. 1.5 Mean basal and GnRH stimulated peak LH and FSH values before and during GnRH analog therapy for 10 girls with central sexual precocity. Estradiol levels before and during treatment are shown on the right.

in all patients with central precocious puberty in whom the etiology is unknown. Although central precocious puberty in females is most commonly associated with no demonstrable abnormality (idiopathic), there may be CNS abnormalities (Table 1.1).

Hypothalamic hamartomas have been identified more frequently since the availability of MRI scans, often among those with onset of puberty at a very young age. Central sexual precocity may occur in association with other CNS tumors, such as astrocytomas and medulloblastomas, or as a consequence of the tumor therapy. More patients are surviving their primary condition, but as a consequence of radiotherapy and chemotherapy, sexual precocity may occur, often in association with hypothalamic–pituitary deficiencies, including human growth hormone. True sexual precocity may develop subsequent to CNS trauma or inflammation and in association with syndromes (e.g., neurofibromatosis with low-grade astrocytomas).

TREATMENT OF CENTRAL SEXUAL PRECOCITY

Indications

Treatment is indicated to prevent or alleviate the physical and psychologic consequences of untimely pubertal development. When central sexual precocity is present, the child can be expected to progress through puberty with a normal sequence with early onset of menses, premature deceleration of growth rate, and completion of growth. Untimely termination of growth may result in foreshortened adult height, because the onset of puberty is accompanied by a pubertal growth spurt with the accelerated growth rate beginning before the child is of normal pubertal height [1,2]. The increased sex steroid levels stimulate a disproportionately rapid maturation of skeletal maturity. This bone maturation, reflected by periodic bone age X-rays, outpaces the expected concomitant height increment. Adult height may be compromised in precocious puberty proportionate to the degree of advanced maturity of bone age.

The early pubertal development, tall stature during childhood, but short stature during adolescent years and adulthood may cause significant psychosocial problems; this is often precipitated by inappropriate reactions or expectations of others, particularly older persons.

Undesirable effects of normal but early puberty then include:

1 early physical pubertal maturation;
2 early menstruation;
3 tall stature for age;
4 diminished stature in adulthood;
5 psychosocial and psychologic problems;
6 increased risk of sexual abuse.

Before therapy is prescribed, however, *nonprogressive puberty* should be ruled out. This entity, an exception to the usual progressive precocious puberty, presents with characteristics of true precocious puberty — early physical development, a mature LH and FSH response to GnRH, rapid development, and growth with bone age advancement. However, this precocious development is not sustained; after a short time there is no further development or regression. To avoid therapy for this self-limiting condition, treatment for sexual precocity should not be begun unless progression has been documented for several months.

Therapy

The indicated treatment for any underlying abnormality associated with pubertal gonadotropin secretion, be it surgery, radiotherapy, or chemotherapy, should be completed before treatment of sexual precocity itself is considered. Decompression of the increased intracranial pressure associated with hyprocephalus may be accompanied by regression of pubertal development. Hypothalamic hamartomas associated with precocious puberty are composed of excessive GnRH-secreting neurons. They present without neurologic abnormalities and are not expected to cause problems other than the stimulatory effect upon episodic GnRH secretion. Because they have no other associated morbidity, no specific treatment is needed other than to treat the sexual precocity. If the tumor is completely pedunculated and the patient very young, surgical removal of the tumor may be a treatment option. Excision of the tumor by experienced neurosurgeons can be expected to be followed by cessation of pubertal hormonal secretion without other sequelae.

Specific treatment is indicated in most instances of progressive central precocious puberty. Indicated therapy is downregulation of pubertal gonadotropin secretion using gonadotropin-releasing hormone analogs (GnRHa) [3–5]. With persistent exposure of the pituitary to GnRHa, the episodic release of LH and FSH is obliterated, mean circulating gonadotropin levels fall, and consequently ovarian sex steroid production drops (Fig. 1.5). Progression of puberty stops; pubertal stages may regress. Menstruation, if present, ceases. Growth rate and skeletal maturity rate decelerate. A prepubertal status is restored.

Treatment ameliorates or precludes the development of psychologic problems and improves or preserves the height potential otherwise diminished if skeletal development exceeds concomitant statural growth.

A variety of GnRHa have been developed which have differing potency and duration of action (Table 1.2). These analogs are available for daily or monthly administration. Downregulation of the hypothalamic–pituitary–gonadal axis should be demonstrated by a minimal LH and FSH response to GnRH stimulation testing and prepubertal estradiol levels (Fig. 1.5) 4–8 weeks after initiating therapy and at 6-month intervals thereafter. Tanner staging, height, and skeletal age must also be monitored.

DIAGNOSIS AND TREATMENT OF PRECOCIOUS PSEUDOPUBERTY

When history, physical, and laboratory findings fail to confirm central precocious puberty or suggest an underlying peripheral cause, each potential etiology (Table 1.1) should be excluded. Levels of sex steroids and other adrenal steroids with visualization procedures (ultrasonography, CT, and MRI) of the adrenal glands and ovaries should identify tumors of these organs, and ovarian cysts. History should indicate exogenous hormone administration. Gonadotropin-producing tumors, exceptionally rare in girls, are suggested by markedly elevated levels of LH, FSH, or human chorionic gonadotropin. The McCune–Albright syndrome — the triad of café-au-lait areas of skin hyperpigmentation, polyostotic fibrous dysplasia, and autonomous endocrinopathies — is diagnosed by verification of these findings on physical examination, skeletal survey X-rays, and pubertal levels of estradiol with low gonadotropin levels before and after GnRH stimulation. The estrogen secretion is characterized by exacerbations which may be accompanied by ovarian cysts and remissions. Withdrawal bleeding may occur, occasionally as the presenting complaint. The exacerbations may be ameliorated by daily medroxyprogesterone therapy to suppress steroidogenesis or testolactone or flutamide by inhibiting aromatase or blocking estrogen synthesis [4]. Therapy for other forms of precocious pseudopuberty is that indicated to eliminate the underlying cause.

Table 1.2 Suppressive dosages of gonadotropin-releasing hormone (GnRH) analogs in true precocious puberty

GnRH analog	Dosages
Buserelin	20 µg/kg per day s.c.
Leuprolide acetate	300 µg/kg per 4 weeks depot
Nafarelin acetate	4 µg/kg per day s.c.

REFERENCES

1 Lee PA. Disorders of puberty. In: Lifshitz F, ed. *Second Edition Pediatric Endocrinology, A Clinical Guide*. New York: Marcel Dekker, 1990: 217–248.

2 Lee PA. Pubertal neuroendocrine maturation: early differentiation and stages of development. *Adolesc Pediatr Gynecol* 1988; 1: 3–12.

3 Loriaux DL. The pathophysiology of precocious puberty. *Hosp Pract* 1989; 55–61.

4 Kaplan SL. Grumbach MM. Pathophysiology and treatment of sexual precocity. *J Clin Endocrinol Metab* 1990; 71: 785–789.

5 Boepple PA. Mansfield MJ. Wierman ME *et al*. Use of potent, long-acting agonist of gonadotropin-releasing hormone in the treatment of precocious puberty. *Endocr Rev* 1986; 7: 24–33.

2

Delayed puberty

GEORGEANNA J. KLINGENSMITH

Puberty is considered to be delayed in the female when breast development or pubic hair has not appeared by 13 years of age and menarche has not occurred by 15.5–16 years. The pubertal process from the beginning of thelarche to menarche usually encompasses 18–36 months.

If this process has not been completed over a 48-month period, puberty is considered arrested and evaluation is recommended. This evaluation should follow the same guidelines as that recommended for delayed puberty.

The evaluation for pubertal delay is frequently initiated by the patient and/or her family because of social discomfort in peer relationships. Since male pubertal development lags behind the female by almost 2 years, physiologically delayed girls generally enter puberty in concert with their male peers. This decreases the social need for evaluation in girls with late pubertal development and frequently delays their presentation for diagnostic evaluation until well into the pathologic range.

The history and physical examination are directed toward elucidation of general health, family history for pubertal timing, eating behaviors, especially directed to symptoms of anorexia nervosa or bulimia, and evaluation for excessive physical training, as well as significant past illnesses and therapies. A review of past growth points plotted on normal growth grids is an important aspect of the initial evaluation. Growth retardation usually is associated with pubertal delay secondary to a physiologic delay of hypothalamic–pituitary–gonadal (HPG) maturation or delayed maturation secondary to chronic illness.

The physical examination should especially note any stigmata associated with syndromes of primary of secondary ovarian dysfunction (Table 2.1). Special attention should be directed to neurologic, ophthalmologic, and endocrine examinations and the documentation of the stage of sexual development according to Tanner.

Helpful initial laboratory evaluation includes an X-ray for skeletal maturation, a complete blood count, and a general chemistry survey that includes thyroxine (T4) and thyroid-stimulating hormone (TSH), and basal luteinizing hormone (LH) and follicle-stimulating hormone (FSH) levels.

CLASSIFICATION OF DELAYED PUBERTY

It is helpful to divide delayed puberty into that associated with low gonadotropin levels (indicative of delayed or absent maturation of the HPG axis) and pubertal delay associated with elevated gonadotropin levels (indicative of primary gonadal failure) (Fig. 2.1).

TEMPORARY GONADOTROPIN DEFICIENCY

Physiologic delay of the maturation of the HPG axis is the most frequent cause of pubertal delay and is a self-limiting problem which usually can be treated with reassurance and expectant waiting. However, the pathologic causes of delayed gonadotropin secretion listed in Table 2.1 must be ruled out, and permanent gonadotropin insufficiency must be excluded.

Excessive physical training is frequently considered in the differential diagnosis of secondary amenorrhea; it is less commonly a cause for delayed pubertal development. The most frequently encountered sport "culprits" at this age are figure-skating, ballet dancing, swimming, and gymnastics. Daily training of over 1 hour is usually required for suppression of hypothalamic maturation.

Anorexia nervosa and/or anorexia bulimia are also less common in this age group but may be associated with more significant psychopathology. Treatment may require a team approach with a dietitian and a medical physician as well as psychologist or psychiatrist.

Table 2.1 Delayed puberty in the female

Hypogonadotropic hypogonadism	Hypergonadotropic hypogonadism
Temporary gonadotropin deficiency	*Abnormalities in ovarian differentiation*
Constitutionally delayed maturation of HPG axis	Turner syndrome
Hypothyroidism	Pure gonadal dysgenesis
Excessive physical training	
Anorexia/malnutrition	*Defects in steroid synthesis and action*
Emotional and psychiatric illness	
Chronic illness	*Secondary defects in ovarian function*
	Surgical removal
Isolated gonadotropin deficiency	Radiation damage
Idiopathic	Infection
Kallmann's syndrome	Autoimmune ovarian failure
Prader—Willi—Lambert	Galactosemia, pseudohypoparathyroidism
Laurence—Moon—Biedl	
Multiple pituitary deficiencies	
Idiopathic	
CNS/pituitary tumor	
Following CNS radiation	
Following CNS trauma	

HPG, Hypothalamic—pituitary—gonadal; CNS, central nervous system.

Depression has been shown to disrupt normal hypothalamic—pituitary functioning. This may be endogenous or situational depression, usually associated with the loss of a family member or significant other through death or divorce. Children who are victims of abuse may have a similarly depressed hypothalamic—pituitary function.

Chronic illness may delay development secondary to the underlying disease process, its therapy, or a combination of the two. Steroid-dependent reactive airway disease is a good example of both the disease process and the therapy contributing to delayed growth and puberty. Many disease processes are amenable to therapy that improves function; this functional improvement is followed by an acceleration in growth velocity, weight gain, and pubertal development. Every attempt should be made to optimize medical management of the underlying chronic illness while pursuing the evaluation of pubertal delay.

PERMANENT HYPOGONADOTROPIC HYPOGONADISM

The differentiation of a temporary, or constitutional, delay in gonadotropin secretion from a permanent gonadotropin deficiency may be difficult. The early pubertal response to gonadotropin-releasing hormone (GnRH) is indistinguishable from that of permanent GnRH deficiency. Even a midpubertal response may not be different from that of a partial GnRH deficiency or partial pituitary insufficiency. Newer, more sensitive assays for LH and FSH may aid in the differentiation of complete GnRH deficiency from constitutionally delayed development, but the diagnosis of partial GnRH deficiency may require continued evaluation over time to document the gradual evolution of a maturing HPG axis.

Findings associated with syndromes with GnRH insufficiency (listed in Table 2.1) are helpful in the differentiation of GnRH deficiency from constitutionally delayed growth and development. Kallmann's syndrome, hereditary GnRH deficiency, and anosmia are discussed elsewhere.

Girls with Prader—Willi—Lambert syndrome are short, with a history of hypotonia and failure to thrive in early infancy, giving way to an excessive appetite and obesity in early childhood. The obesity and hyperphagia may become marked by 9—11 years of age and may be associated with glucose intolerance. In most cases, these patients have mild to marked mental retardation. Prader—Willi—Lambert syndrome is associated with a deletion on the short arm of chromosome 15. Magnetic resonance imaging (MRI) scans are normal.

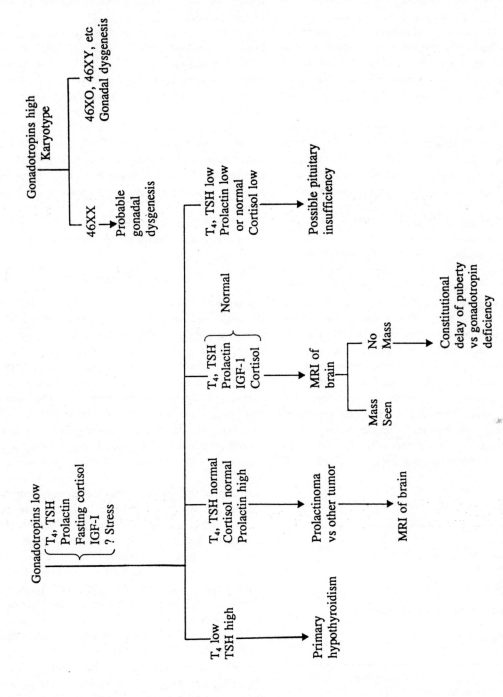

Fig. 2.1 Algorithm of delayed puberty.

CHAPTER 2

MULTIPLE PITUITARY HORMONAL DEFICIENCIES

When pubertal delay is marked, physiologic delay and isolated gonadotropin deficiency may be differentiated only over time. If permanent gonadotropin or GnRH deficiency is suspected, evaluation of other hypothalamic and pituitary hormonal deficits should be undertaken. This may require extensive hormonal testing (Table 2.2) and imaging of the hypothalamus and pituitary.

The history and physical examination in pituitary insufficiency will demonstrate a delay in growth velocity dating back to the onset of the disease process. If there is a history of central nervous system (CNS) irradiation for a CNS tumor or leukemia, complete hormonal evaluation of the hypothalamic–pituitary axis is in order. Eighty percent of such subjects will have some hormonal deficits and 20% will have multiple hormonal deficits. Any history of neurologic symptoms or ophthalmologic findings suggestive of a mass lesion of the hypothalamic–pituitary region should promptly initiate radiographic imaging of the area. At this time, MRI scans offer the best imaging technique for the hypothalamus and pituitary.

Craniopharyngiomas, optic gliomas, and hypothalamic dysgerminomas are the most common tumors causing hypothalamic–pituitary insufficiency in this age group. Rarely, prolactinomas have been reported to cause pubertal delay and primary amenorrhea. The evaluation for a prolactinoma in this age is not different from the evaluation of older patients. One should keep in mind that the stress

Table 2.2 Hormonal evaluation of the pituitary

T₄, free T₄, TSH
    If low T₄ and TSH, consider TRH test
Cortisol (fasting AM)
    ACTH testing if below 20
IGF-I
    Consider GH testing if clinically indicated
LH, FSH
    Consider GRH testing
Prolactin

T₄, thyroxine; TSH, thyroid-stimulating hormone; TRH, thyrotropin-releasing hormone; ACTH, adrenocorticotropic hormone; IGF-I, insulin-like growth factor-1; GH, growth hormone; LH, luteinizing hormone; FSH, follicle-stimulating hormone; GRH, gonadotropin releasing hormone.

of a venipuncture may cause a transient prolactin elevation in a normal subject. In equivocal cases, this may be resolved by drawing several samples from an indwelling line after the stress of the venipuncture has subsided.

The initial evaluation of the hypothalamus and pituitary can include a T4, free T4, TSH, morning cortisol, insulin-like growth factor-1 (IGF-1, somatomedin), and basal LH, FSH, and prolactin values. If abnormal or equivocal values are found, appropriate stimulation or suppression tests can be done (Table 2.2). As noted above, GnRH stimulation testing in the prepubertal subject is not likely to aid in the differentiation of physiologic delay from absolute GnRH deficiency and may not separate hypothalamic from pituitary dysfunction. As we gain more experience with newer and more sensitive assays for LH and FSH, the distinction between primary and secondary or tertiary gonadal failure may become easier.

TREATMENT

The treatment of delayed maturation of the HPG axis is usually reassurance and expectant waiting while directing specific treatment toward any pathologic etiology of delayed maturation. Rarely, very low-dose estrogen therapy is required to provide some physical maturation necessary for normalization of peer relationships and to improve the patient's self-esteem and image. This is usually given as ethinylestradiol, 100 ng/kg per day. Since this low dosage requires special preparation, a dose of 10 μg every other day has been used, but data to support this approach are limited.

If permanent gonadotropin deficiency is demonstrated, either isolated or in combination with other hormonal deficits, then estrogen replacement therapy should be initiated in the appropriate physiologic and psychosocial time frame. This is usually considered to be at a physiologic maturation of 11–13 years of age, as determined by skeletal maturation. When the chronologic age far exceeds the physiologic age, some compromise must be made so that pubertal development does not lag far behind the patient's peer group.

Treatment is best begun with ethinylestradiol, 100 ng/kg per day with increasing doses at 6–12-month intervals until full replacement therapy is achieved. Cyclic progesterone therapy, given as 5–10 mg of Provera for 10–12 days each month, should be initiated when breakthrough bleeding

14

is experienced or when the estrogen dose reaches one-half of the adult replacement level.

Appropriate counseling around issues of fertility needs to be addressed in girls with permanent gonadotropin deficiency. Options may include ovulation induction or *in vitro* fertilization with donor ova, as well as adoption.

PRIMARY GONADAL FAILURE

Elevated gonadotropin levels are the hallmark of primary gonadal failure. However, the rise in LH and FSH usually does not occur until the age of 10–12 years, the usual time for maturation of the HPG axis. In the normal state, as the axis matures, the gradual rise in gonadal estrogen and inhibin maintains a gradually increasing rise in LH and FSH until normal adult levels are achieved. In the absence of gonadal estrogen and inhibin, there is a dramatic rise in LH and FSH as the HPG axis matures until castrate levels of gonadotropins are achieved.

The most common cause for primary gonadal failure is Turner syndrome. Turner syndrome patients most frequently have a single X chromosome instead of the usual 46,XX female pattern. However, they may have a variety of X chromosomal abnormalities or even XO/XY mosaicism (referred to as mixed gonadal dysgenesis). Although the diagnosis may be anticipated by the characteristic phenotype, a confirming karyotype is essential since the presence of a Y chromosome predisposes to gonadoblastoma formation in the streak gonad.

In addition to streak gonads, patients with Turner syndrome have marked short stature, with growth failure usually beginning between 5 and 7 years of age. The findings listed in Table 2.3 are present in 70% or more of Turner syndrome patients, with the exception of the renal and cardiac malformations

Table 2.3 Somatic features of Turner syndrome

Gonadal dysgenesis
Short stature
Webbing of the neck/short, thick neck
High, narrow palate
Low-set, trident hairline
Shield-shaped chest
Cubitus valgus
Renal structural anomalies
Cardiac malformations

which are present in 50% and 25% of patients, respectively.

The renal abnormalities include duplication of the collecting system, a horseshoe kidney and, rarely, dysplastic kidneys. Renal ultrasound can usually identify any renal pathology.

Coarctation of the aorta is the most common cardiac lesion. Bicuspid aortic valve and/or mitral value prolapse occurs in 25–35% of patients. Patients with a bicuspid aortic valve require prophylactic antibiotics to prevent bacterial endocarditis. Teenagers and young adults may develop aortic dilatation which occasionally may progress to an aortic rupture. Careful cardiac follow-up may identify patients at risk for this complication so that appropriate intervention can be recommended.

Limited adult height has been the most consistent finding in Turner syndrome women, affecting 98% of subjects. Recent experiences have documented improved growth potential if recombinant growth hormone is given when growth deceleration occurs. If growth hormone is begun at this time, Turner syndrome girls maintain their height percentile during childhood, and induction of puberty can begin at 11–12 years of age. This allows puberty to progress in concert with peer development.

Lack of spontaneous pubertal development is anticipated in Turner syndrome girls but 5–15% of them will have spontaneous onset of puberty. This is somewhat more likely in mosaic patients but may occur in 45,X subjects. Pubertal arrest, irregular menses, or very early menopause usually follows spontaneous puberty. Thus, these patients need careful follow-up so that estrogen replacement can be given when needed. Rare cases of fertility have been reported.

TREATMENT

Induction of puberty can be accomplished using small doses of estrogen for 1–2 years, followed by a gradual increase until full adult replacement therapy is reached. This therapy should be delayed until maximal height has been achieved with recombinant human growth hormone treatment. Cyclic therapy with estrogen and progestin is important to prevent endometrial hyperplasia. The dose schedule suggested for hypogonadotropic hypogonadism is appropriate for patients with primary gonadal failure as well.

Pure gonadal dysgenesis is diagnosed in patients with streak gonads, normal female external and internal genitalia, a normal somatic phenotype, and either a 46,XX or 46,XY karyotype. Presentation is usually at the time of puberty with lack of pubertal development as the chief symptom. The diagnosis in 46,XY pure gonadal dysgenesis is made by the finding of elevated LH and FSH, low gonadal steroids, and a 46,XY karyotype in a phenotypically normal female. As with all dysgenetic gonads in association with a Y chromosome, malignant degeneration of the streak is common. The most common lesions are gonadoblastoma, dysgerminoma, and embryonal carcinoma. Malignancy can occur in the first decade; thus, complete removal of the streak with a wide margin is indicated at the time of diagnosis. The finding of gonadal steroid production in patients with pure gonadal dysgenesis is highly suggestive of a gonadoblastoma. Pure gonadal dysgenesis with a 46,XX karyotype may be difficult to differentiate from other causes of gonadal failure. Nevertheless, careful evaluation to determine the etiology of gonadal failure is important since there are a few case reports of dysgerminomas in 46,XX pure gonadal dysgenesis patients. In the absence of a clear etiology, laparoscopic examination of the gonads should be considered with removal of the streak gonads, if found.

The etiology of pure gonadal dysgenesis of either the XX or XY variety is unclear. Familial occurrence is not rare, and improved techniques of DNA probing of the XY chromosomes may be informative in some familial cases. Treatment is surgical removal of the streak gonad. Following gonadectomy, estrogen replacement therapy can be instituted. If the patient has reached a satisfactory adult height, the estrogen dose can be increased from an initial low dose to full replacement therapy over a 3–6-month period. Cyclic progestin should be included with the initiation of the estrogen schedule since estrogen may cause rapid maturation of the endometrium. If the diagnosis is made in a younger patient, the low-dose estrogen schedule suggested for patients with other forms of pubertal delay can be initiated at 11–12 years of age.

Defects in gonadal steroid synthesis or action will result in a picture of primary gonadal failure with lack of pubertal development. Defects in 17 α-hydroxylase and 17–20 desmolase will prevent sex steroid synthesis. These are rare disorders. A defect in 17 α-hydroxylase results in increased levels of deoxycorticosterone, a mineralocorticoid. This causes sodium retention and hypertension. When these disorders are present in an XY individual, the testis forms normally and produces Müllerian-inhibiting factor, causing regression of the Müllerian structures. Failure of testosterone synthesis in utero results in female-appearing external genitalia with a blind vaginal pouch. Sex assignment and rearing are almost always female. The 17–20 desmolase deficiency has only been reported in XY subjects.

At puberty, lack of sex steroid production leads to failure of pubertal development. On examination, patients with an XY karyotype will have an absent uterus and the testes are usually intraabdominal. An increase in progesterone is found in both of these disorders. Unless the progesterone level is obtained, these disorders may be confused with pure gonadal dysgenesis in an XX patient.

Complete androgen insensitivity syndrome presents with absent menses, absent or sparse pubic hair, and normal breast development. Androgen insensitivity syndrome and anatomic disorders preventing menses are discussed in Chapter 7.

Other causes of primary ovarian failure which are usually evident from the history include gonadectomy, pelvic irradiation, and rare cases of bilateral ovarian torsion. Likewise, galactosemia is usually a condition that has been known since birth. Since most oral estrogen contains lactose as a filler, replacement therapy in young women with galactosemia is best accomplished with estrogen patch therapy.

CONCLUSION

Pubertal delay is usually a benign, self-limited disorder. However, if the onset of puberty is delayed past the age of 14 years, pathology is common. While most of these disorders are not life-threatening, many result in impaired fertility or infertility. This information should be presented in a thorough, gentle, and sensitive manner to the teenager who is in the midst of developing her sexual identity and plans for family life. Reproductive options available to her should be emphasized. Finally, estrogen replacement therapy, if necessary, should mimic the normal pubertal process in timing and effect as closely as possible.

FURTHER READING

Balfour-Lynn L. Growth and childhood asthma. *Arch Dis Child* 1986; 61: 1049–1055.
Baudier MM, Chihal JH, Dickey RP. Pregnancy and reproductive function in a patient with non-mosaic Turner Syndrome. *Obstet Gynecol* 1985; 65 (suppl): 60A–64S.

Eisenstein TD, Gerson MJ. Psychosocial growth retardation in adolescence. A reversible condition secondary to severe stress. *J Adolesc Health Care* 1988; 9: 436−440.

Garibaldi LR, Picco P, Magier S, Chevli R, Aceto T Jr. Serum luteinizing hormone concentrations, as measured by a sensitive immunoradiometric assay, in children with normal, precocious or delayed pubertal development. *J Clin Endocrinol Metab* 1991; 72: 888−898.

LaPolla JP, Fiorica JV, Turnquist D, Nicosia S, Wilson J, Cavanagh D. Successful therapy of metastatic embryonal carcinoma coexisting with gonadoblastoma in a patient with 46,XY pure gonadal dysgenesis (Swyer's syndrome). *Gynecol Oncol* 1990; 37: 417−421.

Lee PA. Normal ages of pubertal events among American males and females. *J Adolesc Health Care* 1980; 1: 26−29.

Lyen KR, Grant DB. Endocrine function, morbidity, and mortality after surgery for craniopharyngioma. *Arch Dis Child* 1982; 57: 837−841.

Maeyama M, Kagami T, Miyakawa I, Tooya T, Kawasaki N, Iwamasa T. Case report of dysgerminoma in a patient with 46,XX pure gonadal dysgenesis. *Gynecol Oncol* 1983; 16: 405−413.

Rosenfeld RL. Clinical review 6: Diagnosis and management of delayed puberty. *J Clin Endocrinol Metab* 1990; 70: 559−562.

Rosenfeld RG, Hintz RL, Johanson AJ *et al*. Three-year results of a randomized prospective trial of methionyl human growth hormone and oxandrolone in Turner syndrome. *J Pediatr* 1988; 113: 393−400.

3

Vaginal bleeding in the prepubertal child

MARGUERITTE M. WHITE & SUSAN POKORNY

Vaginal bleeding in the prepubertal girl is a source of alarm and great anxiety for parents and caregivers and must be carefully assessed in a thorough and methodic fashion. The differential diagnosis is broad and includes trauma, infection, foreign body, dermatologic lesions, gynecologic and urologic structural anomalies, altered hormonal status, precocious puberty, autoimmune disorders, and rarely, blood dyscrasias (see Fig. 3.1).

To ensure a proper gynecologic evaluation, the examiner must be familiar with the developmental landmarks of each age group, must have available the appropriate diagnostic instruments, and above all, must solicit the trust and confidence of the child (and parent) by providing a relaxed and secure environment for the examination [1]. The importance of "pre-exam" preparation time cannot be overemphasized. The toddler and older child can often times play an active role in their own evaluation, and when possible, efforts should be made to elicit their participation. A careful history must be obtained and parents should be encouraged to bring in evidence of bleeding, should it not be present at the time of the evaluation (i.e., stained panties or diapers). The gynecologic examination should be performed as part of a complete physical. Systematic examination of the vulva, hymen, clitoris urethra, and anus should be performed. Visualization of the entire vagina and cervix is mandatory in virtually all patients with vaginal bleeding. On occasion, this can be accomplished using the frog-leg, knee–chest or lithotomy positions, depending on the child's age. If instrumentation is necessary (i.e., vaginoscopy), it is often advisable to use general anesthesia to ensure a complete and thorough examination. Local application of xylocaine gels, use of oral chloral hydrate, or an injection of demerol may be a reasonable alternative in a few selected cases but the scenario of a screaming, frightened child held down by several assistants must be avoided at all costs.

Judicious use of physical examination, selected laboratory and diagnostic studies, when indicated, will yield an accurate diagnosis in the majority of cases. None the less, the etiology may remain unknown in up to 25% of cases [2].

TRAUMA/FOREIGN BODY

Trauma accounts for up to 8% of referrals for vaginal bleeding [2]. Vulvar hematomas can result from "straddle injuries" or other activities, and often have a seasonal component with many such injuries occurring during the summer months. Circumstances surrounding the injury must be carefully inspected, and the possibility of coital injury must always be entertained. If the latter is suspected or there is inadequate exposure, an examination under anesthesia is mandatory to rule out more extensive injury to the vagina, rectum, and intraabdominal organs [3]. Most vulvar hematomas are self-limiting and can be managed with compresses and analgesics. Evidence of an enlarging hematoma, falling hematocrit, or urethral obstruction requiring prolonged catheterization may necessitate incision under general anesthesia with ligation of actively bleeding vessels.

In a study by Paradise and Willis, 18% of girls under 13 years of age with vaginal bleeding with or without discharge, and 50% of those with vaginal bleeding and no discharge can be expected to have a foreign body [4]. Common offending agents include toilet paper, safety pins, hair pins, and pen tops to name a few. Soft foreign bodies can be removed by gentle irrigation in the knee–chest position, or by twirling a moistened cotton-tipped applicator in the vagina. Application of lubricant and xylocaine jelly at the introitus may facilitate these maneuvers. On occasion, general anesthesia is required for vaginoscopy and/or complete removal of the object(s). General anesthesia is usually required if a child is unable to cooperate with the examination, if there is

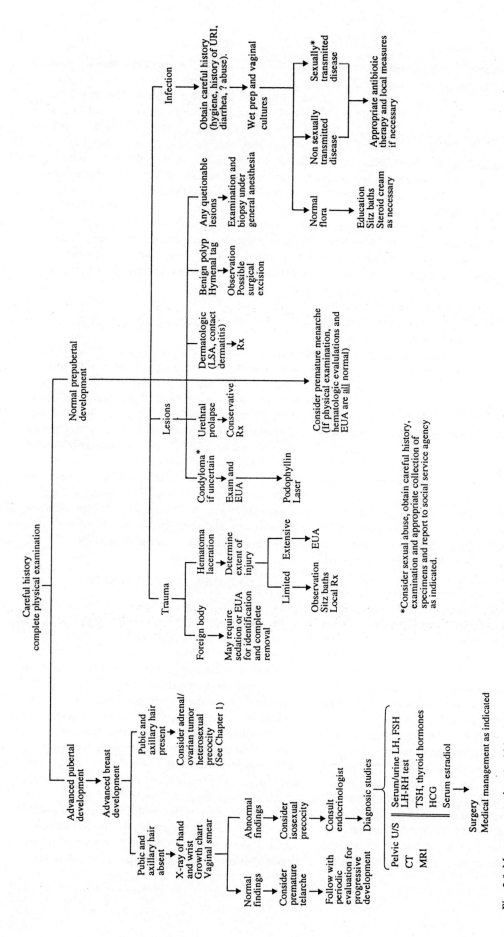

Fig. 3.1 Management of vaginal bleeding in the prepubertal child. EUA, examination under anesthesia.

inadequate visualization, or persistent bleeding or discharge suggests incomplete removal of the object(s).

UROLOGIC STRUCTURAL ANOMALIES

Urethral prolapse defined as complete circular eversion of the urethral mucosa through the external meatus may account for up to 10% of cases of vaginal bleeding [2]. The children commonly have no other symptoms. The peak age of occurrence is between 5 and 8 years old. It is more common in African American girls and seems to be associated with conditions of increased intraabdominal pressure. Methods of treatment include conservative management with sitz baths, estrogen cream, and antibiotics [5]. Surgical correction may, in some circumstances, be necessary. It is important to distinguish between vaginal bleeding and hematuria, which may represent cystitis or upper urinary tract pathology.

INFECTION

Vulvovaginitis, which accounts for 70% of gynecologic complaints in the pediatric age group, accounts for only 6% of cases of vaginal bleeding [2]. The most common cause of hemorrhagic vaginitis is poor perineal hygiene with a large inoculum of bacteria leading to a blood-stained discharge. Treatment consists of detailed education of parent and child regarding proper hygiene techniques, local sitz baths, and topical steroids for pruritus if needed. Vaginal cultures often reveal organisms that may represent colonization and may not be pathogenic. Nonetheless, a colony count of greater than 100 000 organisms should probably be treated with an appropriate antibiotic. Persistent or recurrent cases may require a short course of topical estrogen cream and 2—3 months of a low-dose, broad-spectrum antibiotic for suppression. Estrogen cream can thicken the epithelium making it more resistant to infection but should only be applied for 3—4 weeks at a time because of systemic absorption (nightly for 2 weeks and every other night for the remaining 2 weeks). Common infectious agents that are non-sexually transmitted include *Shigella*, which can cause a bloody purulent discharge and may be preceded by a history of diarrhea. Other causes include pinworms, *Gardnerella vaginalis*, *Candida albicans*, *tinea versicolor*, and *molluscum contagiosum*. A history of a recent upper respiratory tract, ear, or throat infection should alert the physician to the possibility of *Staphylococcus aureus*, hemolytic streptococcus, or β-hemolytic streptococcus as etiologic agents. The possibility of sexual abuse must strongly be considered in girls in whom *Trichomonas*, gonorrhea, *Chlamydia*, syphilis, herpes, and condyloma acuminata are identified. Perinatal transmission of condyloma can occur, but the appearance of lesions after 24 months of age should raise suspicion of sexual abuse [6]. Condyloma of the vulva, vagina, and anus in the prepubertal child can be friable and bleed easily with minimal trauma. All cases of suspected abuse must, of course, be reported to the proper social service agencies. Recommended treatment of specific organisms is outlined in Table 3.1.

NEOPLASMS

Benign polyps, hymenal tags, hemangiomas of the vulva (and rarely clitoris) are examples of neoplasms arising from the vagina that can produce bleeding. Treatment options range from conservative observation to surgical excision. Sarcoma botryoides — embryonal rhabdomyosarcoma — is an aggressive malignant tumor with 90% of cases occurring before age 5. Children typically present with discharge, bleeding, a grape-like mass protruding from the vagina, or a palpable abdominopelvic mass. Aggressive management, including surgery, combination chemotherapy and radiation, is warranted with 90% cure rates reported for localized lesions [8].

DERMATOLOGIC LESIONS

Lichen sclerosis et atrophicus is occasionally a cause of vaginal bleeding. The lesion is characterized by white papules which coalesce into parchment-like plaques. These become wrinkled, inflamed, and ulcerated. Bleeding results from scratching or even friction such as that produced by bike-riding. The vulva and perianal area can both be involved. The etiology is unknown with evidence suggesting an autoimmune disorder. Diagnosis is clinical or via biopsy. The treatment is symptomatic involving sitz baths and local soothing methods. Medicinal treatment involves hydrocortisone cream and occasionally progesterone cream. A few children with severe disease have been treated with laser brushing of the vulva with promising results [9]. The evaluation of vulvar lesions must include the diagnosis of contact dermatitis from bubble baths, perfumes, disposable

Table 3.1 Treatment of vulvovaginitis in the prepubertal child. (Adapted from [7])

Etiology	Treatment
Group A β-streptococcus (*Streptococcus pyogenes*)	Penicillin V potassium, 125–250 mg q.i.d. p.o. ×10 days
Streptococcus pneumoniae	
Chlamydia trachomatis	Erythromycin, 50 mg/kg per day p.o. ×10 days Children ≥8 years of age, doxycycline, 100 mg b.i.d. p.o. × 7–10 days
Neisseria gonorrhoeae	Ceftriaxone, 125 mg i.m. Patients who cannot tolerate ceftriaxone may be treated with spectinomycin, 40 mg/kg i.m. once Children ≥8 years of age should also be given doxycycline, 100 mg b.i.d. p.o. ×7 days Children >45 kg are treated with adult regimens.
Candida	Topical nystatin (Mycostatin), miconazole, or clotrimazole cream
Shigella	Trimethoprim/sulfamethoxazole, 8 mg 40 mg/kg per day p.o. ×7 days
Staphylococcus aureus	Cephalexin (Keflex), 25–50 mg/kg per day p.o. ×7–10 days Dicloxacillin, 25 mg/kg per day p.o. ×7–10 days Amoxycillin-clavulanate (Augmentin), 20–40 mg/kg per day (of the amoxycillin) p.o. ×7–10 days
Haemophilus influenzae	Amoxicillin, 20–40 mg/kg per day p.o. ×7 days
Trichomonas	Metronidazole (Flagyl), 125 mg (15 mg/kg per day) t.i.d. ×7–10 days
Pinworms (*Enterobius vermicularis*)	Mebendazole (Vermox), one chewable 100-mg tablet, repeated in 2 weeks

diapers, etc. A careful history combined with well-focused attention to the problem will often identify the culprit.

HORMONAL

Neonatal estrogen withdrawal
Slight vaginal bleeding within the first week of life is often due to maternal estrogen withdrawal. Bleeding that persists beyond 10 days however must be investigated to rule out the presence of a tumor.

Precocious puberty
Vaginal bleeding can be a sign of precocious puberty with 15–20% of sexually precocious girls menstruating before 2–3 years of age. Sexual precocity is defined as the appearance of breast development before the age of 8 and menarche before the age of 10. Isosexual precocity is the appearance of early sexual development consistent with the sex of the individual and can be divided into true isosexual precocity and isosexual pseudoprecocity. True isosexual precocity is due to premature activation of the hypothalamic–pituitary access resulting in reproductive-age gonadotropin levels, ovarian production of estrogen with subsequent growth spurt, breast development, and on occasion, menses. In isosexual pseudoprecocity, estrogen is produced by an autonomous source, i.e., an ovarian neoplasm or cyst, gonadotropin-producing tumor, and rarely, adrenal adenoma.

Etiology
Though the majority of cases of true isosexual precocity in girls are idiopathic, a number of organic disorders must be considered in the evaluation. Trauma, postirradiation, as well as central nervous system lesions such as congenital brain defects, tuberous sclerosis, prolactinoma, craniopharyngioma, hydrocephalus, postinfectious encephalitis, neurofibromatosis, and suprasellar cysts have all been

associated with sexual precocity. With the advent of newer imaging techniques, the hypothalamic hamartoma — a hyperplastic malformation at the base of the hypothalamus — has been found in up to 30% of girls with reproductive-age gonadotropin levels [10]. These tumors are thought independently to produce gonadotropin-releasing factor, thereby causing pubertal levels of luteinizing hormone (LH) and follicle-stimulating hormone (FSH). Manifestations of sexual precocity may be found in individuals with primary hypothyroidism. This is the only form of sexual precocity in which growth is arrested and not stimulated. Galactorrhea may also be present. A commonly held hypothesis is the "hormonal overlap" theory. It is postulated that a low serum thyroxine level stimulates the hypothalamus to secrete thyrotropin-releasing hormone (TRH). TRH will in turn stimulate pituitary production of thyroid-stimulating hormone (TSH), prolactin and, because of a commonly shared α-subunit, LH and FSH. The development of true isosexual precocity has been described in children with congenital adrenal hyperplasia (CAH). The mechanism is unknown and (1) may involve activation of the hypothalamic–pituitary access by the markedly elevated levels of steroids, (2) the sex steroids may advance the maturational stage to the point where puberty is activated, or (3) abrupt changes in sex steroid levels (i.e., in patients with untreated CAH who receive therapy) may activate the process [11,12].

Irregular vaginal bleeding is more common in isosexual pseudoprecocity. Only 1–2% of girls with precocious puberty have an ovarian tumor. The follicular cyst may be the most common cause of pseudoprecocity, followed by the granulosa theca cell tumor [13]. Teratomas, dysgerminomas and choriocarcinomas can produce gonadotropin which, by its high local concentration, stimulates ovarian hormone production. Girls with McCune–Albright syndrome (polyostotic fibrous dysplasia with multiple cystic bony lesions and irregular café-au-lait spots) have recurrent ovarian cysts which also produce fluctuating levels of estrogen. Premature menarche may be the first sign of this syndrome. Exogenous estrogen in the form of birth control pills, vaginal creams, and tainted water or foods must always be entertained as a possible etiology.

Clinical presentation

When a child presents with vaginal bleeding and premature development of secondary sexual charac-

teristics, a careful history and physical examination must be performed. Clinical presentation will vary depending on the underlying etiology. Ovarian cysts or tumors are often asymptomatic, but may present with pain or abdominal distention. Questions regarding age of onset may be of particular importance, for instance, the hypothalamic hamartoma usually presents by age 3 or 4. Certain exogenous estrogens may cause hyperpigmentation of the nipples and breast areola. Children with CAH often have a long history of virilization and an advanced bone age of at least 10 years.

Diagnostic evaluation

Priority must be to rule out life-threatening disease and determine if there is evidence of progressive changes or if the process is self-limited. On physical examination, a full neurologic evaluation is essential with assessment of visual fields and optic disks. Special attention must be given to the Tanner stages of breast development (Fig. 3.2), the degree of vaginal estrogenization, and presence of pubic or axillary hair. A growth chart to assess linear growth and X-ray films of the hand and wrist to evaluate bone age should be obtained to look for possible estrogen or androgen effect on linear growth rate and osseous maturation. A vaginal smear for maturation index will assess the presence of estrogenization. If this baseline evaluation reveals breast development without any other signs of puberty (normal bone age and growth, age-appropriate maturation index), a diagnosis of premature thelarche is likely. These children can be followed conservatively with periodic evaluations for any signs of progressive sexual development. Conversely, if there is evidence of vaginal estrogenization, acceleration in linear growth and advancing bone age, a complete endocrinologic and radiologic evaluation must be undertaken. The clinician must differentiate between true (central) precocity and pseudoprecocity. A search must be undertaken to rule out the presence of a neoplasm of the central nervous system, ovary, adrenal, or to detect the presence of ectopic trophoblastic tissue. Computed tomography (CT) or magnetic resonance imaging (MRI) scanning will aid in delineating central nervous system and adrenal tumors. Pelvic ultrasound and rectoabdominal examination will often detect ovarian masses. A skeletal survey or bone scan is useful in evaluating the patient for McCune–Albright syndrome.

Endocrinologic evaluation includes a study of

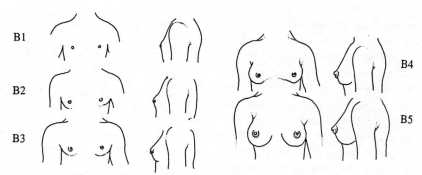

Fig. 3.2 The Tanner stages of human breast development. Stage B1, preadolescent; elevation of the nipple only; Stage B2, breast bud stage; elevation of the breast and nipple as a small mound, enlargement of the areolar diameter; Stage B3, further enlargement of the breast and areola with no separation of the contours; Stage B4, further enlargement with projection of the areola and nipple to form a secondary mound above the level of the breast; Stage B5, mature stage; projection of the nipple only resulting from recession of the areola to the general contour of the breast. (Adapted from [14,15].)

estrogens, androgens, and gonadotropins. Because of fluctuating patterns of secretion, random LH and FSH may not be helpful in differentiating between the various causes of precocious puberty. Timed urine collections of LH and FSH may be of more value [16]. Serum estradiol levels are usually markedly elevated in patients with estrogen-secreting tumors. Elevated serum LH values may represent cross reactivity with human chorionic gonadotropin (hCG) and signal the presence of an hCG-producing tumor. The LH-releasing hormone (LHRH) stimulation test has been widely employed in the diagnosis of precocious puberty. Patients with true precocity have a pubertal response to administration of LHRH analog — LH value should increase 150% above the baseline [17], while patients with pseudoprecocity will have a minimal gonadotropin response. If hypothyroidism is suspected, thyroid hormones including a TSH should be sent along with a prolactin level. Measurement of serum testosterone and dehydroepiandrosterone sulfate (DHEAS) (and/or DHEA) may be valuable in assessing the presence of an adrenal or ovarian tumor as indicated by history and/or physical examination.

Treatment
Ovarian cysts that are purely fluid-filled on ultrasound usually resolve spontaneously. If they persist, enlarge, or become symptomatic they may require aspiration or cystectomy. Because of the low malignant potential of granulosa theca cell tumors, unilateral salpingo-oophorectomy is the treatment of choice with careful follow-up. Ovarian and adrenal neoplasms should be surgically removed. A preoperative serum hCG can be a useful screen for the presence of a gonadotropin-secreting ovarian tumor. Hypothalamic hamartomas are now managed conservatively with serial CT/MRI studies.

LHRH analogs are useful in the management of true (central) precocity. Medical management should only be undertaken when there is *clear* evidence of advancing bone age, impaired height prediction, and progressive changes in secondary sexual characteristics over a 6–12-month period. Such intervention may also be indicated if the child is a risk for significant psychologic trauma. After an initial stimulatory phase, LHRH analogs downregulate LHRH receptors in the pituitary, thereby decreasing gonadotropin production. There may be a regression of secondary sexual characteristics, usually to Tanner stage 1. There may be initial vaginal bleeding from estrogen withdrawal with ultimate cessation of menses, slowing of growth velocity, skeletal maturation, and bone age. Medroxyprogesterone acetate is also useful in suppressing menses and causing resolution of breast development, though the effect on bone maturation is limited. Careful follow-up of all patients under treatment must be done to ensure the appropriate response, including growth charts, vaginal smears, evaluation of bone age, and ultrasounds if necessary. Girls with McCune–Albright syndrome have been successfully treated with testolactone, an aromatase inhibitor which blocks the synthesis of estrogens [16].

CHAPTER 3

Premature menarche (isolated menses)

Premature menarche has been described as vaginal bleeding lasting 2—5 days with no other signs of sexual development or detectable vaginal or uterine anomalies [19]. Bleeding may present as one isolated episode or be cyclic and recurrent for several months. Plasma estradiol levels have been reported to be significantly elevated while gonadotropins have been in the prepubertal range. It is imperative that all other causes of bleeding be thoroughly investigated prior to reaching this diagnosis. The frequency has been reported to be less than 1/10th of cases of isosexually precocity in girls [17].

MISCELLANEOUS

Vaginal bleeding secondary to blood dyscrasias is often associated with other signs of a hematologic disorder, i.e., easy bruisability, epistaxis, petechiae, and should be evaluated with the appropriate laboratory work-up.

CONCLUSIONS

A thorough evaluation must be done to investigate the cause of vaginal bleeding in a prepubertal girl. A combination of history and physical examination will reveal the diagnosis in a majority of cases. A great deal of information can be obtained from visual inspection alone. In some cases, general anesthesia and vaginoscopy should be used to evaluate fully the lower genital tract. The most common causes of vaginal bleeding in this age group include trauma, foreign body, structural lesions, or infection. When there is evidence of advanced secondary sexual characteristics, the rare diagnosis of precocious puberty must be entertained and the work-up pursued diligently.

REFERENCES

1 Gidwani GP. Approach to evaluation of premenarchal child with a gynecologic problem. *Clin Obstet Gynecol* 1987; 30: 643—652.
2 Hill NCW, Oppenheimer LW, Morton KE. The aetiology of vaginal bleeding in children. A 20-year review. *Br J Obstet Gynecol* 1989; 96: 467—470.
3 Muran D, Gale C. Clinical assessment of the sexually abused girl. *Med Aspects Hum Sexual* 1990; 41—48.
4 Paradise JE, Willis ED. Probability of vaginal foreign body in girls with genital complaints. *Am J Dis Child* 1985; 139: 472—476.
5 Richardson DA, Samir N, Herbst AL. Medical treatment of urethral prolapse in children. *Obstet Gynecol* 1982; 59: 69—72.
6 Davis AJ, Emans SJ. Human papilloma virus infection in the pediatric and adolescent patient. *J Pediatr* 1989; 115: 1—9.
7 Bourne R, Masland RP. Vulvovaginal problems in the prepubertal child. In: Emans SJH, Goldstein DP, eds. *Pediatric and Adolescent Gynecology.* Boston: Little, Brown, 1990.
8 Hendren WH, Lillehei CS. Pediatric surgery. *N Engl J Med* 1988; 319: 86—96.
9 Davis AJ, Goldstein DP. Treatment of pediatric lichen sclerosis with the CO_2 laser. *Adolesc Pediatr Gynecol* 1989; 2: 103—105.
10 Kulin HE. Precocious puberty. *Clin Obstet Gynecol* 1987; 30: 714—734.
11 Pescovitz OH, Comite F, Cassorla F et al. True precocious puberty complicating congenital adrenal hyperplasia: treatment with a luteinizing hormone releasing hormone analogue. *J Clin Endocrinol Metab* 1984; 58: 857—861.
12 Pescovitz OH, Hench K, Green O, Comite F, Loriaux L, Cutler GB. Central precocious puberty complicating a virilizing adrenal tumor: treatment with a long-acting LHRH analog. *J Pediatr* 1985; 106: 612—614.
13 Towne B, Mahour G, Wooley M, Isaacs H. Ovarian cysts and tumors in infancy and childhood. *J Pediatr Surg* 1975; 10: 311—320.
14 Ross G, Vande Wiele R. The ovaries. In: Williams R, ed. *Textbook of Endocrinology,* 5th edn. Philadelphia: Saunders, 1974.
15 Marshall WA, Tanner JM. *Variations in Pattern of Pubertal Changes in Girls.*
16 Kulin HE, Bell PM, Santen RJ, Ferber AJ. Integration of pulsatile gonadotropin secretion by timed urinary measurements: an accurate and sensitive test. *J Clin Endocrinol Metab* 1975; 40: 783—789.
17 Lemarchand-Beraud T, Zufferey M, Reymond M et al. Maturation of the hypothalamic-pituitary-ovarian axis in adolescent girls. *J Clin Endocrinol Metab* 1982; 54: 241.
18 Feuillan PP, Foster CM, Pescovitz OH et al. Treatment of precocious puberty in the McCune—Albright syndrome with the aromatase inhibitor testolactone. *N Engl J Med* 1986; 315: 1115—1119.
19 Blanco-Garcia M, Evain-Brion D, Roger M, Job JC. Isolated menses in prepubertal girls. *Pediatrics* 1985; 76: 43—47.

4

Ambiguous genitalia

LISA J. HANSARD & DAVID L. OLIVE

INTRODUCTION

"Is it a boy or a girl?" is usually the first question asked in the delivery room at the birth of a newborn. The inability to answer this question without a second thought upon examination of the external genitalia constitutes a medical emergency. Rapid gender assignment is imperative and must be concordant with the potential anatomic and sexual function. Proper gender assignment depends upon a thorough understanding of embryology, anatomy, life-threatening conditions associated with ambiguous genitalia, as well as knowledge of the potential role of corrective surgery. Ambiguous genitalia presents a diagnostic challenge and requires an aggressive approach. Often a multidisciplinary team is required to assign proper gender. This team may involve pediatricians, gynecologists, urologists, geneticists, and psychiatrists to ascertain which gender role will be most concordant with the appearance of the external genitalia.

GENETIC DETERMINATION OF SEX

Fertilization of a normal ovum by either an X- or Y-bearing sperm establishes genetic sex. Most of the genes for determining gametogenesis and sexual differentiation are located on the X and Y chromosomes. These chromosomes also carry genes which code for somatic characteristics. Female fertility requires the presence of two X chromosomes, although one of these is inactive. However, a portion of the short arm of the inactivated X chromosome is needed for normal development. The inactive X chromosome is thought to be the one which replicates later. Condensed chromatin or Barr bodies may be detected in the inner margin of the nuclear membrane in 15–30% of cells from the buccal mucosa. Barr bodies exist in the number of one less than the total number of X chromosomes in the genotype. The presence of an active X chromosome in the male will lead to abnormal spermatogenesis.

The presence or absence of a Y chromosome determines whether the indifferent gonad will develop into an ovary or a testis. The Y will give rise to male differentiation irrespective of the number of X chromosomes. A gene producing testicular-determining factor has been isolated to the short arm of the Y chromosome. This conclusion was reached after examining individuals lacking the short arm of Y who were female in appearance and possessed bilateral streak gonads. Although not completely understood, the manner in which testicular differentiation occurs seems to be dependent upon a cell surface protein, the H-Y antigen. Genes which regulate the production of H-Y antigen are located on the euchromatic portion of the long arm of the Y chromosome. The H-Y antigen controls spermatogenesis, but not total testis differentiation.

EMBRYOLOGY OF REPRODUCTIVE ORGANS

Although the genetic sex of the embryo is determined at the time of fertilization, the gonads do not differentiate into male or female until the seventh week of gestation. Germ cells appear in the genital ridges at about 6 weeks of development. Shortly before and during the arrival of the primordial germ cells, the coelomic epithelium of the genital ridge proliferates and the cells are incorporated into the indifferent gonad. The primitive duct systems exist in both sexes at this point. The mesonephric or Wolffian system will develop in the male, and the paramesonephric or Müllerian system develops in the female, although remnants of the opposite system can be found in both sexes after sexual differentiation is complete (Table 4.1).

CHAPTER 4

Table 4.1 Embryonic development of male and female structures

Male	Homologous structure	Female

Testes
  Seminiferous tubule
  Sertoli cell
  Leydig cell
	Primitive gonad	Ovary
		  Primordial follicle
		  Granulosa cell
		  Theca cell

Epididymis, vas deferens, seminal vesicles	Wolffian ducts	Gartner's duct
Appendix of testis	Müllerian ducts	Fallopian tubes, uterus, cervix, upper vagina
Glans penis	Genital tubercle	Clitoris
Corpus spongiosum, ventral penis	Urogenital folds	Labia minora
Scrotum	Labioscrotal swellings	Labia majora
Prostate, prostatic utricle	Urogenital sinus	Lower vagina, Skene's glands, Bartholin's glands

Female

In the absence of a Y chromosome or under influence of two X chromosomes, the gonad will differentiate into an ovary. The germ cells which have migrated to the genital ridge have undergone mitosis and are surrounded by a single layer of follicular cells forming primordial follicles. The oocytes in these follicles have arrested in the diplotene stage of meiotic prophase. There are approximately 7 million oocytes at about 20 weeks' gestation. These oocytes undergo atresia, resulting in 2 million oocytes at birth and 300 000−400 000 at menarche. When less than two X chromosomes are present, the oocytes undergo more rapid atresia.

The paramesonephric or Müllerian duct develops into the main genital duct. There are initially three segments to the duct: a cranial vertical part, a mid horizontal part, and a caudal vertical part. The first two parts develop into the uterine tube and the caudal part develops into the uterine canal. The uterine tubes later develop into the fallopian tubes and the fused uterine canal develops into the uterine corpus, cervix, and upper one-third of the vagina.

Starting in the third week of development, mesenchymal cells migrate around the cloaca to form cloacal folds which then unite to form the genital tubercle. The cloacal folds are likewise subdivided into the urethral folds anteriorly which encompass the urogenital sinus and the anal folds posteriorly. At the same time, the genital swellings appear on each side of the urethral folds. In the absence of androgens, the external genitalia differentiates as female. The genital tubercle elongates slightly to form the clitoris; the urethral folds form the labia minora. The urogenital sinus develops into the urethra and the lower two-thirds of the vagina. The genital swellings enlarge, forming the labia majora. Factors controlling development are not entirely clear, but estrogens may also play a role in female differentiation of the external genitalia.

Male

The germ cells are enclosed in tubules under the influence of testis-determining factors. These tubules differentiate into spermatogenic cords and seminiferous tubules. The interstitial cells of Leydig develop and produce testosterone. The testis also secretes Müllerian-inhibiting factor (MIF) by the Sertoli cells. MIF will cause regression of the Müllerian ducts, and may play a role in testicular descent into the scrotum.

Testosterone produced by the Leydig cells acts directly on the ipsilateral mesonephric or Wolffian ducts to stimulate male differentiation. The mesonephric duct forms the main genital duct. At the caudal position, it elongates and convolutes to form the epididymis. Between the tail of the epididymis and the outcropping of the seminal vesicle, the mesonephric duct is surrounded by a thick muscular coat and forms the ductus deferens.

Under influence of fetal androgens, the genital

tubercle elongates, forming the glans penis. As it elongates, the phallus pulls the urethral folds forward and they form the penile urethra. The urethra does not extend to the tip of the glans. The most distal portion of the urethra is formed when ectodermal cells of the glans invaginate and form a short epithelial cord. The genital swellings are initially located in the inguinal area. They migrate caudally, each forming half of the scrotum, and are separated by the scrotal septum (Fig 4.1).

ABNORMAL SEXUAL DIFFERENTIATION

Many diverse etiologies exist for abnormal sexual differentiation. For simplicity and ease of understanding, individuals exhibiting ambiguous genitalia may be divided into those with abnormal gonadal formation or function, female pseudohermaphroditism, male pseudohermaphroditism, and true hermaphroditism.

Abnormal gonadal function can be present in individuals with abnormal or normal karyotypes. Mixed gonadal dysgenesis refers to persons with one streak gonad and with one testis. The testis is often dysplastic, and the most common karyotype is 45,X/46,XY. Phenotypically, the genitalia of these individuals may vary from almost normal female to significantly ambiguous to almost normal male. Those demonstrating female or ambiguous genitalia need removal of the gonads as 15—20% may develop a neoplasm, the most common being a gonadoblastoma with cells of a malignant dysgerminoma. Testicular regression syndrome describes genotypic males who have lost their testicles during embryonic life. The degree of ambiguity of the external genitalia is usually related to the time frame when testicular tissue was lost.

Female pseudohermaphroditism

Female pseudohermaphroditism is a condition in which masculinization of the external genitalia occurs in individuals with a normal 46,XX karyotype. The cause of the masculinization is exposure of the female fetus to abnormally elevated levels of androgens. During early gestation, virilization of the external genitalia occurs, and may be indistinguishable from normal male phenotype except for cryptorchidism if the levels of androgens are high enough. After 12—14 weeks' gestation, clitoromegaly is usually the main manifestation. In almost all cases, the internal organs are female. Female pseudohermaphroditism can be caused by inherited disorders of steroid metabolism, maternal drug ingestion, maternal androgen-producing tumors, or idiopathic causes.

Congenital adrenal hyperplasia (CAH) is the most common cause of female pseudohermaphroditism. This refers to a group of enzymatic disorders in the production of adrenal steroids, inherited as autosomal recessive traits. These disorders lead to decreased synthesis of glucocorticoids which result in increased synthesis of other adrenal hormones such as androgens secondary to increased adrenocorticotropic hormone (ACTH) stimulation. Three of these enzyme deficiencies lead to female pseudohermaphroditism. By far the most common is 21-hydroxylase deficiency. Two forms of this enzyme deficiency exist: salt-wasting and nonsalt-wasting. Neonatal death can occur in the salt-wasting form if it is not identified quickly after birth and glucocorticoid and mineralocorticoid supplementation rapidly initiated. 11β-hydroxylase is a hypertensive form of CAH, and accounts for approximately 3% of all cases. The defect leads to accumulation of 11-deoxycorticosterone (DOC) which has salt-retaining activity. Again, treatment is by replacement of oral glucocorticoids. 3β-hydroxysteroid dehydrogenase deficiency can cause ambiguous genitalia in both females and males. The defect results in accumulation of dehydroepiandrosterone, which is a much weaker androgen than testosterone. This disorder produces severe salt-wasting. These individuals should be treated with oral glucococorticoid and mineralocorticoid replacement therapy (Fig. 4.2).

Certain medications may cause female pseudohermaphroditism when given to pregnant women. The most common are synthetic progestogens administered in the form of oral contraceptives or as agents to prevent early abortion. These progestogens are weak androgens and result in far less genital ambiguity than in cases of CAH. Danazol, a testosterone derivative used commonly in the treatment of endometriosis, crosses the placenta and may cause virilization of the external genitalia in female infants.

Androgen-producing tumors of the ovaries or adrenals can produce varying degrees of female pseudohermaphroditism. There are a large number of tumors which can do this, including arrhenoblastoma, hilar cell tumor, luteoma of pregnancy, lipoid cell tumor, Krukenberg tumor, and others. Fortunately, elevated levels of steroid-hormone-binding globulin as well as significant aromatase capability

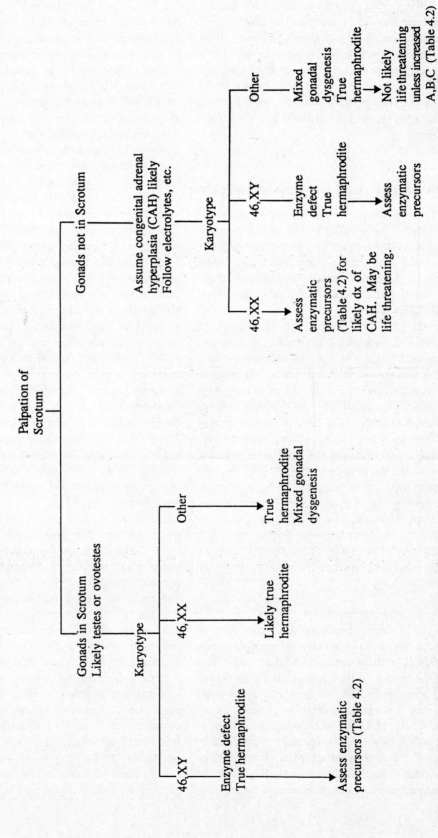

Fig. 4.1 Approach to the child with ambiguous genitalia.

of the placenta may help protect a female fetus from androgenic effects.

Female pseudohermaphroditism has been associated with multiple congenital anomalies, most commonly of the genitourinary or gastrointestinal systems. This association suggests that in some cases the defect in sexual differentiation may not be related to an underlying abnormality of androgen production in the fetus or mother. Precise mechanisms, however, are still unknown.

Male pseudohermaphroditism

Fetuses with a normal 46,XY karyotype and female or ambiguous genitalia are termed male pseudohermaphrodites. External genitalia and, in some cases, internal duct formation are abnormal. These anomalies are usually a result of defects in androgen synthesis or defects in end-organ response. Occasionally, anatomic abnormalities such as severe hypospadias, micropenis, or persistent Müllerian structures make sex assignment difficult.

Several enzymes associated with abnormal androgen synthesis are common to the adrenals as well as the testes, and deficiencies lead to CAH as well as ambiguous genitalia. These enzymes are 20,22-desmolase, 3β-hydroxysteroid dehydrogenase, and 17α-hydroxylase. Two other enzymes are limited to androgen biosynthesis. These are 17,20-desmolase and 17-ketosteroid reductase (Fig. 4.2). All individuals demonstrate Müllerian regression as Sertoli cells are unaffected. The spectrum of ambiguity ranges from totally normal female phenotypes to only mild male anomalies. Most individuals are infertile secondary to low intratesticular levels of testosterone. Those patients raised as females require gonadectomy and estrogen replacement. Individuals raised as males often require testosterone replacement.

Androgen receptor abnormalities are the most common cause of defects in end-organ response. Testicular feminization or androgen insensitivity syndrome usually results in a normal female phenotype with absent Müllerian structures and a blind vaginal pouch. It is inherited as an X-linked recessive or a male-limited autosomal dominant trait. Testes may be located in the abdominal cavity, inguinal canal, or labia. The individuals often present around puberty with the failure to develop menses or axillary and pubic hair. Breast development is usually normal. These patients may retain their gonads through puberty but should have them removed afterwards because of the increased risk of gonadal tumors.

In the incomplete form of testicular feminization, individuals often demonstrate clitoromegaly and labioscrotal fusion. They often masculinize at puberty, so should have their gonads removed before then.

The conversion of testosterone to 5α-dihydrotestosterone (DHT) is critical to the differentiation of the external genitalia. In fetuses with 5α-reductase deficiency, external genitalia are ambiguous, but internal Wolffian structures are normal. Additional virilization with increased penile growth occurs at puberty with the development of a masculine body habitus. This disorder is inherited as an autosomal recessive.

True hermaphroditism

True hermaphrodites are individuals in whom both ovarian follicles and testicular tubular elements are present in one or both gonads. Sixty percent will have a normal female karyotype, and 15% are 46,XY. The remainder are mosaics. Over 50% of these fetuses have a male phenotype, and most patients are raised as males. The most common gonad is the ovotestis. It is most frequently found on the left side of the abdomen but may be in the scrotum. Ambiguous external genitalia is common, Müllerian structures may be present, and menstruation can occur.

DIAGNOSIS AND MANAGEMENT OF AMBIGUOUS GENITALIA

Delivery room management of the fetus with ambiguous genitalia is critical. The obstetrician should avoid an immediate declaration of sex and should inform the parents that the genitalia are incompletely formed, and that further testing is necessary to determine the sex the baby is meant to be. Telling the parents that the baby is part male and part female is inappropriate. The family should examine the genitalia with the obstetrician who can identify the abnormal anatomy. The family may wish to delay naming the infant or choose a name that is appropriate for either a male or female. Documents such as medical records or birth certificates can be delayed until gender assignment is made. Education of the parents is crucial in the immediate neonatal period. Explaining normal sexual differentiation using proper terminology helps parents understand that genital ambiguity results from normal development processes. This can not only alleviate fear, anxiety, and ambivalence in the family, but also helps in understanding the type of evaluation necessary for the baby. A careful family history must be taken to garner clues as to the etiology of the ambiguous genitalia. Questions concerning similarly affected family members or unexplained sibling death can point to genetically linked disorders. A careful review of the mother's prenatal course can give insight into possible androgen-secreting tumors or maternal drug ingestion. Regardless of the cause of the ambiguity, rapid gender assignment will profoundly affect the success of the outcome for the child and family.

Evaluation of the infant should begin with a very careful physical examination aimed at determining if the genital ambiguity is an isolated anomaly or is associated with other malformations. If the infant has multiple defects, the goal becomes identification of the underlying problem. Many of the malformation syndromes which include ambiguous genitalia are life-threatening; therefore, prompt diagnosis is crucial. Assessment of the infant by a geneticist may help diagnose a syndrome and can clarify the natural history as well as outline management options.

If the abnormalities of the genitalia appear to be isolated in an otherwise normal infant, identification of the chromosomal, gonadal, and phenotypic sex is undertaken.

Currently, the only acceptable way to determine chromosomal sex is by chromosome analysis. Buccal smears to look for Barr bodies or fluorescent Y-bodies provide no information about structural defects of the X or Y chromosome or about mosaicism. Chromosome analysis is usually performed on T lymphocytes from peripheral blood. Routine results may take as long as 2–3 weeks, but preliminary results may be available in as few as 5 days. Bone marrow analysis may yield results in 12 hours but involves a painful and invasive procedure. If a normal XY karyotype is obtained, special tests may need to be performed to detect subtle structural abnormalities in the Y chromosome.

Gonadal sex can often be elucidated from the physical examination. Gonads that are palpable in the scrotum or below the inguinal canal contain testicular tissue and are either normal testes or ovatestes. This discovery will rule out simple virilization of a female infant. An ovary may herniate but will be palpable outside the inguinal canal and not in the labioscrotal folds. Occasionally, if tests to determine chromosomal or phenotypic sex have been inconclusive, gonadal visualization and biopsy by laparoscopy or laparotomy may be required. Ultrasonography of the pelvis to evaluate the presence of Müllerian structures

Table 4.2 Diagnosis of enzymatic defects as etiology of ambiguous genitalia

Hormone	Deficient enzyme
All precursors low	20,22-Desmolase
↑ 17-OH Pregnenolone	3β-Hydroxysteroid dehydrogenase
↑ Progesterone, ↑ DOC	17-Hydroxylase
↑ 17-OH Progesterone	21-Hydroxylase
↑ DOC, ↓ deoxycortisol	11-Hydroxylase
↑ Testosterone, ↓ DHT	5α-Reductase

DOC, deoxycorticosterone; DHT, dihydrotestosterone.

is a noninvasive procedure. If a normal uterus and fallopian tubes are present, it can be concluded that normal testicular tissue is absent, and that the gonads are ovaries, streaks, ovatestes, or severely dysgenetic testes.

Laboratory evaluation should be instituted immediately and, in most cases, can be completed within 3 or 4 days. Hormonal studies, especially those that will diagnose possible life-threatening forms of CAH, along with serum electrolytes, should be obtained immediately (Table 4.2). Measurements of serum testosterone, estradiol, follicle-stimulating hormone, and luteinizing hormone may be helpful, but levels vary considerably in the neonatal period.

Gender assignment

The single most important factor in sex assignment is the potential for adequate sexual functioning. The possibility of fertility is also a very important consideration. If the chromosomal and gonadal sex are compatible with fertility, and the external genitalia allows reconstruction for sexual function, gender assignment is made to preserve fertility. If fertility is not possible, sex assignment is usually based on the genital phenotype. For individuals with under- or overvirilization of the genitalia, gender is based on chromosomal and gonadal sex, if the genitalia permits. Infants with incomplete androgen insensitivity or true hermaphroditism may be raised as male if the phallus is of sufficient size at birth that the child has the potential for adequate sexual functioning as an adult; otherwise, the infant should be assigned female gender. Most experts consider the phallus with length of >1.9 cm from the symphysis pubis and/or diameter of 0.5 cm to be necessary for male gender assignment. It is imperative that gender assignment be completed by 18 months of age, the time when gender awareness is established.

Surgical management

A urologist and gynecologist experienced in surgical therapy of infants with ambiguous genitalia is imperative. For infants who are to be raised as male, therapy is aimed at placement of gonads in the scrotum, release of chordee, and correction of hypospadias. More often, surgery is undertaken to reconstruct female genitalia. In general, phallic or clitoral reduction, creation of the labia minora and majora, and gonadectomy, if indicated, are performed at approximately 3−6 months of age. This early genitoplasty ensures that the external genitalia is commensurate with the sex of rearing and can relieve parental anxiety. If the vaginal entry into the urogenital sinus is proximal to the external urethral sphincter and there is adequate drainage of the Müllerian system, vaginoplasty is deferred until age 2 or 3 years to avoid injury to the sphincter. For individuals with an absent vagina, creation of the neovagina is delayed until puberty, when there may be increased estrogen and more fully developed perineal tissues. In addition, chronic use of dilators is often required, and this is generally more successfully accomplished when the patient is more mature.

FURTHER READING

Donahue PA, Berkovitz GD. Female pseudohermaphroditism. *Semin Reprod Endocrinol* 1987; 5: 233.

Herbert CM. Abnormalities of sexual differentiation. *Gynecologic Endocrinology and Infertility for the House Officer*. Baltimore: Williams & Wilkins, 1988; 13−27.

Mastroyannis C, Wallach EE. Male pseudohermaphroditism: inborn errors in testosterone biosynthesis. *Semin Reprod Endocrinol* 1987; 5: 261.

Oesterling JE, Gearhart JP, Jeffs RD. A unified approach to early reconstructive surgery of the child with ambiguous genitalia. *J Urol* 1987; 138: 1079.

Pagon RA. Diagnostic approach to the newborn with ambiguous genitalia. *Pediator Clin North Am* 1987; 34: 1019.

Rock JA, Katz E. Ambiguous genitalia. *Semin Reprod Endocrinol* 1987; 5: 327.

Sadler TW. *Langman's Medical Endocrinology*, 6th edn. Baltimore: Williams & Wilkins, 1990; 260−296.

Simpson JC. Genetic control of sex determination. *Semin Reprod Endocrinol* 1987; 5: 209.

Premature thelarche
(breast development)

MARIA D. URBAN

Premature thelarche is a form of incomplete sexual precocity which presents as isolated breast development in a female child before the age of 8 years.

NATURAL HISTORY OF BREAST DEVELOPMENT

Estrogen levels in the fetal serum are high and are of both fetal and placental origin. Estrogens are responsible for development of breast buds which are present in most full-term newborns of both sexes.

Breast buds are not palpable before 33 weeks of gestation. In a full-term infant, breast buds average 7 mm and they are not only palpable but are readily seen.

In a female newborn, other estrogen effects such as hypertrophy of the labia minora and superficial transformation of the urogenital epithelium are also observed. In some female newborns, withdrawal from the estrogen-rich environment may cause vaginal bleeding or colostrum production ("witch's milk") within several days after delivery.

Postnatally, a transient surge in gonadotropin production causes ovarian stimulation in the female infant which is associated with elevated estrogen levels and a pubertal response to gonadotropin-releasing hormone. This surge of estrogen may be sufficient to sustain breast development through early infancy. However, in most infants breast buds disappear by the sixth month of life. Persistence of significant breast tissue beyond the sixth month of age may be abnormal.

After the short period of gonadal stimulation after birth, a normal child enters a prepubertal period with minimal function of the hypothalamic–pituitary–gonadal axis. During this period, pituitary gonadotropin levels as well as gonadal sex steroids are barely detectable.

Activation of the hypothalamic–pituitary–ovarian axis occurs again at puberty. The time of onset and the speed of progression of pubertal development are highly variable and show significant familial trends. It is generally accepted that normal sexual development in a female child begins between the ages of 8 and 13 years. Development of breast buds is the first sign of puberty in about 90% of females. The average age of onset of breast development (Tanner stage 2) in an American female child is 10.9 ± 1.0 years; the average age of onset of Tanner stage 2 pubic hair is 11.2 ± 1.1 years, and the average age at menarche is 12.7 ± 1.0 years. Breast development before the age of 8 years is considered to be premature.

DEFINITION OF PREMATURE THELARCHE (Tables 5.1 and 5.2)

Premature thelarche is defined as the isolated appearance of breast development in a girl less than 8 years of age. Premature thelarche is a relatively common entity in girls 6 months to 8 years of age.

Although lack of progression of sexual development is typical of premature thelarche, further enlargement and persistence of breast enlargement

Table 5.1 Classification of premature breast development in a girl

Premature thelarche

True precocious puberty
  Idiopathic
  Central nervous system lesion
  Primary hypothyroidism

Precocious pseudopuberty
  Estrogen-producing ovarian tumor
  Estrogen-producing adrenal tumor
  McCune–Albright syndrome

Exogenous source of estrogen

Table 5.2 Differential diagnosis of premature thelarche

	Thelarche	Complete sexual precocity	Pseudoprecocity
Breast	Enlarged	Enlarged	Enlarged
Nipples	Often infantile	Maturing	Maturing
Vaginal mucus	Red	Pink	Pink
Vaginal smear	No or minimal estrogen effect	Estrogenization	Estrogenization
Sexual hair	No	At times	At times
Bone age	Normal	Usually advanced	Usually advanced
Growth rate	Normal	Accelerated	Accelerated
Serum LH and FSH	Normal for age	Normal for pubertal stage	Low or normal for age
Serum estradiol	Normal for age	Normal for pubertal stage	Elevated to very high (serum androgens may be elevated)

LH, luteinizing hormone; FSH, follicle-stimulating hormone.

for several months or even years may occur. Fluctuations in the breast size are not unusual.

The most important characteristic of premature thelarche is that breast development appears as an isolated event with no other signs of sexual development except for occasional mild transient estrogen effects on the vaginal mucosa.

In contrast, *true precocious puberty* occurs in girls younger than 8 years of age and causes progressive development of breasts and pubic hair, growth and bone age acceleration, and earlier than normal epiphyseal fusion leading to a shortened final adult height. Although the exact cause of this condition in the majority of affected girls is not known, the mechanism of central precocious puberty involves activation of the hypothalamic–pituitary–gonadal axis. In this form of precocious puberty, sexual maturation is complete and the pubertal development is appropriate for the sex of the child.

In *precocious pseudopuberty*, sexual maturation is incomplete with only some of the secondary sexual characteristics developing early. Moreover, in some patients, the pubertal development has characteristics of the opposite sex. In this condition, the sexual development in girls is not mediated by the pituitary gland and is usually due to primary ovarian or adrenal disorders.

ETIOLOGY OF PREMATURE THELARCHE

The precise mechanism of premature thelarche is unknown. Several theories have been suggested to explain its development.

1 Since normal prepubertal serum gonadotropin and estrogen levels are found in many girls with isolated breast development, it is believed that premature thelarche may result from increased end-organ sensitivity to normal prepubertal levels of circulating estrogen.

2 Most cases, however, appear to be due to transient or intermittent pituitary secretion of gonadotropins and the subsequent secretion of estrogen by the ovary, resulting in elevation of serum estrogen levels. This precocious but unsustained production of estrogens by the ovaries appears to be responsible for the development of breast tissue and, occasionally, mild estrogenization of the vaginal epithelium.

Further evidence for transient partial activation of the hypothalamic–pituitary–gonadal axis in the etiology of premature thelarche is that sleep-dependent increases in serum gonadotropins with predominance of follicle-stimulating hormone (FSH) secretion during sleep and after luteinizing hormone-releasing hormone (LHRH) stimulation have been observed. Sleep-dependent gonadotropin increases are typically found in the early stages of puberty (Tanner stages 2 and 3). Accordingly, premature thelarche may represent a specific unsustained stage in the maturation of the hypothalamic–pituitary–gonadal axis.

The presence of small follicular ovarian cysts in some patients with premature thelarche is also suggestive that premature thelarche may be caused by transient or intermittent stimulation of ovarian estrogen production by pituitary gonadotropins. Long-term follow-up of affected patients has revealed resolution of the cysts.

3 Premature thelarche may be caused by a larger, possibly autonomous, ovarian cyst which may produce significant amounts of estrogen. Spontaneous regression and recurrences of the cyst and thelarche have been documented.

4 Other authors have suggested that premature secretion of the adrenal androgen, dehydroepiandrosterone (DHEA), and its peripheral conversion to estrogen, may be the cause of premature thelarche. Conversion of DHEA to estradiol in breast tissue or vaginal tissue would allow a significant estradiol level to be present in the target tissue in the absence of its elevation in the serum.

EVALUATION OF A GIRL WITH PREMATURE BREAST DEVELOPMENT

A history should be obtained to exclude an exogenous source of estrogen such as the ingestion of birth control pills, eating food contaminated with estrogen, or the application of an estrogen-containing cream to the child's skin. A recent growth spurt suggests the possibility of true precocious puberty or pseudopuberty rather than premature thelarche.

The presence of neurologic symptoms such as headaches, seizures, deterioration in fine motor skills, and regression of developmental milestones suggest that the breast development is a manifestation of central precocious puberty which is due to an intracranial disorder. In such an instance, computed tomography and/or magnetic resonance imaging of the hypothalamic–pituitary area is indicated.

The *physical examination* should include careful determination of the patient's height. If previous height measurements are available, calculation of the growth rate over the past 6–12 months will be valuable in the differentiation between premature thelarche and precocious puberty or pseudoprecocity. A growth rate of more than 7.5 cm (3 inches) a year

in a child between 3 and 8 years of age and/or the crossing from one percentile to a higher one on the growth curve is very suggestive of an estrogen-mediated pubertal growth spurt. A growth rate of this magnitude is suggestive of either true precocious puberty or pseudopuberty rather than premature thelarche.

The size of the breast and presence of tenderness or nipple discharge should be noted. In premature thelarche, breast enlargement can be unilateral or bilateral. Slight tenderness to touch may be reported by the child. Breast enlargement may be minimal with a breast bud of just several millimeters below the areolae or a well-delineated disk with a diameter of 5–10 cm.

Discharge from the nipples is not observed in patients with premature thelarche and, if present, it should prompt investigation for the possibility of hyperprolactinemia, infection, or pregnancy. Assessment of the development of the nipple and areolae may be helpful in the differential diagnosis. Infantile nipples and areolae are observed in patients with premature thelarche. In contrast, in true precocious puberty or pseudopuberty, the development of the areolae of the nipple occurs as the breast enlargement progresses. Dark pigmentation of the nipples usually occurs in patients with very high estrogen levels, as in children with estrogen-producing tumors. Although enlargement of a breast bud is usually due to breast tissue development, the possibility of a tumor, such as lipoma or neurofibroma, should be considered. Breast carcinoma in a child is extremely rare. Erythema and tenderness of the breast with axillary lymphadenopathy suggest the possibility of an abscess. In a child with unilateral breast enlargement, biopsy of the involved breast is usually unnecessary and contraindicated since the surgical procedure may cause complete destruction of the breast bud with subsequent lack of breast development. In exceptional cases, when either abscess or tumor is highly suspected, careful aspiration or a biopsy may need to be performed.

The genitalia should be examined thoroughly for estrogen and/or androgen effects. In premature thelarche, pubic and axillary hair are not present. Uterine enlargement and ovarian abnormalities, such as granulosa cell tumor or a large ovarian cyst, may be detected by rectal examination in patients with precocious puberty or pseudopuberty.

It is essential to perform a complete neurologic examination including a funduscopic examination in every patient with premature breast development to detect intracranial lesions. The examination is expected to be normal in patients with premature thelarche. Assessment of visual fields should be undertaken in patients with suspected central precocious puberty.

The presence of a ventricular–peritoneal shunt or an arrested hydrocephalus may be an important clue in the evaluation of a child with early breast development. There is an increased frequency of precocious puberty in children with arrested or shunted hydrocephalus as well as those with cerebral palsy and meningomyelocele.

The presence of *café-au-lait* skin pigmentation suggests the possibility that early breast development represents a manifestation of true precocious puberty associated with neurofibromatosis or pseudopuberty, as in patients with McCune–Albright syndrome.

The *laboratory evaluation* of the premature breast development in a female child is summarized in Figure 5.1. The initial diagnostic studies should include bone age and determination of serum gonadotropins and estrogen levels.

In a child with premature thelarche the bone age is normal and levels of randomly determined serum gonadotropin levels are prepubertal and appropriate for the bone age. The estradiol level in serum is usually prepubertal but it may be minimally and transiently elevated. Minimal estrogenization of the vaginal mucosa can be found on vaginal smear. In contrast, children with true precocious puberty have an advanced bone age, elevated serum gonadotropin and estradiol levels, and significant estrogenization of the vaginal mucosa. A child with pseudoprecocity due, for example, to a granulosa cell tumor of the ovary will usually have marked elevations of the serum estradiol level and low prepubertal serum gonadotropin levels.

Pulsatile secretions of serum gonadotropins, predominantly an elevation of the serum FSH level, have been observed in some patients with premature thelarche. Response to LHRH is also prepubertal with a predominant rise in serum FSH levels. In contrast, predominantly LH elevation is seen in patients in true precocious puberty. Although the FSH response to LHRH may be helpful in distinguishing premature thelarche from precocious puberty, the absence of an LH-predominant response should not be taken as assurance that the girl with isolated thelarche will not develop other premature secondary sexual characteristics.

Pelvic ultrasonography performed by experienced radiologists is very helpful in the assessment of uterine and ovarian size. In premature thelarche, pelvic ultrasound reveals prepubertal-size uterus and ovaries with occasional minimal follicular development. Occasionally, a single large follicular cyst can be detected in a child with premature thelarche which in most cases is transient and may be intermittent. In these instances differentiation from a primary ovarian tumor causing pseudoprecocity may be difficult. The serum estradiol level is usually helpful in the diagnosis.

In a child with premature sexual development and growth and bone age retardation and occasionally galactorrhea, primary hypothyroidism should be considered. Measurement of serum thyroxine, thyroid-stimulating hormone, and prolactin allows to make the diagnosis. In this instance central sexual precocity occurs because of hypothyroidism and it is reversed by treatment with thyroid hormone replacement therapy.

MANAGEMENT

The differentiation between premature thelarche, idiopathic central precocious puberty, and pseudoprecocity is important for both prognostic and therapeutic reasons.

Premature thelarche does not require medical treatment. However, it is extremely important to educate the family, care-givers, and if appropriate, the child, that the condition is not permanent. Moreover, the family should be reassured that there will not be any long-term effects from the presence of early breast development. It is also necessary for the physician to observe the child over a period of time to insure that no other pubertal changes occur which would suggest that the early breast development was a manifestation of precocious puberty or pseudopuberty rather than premature thelarche.

Idiopathic true precocious puberty has serious adverse effects such as short final adult height and the psychologic impact of early sexual changes on the child. The affected child can be effectively treated with a LHRH agonist. Patients with precocious pseudopuberty caused by an ovarian or adrenal tumor are treated surgically and usually have a good therapeutic response.

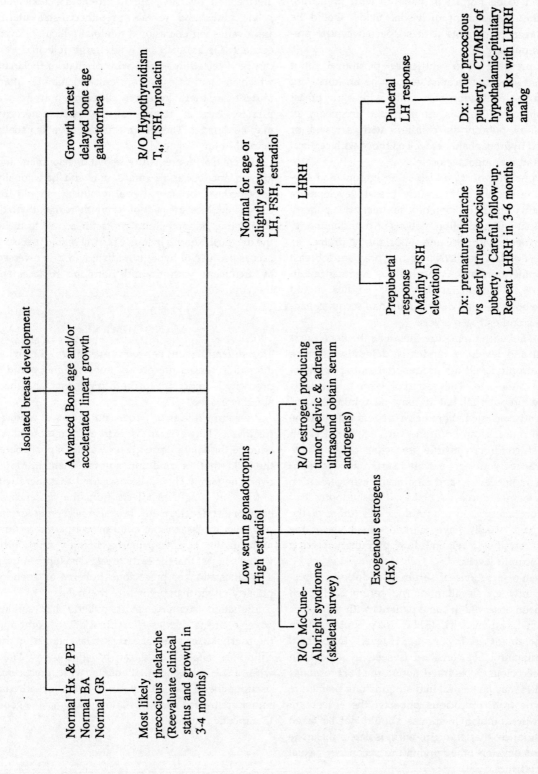

Fig. 5.1 Stepwise approach to evaluation of a girl with premature breast development. Hx, history; PE, physical examination; BA, bone age; GR, growth rate; PT, premature thelarche; E₂, estradiol; R/O, rule out; T₄, thyroxine; TSH, thyroid stimulating hormone; MRI, magnetic resonance imaging; CT, computed tomography; LH, luteinizing hormone; FSH, follicle stimulating hormone; Sx, symptoms; LHRH, luteinizing hormone-releasing hormone; Dx, diagnosis; Rx, treatment.

FURTHER READING

Flicki A, Lewin RP, Kauli R *et al*. Premature thelarche: natural history and sex hormone secretion in 69 girls. *Acta Paediatr Scand* 1984; 73: 756–762.

Forest MG. Function of the ovary in the neonate and infant. *Eur J Obstet Gynecol Reprod Biol* 1979; 9: 145–160.

Rosenfield RL. The ovary and female sexual maturation. In: Kaplan SA, ed. *Clinical Pediatric Endocrinology*. Saunders: Philadelphia, 1990.

Ross GT. Disorders of the ovary and female reproductive tract. In: Wilson JD and Foster DW, eds. *Williams Textbook of Endocrinology*, 7th edn. Saunders: Philadelphia, 1985; 212.

Stenhope R, Abdulwahid NA, Adams J *et al*. Studies of gonadotropin pulsatility and pelvic ultrasound examinations distinguish between isolated premature thelarche and central precocious puberty. *Eur J Paediatr* 1986; 147: 190–194.

6

Precocious adrenarche

GEORGE B. MAROULIS

Precocious pubarche is the result of a premature increase of adrenal or ovarian androgen production or an increased sensitivity to androgens in females younger than 8 years of age.

The evaluation of this problem may be better appreciated if the normal physiology of the onset of adrenarche as well as its relationship to pubarche and normal pubertal development, as it pertains to the female, is reviewed.

NORMAL ADRENARCHE–PUBARCHE

Adrenarche is the increase in adrenal production of the androgens dehydroepiandrosterone (DHEA) and DHEA sulfate (DHEAS) which occurs between ages 6 and 8 years. It is the earliest hormonal manifestation of the onset of normal puberty.

Pubarche is the clinical manifestation of adrenarche; that is, the appearance of axillary and pubic hair which follows the increased production of adrenal androgens. It usually occurs after the age of 8 years, and lags behind adrenarche by about 2 years. Pubic hair precedes axillary hair growth in the majority of cases, but occasionally axillary hair may appear first. An adult axillary odor is often the earliest clinical sign of androgen secretion.

Between the ages of 9 and 11 years adrenarche is followed by an increase in the episodic secretion of follicle-stimulating hormone (FSH) and luteinizing hormone (LH), which leads to ovarian stimulation, increased estradiol secretion (gonadarche), and the onset of breast development (thelarche). Following gonadarche, ovarian androgen production becomes significant at the average age of 11 and contributes to the initiation of axillary hair growth [1]. Pubarche is usually seen when serum DHEA exceeds 1.0 ng/ml and DHEAS levels exceed 400 ng/ml and usually appears after thelarche [2,3]. There is a gradual increase of the mean serum DHEAS levels with advancing pubic hair stages, but there is a significant overlap of the DHEAS levels observed at each stage, which suggests significant individual variation in the biologic effects of androgens (Table 6.1). Adrenarche precedes the beginning of the growth spurt by about 2 years.

Because adrenarche precedes gonadarche by about 2–3 years it has been proposed that adrenarche may be a controlling factor in the onset of puberty; however, this association is not proven and indeed premature adrenarche is not followed by premature gonadarche [5].

Physiology of adrenal androgen production at puberty

The adrenal gland is composed of the cortex and the medulla. The cortex is divided into three zones: the outer zona glomerulosa, the middle zona fasciculata, and the inner zona reticularis.

During fetal life the adrenal gland is markedly enlarged due to enlargement of the zona reticularis, also called the fetal zone. After birth this zone shrinks and remains relatively inactive until adrenarche [3]. At adrenarche, DHEA and DHEAS production increase and continue to do so in relationship to the increasing age and stage of puberty (Table 6.1). This increased production of adrenal androgens is believed to be primarily centered at the zona reticularis, which has the highest concentrations of androstenedione (A), testosterone (T), dihydro-testosterone (DHT), DHEA, and DHEAS [6,7]. The increase in adrenal androgen production observed at puberty parallels the enlargement of the zona reticularis [8].

The stimulus for the initiation of increased adrenal androgen production which signals the onset of puberty is not known. There are, however, a number of theories concerning the postulated mechanism(s) for control of initiation of adrenal androgen production. The first theory proposes that adrenal responsiveness to adrenocorticotropic hormone (ACTH)

Table 6.1 Serum DHEA [2] and DHEAS [4] levels (and ranges) at pubic hair stages of pubarche

Stage	Average age (years)	Serum DHEA (ng/ml)	DHEAS (ng/ml)
I Prepubertal	<8	0.75 (0.19−2.00)	<350
II Labial hair only	9.5	2.93 (0.45−19.04)	1500 (350−1800)
III Labial hair extends over mons pubis	11.2	4.65 (1.25−1.73)	2200 (500−3500)
IV Labial hair extends laterally	12.1	4.50 (1.5−13.2)	2150 (600−3400)
V Further lateral spread to thighs; forms inverse triangle	14.6	5.10 (1.6−16.2)	2150 (600−3400)

DHEA, dehydroepiandrosterone; DHEAS, DHEA sulfate.

changes at puberty. This results in modification of the activity of various adrenal enzymes and results in increased androgens, specifically DHEA [9,10]. A second theory suggests that adrenarche may be caused by the increasing adrenal mass which is a normal process during childhood. This enlargement could result in increased blood flow in the adrenal cortex and higher levels of androgens. Finally, there may be a specific adrenal gland cortical androgen-stimulating hormone (CASH) which may specifically direct adrenal androgen production and be increased at the time of adrenarche [11−13]. Estrogens, gonadotropins, prolactin, and prostaglandins have also been suggested as possible factors stimulating adrenal androgen secretion, but the evidence is not strong [11].

PRECOCIOUS ADRENARCHE−PUBARCHE

The initiation of increased adrenal androgen production before the age of 6 and pubarche before the age of 8 years is considered precocious.

In the majority of cases precocious pubarche is the result of benign precocious secretion of adrenal androgens. It is more frequently seen in girls than in boys and is more often seen in obese children, or in brain-damaged children with or without cerebral palsy [14] who may have an abnormal electro-encephalogram [15]. It is most frequently a benign condition. Yet, despite its usually nonprogressive or slowly progressive nature, it can be of great concern to parents and primary care physicians who may be alarmed, thinking that it may be an early sign of serious problems such as true precocious puberty, adrenal or ovarian tumors, or an attenuated form of congenital adrenal hyperplasia (CAH).

When precocious pubarche is followed by or seen concomitantly with precocious thelarche the underlying problems to be considered should be either true precocious puberty or ovarian or adrenal tumors, where the key findings are a significant elevation of serum DHEAS and/or testosterone, and advanced bone age.

Although pubarche follows thelarche in normal pubertal development, this order is reversed in 15% of children. In such cases precocious pubarche may be the early manifestation of true precocious puberty [16].

CAUSES

True precocious puberty

True precocious puberty should be suspected when precocious pubarche is followed by thelarche and is accompanied by an advancing bone age and height.

CHAPTER 6

It should be suspected when the conditions shown in Table 6.2 are present. The key diagnostic features are the laboratory findings of elevated serum DHEAS, rising serum LH, FSH, and/or a pubertal response to LH-releasing hormone (LHRH) stimulation, a rapidly advancing bone age, and accelerated rate of linear growth.

True isosexual precocity is due to premature maturation of the hypothalamic–pituitary axis resulting

Table 6.2 Causes of pubarche

True precocious puberty

Idiopathic

Congenital anomalies
  Septooptic dysplasia
  Hydrocephalus

Central nervous system tumors

Postinflammatory
  Encephalitis
  Meningitis
  Brain abscess

Neurocutaneous syndromes

Primary hypothyroidism

Associated with early androgen exposure from
  Congenital adrenal hyperplasia
  Ovarian or adrenal tumors

Pseudoprecocious puberty

Ovarian tumors (androgenizing)
  Arrhenoblastoma
  Lipoid cell
  Adrenal rest
  Hilus cell
  Granulosa-theca cell

Gonadoblastoma in
  XY gonadal dysgenesis
  XY testicular dysgenesis

Adrenal tumors

Congenital adrenal hyperplasia

Human chorionic gonadotropin-secreting tumors
  (usually seen only in boys)

Exogenous drug-contaminated sex hormone

Incomplete precocity
Isolated precocious pubarche
  Premature adrenarche
  Atypical congenital adrenal hyperplasia

---

in the premature production of gonadotropins and androgenic as well as estrogenic steroids. Such premature maturation may be idiopathic or may be caused by cerebral problems such as encephalitis, head trauma, hydrocephalus, or other causes as listed in Table 6.2. The clinical presentation in such cases may not follow the normal progression, i.e., thelarche, pubarche, growth spurt, and menses. In some cases isolated precocious pubarche may be the first sign, together with accelerated gain in height and bone age [16].

Pseudoprecocious puberty

Virilizing adrenal tumors
Adrenal adenomas or adenocarcinomas occur most frequently in young girls rather than boys and are often seen under the age of 5 [17]. Such tumors may secrete either androgens exclusively, or may produce excessive amounts of glucocorticoids as well as androgens with an array of symptoms, i.e., hypertension, Cushingoid appearance, excessive fat, hirsutism, and virilization. For these virilizing tumors, serum levels of DHEAS usually exceed 7000 ng/ml. Serum T and A levels may also be elevated either by direct secretion or by conversion of DHEA and DHEAS to T [18]. Rarely such tumors produce only T [18]. Serum cortisol may be entirely normal or elevated, in which case the signs of Cushing's syndrome are observed. Definitive localization of these tumors is accomplished by imaging techniques. Rarely, if these studies are not definitive, the diagnosis is made by measuring levels of DHEA, DHEAS, and T in adrenal vein samples obtained by adrenal vein catheterization [18].

Virilizing ovarian tumors
Virilizing ovarian tumors are rare but have been reported to cause precocious pubarche which is accompanied by precocious thelarche since these tumors may also secrete estrogen. Granulosa-theca cell tumors most frequently cause precocious thelarche, but isolated precocious pubarche or pubarche with thelarche may occasionally be the earliest presenting sign. Arrhenoblastomas, interstitial cell tumors, hilus cell tumors, adrenal rest, and lipoid cell tumors are most frequently associated with high serum T and A levels [18,19].

Children with gonadal dysgenesis or XY testicular dysgenesis who are phenotypically female may also have precocious pubarche due to the development of

40

a gonadoblastoma in the ovarian streak or abnormal gonad [20].

Ovarian cysts have been reported to occur with precocious puberty, possibly due to stimulation of ovarian tissue by DHEAS [21], but in these situations serum T and A levels are usually normal.

If prolonged and not treated, persistent hyperandrogenemia may lead to the onset of true precocious puberty due to persistent exposure of the hypothalamus to androgens, which leads to "maturation" of the normal pubertal mechanism, expressed after the treatment of the primary disorder. This has been described in patients with CAH [22] and adrenal tumors [23], but may theoretically occur in all such patients if they are left untreated. This is more likely to occur when the bone age has increased to more than 12–13 years of age. Most frequently, however, there is no abnormal maturation of the hypothalamic–pituitary–gonadal axis.

Isolated precocious adrenarche
The cause of premature adrenarche is as poorly understood as the control mechanism for adrenarche and could be the result of: (1) premature change of adrenal enzymatic responsiveness to ACTH [9]; (2) premature increased release of CASH [10] or other pro-opiomelanocortin-related peptide; or (3) a precocious increase in adrenal gland mass and thickness which parallels increase in body mass, often observed in children with precocious pubarche. This increase in adrenal mass may in theory lead to an increase in intraadrenal concentrations of steroids which inhibit 3β-hydroxysteroid dehydrogenase activity, leading to increases in DHEA and DHEAS serum levels [10]. This theory may only be a partial explanation of these events since premature adrenarche frequently occurs in children with normal weight and height. The serum level of DHEAS is elevated in more than 85% of cases. Most children have an adult-type axillary odor and are reported to have slightly advanced bone age, but no onset of growth spurt and no other signs of virilization. Occasionally acne, axillary hair growth, and adult-type perspiration may precede pubic hair development [14].

There is no evidence that environmental, dietary, or familial factors play a role in the appearance of precocious pubarche [24]. As an isolated nonprogressive event, precocious pubarche is associated with eventual normal development of secondary sexual characteristics, growth, and fertility. Isolated premature pubarche does not seem to influence the overall height achieved by the individual [25]. In those children in whom DHEAS is normal, the probable cause is an increased sensitivity of the hair follicles.

Atypical CAH
The classic CAH is usually not associated with precocious puberty and is almost always diagnosed at birth, because of genital ambiguity. Atypical CAH can result from similar deficiencies of 21-hydroxylase, 11-hydroxylase, or 3β-hydroxysteroid dehydrogenase enzymes. These deficiencies are mild compared to those in the classic CAH and develop later in childhood [26–28]. The identification of these mild enzymatic defects and their differentiation from simple precocious adrenarche is difficult and requires an ACTH stimulation test, but even then results are not always easy to interpret. An elevation of serum 17-hydroxyprogesterone and adrenal androgens suggests the diagnosis of 21-hydroxylase deficiency; an elevation of 11-deoxycortisol makes us suspicious of diagnosis of an 11-hydroxylase deficiency and an elevation of 17-OH-pregnenolone : 17-OH-progesterone ratio suggests diagnosis of 3β-hydroxysteroid dehydrogenase deficiency. The clinical presentation of these problems — bone age, height, or chronologic age — is similar to that seen in precocious adrenarche. The incidence of atypical CAH is reported to be high in blacks [24] and Hispanics [26], but other studies have failed to show such an increase in Hispanics, blacks, or Jews [29].

DIFFERENTIAL DIAGNOSIS – DIAGNOSTIC EVALUATION

Despite the fact that isolated precocious pubic hair growth is generally a benign condition, a careful and thorough evaluation is needed to rule out the possibility that this is the first sign of a more significant underlying problem, such as: (1) true precocious puberty; (2) CAH; or (3) virilizing tumor.

The main concerns are to rule out a life-threatening condition such as adrenal or ovarian tumors, and to establish the rate of progression of pubic hair stages and accompanying signs or symptoms. The management depends on whether the process is advancing or stabilized, and whether thelarche and an increase in bone age and height are present.

During evaluation particular attention should be addressed to the following.
1 *History*: Exogenous hormone exposure, family

history, growth pattern, type of hair growth pattern, neurologic symptoms.

2 *Physical examination*: Record growth, establish Tanner stages of pubic hair and breast development; measure height carefully; look for axillary hair growth; pelvic examination (if tumor is suspected); neurologic examination.

3 *Laboratory evaluation* (in order of increasing seriousness): Left hand and wrist for bone age, serum DHEAS, serum T; serum estradiol, LH, FSH basal and stimulated after LHRH stimulation, ACTH stimulation, abdominal computed tomography (CT) or ultrasound to rule out adrenal or ovarian tumors, thyroid function test (thyroxine, thyroid-stimulating hormone). In the majority of cases isolated pubarche is a benign condition characterized by predominantly pubic hair development which does not progress. In such cases we recommend that the patient should be evaluated carefully to (1) rule out the presence of virilization, (2) rule out the presence of thelarche, (3) measure serum DHEAS, (4) measure height, and (5) measure bone age.

If pubarche is an isolated event with only a mild elevation of DHEA (higher than 1.0 ng/ml) and DHEAS (>400 ng/ml) and only mild or no advancement in the bone age, then the recommended management is continued observation with reevaluation of height, bone age, and DHEAS every 6–12 months. If DHEAS is elevated but not in the tumor range (>400 ng/ml but <7000 ng/ml), the bone age is slightly advanced, and the height is near or exceeds the 95th percentile and no other evidence of isosexual precocity exists, the underlying cause is either precocious adrenarche or a mild form of atypical CAH. The incidence of such CAH abnormalities is low, and only an ACTH stimulation test can reveal such an abnormality [24,27]. This necessitates elaborate testing and measurement of 17-OH-progesterone, 17-OH-pregnenolone, 11-deoxycorticosterone, and cortisol in order to diagnose a 3β-hydroxysteroid dehydrogenase, 21-OH hydroxylase, or 11-hydroxylase enzyme deficiency. At the present time the need for the diagnosis of such CAH — other than for investigational purposes — is debatable. Indeed since

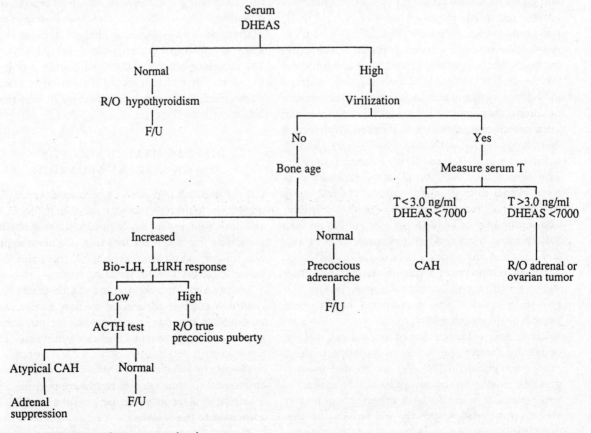

Fig. 6.1 Algorithm of premature pubarche.

clinically these entities — precocious adrenarche and subtle CAH — are almost indistinguishable, it is debatable as to whether such evaluation is necessary, particularly since treatment and follow-up depend more on clinical presentation than on the results of ACTH testing. The author does not recommend measuring 17-OH-pregnenelone or deoxycorticosterone or an ACTH stimulation test unless the child has an advanced bone age. As long as the child has a normal bone age and shows normal growth, no further evaluation or treatment is necessary, because in the majority of these children the elevation of DHEAS is not followed by a premature growth spurt and the remainder of the pubertal development is normal.

If pubarche advances and other signs, such as advancing bone age, suggest isosexual precocity, then true precocious puberty can be ruled out by measuring estradiol, FSH, LH, bioactive LH, and performing an LHRH stimulation test. The FSH and LH levels may actually be at prepubertal levels at this early stage of isosexual precocity and increase with age, but the bioactive LH is increased in patients with isosexual precocity [30]. Similarly, the response of FSH and LH levels to LHRH are usually diagnostic of true precocious puberty, but occasionally the response is incomplete or absent [31].

If serum DHEAS is significantly elevated or the bone age is rapidly advancing and the patient is virilized, the possibility of an adrenal or ovarian tumor or CAH should be ruled out. In these situations we recommend that in addition to serum DHEAS, serum levels of T should be evaluated. An adrenal tumor should be particularly suspected when the child is less than 5 years of age and the serum level of DHEAS exceeds 7000 ng/ml or the T level exceeds 3.0 ng/ml [18]. Most adrenal tumors have elevated serum levels of DHEAS and T but there are occasional adrenal tumors with isolated T secretion and normal DHEAS levels [18]. If an adrenal tumor is suspected an ultrasound or CT scan of the adrenal should be done. If these are normal an adrenal–ovarian vein catheterization should be done. Dynamic adrenal tests are not useful in ruling out a tumor. If the adrenal vein level of T or DHEAS level is very elevated in only one of the adrenal veins, a tumor is suspected [18]. If the levels are equally elevated in both adrenal veins, CAH is most likely the underlying cause.

If the serum T level exceeds 3.0 ng/ml an ovarian tumor is most likely present but an adrenal tumor cannot be ruled out [18]. If a physical examination done under anesthesia reveals a pelvic mass, an ovarian tumor can be confirmed by other proper studies such as pelvic ultrasound, a CT scan or a nuclear magnetic resonance (NMR) study. If a pelvic mass is not present, further abdominal CT scans are necessary to rule out an adrenal tumor. If in doubt an ovarian vein catheterization and sampling of both ovarian veins' blood may be necessary. A significant elevation of serum T in one vein with levels usually 5–10 times higher than that of peripheral circulation is diagnostic of a tumor; if the levels are elevated bilaterally a tumor is not present, and the most likely diagnosis is a variant of polycystic ovarian disease.

If pubarche is accompanied by thelarche then the differential diagnosis should include: (1) feminizing and/or androgenizing ovarian tumors; (2) true precocious puberty; and (3) hypothyroidism.

In certain situations ultrasonographic evaluation of uterus ovaries and adrenals may be of help. The ovarian size in young women is 0.7–0.9 ml, while after puberty it exceeds 3.0 cm [32]. In true precocious puberty the ovaries are not only enlarged but show follicular development. Ovarian cysts can also be identified by ultrasound. In suspected cases of CAH or adrenal tumors ultrasonographic studies will show enlarged adrenals. In such cases ovarian size is normal [32].

If pubarche is associated with delayed bone age primary hypothyroidism should be ruled out, by measuring thyroxine and thyroid-stimulating hormone levels. In these girls serum FSH and LH levels may be elevated in the pubertal range and will be reduced when the patient is treated.

TREATMENT

Isolated pubarche

In the absence of advanced bone age, virilization, or a significant increase of serum DHEAS levels, the child should be followed every 6 months and the parents should be appropriately informed to alleviate their concerns. As long as the child has a normal bone age and shows normal growth no further evaluation or treatment is necessary. In the majority of these children the elevation of DHEAS is not followed by a premature growth spurt and the remainder of pubertal development is normal.

If the bone age is slightly advanced but there is no other evidence of isosexual precocity or tumor, a closer follow-up is required. As long as the bone age does not rapidly advance, the eventual growth and height are normal and so is the sexual development. It has been stated that in the experience of some investigators such girls may develop the hirsutism—polycystic ovarian syndrome, but more studies are needed to confirm such an impression [33]. This concern may be more likely in girls in whom atypical CAH is diagnosed.

Atypical CAH

Such patients may be treated with adrenal suppression, particularly if there is significant acne, hirsutism, or advancing bone age, but at the present time there is no study to support the routine use of such therapy. Most such patients may have a slightly advanced bone age but their eventual height and sexual development are normal. More studies are needed to clarify this, and in particular whether the eventual height is normal.

CAH

Adrenal suppression with glucocorticoids is necessary; however, such a diagnosis is extremely rarely made at this late age. Such cases are diagnosed at birth.

Ovarian—adrenal tumors

If an ovarian cyst is present it is important to determine whether the cyst is the source of the androgens or whether it is secondary to gonadotropin stimulation or secondary to stimulation by DHEAS [21]. In such situations surgery should be avoided. Ultrasonographic studies offer help in clarifying the issue. If the cysts are multiple and bilateral they are usually secondary to gonadotropin stimulation but if they are solitary or solid they are probably virilizing tumors. Surgical therapy is the only recommended therapy of such virilizing tumors. A conservative approach with conservation of the ovary and removal only of the cyst or tumor, if small, should be considered. If the tumors are malignant appropriate therapy will depend on the exact nature and stage of the ovarian tumor [18].

Adrenal tumors are frequently malignant and need very careful excision and possibly subsequent chemotherapy [18].

True precocious puberty

Treatment with gonadotropin-releasing hormone analogs is the most promising therapy. In these girls the bone age advance and increased height are slowed [34,35]. Many other therapies for precocious puberty are discussed fully in Chapter 1.

REFERENCES

1 Korth-Schultz S, Levine L, New M. Evidence for the adrenal source of androgens in precocious adrenarche. *Acta Endocrinol (Copenh)* 1976; 82: 342.
2 Simonenko PC, Paunier L. Hormonal changes during puberty III. Correlation of plasma dehydroepiandrosterone, testosterone, FSH and LH with stages of puberty and bone age in normal boys and girls and in patients with Addison's disease or hypogonadism or with premature or late adrenarche. *J Clin Endocrinol Metab* 1975; 41: 894.
3 Reiter EO, Fuldauer VC, Root AW. Secretion of the adrenal androgen dehydroepiandrosterone sulfate during normal infancy, childhood and adolescence, in sick infants, and in children with endocrinologic abnormalities. *J Pediatr* 1977; 90: 766.
4 Rosenfield RL, Rich BH, Lucky AW. Adrenarche as a cause of benign pseudopuberty in boys. *J Pediatr* 1982; 101: 1005.
5 Lee PA, Gareis F. Gonadotropin and sex steroid response to luteinizing hormone-releasing hormone in patients with premature adrenarche. *J Clin Endocrinol Metab* 1976; 43: 195.
6 Dickerman Z, Grant DR, Faiman C, Winter JS. Intradrenal steroid concentrations in man: zonal differences and developmental changes. *J Clin Endocrinol Metab* 1984; 59: 1031.
7 Maroulis GB, Abraham GE. Concentration of androgens and cortisol in the zones of the adrenal cortex. In: Genazzani A, Thijssen T, Siiteri P, eds. *Adrenal Androgens*. New York: Raven Press, 1980: 49.
8 Grumbach MM, Richards HE, Conte FA, Kaplan SL. Clinical disorders of adrenal function and puberty: an assessment of the role of the adrenal cortex in normal and abnormal puberty in man and evidence for an ACTH-like pituitary adrenal androgen stimulating hormone. In: Serio M, ed. *The Endocrine Function of the Human Adrenal Cortex*. New York: Academic Press, 1977.
9 Rich BH, Rosenfield RL, Lucky AW, Heke JC, Otto P. Adrenarche: changing adrenal response to adrenocorticotropin. *J Clin Endocrinol Metab* 1981; 52: 1129.
10 Byrne JSD, Perry GC, Winter YS. Steroid inhibitory effects upon human adrenal 3β-hydroxysteroid dehydrogenase activity. *J Clin Endocrinol Metab* 1986; 62: 113.
11 Parker LN. Control of adrenal androgen secretion. In: *Adrenal Androgens in Clinical Medicine*. San Diego: Academic Press, 1989; 30.
12 Parker L, Lifrak E, Shively J et al. Human adrenal gland cortical androgen-stimulating hormone (CASH) is identical with a portion of the joining peptide of pituitary pro-opiomelanocortin (POMC). Program 71st Annual Meeting, Endocrine Society 1989. Abstract 299, 97.

13 Genazzani A, Facchinetti F, Pintor C et al. Propiocortin-related peptide plasma levels throughout prepuberty and puberty. J Clin Endocrinol Metab 1983; 57: 56.

14 Voutilainen R, Perheentupa J, Apter D. Benign premature adrenarche: clinical features and serum steroid levels. Acta Paediatr Scand 1983; 72: 707.

15 Lin N, Grumbach MM, de Napoli RA, Morishima A. Prevalence of electroencephalographic abnormalities in idiopathic precocious puberty and premature pubarche bearing on pathogenesis and neuroendocrine regulation of puberty. J Clin Endocrinol Metab 1965; 25: 1296.

16 Marshall WA, Tanner TM. Variations in pattern of pubertal changes in girls. Arch Dis Child 1969; 44: 291.

17 Lee PDK, Winter RT, Green OG. Virilizing adrenocortical tumors in childhood: eight cases and a review of the literature. Pediatrics 1985; 76: 437.

18 Maroulis GB. Evaluation of hirsutism and hyperandrogenemia. Fertil Steril 1981; 36: 273.

19 Towne BH, Mahour GH, Wooley MM, Isaacs H. Ovarian cysts and tumors in infancy and childhood. J Pediatr Surg 1975; 10: 311.

20 Frasier SD, Bashore RA, Mosier HD. Gonadoblastoma associated with pure gonadal dysgenesis in monozygous twins. J Pediatr 1964; 64: 740.

21 Chasalow FI, Granoff AB, Tse TF, Blethen SL. Adrenal steroid secretion in girls with pseudoprecocious puberty due to autonomous ovarian cysts. J Clin Endocrinol Metab 1986; 63: 828.

22 Pescovitz OH, Comite F, Cassorla F et al. True precocious puberty complicating congenital adrenal hyperplasia. Treatment with luteinizing hormone-releasing hormone analogue. J Clin Endocrinol Metab 1984; 58: 857.

23 Pescovitz OH, Hench K, Green O, Comite F, Loriaux DL, Cutler GB Jr. Central precocious puberty complicating a virilizing adrenal tumor. Treatment with a long acting LH-RH analog. J Pediatr 1985; 106: 612.

24 Kaplowitz PB, Cockrell JL, Young RB. Premature adrenarche. Clin Pediatr 1986; 25: 28.

25 Sigurjonsdottir TJ, Hayles AB. Premature pubarche. Clin Pediatr 1968; 7: 26.

26 Oberfield SE, Darrel MM, Leving LS. Adrenal steroidogenetic function in a Black and Hispanic population with precocious pubarche. J Clin Endocrinol Metab 1990; 70: 76.

27 Temeck JW, Pang S, Nelson C, New MI. Genetic defects of steroidogenesis in premature pubarche. J Clin Endocrinol Metab 1987; 64: 609.

28 Zackman M, Tassinari D, Prader A. Clinical and biochemical variability of congenital adrenal hyperplasia due to 11-hydroxylase deficiency. A study of 25 patients. J Clin Endocrinol Metab 1983; 56: 222.

29 Morris AH, Reiter ED, Geffner ME, Itami RM, Mayes D. Absence of non-classical congenital adrenal hyperplasia (CAH) in patients with precocious adrenarche (PA): (Abstract) 70th Annual Meeting Endocrine Society 1988.

30 Lucky AW, Rich BH, Rosenfield RL, Farig VS, Roche-Bender N. Bioactive LH: a test to discriminate true precocious puberty from premature thelarche and adrenarche. J Pediatr 1980; 97: 214.

31 Reiter EO, Kaplan SL, Conte FA, Grumbach MM. Responsivity of pituitary gonadotropes to luteinizing hormone releasing factor in idiopathic precocious puberty, precocious thelarche, precocious adrenarche and in patients treated with medroxyprogesterone acetate. Pediatr Res 1975; 9: 11.

32 Fleischer AC, Shawker TH. The role of sonography in pediatric gynecology. Clin Obstet Gynecol 1987; 30: 735.

33 Root AW, Shulman DI. Isosexual precocity. In: Wallach EE, Kempers RD, eds. Modern Trends in Infertility and Conception Control, Vol 4. Year Book Medical Publishers, 1988.

34 Styne DM, Harris DA, Egli CA et al. Treatment of true precocious puberty with a potent luteinizing hormone-releasing factor agonist: effect on growth, sexual maturation, pelvic sonography and the hypothalamic-pituitary gonadal axis. J Clin Endocrinol Metab 1985; 61: 142.

35 Boepple PA, Mansfield MJ, Crawford JD, Crigler JF, Blizzard RM, Crowley WF. Gonadotropin-releasing hormone agonist treatment of central precocious puberty: an analysis of growth data in a developmental context. Acta Paediatr Scand 1989; 367 (suppl): 38.

Part II
Menstrual abnormalities

7

Primary amenorrhea

SANTIAGO L. PADILLA

Primary amenorrhea is classically defined as absence of menses by chronologic age 16. Since pubertal development follows a normal sequence, absence of menses for 2 years after the initiation of breast development should also follow the diagnostic evaluation of primary amenorrhea. Primary amenorrhea may be caused by serious and life-endangering illness, therefore it is essential to make a prompt and accurate diagnosis.

ETIOLOGY

In general, amenorrhea may be caused by central, systemic, gonadal, or anatomic pathology. The degree of sex steroid production by the gonads divides these individuals into two main groups: hypogonadal and eugonadal.

Hypogonadism

Hypergonadotrophic hypogonadism
Individuals with no sex steroid production may have low or high gonadotropins (Table 7.1). Hypergonadotrophic hypogonadism is most commonly caused by chromosomal accidents that result in the deletion of ovarian determinant genes. Classically, these patients have a 45,X cell line (Turner's syndrome), although mosaic gonadal dysgenesis is probably more frequent than the single cell line. Patients with Turner's syndrome have short stature, and complete or partial expression of the Turner phenotype — webbed neck, high arched palate, short fourth metacarpal, cubitus valgus, widely spaced nipples, pigmented nevi, etc.

When the mosaic line involves a Y cell line (i.e., 45,X/46,XY), these patients are categorized as mixed gonadal dysgenesis. Phenotypically they may be indistinguishable from other Turner syndrome patients or may have varying degrees of sexual ambiguity [1]. The presence of a Y chromosome and streak gonads predisposes 30% of these patients to gonadal ridge tumors, like gonadoblastomas, yolk sac tumors, and dysgerminomas. Extirpation of the gonads of these patients is indicated as soon as the diagnosis is made. Thirty percent of these patients with chromosomally incompetent ovarian failure have cardiovascular and renal anomalies. Coarctation of the aorta and horseshoe kidney are the most common. Gonadal dysgenesis patients may be at risk for glucose intolerance. Patients with isochromosome of the

Table 7.1 Hypergonadotrophic hypogonadism

Chromosomally incompetent ovarian failure	Chromosomally competent ovarian failure
X chromosome deprivation	*46,XX*
45,X (classic Turner syndrome)	Autosomal recessive
45,X/46,XX	Autoimmune
45,X/46,X,i(Xq)	Environmental (e.g., viral)
46,X,i(Xq)	Neoplastic therapy (e.g., chemotherapy and radiation)
	17-Hydroxylase deficiency
Mixed gonadal dysgenesis	Ovarian infiltration (tuberculosis, mucopolysaccharidosis)
45,X/46,XY	Gonadotropin resistance (Savage or Jones' syndrome)
	Galactosemia
	46,XY gonadal dysgenesis (Swyer's syndrome)

long arm of X are at risk for developing Hashimoto's thyroiditis.

Hypergonadotrophic hypogonadism also occurs in patients with intact X chromosomes (chromosomally competent ovarian failure). Etiologic factors may include autosomal recessive genes, environmental agents (e.g., mumps), chemotherapy or radiation therapy, autoimmune disorders, galactosemia, ovarian infiltrative processes (e.g., tuberculosis) and mucopolysaccharidosis. Although the majority of these patients present with primary amenorrhea, 46% will have a few follicles and have some menses before the ovarian failure [2]. Individuals with 17-hydroxylase deficiency will have normal ovarian structure but lack steroidogenesis. If the 17-hydroxylase deficiency occurs in a 46,XX individual, the phenotype will be female and the cervix and uterus will be present. If this deficiency occurs in a 46,XY individual, the testis will produce Müllerian-inhibiting factor, but no sex steroids except for progesterone and pregnenolone. The phenotype will be female but the cervix and uterus will be absent.

Patients with 46,XY gonadal dysgenesis (Swyer's syndrome) have hypergonadotrophic hypogonadism. Testicular development is arrested early in embryogenesis, resulting in streak gonads that do not produce any androgens or Müllerian-inhibiting factors. They develop as phenotypic females with cervix and uterus. These dysgenetic gonads are at risk for germ cell tumor formation and need to be removed as soon as the diagnosis is made. The mode of inheritance is X-linked recessive. Another group of individuals with gonadotropin resistance (Savage or Jones' syndrome) have ovarian follicles, but lack steroidogenesis and will have high gonadotropins. Patients with chromosomally competent ovarian failure may have normal or tall stature, because they have intact growth determinant genes and their epiphyses remain open in the absence of sex steroid production.

Hypogonadotrophic hypogonadism

Hypogonadotrophic hypogonadism results from hypothalamic failure to secrete gonadotropin-releasing hormone (GnRH) adequately or from pituitary disease affecting production and/or release of gonadotropins (Table 7.2). Physiologic delay of puberty is one of the most frequently occurring syndromes in this category. This diagnosis is made by exclusion. GnRH deficiency (Kallmann's syndrome) is the second most common hypothalamic cause and is associated with anosmia and other midline facial defects. These pa-

Table 7.2 Hypogonadotrophic hypogonadism

Physiologic delay

Endocrine diseases
  GnRH deficiency (e.g., Kallmann's)
  Hypopituitarism
  Hypothyroidism
  Cushing's syndrome
  Hyperprolactinemia
  Congenital adrenal hyperplasia

Anatomic disorders
  Craniopharyngioma
  Pituitary adenoma
  CNS tumors
  Histiocytosis X
  Tuberculosis
  Sarcoidosis
  Hydrocephaly
  Post-CNS infections

Systemic disorders
  GI malabsorption
  Anorexia and weight loss
  Excessive exercise
  Chronic pulmonary or renal disease
  Neoplasia
  Collagen vascular disease
  Laurence–Moon–Bidle syndrome
  Prader–Willi syndrome

GnRH, gonadotropin-releasing hormone; CNS, central nervous system; GI, gastrointestinal.

tients invariably are sexually infantile. Neoplasms involving the hypothalamic or pituitary area must be eliminated as a possible cause. Craniopharyngiomas commonly develop between age 6 and 14 and grow rapidly with interference of pituitary function early. Pituitary adenomas, unlike craniopharyngiomas, tend to develop later and grow slowly. They usually interrupt the pubertal process after thelarche.

Some endocrine disease processes like hypothyroidism, adrenal insufficiency, and Cushing's syndrome, as well as systemic diseases like ulcerative colitis and regional enteritis, weight loss, psychologic dysfunction, stress, and excessive exercise may have a suppressive effect on the hypothalamus and pituitary gland.

Eugonadism

Anatomic causes

Eugonadal patients with primary amenorrhea most

Table 7.3 Eugonadal causes of primary amenorrhea

Anatomic causes
  Congenital absence of the uterus and vagina
    (Rokitansky's syndrome)
  Transverse vaginal septum
  Imperforate hymen
Testicular feminization syndrome
Polycystic ovarian syndrome
Hyperprolactinemia
Hypothyroidism

---

commonly have an anatomic cause (Table 7.3). Congenital absence of the uterus and vagina (Rokitansky's syndrome) is the most common anatomic abnormality encountered, followed by imperforate hymen, transverse vaginal septum, and testicular feminization syndrome (androgen insensitivity). In Rokitansky's syndrome, pubertal landmarks occur at the appropriate age and secondary sexual characteristics are normal. Most commonly there is a fusion failure of the two Müllerian anlagen with bilateral hypoplastic uterine remnants and vaginal agenesis. Fallopian tubes and ovaries are present. Variations may occur with different degrees of Müllerian development, which range from a complete absence of the fallopian tubes, to some degree of a functional uterus and endometrium. Congenital absence of the cervix may occur, but is extremely rare. The incidence of the Rokitansky's syndrome is 1:4000 female births. Renal abnormalities occur in one-third of the patients, especially unilateral renal agenesis. Major skeletal abnormalities such as phocomelia, digital agenesis, and scoliosis may also occur. The external genitalia are normal. Frequently there is a very short vaginal pouch. These patients have normal ovarian function and ovulation has been documented. In the instance of functional endometrium, different degrees of hematometra can occur and the clinical presentation will vary accordingly.

Transverse vaginal septum and imperforate hymen are two other anatomic causes of primary amenorrhea. Accumulation of blood behind these obstructions (hematocolpos) will cause cyclic pain and irritability. These individuals may present with a pelvic and/or abdominal mass. Further blood backup may result in reflux into the pelvis and potentially induce formation of endometriosis. In cases of imperforate hymen or low vaginal septum, clinical diagnosis is not difficult because protrusion of the hymen or septum can be

found. These obstructed mucosal membranes should not be pierced by needles in the office because of the possibility of inducing formation of a pyocolpos. If a needle is inserted, surgical repair should be done immediately to evacuate the accumulation of blood and repair the defect. Prognosis for adequate menstrual and sexual function is excellent.

In cases of transverse septum of the middle or upper vagina, the diagnosis and operative approach is more difficult. Vaginal constriction rings can occur after surgical repair. The surgical approach should be carefully tailored to the patient's anatomic abnormality [3]. Prognosis for adequate sexual and reproductive function is guarded.

Testicular feminization (androgen insensitivity syndrome)
Testicular feminization or androgen insensitivity syndrome consists of a 46,XY individual with a female phenotype. These patients are eugonadal because there is testicular production of androgens. A lack of an androgen receptor in the target cell prevents phenotypic expression of the androgen production. The uterus, vagina, and fallopian tubes are absent because the testes secrete normal amounts of Müllerian-inhibiting factor. In the complete form axillary and pubic hair is absent or minimal. Breast development is normal. Incomplete forms with varying degrees of masculinization have been reported [4]. Serum levels of gonadotropins are normal, although the luteinizing hormone (LH) may be elevated. The testes are usually intraabdominal, although they can be found in the inguinal canals or in the labioscrotal folds. Neoplasia is rare; therefore surgical removal is deferred until after puberty to allow for growth and breast development.

Polycystic ovarian syndrome
Polycystic ovarian syndrome (PCOS) classically presents with postmenarchal menstrual disorders such as dysfunctional uterine bleeding or secondary amenorrhea, but can present as primary amenorrhea also. Steroidogenesis is present in these patients with adequate pubertal development. Hirsutism is found as a common complaint. Congenital adrenal hyperplasia usually presents at birth, but the nonclassical form may present at puberty with a PCOS-like syndrome. Hyperprolactinemia and hypothyroidism can present as a eugonadal condition. These conditions are described in more detail elsewhere.

CHAPTER 7

CLINICAL EVALUATION

Figure 7.1 describes the evaluation scheme for these patients. An accurate history is paramount in evaluating these patients. Particular attention should be paid to family history and pubertal development. Patient prenatal history, ingestion of drugs, and exposure to chemicals and radiation should be noted. Lack of breast development or suboptimal breast development suggests hypogonadism. History of associated congenital abnormalities, dietary habits, weight changes, exercise history, and psychosocial history are of importance to evaluate the hypogonadal states. The chronology of pubertal changes is critical. Normal thelarche will point toward the eugonadal conditions. If they have pubarche along with thelarche, anatomic abnormalities like Rokitansky's syndrome, transverse vaginal septum, and imperforate hymen will be the most likely etiologies. Presence of thelarche with lack of axillary and pubic hair suggests testicular feminization.

Complete physical and pelvic examination is essential. Tanner staging of the breast is used to assess the degree of development [5]. Current and past height and weight should be assessed on a growth chart. Attention should be paid to hirsutism, abdominal striae, central obesity, galactorrhea, short stature, musculoskeletal anomalies, sexual ambiguity, signs of Turner's syndrome, hypothyroidism, and Cushing's syndrome. Many of these patients may have never been examined gynecologically; therefore special attention must be given to make the examination as atraumatic as possible and, if necessary, done under anesthesia or sedation.

Pertinent laboratory tests complement the clinical evaluation. All patients with intact Müllerian systems need a prolactin level and a thyroid-stimulating hormone (TSH) level. A vaginal maturation index or a progestational challenge test will determine if the patient is hypogonadal. A progestational challenge consists of a progestin, like medroxyprogesterone acetate 10 mg for 5 days. If the patient has endogenous estrogen production, vaginal bleeding will start within 2 weeks. If congenital absence of the uterus and vagina is suspected, a karyotype analysis is obtained to rule out testicular feminization syndrome. If the patient is hirsute, serum testosterone, dehydroepiandrosterone sulfate and 17-OH-progesterone should be evaluated. If the patient is hypogonadal or has suboptimal breast development, a serum follicle-stimulating hormone (FSH) should be obtained. If

the serum FSH is elevated or the patient has Turner's stigmata, a peripheral blood karyotype is indicated. Patients with autoimmune ovarian failure are at risk for other autoimmune disorders and should have serum assays for calcium and phosphorus levels, a.m. cortisol, antinuclear antibodies, thyroid antibodies, and rheumatoid factor. If the FSH level is low or normal, other endocrine tests should be obtained as indicated and pituitary or hypothalamic tumors ruled out with computed tomography scan or magnetic resonance imaging. A GnRH challenge test will follow if the radiologic and endocrine evaluation is normal.

Some investigators have suggested the utilization of Y-specific DNA probes to identify the presence of Y chromosome material which may predispose some of the gonadal dysgenesis patients to tumor formation [6]. If there is a hypergonadotrophic hypogonadal patient with high blood pressure, she should be evaluated for 17-hydroxylase deficiency with a serum progesterone which will be markedly elevated.

TREATMENT

The treatment of primary amenorrhea depends on its cause. The hypergonadotrophic hypogonadal patients ultimately need estrogen replacement therapy for initiation or completion of pubertal development and long-term preservation of bone structure. Patients with dysgenetic gonads and a Y chromosome should have their gonads removed as soon as the diagnosis is made. In cases of testicular feminization, surgical removal of the gonads can be postponed until after puberty is completed to allow for adequate growth.

Many of the hypogonadotrophic hypogonadism patients will need careful assessment of their diet, exercise, and stress factors. When reproduction becomes a question, ovulation induction may be necessary. In the meantime, estrogen replacement is indicated. Patients with hormonal disorders should be treated accordingly. A patient with physiologic delay of puberty can be reassured that puberty will soon progress. The patient with PCOS should undergo monthly withdrawal with progestins.

Imperforate hymen and transverse vaginal septa need to be repaired as soon as possible to avoid consequences of retrograde flow of the menstrual blood. Imperforate hymen is repaired with radial incisions on the hymen. A transverse vaginal septum needs to be repaired carefully with special attention to the possibility of vaginal constriction rings. The wider the wall of the septum, the higher the risk for

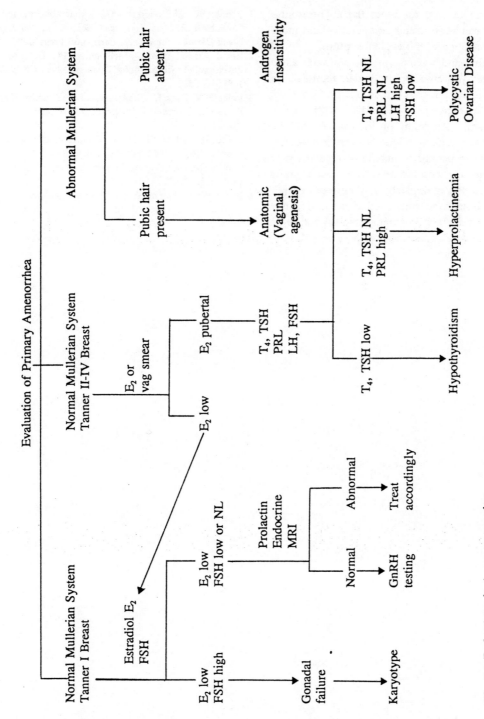

Fig. 7.1 Evaluation of primary amenorrhea.

constriction rings. To prevent vaginal constriction rings, the vaginal mucosa covering the septum is preserved and utilized to create flaps. Ultrasound examination can assist in the preoperative and intra-operative evaluation of the vaginal septum.

If the uterus and vagina are absent, such as in Rokitansky's syndrome or testicular feminization syndrome, vaginal pouches can be created by vaginal dilatation with progressively larger dilators [3]. Careful instruction and motivation of the patient by the physician make vaginal dilatation very successful. Occasionally the patient is unable to create a new vagina adequately and split-thickness skin grafts like the McIndoe vaginoplasty may be required [3]. Vaginal molds are commonly used after vaginoplasty as well as after the repair of transverse vaginal septa to prevent stricture and scarring.

REFERENCES

1 Padilla SL, McDonough PG. Sexual abnormalities. In: Greenblatt RB, ed. *Unwanted Hair — Ancestral Curse or Gland Disorder*. New York: Parthenon Press, 1985.
2 Reindollar RH, Byrd JR, McDonough PG. Delayed sexual development — a study of 252 patients. *Am J Obstet Gynecol* 1981; 140: 371.
3 Jones HW, Rock JA. *Reparative and Constructive Surgery of the Female Generative Tract*. Baltimore: Williams & Wilkins, 1983.
4 Griffin JE, Wilson JD. The syndromes of androgen resistance. *N Engl J Med* 1980; 302: 198.
5 Tanner JM. *Growth at Adolescence*, 2nd edn. Oxford: Blackwell Press, 1962.
6 Butler WJ, McDonough PG. The new genetics: molecular technology and reproductive biology. *Fertil Steril* 1989; 51: 375.

8

Secondary amenorrhea

SUZAN A. AYDINEL & JAMES A. SIMON

Secondary amenorrhea is a clinical symptom which results from a wide variety of etiologic factors (Table 8.1). The physician must be concerned with an array

Table 8.1 Common causes of secondary amenorrhea

Pregnancy

Idiopathic

Hypothalamic
  Psychogenic: stress, anxiety, anorexia nervosa, pseudocyesis
  Organic brain disease
  Strenuous exercise
  Chronic disease

Anovulation
  Cushing's disease or syndrome
  Late-onset congenital adrenal hyperplasia
  Stein–Leventhal syndrome
  Adrenal tumor
  Idiopathic

Pituitary
  Sheehan's syndrome
  Tumors
  Idiopathic
  Cushing's disease

Thyroid Disease

Ovarian
  Hermaphroditism
  Premature ovarian failure
  Destructive lesions: surgical, trauma, neoplasms, irradiation

Uterine
  Sclerosis of the uterine cavity: destructive lesions, vaginal, or cervical obstructions, scarring of the endometrium

Other
  Iatrogenic
  Liver cirrhosis
  Malnutrition
  Thyroid disease

of potential physiologic and pathologic causes. In order to maximize diagnostic accuracy and minimize office time, this chapter provides a simple mechanism to further define possible causes. The basic approach described is not new; an assessment of estrogenicity forms the working diagnosis. However, we emphasize the use of clinical judgment over the progestogen challenge test to determine estrogen status. The high frequency of false-positive and false-negative results associated with the progestogen challenge test commonly confuses rather than clarifies the actual diagnosis [1].

Estrogens are necessary for menstrual function, vasomotor stability, breast development, and support of vaginal and vulvar tissues. One can use the presence or absence of these physical criteria to broadly classify a patient with secondary amenorrhea into those who are estrogenized and those who are not. Armed with information gathered from the medical history and a complete physical examination, one should be able to pinpoint potential etiologic factors and reduce laboratory tests to a minimum. As a result, the patient receives the most reliable diagnosis at the minimal cost.

Diagnosis and management of abnormal menstrual function must be based upon an understanding of normal menstrual cycle variation. To this end, normal menstruation will be considered before presenting the diagnostic work-up for secondary amenorrhea. A clearer delineation of what is actually abnormal can aid the physician in making rational clinical judgments.

DEFINITION

Amenorrhea is a general term used to denote the absence of menses. It is described as secondary if a woman ceases to menstruate after the initial menarche. In actual usage, however, secondary amenorrhea refers to a clinical entity where menses have ceased after a "normal" pattern of menstrual function previously existed. It should be evaluated if there are no menses for three previous cycles in a female who has achieved menarche. This chapter will focus on secondary amenorrhea in women of reproductive age. Obviously, menopause is usually a normal physiologic event leading to secondary amenorrhea.

NORMAL CYCLE VARIABILITY

In order to facilitate an accurate diagnosis of secondary amenorrhea, it is necessary to have a clear understanding of normal variations in the menstrual cycle. Healthy women menstruate in cyclic intervals from menarche to menopause. To the physician, the 28-day menstrual cycle has long been accepted as a diagnostic criterion of normal menstrual performance in women of reproductive age. With advances in our

knowledge of the physiologic mechanisms by which a menstrual flow is produced and appreciation of correlative laboratory data, the length of the menstrual cycle is more accurately described as ranging in length between 24 and 32 days [2].

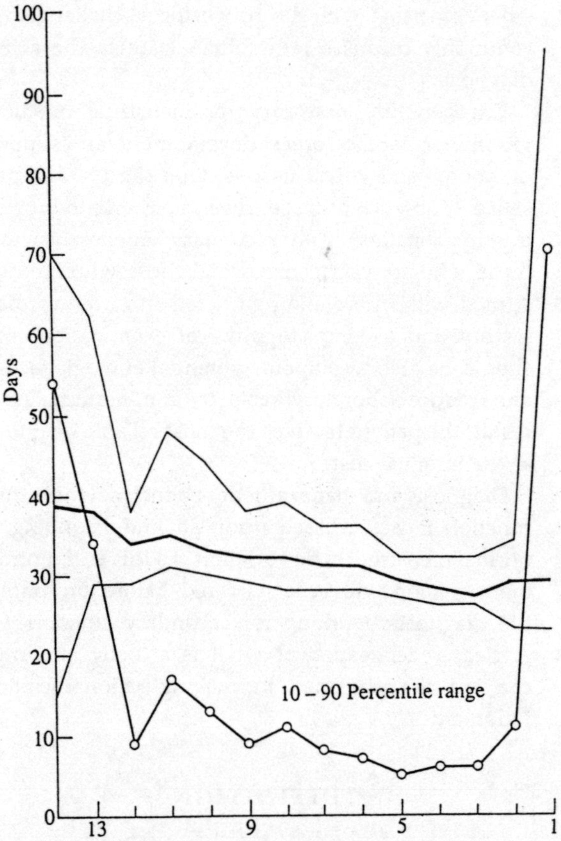

The length of the menstrual cycle varies according to a predictable pattern as a young woman matures. The mean cycle length drops from 35.1 days at age 12 to 27.1 days at age 43, and then rises to a maximum interval of 51.9 days at 55 years of age in those women still menstruating [3]. Variability in menstrual cycle length also demonstrates a common pattern from menarche to the climacteric phase (Fig. 8.1). The pattern follows a U-shaped curve with the range of variability dropping precipitously during the adolescent phase and rising abruptly in the climacteric phase. After childbirth, there are great irregularities as well. In addition, a variety of chronic diseases and psychologic factors, nutritional deficiencies, and endocrine dysfunctions may interfere with menstrual function (see below).

SIGNIFICANCE OF SECONDARY AMENORRHEA

In reference to clinical significance, amenorrhea *per se* may be considered a completely innocuous state for women. Its occurrence should not be disregarded, however, since it is associated at times with serious endocrine defects or systemic diseases and can be closely related to fertility. Pregnancy, while possible, is improbable during the amenorrheic state and in fact is often the most likely cause. It is for this reason that the majority of patients come to their physician.

DIAGNOSIS OF SECONDARY AMENORRHEA

Secondary amenorrhea is often the result of multiple causes. For instance, amenorrhea due to physiologic causes may have emotional elements as well. As a result, it may be difficult to pinpoint an exact etiologic factor. Despite this limitation, a rational approach to the diagnosis of secondary amenorrhea is based on the determination of estrogen status. The basic principles underlying the physiology of menstruation permit classification of etiologic factors on the basis of estrogenicity as presented in Table 8.2. Determination of estrogenicity reduces the number of potential causes to be evaluated. Armed with information gathered from a detailed history and physical

Fig. 8.1 The median length and the 10 to 90 percentile range of variability in successive scores of cycles from maturity to menopause (gynecologic age 11 to 39). Case 539 : 1908 : 15, age 26 to 54 years. (From Vollman.)

Table 8.2 Evaluation of secondary amenorrhea

History and physical examination
Cervical mucus study
Additional diagnostic measures
  Neurologic and ophthalmologic examinations
  Evaluation of the chest or sella turcica
  Electroencephalogram hematology (complete blood
    count) with sedimentation rate
  Liver and kidney function studies
  Thyroid function studies
  Glucose tolerance test
  Hormonal analysis (i.e., DHEAS, serum estradiol,
    testosterone)
  Gonadotropin assays
  Basal body temperature charts

DHEAS, dehydroepiandrosterone sulfate.

Table 8.3 Possible diagnoses of secondary amenorrhea according to estrogen status

Euestrogenic Causes
  Cushing's disease
  Late-onset congenital adrenal hyperplasia
  Stein–Leventhal syndrome (polycystic ovarian disease)

Hypoestrogenic causes
  Organic brain disease
  Chromophobe adenoma
  Sheehan's syndrome
  Strenuous exercise
  Anorexia nervosa
  Malnutrition
  Premature ovarian failure
  Severe hypothyroidism
  Hyperprolactinemia states

Variable
  Iatrogenic
  Acidophilic adenoma
  Psychogenic
  Chronic disease
  Thyroid disease
  Adrenal tumor
  Liver cirrhosis
  Ovarian tumors
  Hermaphroditism
  Sclerosis of the uterine cavity

Undetermined
  Diabetes mellitus

examination, the clinician can determine and select tests necessary to confirm a preliminary clinical diagnosis. The evaluation should proceed as outlined in Figures 8.2 and 8.3.

EVALUATION OF SECONDARY AMENORRHEA

Patient history

A careful history should obtain the following information: history of emotional disturbance; vasomotor symptoms; dietary history; gain or loss of weight; acute or chronic illnesses; surgery or trauma to the uterus; relationship to pregnancy or possibility of unsuspected pregnancy; symptoms characteristic of thyroid disease; and the family history relating to menstrual characteristics, fertility, metabolic disease, and tuberculosis. Specific questions as to the use of therapeutic or recreational pharmaceuticals must also be asked.

Physical examination

The physician should investigate for clinical signs and symptoms that point toward a specific diagnosis and appropriate tests should follow. Special attention to height, weight, abnormal hair growth, and the status of estrogen-dependent tissues such as the breast, vagina, cervix, and vulva are important. It is necessary to exclude physiologic causes of amenorrhea, such as pregnancy, postpartum lactation, hyperprolactinemia, and the amenorrhea associated with the normal menopause before proceeding with an extensive evaluation. Also, a cervical mucus evaluation should be obtained at the preliminary exam-

ination. Cervical mucus appearance on physical examination is a reliable index of estrogenicity as well as the single best predictor of clinical response to the progestogen challenge test [4]. Additional diagnostic measures will depend upon the specific problems involved and may include special examinations, such as those listed in Table 8.2.

Information gathered from the history and physical examination is utilized as the primary diagnostic criteria. In further defining possible causes, it is useful to categorize patients into one of four diagnostic groups based on estrogen status and investigate for clinical signs and symptoms of the various causes within each group (Table 8.3).

Estrogenic causes

The absence of vasomotor symptoms and vulvovaginal atrophy in women with normal breast development indicates endogenous estrogen production. Estrogenicity is further confirmed by estrogenic cervical mucus. Estrogenic cervical mucus characterizes the estrogenic patient with secondary amenorrhea. Cer-

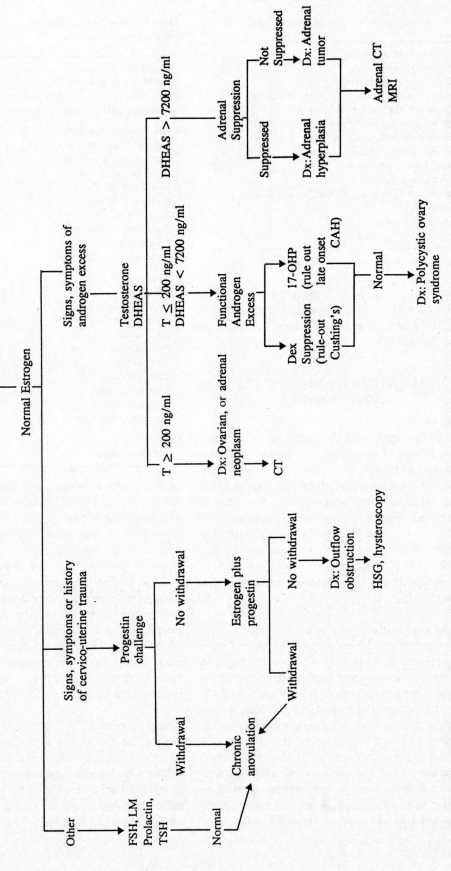

Fig. 8.2 Evaluation of secondary amenorrhea. FSH, follicle stimulating hormone; TSH, thyroid stimulating hormone; LH, luteinizing hormone; T, testosterone; DHEAS, dehydroepiandrosterone sulfate; 17-OHP, 17-hydroxyprogesterone.

vical mucus is described as estrogenic if it is thin, watery, clear, and profuse. Although a variety of factors can adversely affect cervical mucus production (i.e., vaginitis, prior cervical laser or cryosurgery, or cone biopsy), cervical mucus is a reliable measure of estrogenicity [4]. Occasionally, a woman with estrogenic secondary amenorrhea will spontaneously ovulate prior to her examination. In these instances, pelvic tissues will be well estrogenized but cervical mucus will be progestational. The patient will report menses within 2 weeks. The use of progestational agents will cause similar responses.

A variety of etiologic factors are associated with euestrogenicity. The physician must examine the patient for additional signs and symptoms to differentiate further the cause of secondary amenorrhea. This is outlined in Figure 8.2.

Cushing's syndrome or disease
Cushing's syndrome is characterized by excessive secretion of cortisol. It may be caused by an autonomous adrenal overproduction (i.e., adenoma carcinoma or Cushing's syndrome) or by excessive stimulation from the pituitary gland (basophilic adenoma — Cushing's disease). The physical characteristics of Cushing's are often so striking that the diagnosis is obvious: truncal obesity, moon face, hirsutism, hypertension, purple abdominal striae, erythemic acne, and easy bruisability. The pelvic organs are usually normal. The laboratory findings which confirm the diagnosis of Cushing's syndrome/disease indicate an elevation of urinary and/or serum corticosteroids.

Late-onset congenital adrenal hyperplasia
Congenital adrenal hyperplasia (CAH) an autosomal recessive disorder characterized by excessive androgen production, is usually diagnosed in infancy. However, a mild block in adrenal steroid synthesis may appear after puberty as progressive hirsutism or virilization. These patients may have mild deficiencies of 21-hydroxylase, 11β-hydroxylase, and 3β-hydroxysteroid dehydrogenase. Clinical features that are associated with late-onset CAH may include short adult height, acne, oily hair, temporal balding, clitoromegaly, hirsutism, and oligo- or amenorrhea, although features are highly variable. Accurate identification of patients with late-onset CAH may be obtained with an elevated serum assay of 17-hydroxyprogesterone, particularly following adrenocorticotropic hormone (ACTH) stimulation. Almost all individuals with late-onset CAH are characterized by deficient 21-hydroxylase activity [5].

Stein—Leventhal syndrome
Also known as polycystic ovary syndrome (PCOS), Stein—Leventhal syndrome is characterized by disturbed ovarian steroid feedback to the hypothalamus and pituitary. Luteinizing hormone (LH) stimulation results in excessive production of androgenic hormones androstenedione and testosterone. These androgens are converted peripherally to estrone, resulting in excessive estrogen levels. The result is failure of normal follicular development and secondary oligo- or amenorrhea. These patients tend to be obese and hirsute and enlarged ovaries may be palpated at physical examination. The gonadotropin pattern is one of persistent pulsatile elevation of LH above the expected normal range for the follicular phase of the cycle and a normal or occasionally suppressed follicular-stimulating hormone (FSH) level. Some authors have reported LH:FSH ratios typically greater than or equal to 3:1, however, this finding may be lightly variable. The differentiation of PCOS from late-onset CAH may be extremely difficult with ACTH testing (see above).

Hypoestrogenic causes
Atrophy of the mucosal surfaces, notably those of the vagina and vulva, indicate estrogen deficiency. Estrogen deficiency may also be associated with dryness of the skin and hair, a decrease in breast size, vasomotor symptoms (hot flashes), and dyspareunia. The diagnosis of hypoestrogenicity is further confirmed by cervical mucus that is absent, scanty, white, or opaque. These patients may have one of a variety of disorders. The following is a description of the clinical signs and symptoms that characterize the various causes of secondary amenorrhea associated with hypoestrogenicity. This is also outlined in Figure 8.3.

Organic brain disease
A history of encephalitis or related infections, accidents, injuries, or exposure to toxic substances such as lead or carbon monoxide is associated with organic brain disease. Laboratory findings are characterized by low gonadotropin concentrations, lowered serum estrogen levels, or urinary estrogen excretion, and a moderately atrophic vaginal smear. The neurologic examination and electroencephalogram are frequently valuable diagnostic aids.

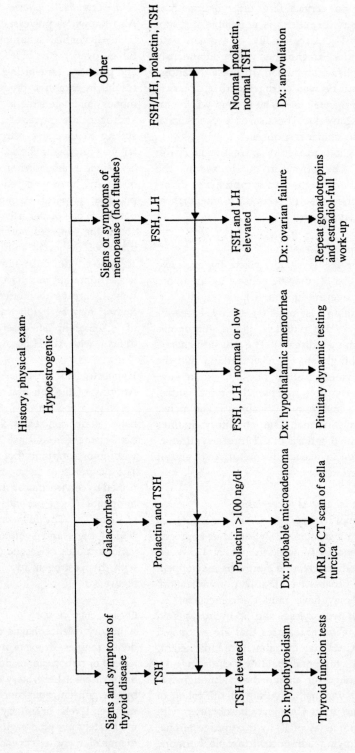

Fig. 8.3 Evaluation of secondary amenorrhea.

Chromophobe adenoma

A pituitary tumor is suspected if the patient reports a history of headaches and visual disturbances. The most common type of pituitary tumor, chromophobe adenoma, often has no specific endocrine symptoms and produces amenorrhea through gross destruction of pituitary tissue or functional disconnection from the hypothalamus. As indicated, evaluation of the sella turcica is the chief diagnostic aid. In the absence of a defect in the sella turcica, a prolactin-producing adenoma must be ruled out. These are often characterized by persistent galactorrhea or lactation in the absence of a previous pregnancy. Extreme atrophy of the uterus and vaginal mucosa and small ovaries with hyperprolactinemia complete the syndrome. When these symptoms occur following pregnancy, this condition is referred to as the Chiari—Frommel syndrome, a distinction no longer offering additional diagnostic importance.

Sheehan's syndrome

Severe postpartum hemorrhage can cause necrosis of the anterior lobe of the pituitary. This results in partial or complete absence of trophic hormone secretion. The initial physical signs of pituitary insufficiency due to Sheehan's syndrome may be failed lactation postpartum, uterine and vaginal atrophy, and a slight or occasionally marked gain in weight. Signs characteristic of late stages are loss of axillary and pubic hair, lowered blood pressure, and weight loss. Laboratory findings are characterized by lowered or absent gonadotropin concentrations.

Strenuous exercise

Persistent strenuous exercise such as running, dancing, and body-building may play a role in amenorrhea. The development of amenorrhea in women athletes appears to be related to a low percentage body fat, high level of training, and competitive stresses. According to Frisch [6], the regularity of menstrual function necessitates maintaining a composition above 22% body fat. Some amenorrheic women athletes are markedly estrogen deficient. Most women who develop this amenorrheic syndrome are under the age of 20, have had previous menstrual problems, and weighed less than 52 kg (115 lb) before beginning their training programs. Low gonadotropins in the face of hypoestrogenicity along with the appropriate history and physical examination can be diagnostic.

Anorexia nervosa

The physical signs of anorexia nervosa include emaciation (weight 15% below normal), a fine lanugo body hair, normal axillary and pubic hair, and atrophy of the internal and external genitalia. Constipation, low metabolic rate, bradycardia, and low blood pressure are common symptoms. Laboratory findings indicate low levels of FSH and LH, elevated serum cortisol, normal prolactin, thyroid-stimulating hormone (TSH) and thyroxine (T_4) levels, but the 3,5,3-triiodothyronine (T_3) level is low and reverse T_3 is high. A persistent feeling of well-being in spite of profound weight loss and the inability of the patient to give an accurate account of her food intake or body image distinguish the condition from other hypothalamic causes.

Malnutrition

The importance of malnutrition in reproductive function has been demonstrated in documents of concentration camp victims of World War I. Although emaciation is often characteristic of patients with nutritional deficiencies, exogenous obesity can also be associated with malnutrition. A careful dietary history will reveal specific caloric, protein, or vitamin deficiencies, which may be diagnostic. Other more common causes of secondary amenorrhea in a US based population must be excluded.

Premature ovarian failure

A history of hot flushes is suggestive of premature ovarian failure. The etiology of premature ovarian failure can be congenital or acquired. Some factors which interfere with oogenesis or cause damage include anomalies of the X chromosomes, abscess formation in the ovary including tuberculosis, neoplasms, irradiation, surgical trauma, or an autoimmune process. The absolute diagnostic criterion of premature ovarian failure is the laboratory finding of elevated gonadotropin concentrations in the face of extremely low estrogens. While levels vary depending on assay parameters and standard used, levels of FSH in excess of 40 mIU/ml on more than one occasion usually represent postmenopausal or ovarian failure concentrations.

Variable estrogenicity

A number of etiologic factors can be associated with varying degrees of estrogenicity. As indicated, the patient's history and the physician's clinical judgment are the most reliable indicators of how the diagnosis should best proceed.

Iatrogenic

A history of oral contraceptives, phenothiazines, tricyclic antidepressants, and some antihypertensives may cause secondary amenorrhea. While mechanisms vary, centrally mediated, hypothalamic gonadotropin-releasing hormone (GnRH) effects predominate. The occurrence of iatrogenic secondary amenorrhea is sufficiently rare that other causes must always be ruled out.

Acidophilic adenoma

This type of pituitary tumor is associated with the signs and symptoms of acromegaly such as excessive growth of distal extremities and coarsening of facial features. There may be unusual muscular weakness, polyuria, and polydipsia. The laboratory findings indicate an increase in serum growth hormone and decreased gonadotropin excretion, and a "diabetic" glucose tolerance test. An increased metabolic rate may also be evident.

Table 8.4 Pharmacologic agents associated with secondary amenorrhea

Proposed mechanism	Agents
Elevation of serum prolactin	Calcium channel blockers
	Cimetidine
	Methyldopa
	Narcotics
	Phenothiazines
	Reserpine
	Tricyclic antidepressants
Intrinsic estrogenic activity	Dicoumerol
	Digitalis
	Flavenoids
	Marijuana
	Oral contraceptives
Direct ovarian toxicity	Busulfan
	Chlorambucil
	Cisplatinum
	Cyclophosphamide
	Etoposide
	5-Fluorouracil (5-FU)
	L-phenylalanine mustard (L-PAM)
	Methclorethamine
	Melphalan

Psychogenic

Psychosis, severe emotional shock, and pseudocyesis are psychogenic causes of secondary amenorrhea associated with varying degrees of estrogenicity. After ruling out all other etiologic factors in an emotionally unstable patient, the diagnosis of psychosis is made on the basis of the patient's psychiatric history. The diagnosis of severe emotional shock is relatively easier since the amenorrhea immediately follows an unfortunate emotional experience. Pseudocyesis is a psychogenic condition characterized by an obsession with pregnancy. Weight gain, normal secondary sexual characteristics and pelvic organs, lactation, and anovulation appear in the absence of pregnancy. Laboratory findings indicate a low normal gonadotropin secretion, estrogens in the normal range, and a midzone shift in the vaginal smear.

Chronic disease

A variety of chronic diseases such as tuberculosis may cause secondary amenorrhea. Tuberculosis may cause amenorrhea by destruction of the ovary (hypoestrogenic) or endometrium (euestrogenic). The chief diagnostic aid of chronic disease is an increased sedimentation rate and specific test for the disease entities suggested by the history.

Thyroid disease

Hypothyroidism may be associated with secondary amenorrhea. The classic signs of hypothyroidism are sensitivity to cold, a tendency to constipation, dryness of the skin and hair, and slow reaction time. The patient with severe primary hypothyroidism will usually have hyperprolactinemia, as thyrotropin-releasing hormone (TRH) may act as a prolactin-releasing hormone. The diagnosis of a thyroid disturbance must be made by specific tests of thyroid function.

Adrenal tumor

Adrenal tumors are frequently associated with menstrual abnormalities. Physical signs that characterize adrenal tumors in women are usually related to androgen excess. Marked hirsutism, enlargement of the clitoris, breast changes, and temporal balding are common. The chief diagnostic criterion is an elevated serum cortisol level that is not suppressed with dexamethasone. Dehydroepiandrosterone sulfate and testosterone may also be increased and their levels tend to parallel, albeit imprecisely, the masculinizing symptoms of this problem (see also Cushing's syndrome or disease, above).

Liver cirrhosis

In severe biliary cirrhosis, impairment of estrogen metabolism, particularly conjugation, leads to excess circulating active estrogens. This may result in episodes of secondary amenorrhea. Depending on the overall level of disease, estrogenicity can be variable. The diagnosis is made on the basis of physical findings and obvious derangements of liver function tests.

Ovarian tumors

Androgen-producing tumors (arrhenoblastoma, hilus cell, and adrenal rest), estrogen-producing tumors (granulosa and theca cell), and nonspecific varieties with steroidogenic stroma can cause secondary amenorrhea. A history of rapidly progressive masculinization is characteristic of an androgen-producing tumor. The chief laboratory finding is a testosterone level greater than 200 ng/dl. Although estrogen production by granulosa-theca cell tumors is the norm, virilization as a result of androgenic function may rarely occur. A history of abnormal uterine bleeding, including amenorrhea, may be the most striking symptom in patients with ovarian tumors.

Hermaphroditism

A true hermaphrodite possesses both ovarian and testicular tissue. The diagnosis of hermaphroditism can be suspected in patients who demonstrate ambiguous external genitalia associated with breast development. This condition may also be characterized by minimal hirsutism. Laboratory findings vary to a large degree, depending on the relative functional level of gonadal tissue from each sex, and are of little diagnostic assistance.

Sclerosis of the uterine cavity (Asherman's syndrome)

Lesions on the uterine cavity may be associated with previous dilatation and curettage or some other intracervical or intrauterine procedure which has been extremely traumatic. Most of these lesions occur in association with pregnancy or a pregnancy complication, infection, or both. Diagnosis of secondary amenorrhea associated with destructive lesions in the uterine cavity is made on the basis of a suggestive history, physical examination, hysterosalpingogram, and/or hysteroscopy. Curettage which demonstrates vaginal or cervical obstruction or scarring of the endometrium may also be diagnostic.

Undetermined estrogenicity

Some etiologic factors of secondary amenorrhea have yet to be identified or have unknown estrogenic characteristics. Diabetes mellitus, for instance, is occasionally associated with secondary amenorrhea. Amenorrhea may result from insulin deficiency or nutritional deficiencies and emotional disturbances commonly associated with this disease. The classic signs and symptoms of diabetes mellitus are obesity followed by weight loss, polyuria, polydipsia, and nocturia. Laboratory findings are characterized by an elevated fasting blood sugar.

CONCLUSIONS

Numerous etiologic factors can cause secondary amenorrhea. Since most of these can be classified on the basis of estrogenicity, an attempt to group patients with secondary amenorrhea based on their clinical signs of estrogenicity is the approach emphasized here. Emphasis on clinical judgment facilitates a correct diagnosis of secondary amenorrhea at minimal cost and maximal convenience to the patient by limiting laboratory tests and reducing the number of office visits. Although other diagnostic schemata for secondary amenorrhea have relied on the progestogen challenge test, we have found the results of this test to be too variable to be of value. Armed with information gathered from the patient history and physical examination, good clinical judgment can guide the physician toward an accurate diagnosis without unnecessary tests.

Once the etiology of secondary amenorrhea has been determined, treatment should be based upon the etiologic factor and reproductive desires of the patient. It is important to note that most estrogenic patients require cycling with a progestational agent to prevent endometrial hyperplasia and possibly carcinoma. Hypoestrogenic patients who are not candidates for ovulation induction require hormone replacement therapy to prevent symptoms associated with estrogen deficiency and its late nonreproductive sequelae, including cardiovascular disease and osteoporosis. The reader can refer to adjoining chapters for information regarding the specific management of the various etiologic factors associated with secondary amenorrhea.

CHAPTER 8

REFERENCES

1 Shangold M, Tomai T, Chin S, Zinaman M, Cook J, Simon J. Factors associated with withdrawal bleeding following administration of oral micronized progesterone in women with secondary amenorrhea. *Fertil Steril* 1992; 56: 1040–1047.

2 Chiazze L, Brayer FT, Micisco JJ, Parker MP, Duffy BJ. The length and variability of the human menstrual cycle. *JAMA* 1968; 203: 337.

3 Vollman RF. The menstrual cycle. Philadelphia: WB Saunders, 1977.

4 Rarick LD, Shangold M, Ahmed SW. Cervical mucus and serum estradiol as predictors of response to progestin challenge. *Fertil Steril* 1990; 54: 353.

5 Brodie BL, Wentz AC. Late onset congenital adrenal hyperplasia: a gynecologist's perspective. *Fertil Steril* 1987; 48: 175.

6 Frisch RE. Body fat, menarche, and reproductive ability. *Semin Reprod Endocrinol* 1985; 3: 45.

9

Hypermenorrhea

RONALD M. NELSON & EDROY McMILLAN

INTRODUCTION

Abnormal menstrual flow with excessive and prolonged bleeding is one of the most common gynecologic complaints encountered in practice. From 10 to 35% of patients in a gynecologic practice will present with hypermenorrhea. Prevalence rates of hypermenorrhea have been reported at 20.4 per 1000 women or 2% of the general population [1]. It is estimated that 20% of women will experience excessive bleeding during their reproductive lifetime.

The mean duration of menstrual flow in women is 4 days. Any bleeding that occurs for greater than 7 days or is excessive is considered abnormal. Studies objectively measuring menstrual blood loss have demonstrated that the average blood loss with menstruation is 35 ml and 90% of women will bleed less than 80 ml. Blood loss of greater than 80 ml is considered abnormal and defines hypermenorrhea [2].

Patients with hypermenorrhea will complain of increased menstrual flow and duration. The passing of clots is highly suggestive of excessive bleeding. The amount of menstrual flow is subject to considerable individual variations. The diagnosis of hypermenorrhea is based primarily on the subjective description of the patient since it is difficult to objectively quantitate menstrual blood loss. However, in cases of severe blood loss the patient may have physical findings consistent with hypovolemia and laboratory findings consistent with iron-deficiency anemia.

DIFFERENTIAL DIAGNOSIS

A differential diagnosis and diagnostic approach to hypermenorrhea is detailed in Figure 9.1. The differential diagnosis of hypermenorrhea can be divided into five general categories. These categories are pregnancy complications, local pelvic pathology, systemic pathology, iatrogenic causes, and dysfunctional uterine bleeding (DUB). A brief review of these categories follows.

Complications of pregnancy

Pregnancy complications are the most common causes of abnormal uterine bleeding in the reproductive years. Therefore a complication of early pregnancy should always be suspected with hypermenorrhea in an acute setting. The more common pregnancy complications encountered include various stages of the abortion process, trophoblastic disease, and ectopic pregnancy. A pregnancy test should always be a part of the work-up of a patient who is being evaluated for hypermenorrhea. If the β-human chorionic gonadotropin is positive, serial quantitative levels and a pelvic ultrasound will be helpful in establishing the reason for the uterine bleeding. The physician must exclude the possibility of ectopic pregnancy in any patient with hypermenorrhea and pelvic pain since potentially fatal hemorrhage could result if this diagnosis is missed.

Local pathology

Local conditions that can present with hypermenorrhea include benign and malignant disease of the vagina, cervix, uterus, fallopian tubes, or ovaries. Benign conditions include adenomyosis, leiomyomas, and endometrial polyps. Inflammation of the uterus and tubes in addition to other physical and chemical trauma of the vagina can present with abnormal menstrual bleeding.

Systemic pathology

Systemic disease is an uncommon but important cause of hypermenorrhea. Hematologic derangements are among the most commonly encountered of the systemic problems that may present in adolescents with abnormal uterine bleeding. Up to 10% of women with blood dyscrasia will have hypermenorrhea.

The more common coagulation disorders that may

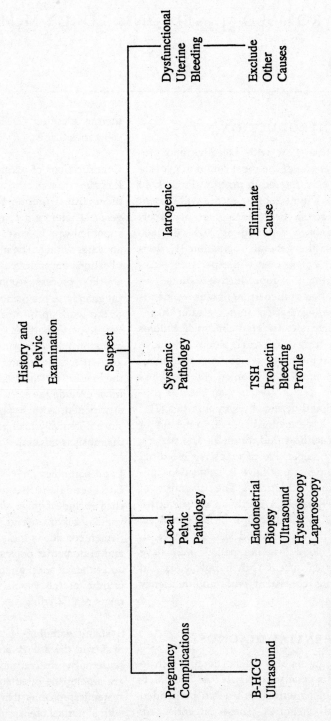

Fig. 9.1 Diagnostic approach to hypermenorrhea.

present with hypermenorrhea include acute leukemia, idiopathic thrombocytopenia purpura, and von Willebrand's disease. Twenty-five percent of adolescents who present with anemia associated with severe hypermenorrhea at the time of menarche may have a coagulation disorder [3]. A history of other bleeding problems or the finding of unexplained bruises on examination should alert the physician to the possibility of an underlying bleeding disorder.

Clinical hypothyroidism is an uncommon cause of abnormal uterine bleeding. However, a report by Wilensky and Greisman has suggested that subclinical hypothyroidism may be found in 22% of patients with severe hypermenorrhea [4]. The demonstration of early hypothyroidism was made only by an abnormal thyroid-stimulating hormone (TSH) response to thyrotropin-releasing hormone stimulation. Other endocrine diseases associated with chronic anovulation may cause hypermenorrhea but more often produce amenorrhea.

Iatrogenic causes of hypermenorrhea

Some of the more common iatrogenic causes of hypermenorrhea include sex steroid hormone therapy, the intrauterine device, anticoagulants, and phenothiazines. The elimination of the suspected cause should result in a return of normal menstrual flow.

DUB

DUB is defined as bleeding from the uterus, unrelated to pelvic or systemic pathology. A diagnosis is made only by the exclusion of all other causes. Chronic anovulation is found in 90% of women with DUB. DUB is usually seen at the extremes of reproductive life and commonly affects postmenarchal and premenopausal women. Because of anovulation, the corpus luteum fails to form and progesterone is not produced. Progesterone has a stabilizing effect on the endometrial stroma and inhibits endometrial proliferation. In the absence of progesterone and in the presence of continuous estrogen stimulation, the endometrium will have increased volume, glandularity, and vascularity. Because the endometrium lacks progestational stromal support, it tends to be unstable and develops frequent and irregular breakdown, resulting in prolonged and often heavy uterine bleeding.

EVALUATION

In the evaluation of hypermenorrhea, a complete medical and gynecologic history is particularly important. A detailed menstrual history should be taken and includes the age of menarche, the usual duration, and frequency of menses. An estimate of the amount of bleeding is made by a description of the number of pads used by the patient. The gynecologic history should include questions regarding sexual activity, the use of contraception, and exposure to sexually transmitted diseases.

Other inquiries in the history include questions pertaining to a family history of blood dyscrasia, other abnormal bleeding episodes, history of medical illnesses, all current medications, dietary habits, visual changes, headaches, galactorrhea, hirsutism, premenstrual symptomatology, and symptoms of hypothyroidism.

A thorough physical examination is necessary in confirming impressions gathered from the history, and in determining the amount and source of the bleeding. The general condition and vital signs of the patient are helpful in quantitating the acute nature of the bleeding. The presence of enlarged lymph nodes, liver, or spleen would suggest a blood dyscrasia. Pelvic examination is an essential part of the examination. A detailed explanation, gentleness, and reassurance are important ingredients, particularly in the successful pelvic examination of the adolescent patient. Local pelvic causes of bleeding are usually determined by the abdominal and pelvic examination.

The laboratory evaluation of abnormal uterine bleeding should be relatively simple and inexpensive in most patients. A complete blood count is required. The hemoglobin concentration is a helpful indicator of the severity of the bleeding. Anemia suggests a history of prolonged and/or excessive blood loss. Other measurements of the complete blood count may indicate the possibility of a blood dyscrasia (e.g., leukemia or idiopathic thrombocytopenic purpura). Thyroid function studies and a bleeding profile are not necessary routinely in the absence of suggestive findings from the history or examination. However, they should be obtained when there is a history of recurrent, severe, or refractory bleeding and in the presence of marked anemia. A serum pregnancy test will rule out the possibility of a pregnancy complication.

Elaborate endocrine studies are rarely indicated in a patient with DUB. The determination of plasma follicle-stimulating hormone (FSH), luteinizing hormone (LH), estradiol, or progesterone is unnecessary as the results can easily be predicted if the pathophysiology of the problem is considered. These studies will not influence the management of the problem and present an unnecessary expense to the patient.

Endometrial samplings and possible hysteroscopy should be performed on all patients over the age of 35 in the presence of abnormal uterine bleeding. The incidence of intrauterine pathology significantly increases with advancing age and a normal pelvic examination is not sufficient to rule out intrauterine pathology in the older patient [5]. Endometrial sampling should be performed on women under the age of 35 when the examiner is unable to do an adequate pelvic examination, when there is an abnormal examination, a chronic history of anovulatory cycles, or when there is recurrent or uncontrolled bleeding in spite of adequate therapy.

THERAPY

The treatment approach will depend on the underlying cause. A specific cause will indicate a specific therapy. This section will consider the management of hypermenorrhea associated with DUB.

The first therapeutic decision by the physician is to determine whether the patient can be treated on an inpatient or outpatient basis. The general condition of the patient and the results of the complete blood count are helpful in making the decision. The patient who is actively bleeding and exhibits a hemoglobin of less than 9 g% should be admitted to the hospital for observation and therapy. Any patient who is symptomatic from acute blood loss or demonstrates tachycardia or postural changes in cardiovascular status should be managed in the hospital.

The immediate goal in the treatment of DUB is obtaining hemostasis as soon as possible. Potent orally effective progestin hormones will almost invariably stop excessive bleeding within a short time if administered in sufficient and frequent dosage. When the administered dose is too small or infrequent, bleeding will continue and may be mistakenly attributed to medical failure to control the bleeding. Surgical intervention by dilatation and curettage or hysterectomy is rarely necessary as the primary mode of therapy for DUB.

Many preparations and treatment programs of progestins can be successfully used. Norethindrone acetate (Norlutate) 5 mg or Ovral every 4 hours is quite effective. Bleeding subsides promptly on initiation of therapy and is completely controlled within 12–24 hours. Intravenous conjugated estrogen (Premarin) 25 mg intravenously every 4 hours has been used for many years in the immediate therapy of an acute bleeding problem.

After 72 hours, progestin therapy at a reduced dosage of twice daily should be continued for at least 2–3 weeks. Controlled, menstrual-like withdrawal bleeding can be expected on cessation of therapy. Iron replacement therapy should be started when the patient is first seen and continued for some time after the control of the menstrual cycle has been established. These patients will invariably demonstrate iron-deficiency anemia or at least be deficient in iron reserves. Parenteral iron therapy has no advantage over oral iron and is rarely indicated. It is easy for the physician to overlook iron therapy when concerned about the management of the bleeding episode.

The follow-up therapy goal in these patients is to prevent recurrence of bleeding. As in other endocrine-deficiency problems, specific replacement therapy is mostly physiologic. Cyclic progestin therapy with oral medroxyprogesterone (Provera) 10 mg daily for 10–14 days each month will allow normal progestin-based withdrawal bleeding. Cyclic oral contraceptive pills will also prevent recurrent abnormal cycles, and have the added advantage of providing effective contraception.

Empiric thyroid hormone therapy has been used frequently in the past in the treatment of menstrual dysfunction. Hypothyroidism is an unusual cause of menstrual abnormalities. Thyroid hormone should not be used without documented laboratory evidence of hypothyroidism. Too many patients with a history of DUB are taking lifetime thyroid hormones unnecessarily.

PROGNOSIS IN ADOLESCENTS

The prognosis for the development of normal ovulatory menstrual function in adolescents with DUB is not clear. Relatively few long-term studies have been undertaken. Southam and Richart reported in 1966 a retrospective study of 538 adolescents who had either DUB or oligomenorrhea in an attempt to characterize the natural history of adolescent menstrual abnormalities [6]. They found that only 50% of the young patients with DUB had reverted to normal menstrual cycles within 4 years. In those young women who continued to have abnormal periods after 4 years, very few developed normal cycles. Similar findings were found for the women with oligomenorrhea. These patients will present in later years with significant problems in reproduction and increased gynecologic morbidity.

REFERENCES

1 Mishell D Jr, Fisher H, Haynes P, Jones G, Smith R. Menorrhagia — a symposium. *J Reprod Med* 1984; 29 (suppl): 763–782.

2 Hallberg L, Hagdahl A, Nilsson L, Rybo G. Menstrual blood loss — a population study. *Acta Obstet Gynecol Scand* 1966; 45: 320.

3 Claessens E, Cowell C. Acute adolescent menorrhagia. *Am J Obstet Gynecol* 1981; 139: 277–280.

4 Wilensky D, Greisman B. Early hypothyroidsim in patients with menorrhagia. *Am J Obstet Gynecol* 1989; 160: 673–677.

5 Kaminski P, Stevens C. The value of endometrial sampling in abnormal uterine bleeding. *Am J Gynecol Health* 1988; II: 33.

6 Southam A, Richart R. The prognosis for adolescents with menstrual abnormalities. *Am J Obstet Gynecol* 1966; 94: 637.

Management of dysmenorrhea

RICHARD E. BLACKWELL

INTRODUCTION

Dysmenorrhea is a symptom complex that is thought to be due to an alteration in prostaglandin production. It consists of severe cramping associated with menstruation, breast tenderness, abdominal bloating, mood alterations, edema, headache, and occasionally excess menstrual flow. Dysmenorrhea affects approximately 50% of all postpubescent women, and is classified as either primary or secondary. Anatomic pathology is not commonly identified in the case of primary dysmenorrhea, though secondary dysmenorrhea has been thought to be associated with endometriosis, pelvic inflammatory disease, congenital anomalies of the genital tract, and cervical stenosis.

For years dysmenorrhea was considered to be a neglected syndrome, although its presence has been recorded since early history. Various menstrual taboos have existed in many cultures. Menstruating women were often separated from others, and were subjected to ritualistic cleansing procedures, some of which are still followed in various cultures today (Orthodox Jews, Navajo Indians). At times, dysmenorrhea has been regarded as an illness. Historically, it was recommended that women remain at home, rest, and avoid social contact. Bathing was to be avoided until menstruation was completed [1].

In the twentieth century there was a change in attitude toward the etiology of dysmenorrhea. In the past, dysmenorrhea had been felt associated with epilepsy, hysteria, and various forms of mania, and it was suggested that patients with dysmenorrhea show "resentment for the feminine role." However, in 1940 suppression of ovulation was shown to prevent primary dysmenorrhea, thus refuting the psychodynamic theory. Unfortunately, textbooks of the 1950s and 1960s still referred to dysmenorrhea as being related to conflicts regarding childbearing, sexuality, and a dislike for the feminine role.

More recently, as increased numbers of women have begun entering the work force, dysmenorrhea has come to be perceived by society as an important medical problem. In 1980, it was estimated that 140 million work hours were lost as a result of two or more working days per month lost per female employee. It was also estimated that 10% of female college students missed 2−3 days of classes each month, and that up to 20% of high school adolescents missed as least 1 day annually because of dysmenorrhea. This stimulated a renewed interest in defining the pathophysiology of dysmenorrhea and developing new therapeutic modalities to manage this problem.

Physiology of dysmenorrhea

In 1934, Macht and Davis demonstrated that lipid-soluble extracts of menstrual fluids could potentiate adrenalin-induced contractions of smooth muscle from rat vas deferens *in vitro*. In 1957, Pickles demonstrated the presence of a menstrual stimulant which could produce contractions of uterine smooth muscle. This stimulant was later demonstrated to be the family of prostaglandins. Pickles observed that patients with primary dysmenorrhea had higher prostaglandin $F_{2\alpha}$ ($PGF_{2\alpha}$) concentrations than those patients who did not have the symptoms, and that these patients had an increase in the $PGF_{2\alpha}$:prostaglandin E (PGE) ratio [2]. Subsequently, it was demonstrated that long-term infusion of $PGF_{2\alpha}$ duplicated typical menstrual pain.

Prostaglandins are unsaturated hydroxy fatty acids that contain 20 carbons, configured as a cyclopentane ring with two side chains. Prostaglandins are derived from membrane arachidonic acid and are related to both the thromboxanes and the leukotrienes. The precursor of the prostaglandins, arachidonic acid, is released from the cell membrane by the action of lysosomal phospholipases and acid phosophatases (Fig. 10.1). Phospholipase A_2 is facilitated by calcium

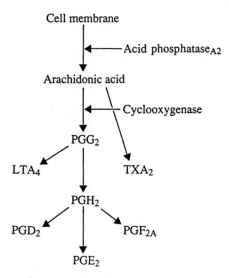

Fig. 10.1 The release of arachidonic acid from the cell membrane by the action of lysosomal phospholipases and acid phosphatases.

ionophores and inhibited by glucocorticoids and local anesthetics. The conversion of arachidonic acid to the cyclic endoperoxide prostaglandin G_2 (PGG_2) is catalyzed by cyclooxygenase which is inhibited by aspirin-like compounds. PGG_2 is an unstable compound and is immediately catalyzed to prostaglandin H_2 and subsequently to PGE and $PGF_{2\alpha}$ by endoperoxide isomerase and endoperoxide reductase.

$PGF_{2\alpha}$ and PGE_2 are important in reproduction and have been measured in menstrual blood and endometrium. Though prostaglandins are rapidly metabolized, they are found to be elevated in secretory endometrium when compared to tissues

harvested during the follicular phase. Assay of menstrual fluid has suggested that prostaglandin levels are elevated in dysmenorrheic women when compared to controls. $PGF_{2\alpha}$ destabilizes lysosomal membranes causing release of the acid phosphatases which result in endometrial necrosis and initiation of menstruation. Simultaneously, $PGF_{2\alpha}$ produces constriction of endometrial arterioles and contraction of the myometrium. These contractions have been measured directly and have been shown to increase intrauterine pressure from 0 to 10 mmHg to more than 100 mmHg. The contractions thus produced are frequently described as "labor-like." Thus, the pain associated with dysmenorrhea is due to increased uterine contractility and uterine ischemia, both likely a function of prostaglandin endoperoxidases (Fig. 10.2).

Treatment of dysmenorrhea

While Pickles had suggested in the 1960s that prostaglandins could be the precipitating factor of dysmenorrhea, Chauncey D. Palmer had observed as early as 1895 that "experience has taught us that drugs used in chronic rheumatism may be admirably adapted to dysmenorrhea." He is credited with being one of the first to use salicylates in the treatment of dysmenorrhea, the primary treatment for almost 8 years. In 1971, Vane proposed that other aspirin-like compounds could inhibit prostaglandin synthetase [3]. Subsequent clinical observations led to the development of the nonsteroidal antiinflammatory agents ibuprofen, naproxen, mefenamic acid, and meclofenamate sodium. These compounds produced dramatic pain relief in the majority of cases. Furthermore, some compounds have also

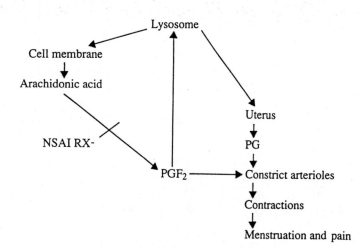

Fig. 10.2 Illustration of the causes of pain associated with dysmenorrhea.

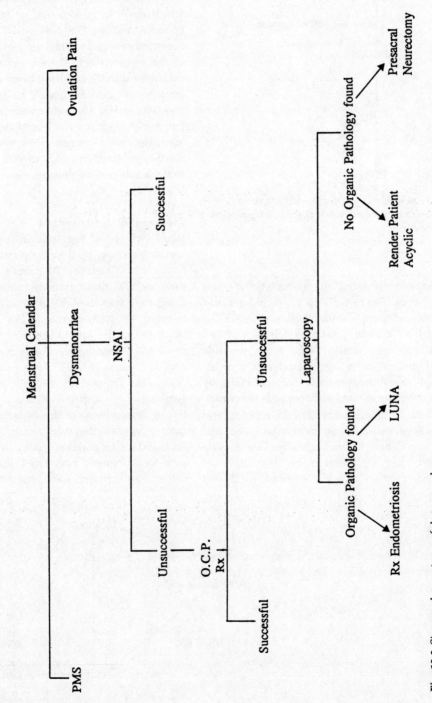

CHAPTER 10

Fig. 10.3 Signs and symptoms of dysmenorrhea.

been demonstrated to decrease the magnitude of menstrual flow by as much as 75% [4].

An alternate approach to treatment grew out of the recognized association between ovulation and dysmenorrhea, described as early as 1930. At first, systemic estrogens were used to block ovulation and reduce dysmenorrhea. Subsequently, it was recognized that contraceptive agents reduced menstrual fluid, $PGF_{2\alpha}$, uterine motility, and the sensitivity of the myometrium to exogenously administered prostaglandins. These facts, combined with the contraceptive properties of the birth control pill, justify the utilization of this approach among young reproductive-aged women [5]. Given these observations, it is apparent that nonsteroidal antiinflammatory agents and oral contraceptive pills are the first two approaches which might be considered in the treatment of the patient with dysmenorrhea. Alternately, systemic analgesics such as occasional treatment with codeine with or without aspirin or tylenol may be considered.

A difficult dilemma arises in the patient who has persistent dysmenorrhea despite the optimal doses of the above medications, or who is unable to tolerate any or all of them. In such cases, a careful reassessment of physical findings should be performed to exclude new pelvic pathology. A specific diagnosis should be sought by laparoscopy before consideration of other, more expensive therapies which have relatively high rates of unpleasant side-effects. Should endometriosis be found at laparoscopy, treatment with danazol or a gonadotropin-releasing hormone analog would be considered. Should other pathology such as pelvic adhesions or mass be seen, more specific surgical therapy could be provided.

CONCLUSIONS

Patients who present with signs and symptoms of dysmenorrhea should be asked to keep a menstrual calendar to determine whether their symptoms are due to dysmenorrhea, premenstrual syndrome, or ovulation (Fig. 10.3). If contraception is not an issue, nonsteroidal antiinflammatories should be employed as a first-line therapy. If the patient fails to respond satisfactorily to prostaglandin synthetase suppression, oral contraceptive therapy should be instituted, sometimes simultaneously. Failure to respond to either of these modes of therapy or their combination should be highly suggestive of underlying pelvic pathology. It is suggested that laparoscopy be carried out to rule out endometriosis or other forms of pelvic pathology. If no pathology is found at the time of endoscopic examination, patients can be rendered acyclic with agents such as norethindrone acetate or medroxyprogesterone acetate, and undergo laser uterine nerve ablation (LUNA) at the time of laparoscopy, or perhaps presacral neurectomy. It should be pointed out that the LUNA procedure does not produce permanent pain control and despite its long-standing use, presacral neurectomy for the control of midline pain of various pelvic etiologies is still considered an appropriate surgical alternative.

REFERENCES

1 Sobczyk R. Dysmenorrhea: the neglected syndrome. *J Reprod Endocrinol* 1980; 25: 198.
2 Pickles VR, Hall WG, Best FA *et al*. Prostaglandins in endometrium and menstrual fluid from normal and dysmenorrheic subjects. *Br J Obstet Gynaecol* 1965; 72: 185.
3 Vane JR. Inhibition of prostaglandin synthesis as a mechanism of action for aspirin-like drugs. *Nature New Biol* 1971; 321: 232.
4 Anderson ABM, Haynes PJ, Guillebaud J, Turnbull AC. Reduction of menstrual blood-loss by prostaglandin synthetase inhibitors. *Lancet* 1976; 1: 744.
5 Ylikorkala O, Dawood MY. New concepts in dysmenorrhea. *Am J Obstet Gynecol* 1978; 130: 833.

11

Premenstrual syndrome

WILLIAM R. KEYE JR

INTRODUCTION

Despite the fact that many women will seek medical care for recurring premenstrual symptoms, our understanding of this enigmatic condition is very limited. As a result, most of the scientific literature dealing with premenstrual syndrome (PMS) has been devoted to an attempt to determine its cause. In contrast, very little has been written about the practical management of women with premenstrual symptoms. Thus the physician is left with a confusing array of negative scientific data and little to guide him or her in the care of women who present with premenstrual symptoms. It is therefore not surprising that there are many untested or unproven approaches to the evaluation and treatment of women with premenstrual symptoms. Each practitioner is left to his or her own interpretation of the literature and his or her own limited experience with this problem.

To simplify the clinical approach to the evaluation and treatment of women with PMS, I will outline in this chapter a six-step approach that can be applied by an individual practitioner in his or her office. This simple approach is based on the experience of a multidisciplinary team with treating more than 2000 patients over a 10-year span. It is empirically derived and based on the assumption that premenstrual symptoms are the result of the interaction of biologic, psychologic, and social factors. It is an approach that can be easily modified as we gain new information and insight into the etiology, pathopsychology, and pathogenesis of PMS.

DEFINITION

While there have been many attempts to establish a definition of premenstrual syndrome and the DSM-III-R has established criteria for a variant of PMS known as late lutealphase dysphoric disorder (LLPDD) [1], there is no universally accepted set of criteria for the diagnosis of PMS. From the clinician's standpoint, PMS exists when a woman presents with any recurring set of symptoms which appear at or after the onset of the luteal phase (that is, at the time of ovulation) and ends at or soon after the onset of menstrual flow. In addition, these symptoms must be severe enough to interfere with the functional level of the individual and/or significantly alter the woman's quality of life. These must also be recurring symptoms and they must not be the result of any underlying psychiatric or physical disease. The important features of this definition are that it does not state specifically the symptoms that must occur but emphasizes the timing of symptoms and their severity. Premenstrual *syndrome* is indeed just that. It is a syndrome and not a specific disease. This implies that there may be a number of underlying disorders that at our present stage of understanding all appear to be identical and present in a similar clinical fashion. In the future, we may be able to establish a specific diagnosis and understand the specific etiology of premenstrual symptoms for each woman just as we have for the syndromes amenorrhea/galactorrhea.

PREVALENCE

The literature suggests that PMS may be present in as many as 95% of women of reproductive age. However, more careful epidemiologic studies have reported that only 5% of women of reproductive age are experiencing significant premenstrual symptomatology at any one time. Reports which suggest that 50−95% of women suffer from PMS are generally retrospective reports that do not require specific diagnostic criteria nor specify a certain degree of severity to make the diagnosis. In most of these cases, women with mild premenstrual molimina will be included with those who have more severe symptoms and thus, PMS. While the majority of women can often predict the impending onset of menstruation because of subtle changes in mood, behavior, or physical sensations, most of these women do not have PMS by the criteria established above. Only 5—10% of women of reproductive age will seek medical care for their symptoms.

ETIOLOGY

Since Frank's original description of PMS in 1931 [2], there has been a long list of proposed etiologies. Social scientists have suggested that PMS exists to discourage multiple sexual contacts following ovulation. The behavioral scientists have suggested that PMS may be a variation of more common forms of affective disorders. Skeptics have claimed that PMS does not exist at all but has simply been created by the media and health care professionals who may profit from such a concept. Scientists and physicians using the medical model have suggested a number of biologic etiologies which may either act alone or in concert with psychologic and social factors. Unfortunately, none of these theories has withstood the test of time nor close scientific scrutiny. Thus, it does not appear that the excessive production of estradiol, aldosterone, prolactin, antigen/antibody complexes, or toxins can account for PMS. Similarly, there is no convincing evidence that deficiencies in vitamins, essential fatty acids, trace minerals, progesterone, adrenocorticotropic hormone, or β-endorphins are responsible for premenstrual symptoms. Skeptics claim that without a thorough understanding of the etiology and pathophysiology of PMS we really have very little to offer these women. However, they need only look at pregnancy-induced hypertension, a disorder for which we have developed effective therapies despite a lack of understanding of the etiology or pathogenesis of the disorder. The situation currently with regard to PMS is much the same. Despite a lack of understanding about the etiology of PMS, it is still possible systematically and logically to evaluate women with premenstrual symptoms and to provide effective therapy.

CLINICAL FEATURES

Although there may not be general agreement as to the etiology and pathophysiology of PMS, there is agreement as to its clinical features. Women with PMS are usually in the third or fourth decade of life. They commonly report 10—15 years of symptoms prior to seeking medical care and usually report

increasing severity of symptoms following pregnancy, use of oral contraceptives, or the onset of puberty.

The symptoms that are most common and troublesome are those of anxiety, depression, and irritability. While many women with PMS also complain of fatigue, headache, dizziness, palpitations, joint pain, breast tenderness, and of bloating, they more commonly seek care for their emotional symptoms than these physical symptoms. In addition some women will experience feelings of paranoia, increased sensitivity, decreased self-confidence, displeasure with their appearance, sensitivity to rejection, desire to be alone, impaired judgment or memory, or a decreased ability to concentrate.

Women who have long-standing and moderate or severe premenstrual symptoms may also experience significant disturbance in interpersonal relationships, particularly with other family members. PMS has in many cases led to divorce from one's spouse or confusion on the part of one's children. In addition, PMS may interfere with schooling or effective performance on the job. As a result, some women with severe PMS may seek family or marriage therapy or individual psychotherapy for these complications of PMS and yet be completely unaware of the fact that it is the PMS that is the underlying cause of these psychosocial disorders. Thus, the mental health care professional or family or marriage therapist should be aware that PMS is among those conditions that may cause psychosocial problems.

EVALUATION

Typically, the health care practitioner is overwhelmed by the woman who presents with a list of 10—15 physical and psychologic symptoms. Even if these symptoms follow a predictable premenstrual pattern, the mere number and severity of these symptoms discourage even the most dedicated clinician. However, the evaluation of the woman with multiple premenstrual symptoms can be broken down into three essential steps. These three steps, as seen in Figure 11.1, can be applied to any woman who presents with premenstrual symptoms and can be performed easily in an outpatient setting.

Step 1: Obtaining a history
Because of the widespread popularity of PMS in the public press, increasing numbers of women have presented for the evaluation of what they believe

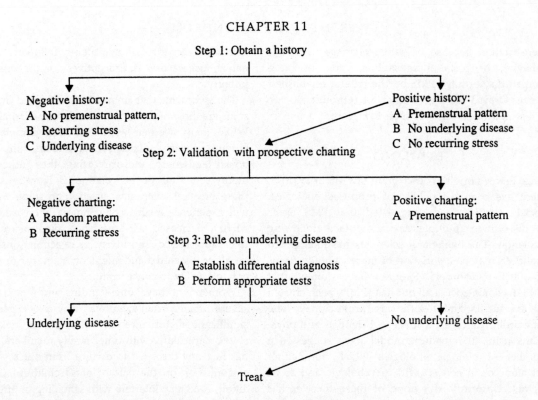

Fig. 11.1 A decision tree for the evaluation of women with premenstrual symptoms.

to be PMS. Often women will read about it and recognize symptoms that they may share in common with those women who do experience PMS. As a result, they may present to the health care practitioner with a self-made diagnosis of PMS. Unfortunately, many women focus on the symptoms and not on the timing of the symptoms: thus, many women with chronic physical and emotional disorders have sought help for what they believe to be PMS. Thus it is important to take a very careful history at the initial visit.

The history should include questions regarding the onset of menstruation, the timing of menstruation, the nature of menstrual flow, the use of exogenous hormones, including birth control pills, a reproductive history, a general medical history, a review of symptoms, and review of familial disease patterns. In addition to these general background questions, a history should be obtained regarding the specific symptoms that the woman experiences and the specific timing of those symptoms within the menstrual cycle. Thus it is important to determine how many days before the onset of menstruation symptoms typically begin and how soon after the onset of menstruation these symptoms end. In addition the social history of the patient should

be obtained to determine that there are no recurring environmental stressors that may be creating premenstrual emotional distress on a monthly basis.

If the history is one of intermittent or continuous symptoms that bear no relationship to the luteal phase of the menstrual cycle, it is unlikely that the woman has PMS. Similarly, if the woman complains primarily of pain, it is likely that she is suffering from a chronic underlying disease that may be symptomatic only during the luteal phase of the menstrual cycle. On the other hand, if the history suggests that the symptoms are present only during the luteal phase of the menstrual cycle beginning at or after ovulation and ending at or soon after the onset of menstruation and there are no underlying diseases or recurring environmental or social stressors, it is likely that the woman is experiencing PMS. However, histories are notoriously incomplete or misleading. Because of selective recall and the tendency to remember events that occur together (that is, symptoms that occur in association with menstruation are more likely to be remembered than symptoms that occur at times remote from menstruation), it is important to validate the history through the gathering of data in a more prospective fashion.

Step 2: Evaluation of the history with prospective data-gathering

There are a number of ways to gather of data regarding symptoms in a prospective fashion. One may simply suggest that the woman keep a daily diary of how she feels and return to the physician after a month or two to review the diary. Unfortunately, the review of such a diary is often times very painstaking and laborious and one frequently gets lost with all the details. Thus there have been many attempts to create a simplified chart or calendar for the recording of daily symptoms so that the pattern may be easily and quickly ascertained. Some women may simply note the occurrence of symptoms on a standard wall calendar, thus allowing the health care practitioner to see the relationship between symptoms and the phase of the menstrual cycle. For many women this is the most practical and easiest way to gather this prospective data. Other more elaborate means include the PRISM calendar and the Utah Premenstrual Syndrome Calendar. A sample calendar is seen in Figure 11.2. As you can see, the calendar consists of a grid with the days of the menstrual cycle listed across the top and the symptoms listed along the left-hand side of the calendar. At the end of each day, the woman simply notes the presence or absence of each symptom and its severity, using a scale of 1 through 10 (1 = mild symptoms and 10 = severe symptoms). In addition the woman notes on the calendar whether there are any specific or severe stressors in her life on that day which may account for significant symptoms. Despite the self-report nature of this calendar, it has been established to be a valid means of documenting the pattern of symptoms throughout the month [3]. In addition it only takes a matter of seconds for the clinician to ascertain whether symptoms occur only in the luteal phase of the menstrual cycle. A variation on this calendar would include information regarding the basal body temperature which would provide a marker for ovulation and the onset of the luteal phase.

This calendar can be presented to the patient at the end of the initial visit and following the initial history. The patient is instructed to return in 1 or 2 months after having completed 1–2 cycles of the calendar. At this time the clinician determines whether there is a premenstrual pattern to the symptoms. If all of the symptoms occur randomly throughout the month, then it is unlikely that the patient has PMS. If the symptoms occur only on days in which there is significant or environmental stress, it is unlikely

that the patient has PMS. Usually the patient will return with 10–15 symptoms that have been charted. A careful examination will determine that some of those symptoms occur randomly, while others occur continuously throughout the menstrual cycle. However, other symptoms may occur only during the luteal phase of the menstrual cycle; therefore, the woman may indeed have premenstrual syndrome superimposed upon more chronic symptoms. If all of her symptoms occur only during the premenstrual part of the menstrual cycle and are rated as moderate or severe (that is, scored between 5 and 10 by the patient), it is likely that she is experiencing PMS. However, it appears that some psychiatric and physical conditions may in their early subclinical stages present only as symptoms during the luteal phase of the menstrual cycle. Therefore, even a positive prospective charting of symptoms — that is, a premenstrual pattern to symptoms — may not be the result of PMS but may be secondary to chronic underlying physical or psychiatric disease. Therefore, the diagnosis of PMS is a diagnosis of exclusion that can only be made after underlying diseases have been ruled out.

Step 3: Rule out underlying diseases

Once the prospective calendar has been completed and a premenstrual pattern to the symptoms has been established, it is still important to rule out underlying disease that may mimic PMS. The approach to ruling out underlying disease as a cause of premenstrual symptoms is identical to the process used by any physician to establish the presence or absence of a disease. Thus each individual symptom is evaluated independently. A differential diagnosis for that symptom is established and appropriate tests are done to rule in or rule out the underlying possible disorders. Ruling out the underlying diseases after establishing a differential diagnosis for the symptoms generally begins with a detailed physical examination. This examination is directed specifically at determining the presence or absence of the underlying diseases, as established in the differential diagnosis. Based on the specific symptoms and physical findings, additional laboratory and X-ray tests may be performed. There is unfortunately no biochemical marker for PMS; thus, there is no specific test that is appropriate for all women with premenstrual symptoms. Thus, some women may require a hemocrit while others may need tests of thyroid function.

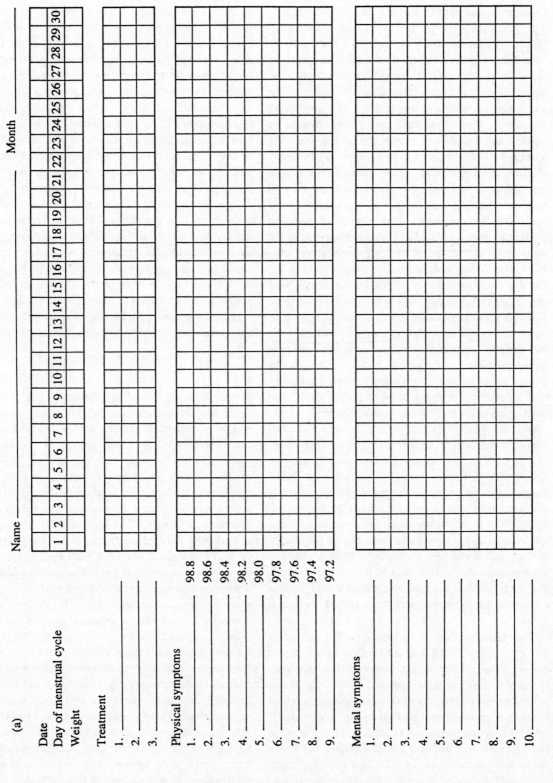

Fig 11.2 (a) Utah premenstrual calendar.

(b)

INSTRUCTIONS

The PMS calendar is essential for the diagnosis of PMS. In addition, it is the only way to monitor your response to treatment. The PMS calendar should be completed according to the following instructions.

1 Begin your chart with the first day of your menstrual period (the first day of bleeding). That will become the first day of your cycle or "Day 1". If you do not have periods, simply begin with the first day of each month.

2 Each morning before arising, take your temperature orally with an oral thermometer. Using the calendar section under "Physical symptoms" as a temperature graph, locate your current temperature and put a dot along the horizontal line next to it below the appropriate date.

3 Weigh yourself unclothed each morning before you eat or drink and after you empty your bladder and, if possible, your bowels. Record the results.

4 Note any medications taken or dietary changes made under the heading "Treatment". Write the name and dose of medication (e.g., progesterone suppositories, 200 mg). Note the number of times that medication was taken on a given day by writing the appropriate number in the box opposite the medication and below the date.

5 Choose the most common or severe physical and emotional symptoms that you experience with PMS from the symptom list below and write them in the blanks on the PMS calendar. (Remember, the list below is not complete. Add any other recurring symptoms you can identify to your calendar.)

6 At the end of each day, note any of the physical or mental symptoms. If you have experienced a symptom, determine the severity of that symptom from 1 (mild) to 7 (severe) and write the number in the box opposite the symptom and below the appropriate date.

7 Bring this calendar with you to each appointment or mail a copy to the PMS center at which are being treated.

8 Also, bring or send a written description of how severe your PMS was during the month, how effective the treatment was and suggestions or any questions you wish to have answered.

Physical symptoms

Abdominal bloating	Increased appetite	Herpes "cold sores"
Breast tenderness	Sensitivity to light	Nasel congestion
Headache	Joint pain	Dizziness
Leg cramps	Incoordination or clumsiness	Fainting spells
Breast swelling	Constipation	Craving for sweets or salty foods
Heart palpitations	Acne	Leg heaviness or swelling
Chest pain	Eye problems	Backache
Sharp one-sided ovarian pain	Hives or rash	Accidents
Decreased alcohol tolerance	Sinusitis	Increased thirst
Increased alcohol consumption	Itching	
Seizures	Sensitivity to noise	

Emotional symptoms

Intolerance	Inability to cope	Insecurity	Suicidal thoughts
Hostility	Tearfulness	Sense of being out of control	Mania
Depression	Decreased self-esteem	Inefficiency	Desire to leave home
Anger	Physical aggression	Guilt feelings	Weakness
Fatigue	Mental aggression	Desire to stay home	Increased sex drive
Sadness	Decreased sex drive	Dissatisfaction with appearance	Irritability
Paranoia	Forgetfulness	Poor judgement	Physical violence
Fear	Loneliness	Indecision	Absence from work
Panic	Poor concentration or	Insomnia	Tension
Restlessness	distractability	Desire to be alone	Anxiety

Fig. 11.2 (b) Instructions for completing the Utah premenstrual calendar.

The testing of women with premenstrual symptoms should be individualized and the test justified on the basis of the symptoms and physical findings. In this way the cost of the evaluation of PMS will be minimized. In some cases the symptoms and physical findings are of such a nature that the patient must be referred to a specialist. For example, patients with recurring and severe headaches may require neurologic evaluation by a neurologist. Similarly, a patient with recurring suicidal ideation and severe depression during the luteal phase may benefit from evaluation by a psychologist or psychiatrist.

The psychologist or psychiatrist may on the basis of the history elect to perform psychometric tests. If psychometric testing is done, however, it is important that they be performed once in the follicular and once in the luteal phase of the menstrual cycle. Numerous studies have now shown that standard psychometric tests may be well within the normal limits during the follicular phase of the menstrual cycle but be clearly abnormal during the luteal phase of the menstrual cycle. Therefore, unless one performs a psychometric test in both phases of the menstrual cycle, the tests will be of limited value and an erroneous conclusion may be drawn by the psychologist or psychiatrist.

If additional testing demonstrates the presence of an underlying disease, then it is important that appropriate therapy for that disease be initiated and the diagnosis of PMS be discarded. If however the testing is negative and there appears to be no evidence of an underlying disease, the presumptive diagnosis of PMS can be made and therapy initiated.

TREATMENT OF PMS

The treatment of PMS also consists of three steps (Fig. 11.3). Unfortunately, there is no single therapy that is universally effective for all women with premenstrual symptoms. Therefore the approach to therapy is empiric and it may take several months to establish the most effective therapy.

Step 1: Education and lifestyle changes

Therapy can be initiated at the time of the initial visit. Many women with premenstrual symptoms will respond to simple lifestyle changes that include

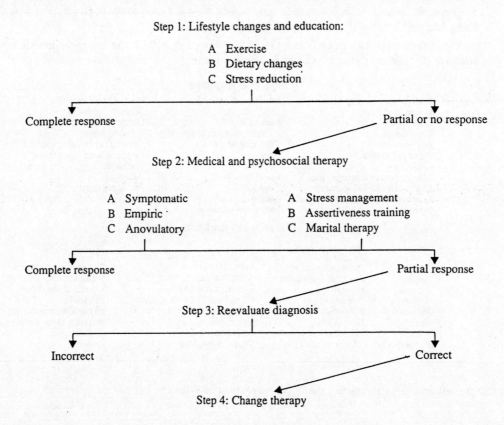

Step 1: Lifestyle changes and education:

    A Exercise
    B Dietary changes
    C Stress reduction

Complete response   Partial or no response

Step 2: Medical and psychosocial therapy

  A Symptomatic   A Stress management
  B Empiric   B Assertiveness training
  C Anovulatory   C Marital therapy

Complete response   Partial response

Step 3: Reevaluate diagnosis

Incorrect   Correct

Step 4: Change therapy

Fig. 11.3 A decision tree for the treatment of women with premenstrual symptoms.

exercise and dietary management. Women with premenstrual symptoms may experience marked reduction in their symptoms if they engage in a program of daily aerobic exercises lasting 30–60 min. This may take the form of jogging, bicycling, treadmill or low- or medium-impact aerobic exercises. Exercises perform several functions which include distraction, release of anxiety and tension, and perhaps even biochemical changes involving changes in neurotransmitter levels. In addition to these exercise programs, minor dietary changes may also markedly reduce the severity of symptoms. Women may experience relief in response to the following dietary changes:

1 The elimination of fasting for more than 4–6 hours at a time.
2 A decrease in the ingestion of simple sugars and their replacement by complex carbohydrates.
3 Reduction or elimination of caffeine from the diet.
4 Reduction of salt in the diet.
5 The reduction or elimination of alcohol in the diet.

However, there is no predictable response to these specific recommendations and thus each woman will have to decide for herself which, if any, of these dietary recommendations is of benefit. While some women may benefit from the elimination of caffeine in their diet, other women may find they actually feel better after taking caffeine for it may overcome some of the feelings of fatigue and drowsiness that they commonly experience.

In addition to exercise and dietary changes, women with premenstrual symptoms should realize that not all uncomfortable emotional symptoms or behaviors are necessarily the result of PMS. Often in the life of men and women there are events which will and should provoke anxiety or depression. In addition the woman with PMS should become aware that others may use her premenstrual symptoms as a scapegoat and blame their own failure on her symptoms. Thus, neither the woman nor those with whom she lives and works should use her premenstrual symptoms as an excuse for unacceptable behavior. Nor should the woman feel that she does not have the right to feel angry or depressed under appropriate circumstances.

Step 2: Medical therapy

Symptomatic therapies
After the diagnosis of PMS has been made, there are a number of medical therapies that can be instituted. Most will fall into one of three categories. The first of those categories is symptomatic therapies. These therapies are designed to reduce or eliminate specific symptoms in those women who are troubled by only a few symptoms. Thus, the woman who has premenstrual mastalgia may benefit from the use of bromocriptine or danazol. Likewise a woman with premenstrual anxiety may benefit from intermittent therapy with alprazolam (Xanax) and the woman with premenstrual depression may benefit from the intermittent administration of fluoxetine hydrochloride (Prozac). However, the administration of psychotropic drugs on an intermittent basis for premenstrual symptoms should generally be discouraged and, when used, should be prescribed by a health care professional with extensive experience with the use of these medications. Unfortunately, some psychotropic medications may have addictive properties and thus their use for PMS may be inappropriate.

Therapies based on theory
An alternative approach to therapy involves the use of medications based on one of several theories regarding the etiology of PMS. An example is the use of dietary supplements such as amino acids, multiple vitamins rich in magnesium, and vitamin B₆. However, it is important that megadose vitamin therapy is not instituted, for serious side-effects may occur. Recent examples include the occurrence of the eosinophilia-myalgia syndrome following the ingestion of contaminated tryptophan or neurologic symptoms associated with excessive use of pyridoxin (vitamin B₆).

Perhaps the most common and popular approach to therapy during the last decade has been the administration of supplemental progesterone in the luteal phase of the menstrual cycle. The use of progesterone is based on the work and suggestions of Dr Katharina Dalton of England [4] who has prescribed progesterone for PMS for nearly 40 years. She has reported significant reduction in premenstrual symptoms after the administration of vaginal or rectal suppositories of progesterone in doses ranging from 400 to 1600 mg a day given in divided doses during the luteal phase. Recently micronized progesterone in the form of 100 mg capsules has been used in doses of 200–300 mg/day with significant reduction of symptoms. For specific information regarding therapy, the reader is referred to references [3–6].

Anovulatory therapy

The last category of medications that may be effective in the treatment of premenstrual symptoms are those medications designed to eliminate ovulation and menstruation. Some adolescents with significant behavior changes and symptoms during the luteal phase of the menstrual cycle may benefit from the administration of combination oral contraceptives. Unfortunately, over half of the women with PMS may have no benefit or an actual worsening of their premenstrual symptoms on combination oral contraceptives. Therefore, the minipill (progestin-only birth control pill) or the use of medroxyprogesterone acetate, 30 mg/day on a continuous basis, to eliminate ovulation and menstruation may be effective.

For those women who have significant gynecologic disease and are contemplating hysterectomy, it is possible to predict their response to ovariectomy and subsequent estrogen replacement therapy by placing these women on danazol or a gonadotropin-releasing hormone (GnRH) agonist to create a pseudomenopause-like state. If severe premenstrual symptoms are eliminated completely by the GnRH agonist or danazol and do not recur with the use of hormone replacement therapy, then ovariectomy at the time of hysterectomy may be considered. This approach should be truly considered as a last resort and is only applicable in those women who have severe, unrelenting, and unresponsive PMS that is disabling. The routine use of ovariectomy for the treatment of more mild and moderate PMS or PMS that readily responds to other therapies is inappropriate.

Step 3: Reevaluation of the diagnosis

If the response to therapy is incomplete or the patient fails to respond to the initial therapy, then the working diagnosis should be reevaluated. It is not rare for additional psychosocial problems to come to the surface during the course of evaluation and treatment of women with PMS. The woman who is unresponsive to medication may be suffering from more chronic affective disorders, she may be in an abusive relationship, or she may be suffering from the effects of chronic alcohol abuse. A failure to respond to the therapies listed above should result in an in-depth reevaluation of the patient. If the diagnosis of PMS is still entertained and thought to be correct, then another approach to therapy from the list above is appropriate. The process may be a matter of trial and error, with a several-month trial of a specific approach to medical therapy and the use of an alternative therapy if the initial therapy is unsuccessful. Fortunately, using this approach the vast majority of women with PMS will eventually find significant and marked reduction of their symptoms.

CONCLUSIONS

This chapter has summarized and outlined a simple, direct approach to the evaluation of women with premenstrual symptoms. Unfortunately, we do not have an understanding of the etiology and pathogenesis of PMS. However, if one uses this straightforward and simple approach, one can make the diagnosis of PMS and provide an effective therapy for these women. At the same time, one can determine that the premenstrual symptoms are not the result of underlying diseases that need to be evaluated and treated in a more specific fashion. The diagnosis of PMS is clearly a diagnosis of exclusion and its treatment is empiric. Hopefully in the future we will be able to discard the label of PMS for more specific disease entities and more specific and effective approaches to therapy.

REFERENCES

1 American Psychiatric Association. *Diagnostic and Statistical Manual of Mental Disorders*, 3rd edn. Washington, DC: American Psychiatric Press, 1987.
2 Frank RT. The hormonal causes of premenstrual tension. *Arch Neurol Psych* 1931; 26: 1053–1057.
3 Keye WR Jr. *The Premenstrual Syndrome*. Philadelphia: WB Saunders, 1988.
4 Dalton K. *Once a Month*. Claremart: Hunter House, 1990.
5 Dennerstein L, Spencer-Gardner C, Gotts G. Progesterone and the premenstrual syndrome: a double-blind crossover trial. *Br Med J* 1985; 290: 1617.
6 Maxson WS. The use of progesterone in the treatment of PMS. In: Johnson SR, ed. *Clinical Obstetrics and Gynecology*. Hagerstown: JB Lippincott, 1987: 464–478.

FURTHER READING

Bender SD, Kelleher K. *PMS: A Positive Program to Gain Control*. Tucson: The Body Press, 1986.
Berger G. *PMS: A Guide for Young Women*. Claremart: Hunter House, 1988.
Gise LH. *The Premenstrual Syndrome*. New York: Churchill, Livingstone, 1988.
Halas C. *Relief from Premenstrual Syndrome*. New York: Frederick Fen, 1984.
Harrison M. *Self-Help for Premenstrual Syndrome*. New York: Random House, 1982.

PREMENSTRUAL SYNDROME

Johnson SR. *Clinical Obstetrics and Gynecology: Premenstrual Syndrome*. Hagerstown: JB Lippincott, 1987.

O'Brien PMS. *Premenstrual Syndrome*. Oxford: Blackwell Scientific Publications, 1987.

Severino SK, Moline ML. *Premenstrual Syndrome: A Clinician's Guide*. New York: Guilford Press, 1989.

12

Premenstrual spotting

SEZER AKSEL

INTRODUCTION

Premenstrual spotting is defined as a minimal amount of bleeding observed in the late luteal phase prior to onset of menses. In a large number of women, premenstrual staining precedes the actual onset of menstrual flow by 3 hours [1]. Sporadic or recurrent episodes of spotting of longer duration (2–7 days), during the periovulatory or mainly during the premenstrual days, are frequent complaints that bring the patient to the gynecologist. Although this type of bleeding involves insignificant blood loss, it is of utmost nuisance to the patient when it recurs on a monthly basis.

MECHANISM

Any factor that disrupts the endometrial integrity independent from the chain of events that results in actual menstrual bleeding may initiate spotting or light bleeding episodes. Endometrial tissue obtained during premenstrual spotting may show focal stromal disintegration or disruptive lesions of the blood vessels without a notable hemostatic reaction [2]. To understand these changes, a brief review of Henzl's electron microscopic studies of menstrual endometrium and the lysosomal concept of menstrual bleeding is helpful [3].

During the follicular phase of the cycle, under the influence of estrogens, lysosomes containing phosphatase and hydrolase enzymes increase in the cytoplasm of the endometrial cells. Progesterone, secreted in high concentrations during the luteal phase, augments the lysosomal contents. Alteration in the concentration of estrogen and progesterone causes disruption of the lysosomal membranes, resulting in leakage of these destructive enzymes into the cytoplasm, and inducing a breakdown of tissues. Also endometrial prostaglandins, mainly prostaglandin $F_{2\alpha}$, increase during the luteal phase

of the cycle, causing vasoconstriction and breakage of the arterioles. The hemostatic mechanism in these endometrial arterioles is achieved by aggregation of platelets at points of vascular breaks. These platelet plugs are reinforced with fibrin, which in turn are lysed by fibrinolytic enzymes. Therefore, a focal and premature activation of this mechanism in the endometrial tissues may cause spotting or light bleeding. For example, superficial trauma induced by an endometrial biopsy or irritation and trauma to the endometrial lining by the insertion of an intrauterine device may result in spotting. This will occur more commonly during the luteal phase of the cycle. In these circumstances, fewer platelet plugs may form locally, as a result of less available fibrin, and the fibrinolytic activity may disrupt the orderly shedding pattern of the endometrium, resulting in premenstrual spotting.

Table 12.1 lists the causes of premenstrual spotting based on the frequency of occurrence, the origin and etiology of bleeding.

When spotting is of a sporadic nature, occurring three or four times a year, the etiology may be simple and easily curable. Vaginal lesions such as infections or condylomas are clearly evident during a careful speculum examination. A wet smear identifies the cause of infection and appropriate treatment may resolve the spotting. Condylomatous lesions in the vagina or on the cervix may also bleed easily when traumatized during coitus or in the use of tampons. Diaphragms or sponges left in the vagina over 24 hours may produce spotting and a foul odor due to local irritation and excess amount of anaerobic organisms, both of which will be alleviated once the intravaginal item has been removed.

Sometimes spotting may originate from the urethra and may be easily confused with vaginal bleeding. If the perineal examination is carried out carefully, a urethral diverticulum or a caruncle, which may bleed with pressure or contact, may be observed. Cervical

Table 12.1 The causes of premenstrual spotting

Sporadic	Recurrent
Vaginal	Urethral
Vaginitis	Caruncle
Condylomas	Diverticula
Trauma	Hemorrhagic cystitis
Urethral	Cervical
Caruncle	Cervicitis
Diverticula	Polyp
Cervical	Endometrial
Cervicitis	Pelvic inflammatory disease
Eversion	Polyps
Condyloma	Leiomyoma
Polyp	Ovulatory dysfunction
Carcinoma	Adenomyosis
Endometrial	Endometriosis
Endometritis	Rectal
Pregnancy-related	Hemorrhoids
Persistent corpus luteum	Iatrogenic
Irregular shedding	Intrauterine device
Rectal	Oral contraceptives
Hemorrhoids	Progestational agent
Iatrogenic	Anticoagulants
Endometrial biopsy	
Tampons	
Diaphragm/sponge	

lesions such as eversion, polyp, condyloma, or dysplastic changes are prone to contact bleeding and frequency of these episodes are usually based on the frequency of coitus, usage of diaphragm, sponge, or tampons.

Hemorrhoids may not be easy to visualize or feel during a rectal examination. These lesions will cause spotting more frequently after bowel movements. Sporadic spotting accompanied with pelvic pain, menstrual cramps, or low-grade fever may be due to endometritis of bacterial origin. In these instances pelvic inflammatory disease should be considered and, after endocervical cultures for gonorrhea and *Chlamydia* are obtained, antibiotic treatment should be started.

Spotting of endometrial origin, not associated with menstrual cramps or fever, may be pregnancy related. Implantation bleeding shortly before anticipated menses or onset of spotting instead of the expected menstrual flow with ectopic implantation may occur. More prolonged episodes of spotting

may be observed when irregular endometrial shedding develops. Usually, premenstrual spotting may continue postmenstrually. The histology of tissue obtained from the endometrial cavity may show a combination of proliferative and secretory endometrium and an aggressive four-quadrant biopsy or a "mini" dilatation and curettage in the office may cure the spotting episode completely. Also, a rare cause of premenstrual spotting may be a persistent corpus luteum (Halban's disease). It is assumed that progesterone production from the corpus luteum does not cease at the end of the 2-week life span. However, the level of estrogen and progesterone produced by the corpus luteum is not adequate to maintain the integrity of the endometrium and spotting ensues. Although the exact etiology of a persistent corpus luteum is unknown, a decrease in prostaglandin $F_{2\alpha}$ synthesis in the active ovary has been hypothesized [4].

Recurrent premenstrual spotting (Table 12.1) is inherently a chronic condition. Since it occurs every month, there is compelling reason to find a treatable cause. The iatrogenic basis of recurrent spotting due to intrauterine devices, usage of oral contraceptives, progestins, and anticoagulants may be easily resolved. Removal of the intrauterine device, changing the kind of oral contraceptive, or stopping the progestational agent will usually cure the spotting episodes. For lesions of the urethra, cervix and rectum observed during a pelvic examination, a ready cure may be offered on the spot, as discussed for lesions found in sporadic bleeders.

Recurrent premenstrual spotting from the endometrium may be caused by a variety of factors. Chronic pelvic inflammatory disease is often characterized by specific patient complaints, including premenstrual spotting and pelvic pain. Although small submucous leiomyomas or placental polyps may on occasion produce spotting of a recurrent nature, usually the presence of these benign uterine tumors is associated with heavy, prolonged uterine bleeding which is only relieved after the myoma or polyp is removed.

Ovulatory dysfunction such as luteal-phase insufficiency, luteinized unruptured follicle syndrome, and anovulation may be infrequently associated with premenstrual spotting. In some patients, premenstrual spotting may be directly attributed to adenomyosis or endometriosis. A direct causal relationship between premenstrual spotting and adenomyosis can only be established by evaluating the

CHAPTER 12

uterine pathology after a hysterectomy. It has been reported that in a small group of infertility patients with endometriosis, one-third experienced recurrent premenstrual spotting [5]. The exact mechanism of spotting in these women with endometriosis or adenomyosis is unclear.

DIAGNOSIS AND TREATMENT

Some patients with premenstrual spotting accept this condition as inherently transient and may not require a diagnosis nor desire any treatment. However, for those patients who consider this ailment totally undesirable, Figure 12.1 outlines a simple plan in evaluation and treatment of premenstrual spotting.

The history obtained should include a description of the menstrual bleeding, onset and duration of premenstrual spotting, and the association of dysmenorrhea or pelvic pain. Presence of an intrauterine device, frequency of use of contraceptive sponge or diaphragm and chronic use of tampons for discharge during the periovulatory phase of the menstrual cycle should be queried. A thorough drug history should be obtained, listing the dosage of salicylates and anticoagulants. Previous treatments to the vagina, urethra, rectum, and cervix for persistent infections,

condylomas, dysplasias, and persistent bleeding episodes should be outlined. A careful physical examination should be performed and a Pap smear obtained. Once the vaginal, urethral, rectal, and cervical causes are evaluated and excluded, then the endometrial cavity remains as the sole source for spotting and must be evaluated. The investigational plan may be as rigorous as the patient desires. At this stage of the work-up it is worthwhile determining if the patient is ovulatory. This information may be easily obtained from a basal body temperature record or a midluteal-phase progesterone. An endometrial biopsy may also provide information on the ovulatory status of the patient as well as the adequacy of progesterone production during the luteal phase.

Corrective measures include progesterone supplementation versus ovulation induction, based on the patient's desire for fertility. Induction of ovulatory cycles in anovulatory women will usually alleviate spotting if a myoma or a polyp does not coexist with the anovulatory state. Also, stimulating withdrawal bleeding with progestins will achieve the same result. In these patients, withdrawal therapy with medroxyprogesterone acetate 10 mg for 7–10 days, norethindrone or norethindrone acetate 2.5 or 5 mg daily for the same duration will cure the recurrent incidences of spotting. Use of oral contraceptive pills may be

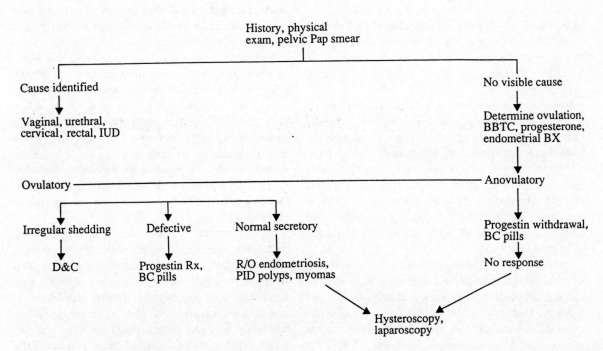

Fig. 12.1 Evaluation and treatment of premenstrual spotting.

equally effective. However, if the endometrial biopsy is secretory, without any indication of ovulatory dysfunction, hysteroscopy alone or combined with laparoscopy may assist in the diagnosis and removal of intrauterine polyps or submucous myomas.

Laparoscopy is essential in diagnosis of endometriosis. During this invasive procedure, it is possible to remove endometrial implants and cysts by cautery or vaporize these lesions by laser. Suppression of ovarian steroids by danocrine or the gonadotropin-releasing hormone analogs may render the patient amenorrheic and cure the premenstrual spotting for the duration of therapy. There is no current information on whether the surgical or medical intervention for endometriosis cures premenstrual spotting.

REFERENCES

1 Donald JL, Fraser IS, Duncan L, McCarron G. Analysis of the time or day of onset of menstruation. *Clin Reprod Fertil* 1987; 5: 77–83.
2 Christiaens GC, Sixma JJ, Haspels AA. Morphology of haemostasis in menstrual endometrium. *Br J Obstet Gynaecol* 1980; 87: 425–439.
3 Henzl MR, Smith RE, Boost G, Tyler, ET. Lysosomal concept of menstrual bleeding in humans. *J Clin Endocrinol* 1972; 34: 860–874.
4 Aksel S, Schomberg DW. Prostaglandin $F_{2\alpha}$ levels in human ovarian plasma in pregnancy and in a case of Halban's disease. *Obstet Gynecol* 1978; 52: 421–423.
5 Wentz AC. Premenstrual spotting: its association with endometriosis but not luteal phase inadequacy. *Fertil Steril* 1980; 33: 605–607.

13

Midcycle spotting

GARY FRISHMANN & ANTHONY A. LUCIANO

INTRODUCTION

One of the most common problems presenting to the practicing gynecologist is abnormal uterine bleeding which may result from an imbalance of sex hormones, organic pathology, or hematologic disorders. The bleeding pattern, the amount, duration, and timing of flow, as well as the patient's age and medical history have important etiologic and therapeutic implications.

The most common manifestation of abnormal bleeding is dysfunctional uterine bleeding (DUB), which occurs most frequently at the two extremes of a woman's reproductive life. Of patients with DUB, roughly 50% are over 45 years of age, 20% are adolescents, and 30% are in the midreproductive years. Eighty percent of patients with DUB are anovulatory, as evidenced by proliferative or hyperplastic endometrial biopsies.

With the many different manifestations of abnormal uterine bleeding, a variety of terms have been used to describe these abnormal menstrual patterns. To avoid confusion, it is important to have precise definitions of them.

DEFINITIONS

DUB is not a symptom but a well-defined diagnosis of abnormal uterine bleeding not associated with pregnancy or an organic pathology. Thus, DUB is a diagnosis of exclusion, resulting from an imbalance of sex steroid hormones acting upon an otherwise normal uterus.

Metrorrhagia — uterine bleeding, of variable amounts, occurring at irregular intervals. Metrorrhagia is the most commonly reported abnormal bleeding pattern in women with DUB due to anovulation.

Menometrorrhagia — uterine bleeding that is excessive in both quantity and duration, occurring at irregular intervals.

Menorrhagia — uterine bleeding that is excessive in both quantity and duration, occurring at regular intervals.

Hypermenorrhea — excessive uterine bleeding that is of normal duration and occurs at regular intervals. Hypermenorrhea is frequently used synonymously with menorrhagia.

Polymenorrhea — uterine bleeding that is normal in duration and quantity but is abnormally frequent, occuring at less than every 21-day intervals.

Oligomenorrhea — uterine bleeding that is normal in duration and quantity, occurring in abnormally infrequent intervals of greater than 35 days.

Midcycle spotting — bleeding, of any amount, in the middle of the cycle, in patients who are usually ovulatory and have regular menses. Bleeding at the middle of the menstrual cycle is a less common presentation of abnormal bleeding. Some 60–90% of ovulating women have at least microscopic periovulatory uterine bleeding while 20% of all women with mittelschmerz pain experience macroscopic intermenstrual bleeding.

The rest of this chapter will review the pathophysiology, evaluation, and treatment of midcycle spotting which may be due to a variety of hormonal and organic dysfunctions.

HORMONAL DYSFUNCTIONS

Estrogen withdrawal

The normal uterine endometrium consists of three distinct layers. The most superficial (stratum compactum) and middle (stratum spongiosum) layers are sloughed each month with menstruation, while the innermost (stratum basalis) layer is retained and plays a key role in the regeneration of the postmenstrual endometrial lining. The postmenstrual endometrium lining is only 0.5 mm thick. During the proliferative phase, repair of glands, stroma, and vasculature occurs under estrogen stimulation and regulation, so that by the end of the proliferative phase, the height of the endometrium increases 10-fold, up to 5.0 mm. This is the peak height achieved throughout the menstrual cycle with no further growth obtained during the secretory phase. If estrogen support ceases or is diminished, areas of fragile endometrium may be shed in variable amounts, resulting in estrogen withdrawal bleeding. Estrogen withdrawal bleeding occurs iatrogenically following surgical (oophorectomy) or medical (gonadotropin-releasing hormone agonist) castration or with cessation of estrogen replacement therapy. Physiologically, estrogen withdrawal occurs during the late follicular phase of the menstrual cycle. Following the estradiol surge that stimulates the midcycle luteinizing hormone (LH) surge, a precipitous decline in serum estradiol levels occurs, from a peak level of 300–500 pg/ml to 100–125 pg/ml, over a 24-hour period. This abrupt drop in circulating estrogen levels frequently leads to some endometrial shedding of variable amounts and duration. This type of midcycle bleeding has also been referred to as ovulation bleeding or pseudopolymenorrhea, which in most women is not significant enough to warrant intervention. However, in some women the midcycle bleeding may be moderate, lasting up to 5 days, and may interfere with periovulatory coital activity. In such cases, medical intervention may be successfully implemented by the use of estrogen (micronized estrogen 2.0 mg or conjugated estrogens 1.25 mg) daily from day 10 through day 16 of the cycle.

Progesterone breakthrough bleeding

Breakthrough bleeding related to progesterone insufficiency or withdrawal may occur at any point during ovulatory cycles and may mimic estrogen withdrawal bleeding in both amount and timing in the cycle. However, it is seldom persistent from cycle to cycle. Occasionally, midcycle bleeding may be associated with Halban's disease, a condition whereby the corpus luteum has a prolonged life span and may continue to secrete progesterone, even if at lower levels into the subsequent menstrual cycle. Areas of well-developed secretory endometrium may persist past the normal cessation of menses, resulting in irregular endometrial shedding. Four-quadrant endometrial biopsies may reveal mixed histology with both proliferative and secretory endometrium. Halban's disease is uncommon and rarely persistent. When it does require therapy, this may be easily corrected with oral contraceptives.

Exogenous hormones

Various steroidal or nonsteroidal medications may cause abnormal endometrial shedding which may present as midcycle spotting. One of the most frequent of these is oral contraceptives which commonly cause spotting and breakthrough bleeding in the first few months of use. Spironolactone, an antihypertensive diuretic with antiandrogenic properties, has been reported to cause metrorrhagia in up to 58% of women treated for hirsutism. Ginseng facial cream, which contains estrogen-like compounds, may also interfere with the normal menstrual cycle and cause abnormal uterine bleeding which may occur at midcycle.

Nonsteroidal etiologies

Any endocrinopathy that leads to ovulatory dysfunction or alterations in sex hormone metabolism may lead to abnormal uterine bleeding which may manifest as midcycle spotting or bleeding. Hyperprolactinemia and thyroid abnormalities are common endocrinopathies in women of reproductive age and should be evaluated in all women with menstrual disorders.

FUNCTIONAL ETIOLOGIES OF MIDCYCLE SPOTTING

Midcycle vaginal bleeding may result from a variety of organic dysfunctions which may or may not be of uterine origin. Table 13.1 presents an extensive list of possible etiologies of vaginal bleeding with the most common causes of midcycle spotting in bold type.

EVALUATION

History

The first step in the evaluation is to take a thorough medical history with special emphasis on the timing and amount of bleeding. The relationship of the abnormal bleeding to menses or time of ovulation, and the duration of the symptoms may give important clues as to the underlying disorder. Abnormal bleeding over 6 months is more likely to be a variant of DUB, while abnormal bleeding less than 3 months may reflect acute hormonal imbalances or organic pathology such as a polyp or endometritis. Bleeding following coitus may reflect a friable cervix and/or cervicitis due to dysplasia or infection. Metrorrhagia and other bleeding abnormalities have been found

Table 13.1 Causes of vaginal bleeding

Vulvar origin	Uterine origin
Infection, ulcers	**Hormonal-related (estrogen**
Trauma	**withdrawal bleeding)**
Neoplasms (benign and malignant)	**Foreign body (intrauterine device)**
	Polyp
Cervical origin	**Fibroid**
Polyp	Infection (pelvic inflammatory disease/**endometritis**)
Cervicitis/infection	Malignancy
Erosion/trauma	Atrophic endometrium
Malignancy	
	Tubal/ovarian disease
Pregnancy complications	Neoplasm (thecoma/granulosa cell tumor)
Abortion	Fallopian tube malignancy
Ectopic pregnancy	
Trophoblastic disease	Nongynecologic bleeding
Retained products	Urinary tract origin
	Gastrointestinal tract origin
Vaginal origin	
Foreign body (tampon, pessary, diaphragm)	Systemic disease
Adenosis	Coagulopathies/blood dyscrasias
Endometriosis	Liver cirrhosis
Malignancy	
Vaginitis	Medications
Trauma	Warfarin
	Spironolactone
	Oral contraceptives
	Over-the-counter medications (facial creams)

Bold type indicates the most common causes of midcycle spotting.

more often in adolescents with *Chlamydia* than those with negative genital cultures. However, with adolescent patients, a complaint of spotting or other bleeding abnormality may merely be an excuse to seek the physician's care in obtaining contraception or reproductive counseling. Finally, it is important to enquire as to any family history of bleeding disorders, problems prior to surgery, or easy bruising in order to evaluate for any hematologic abnormalities.

A menstrual calendar with the basal body temperature chart on which the patient records bleeding episodes, spotting, and coital activity, is the most informative and cost-effective way to evaluate abnormal bleeding, including midcycle spotting. One common patient complaint is of having periods every 2 weeks, with one being lighter than the other. This may be suggestive of polymenorrhea associated with either a short luteal phase (as in postmenarchal girls) or very short follicular phases, as may occur in perimenopausal women. The clinician may differentiate anovulatory from periovulatory bleeding and suspect organic or hematologic disorders by determining the temporal relationship of the ab-

normal bleeding to basal body temperature changes, coitus, and other potentially precipitating events. By the use of the basal body temperature chart, polymenorrhea may be easily differentiated from midcycle bleeding which occurs prior to or at the time of the temperature rise instead of following a temperature drop, as occurs with polymenorrhea.

Physical examination

A physical examination is essential to rule out any significant organic abnormalities. Evaluation of the vulva, vagina, cervix, and uterus will search for infectious etiologies (such as a vaginal infection or cervicitis), evidence of coital trauma, cervical polyps, an enlarged myomatous uterus, etc. A Pap smear and cultures for *Chlamydia* and gonorrhea are taken at the time of examination.

Laboratory tests

These can be selected according to the severity of symptoms and the index of suspicion of an organic etiology. With classic light spotting that consistently occurs at midcycle, no laboratory tests are needed

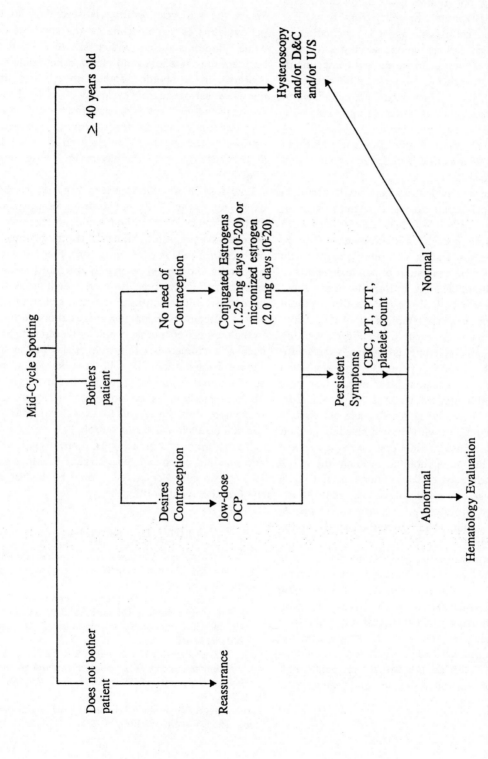

Fig. 13.1 Flowchart for management of midcycle spotting. OCP, oral contraceptive; PT, prothrombin time; PTT, partial thromboplastin time; CBC, complete blood count; U/S, ultrasound.

and the patient may be reassured. With moderate to severe spotting, obtain a complete blood count with platelets and PT/partial thrombaplastin time. The complete blood count will assist in evaluation of hematologic disorders as well as serving as a baseline for future reference. If the patient complains of "hemorrhaging" each month, but has no change in her hematocrit, she can be reassured from a hematologic viewpoint. A low hematocrit should be an indication for iron supplementation.

With severe irregular bleeding, obtain a bleeding time. Other tests to consider include pregnancy and thyroid function studies.

Ultrasonographic evaluation may prove useful in the search for pelvic pathology such as fibroids, endometrial polyps, hyperplasia, and malignancy with depth of invasion. Because of its excellent resolution, transvaginal ultrasound is becoming progressively more utilized in the evaluation of pelvic disorders.

With recalcitrant bleeding and/or advanced patient age, further evaluation of the endometrium should be done by endometrial sampling or hysteroscopy. While cancer in a patient with true midcycle spotting is extremely rare, bleeding is always a cause for concern. More than 90% of patients with endometrial cancer present with vaginal bleeding as their only symptoms. Although only 2.9% of endometrial cancers occur in women under 40 years old, 81% of these patients present with vaginal bleeding as their chief complaint. In a perimenopausal patient, there should be a low threshhold to evaluate the endometrium which may easily be done in the office with the Pipelle or a similar device. In general, any patient over 40 years of age should have an assessment of her endometrium performed early in the evaluation.

Hysteroscopy is an extremely useful tool to evaluate the endocervical canal and uterine cavity for organic pathology and to obtain adequate tissue sampling under direct visualization. With experience, diagnostic hysteroscopy can be successfully utilized in an office setting. However, hysteroscopy does not obviate the need for endocervical and endometrial sampling to obtain an appropriate histopathologic evaluation of the endometrium and endocervical epithelium.

TREATMENT

When the midcycle spotting is secondary to the periovulatory estrogen decline, no therapy is needed if the symptoms are not bothersome to the patient. Furthermore, it should not impair her ability to conceive. If the spotting bothers the patient, then the use of estrogens from cycle day 10 to day 16 will be adequate to prevent estrogen withdrawal. Estrogen preparations commonly used include conjugated estrogens (1.25 mg daily), micronized estradiol 17β (2.0 mg daily), and ethinylestradiol (20 μg daily) (Fig 13.1).

Low-dose oral contraceptives are an excellent choice for any patients not desirous of pregnancy in the absence of contraindications to the use of estrogen or progestin. Midcycle spotting while on birth control pills is common during the first cycles of therapy and should resolve by the fourth cycle of medication. If the breakthrough bleeding persists beyond the initial months of therapy, switch to a pill with a different estrogenic or progestational activity. In the presence of another condition requiring therapy such as endometriosis or leiomyomas, one should choose a medication that will treat both problems, such as danazol, progestins, or a GnRH analog. Some of these medications do not afford adequate contraception; thus, be careful to alert the patient that she still needs to use birth control.

If the hormonal approach fails, then surgical evaluation should be considered. Surgical therapy, such as a dilatation and curettage, should be the last, not the first therapeutic option.

FURTHER READING

Crissman JD, Azoury RS, Barnes AE, Schellhas HF. Endometrial carcinoma in women 40 years of age or younger. *Obstet Gynecol* 1981; 57: 699.

Fleischer AC, Kalemeris GC, Machin JE, Entman SS, James AE. Sonographic depiction of normal and abnormal endometrium with histopathologic correlation. *J. Ultrasound Med* 1986; 5: 445.

Loffer FD. Hysteroscopy with selective endometrial sampling compared with D&C for abnormal uterine bleeding: the value of a negative hysteroscopic view. *Obstet Gynecol* 1989; 73: 16.

Scommegna A, Dmowski WP. Dysfunctional uterine bleeding. *Clin Obstet Gynecol* 1973; 16: 221.

14

Postpill amenorrhea

JULIA V. JOHNSON

OVERVIEW

In 1966, Whitelaw and colleagues [1] described a delay in the resumption of menses following use of synthetic progestins. Soon thereafter, Shearman [2] documented a series of 86 women who had at least 12 months of amenorrhea after stopping birth control pills. This "postpill" amenorrhea raised concerns regarding the effect of oral contraceptive agents on the hypothalamic–pituitary–ovarian axis and subsequent fertility. As Whitelaw *et al.* stated: "we are dealing with a small but definite group of women whose pituitary gonadotropic function is temporarily blocked by oral contraceptives" [1].

There is debate whether this disorder exists. When amenorrhea follows oral contraceptive use, conventional evaluation will identify known causes of amenorrhea in most women. Many believe that normogonadotropic amenorrhea following pill use is indistinguishable from that which occurs independent of oral contraceptives. In patients with hypogonadotropic anovulation, the question remains as to whether this condition is caused by oral contraceptives or is coincidental to pill use. Even when there is no other etiology for postpill amenorrhea, it has been documented that these women respond well to ovulation induction. Therefore, concern regarding future fertility should not prevent the use of oral contraceptive agents. It is also known that the length of contraceptive use is unrelated to the incidence of postpill amenorrhea, suggesting that there is no benefit in "resting" patients on the pill.

This chapter will consider the incidence of postpill amenorrhea and discuss whether it is a distinct entity. Proposed pathophysiologies for postpill amenorrhea will be briefly discussed. Evaluation of secondary amenorrhea in these women will be reviewed, as well as the treatment of patients with unexplained amenorrhea. This chapter cannot resolve the debate regarding postpill amenorrhea, but will review the knowledge to date, and outline a plan for its diagnosis and treatment.

INCIDENCE

Postpill amenorrhea has been reported to affect between 0.2 and 3.1% of all contraceptive users. The largest series, with more than 20 000 women, established a rate of only 0.22% [3]. The variations in the reported incidence of this disorder may reflect differing referral patterns to the authors and absence of a standard definition of the disorder. While Shearman [2] required 12 months without menses prior to diagnosing postpill amenorrhea, others have considered intervals of 3, 4, or 6 months.

Because the true rate of postpill amenorrhea is unknown, it is difficult to know if it exceeds the rate of secondary amenorrhea in all women. The reported incidence of secondary amenorrhea of greater than 6 months' duration is between 0.7 and 1% [4]. This incidence is even higher in select populations, such as postmenarcheal teenagers and college students, that are likely to use oral contraceptives. It can be argued that postpill amenorrhea is simply a reflection of the usual occurrence of menstrual disorders in these women.

When amenorrheic oral contraceptive users and nonusers are compared, no specific diagnostic findings have been associated with pill use. It is interesting to note that the strongest positive correlation with the development of postpill amenorrhea is a history of menstrual irregularities prior to pill use [3]. This suggests there is a preexisting condition that was temporarily masked by the use of oral contraceptives. However, there remains a subset of women whose use of birth control pills constitutes the only apparent explanation of the development of amenorrhea.

CHAPTER 14

PATHOPHYSIOLOGY

Oral contraceptive agents interfere with reproduction at several levels. Birth control pills interfere
with the normal release of gonadotropins by direct
effects on the hypothalamus and pituitary [5]. Oral
contraceptives also create an atrophic, inactive endometrium. It has been suggested that postpill amenorrhea may reflect a prolonged suppression of the
hypothalamus and/or pituitary. This is in contrast
to the normal response to the withdrawal of contraceptive agents, which results in a return to usual
basal gonadotropin levels within several days and
normal gonadotropin-releasing hormone (GnRH)
response within 2 weeks. Several authors have noted
that a group of women with postpill amenorrhea
have decreased basal follicle-stimulating hormone
(FSH)/luteinizing hormone (LH), although this
may merely reflect an unrelated pituitary or hypothalamic disorder.

Birth control pills may alter the secretion of other
pituitary hormones as well. There appears to be
no effect on thyroid-stimulating hormone (TSH)
production, but an alteration in growth hormone
secretion has been suggested. Although basal prolactin levels are unchanged, prolactin response to
thyrotropin-releasing hormone (TRH) and hypoglycemia is elevated in women on contraceptive
agents. This exaggerated response to stimuli may
cause periodic hyperprolactinemia [5]. As a clinical
corollary to this theory, it has been suggested that
the incidence of galactorrhea is increased following
the use of oral contraceptives. In contradiction,
however, there is no difference in the rate of hyperprolactinemia or prolactinomas in these patients as
compared to all women with secondary amenorrhea.
Early concerns that oral contraceptives cause a prolonged elevation in prolactin levels are unfounded.

A direct effect on the endometrium was also considered as a cause of postpartum amenorrhea. Biopsies
from more than 50% of women with postpill amenorrhea revealed atrophic or resting endometrium.
This finding, however, probably reflects a disorder
in the hypothalamic—pituitary—ovarian axis. Our
knowledge of endometrial development argues
against an isolated endometrial etiology for postpill amenorrhea.

It is also important to consider the effect of the
patient's body habitus on postpill amenorrhea.
One study suggested that low body weight was a
consistent finding in women who developed amen-

orrhea. Although the precontraceptive weight was
not reported, it is possible that interval weight loss
influenced postpill menstrual patterns. Significant
weight gain during the use of birth control pills may
also affect menstrual regularity. Since weight gain
is a reported side-effect of oral contraceptives, the
medication may be contributing to amenorrhea by
an indirect mechanism.

DIAGNOSIS AND TREATMENT

Because the cause of amenorrhea following oral
contraceptives is usually unrelated to pill use, it is
important to evaluate each patient for the etiology
of her menstrual disorder. The diagnosis of postpill amenorrhea can only be made when all other
etiologies have been eliminated. The timing of
this work-up may vary with the practitioner, as the
recommended interval prior to the evaluation of
secondary amenorrhea ranges from 3 to 12 months.
Because normal cycle length returns within 3 months
of pill use, this is an appropriate time to begin the
evaluation. Spontaneous menses after 12 months of
postpill amenorrhea is rare, so there is no reason to
delay the evaluation beyond this point. If the patient
has symptoms which suggest a specific disorder, e.g.,
galactorrhea, there is no need to delay the work-up
for any period of time.

A thorough history and physical examination may
suggest the etiology for the amenorrhea. A history of
previous menstrual disorders suggests a preexisting
problem. Weight loss, extremes of exercise or stress,
or poor nutrition may suggest a hypothalamic disorder. Heat/cold intolerance, changes in bowel habits,
changes in hair or skin, and alterations in energy
level suggest thyroid disease. Galactorrhea, with or
without headache and visual changes, may indicate
a prolactin (PRL)-secreting adenoma. Perimenopausal
symptoms, such as hot flushes, may be present.
Medications such as phenothiazines, anabolic steroids, or diet pills can contribute to amenorrhea.
History of recent uterine surgery may indicate an
anatomic cause of amenorrhea.

Physical signs are also important to consider.
Abnormal body habitus with obesity or anorexia
may be present. Expressible galactorrhea suggests
possible hyperprolactinemia. Breast or genital atrophy
may suggest a hypoestrogenic state. Eye changes
are noted with hyperthyroidism, as well as skin
and hair changes. A thyroid examination should be
performed and hypo-/hyperreflexia noted. Signs of

androgen excess, such as hirsutism and acne, should be sought. The pelvic examination can aid in ruling out pregnancy.

If no obvious etiology for amenorrhea is found, the laboratory evaluation can proceed as noted in the flow chart (Fig. 14.1). If the pregnancy test is negative, TSH, PRL, and FSH/LH levels will evaluate for pituitary disease. Elevated FSH/LH indicates ovarian failure. The Provera withdrawal test has been recommended to evaluate end-organ function and also suggests that there is ovarian stimulation by gonadotropins. Alternately, if the FSH:LH ratio is reversed, the Provera withdrawal can be eliminated, as these patients usually have polycystic ovarian disease. If fertility is desired, this group may be successfully treated with clomiphene citrate and ovulation monitoring. If fertility is not desired, monthly Provera withdrawal will prevent over-

development of the endometrium and reduce the patient's risk for endometrial hyperplasia.

Low or normal gonadotropins can be further evaluated with estrogen, followed by progestin withdrawal. If this test is negative, an anatomic problem is suggested. However, when there is no history of uterine manipulation, the estrogen/Provera withdrawal test is rarely helpful. Patients with low levels of FSH and LH usually have a hypothalamic or pituitary disorder. A radiographic evaluation (magnetic resonance imaging or computed tomography) will rule out a central nervous system lesion. If there is any suggestion of pituitary failure, appropriate stimulatory testing should be performed. If pregnancy is desired, patients with hypothalamic or pituitary amenorrhea can be treated with human menopausal gonadotropins and human chorionic gonadotropin to induce ovulation. If these patients

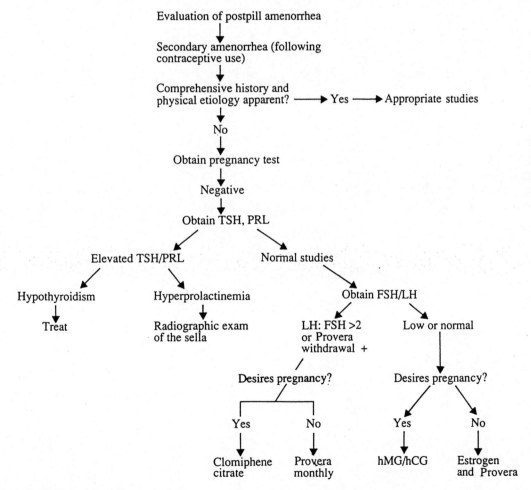

Fig. 14.1 Evaluation of postpill amenorrhea.

95

CHAPTER 14

remain amenorrheic, and do not desire fertility, cyclic estrogen and progesterone should be prescribed to prevent osteoporosis and genital atrophy.

Because the diagnosis of postpill amenorrhea is still in question and its etiology unknown, it is wise to evaluate and treat these women as you would any patient with secondary amenorrhea. If no etiology for the menstrual irregularity is found and the patient does not desire pregnancy, expectant management for up to 6 months may be reasonable. If, however, the patient does not spontaneously cycle during this time, she should be treated appropriately with progestin or estrogen/progestin therapy.

REFERENCES

1 Whitelaw MJ, Nola VF, Kalman CF. Irregular menses, amenorrhea, and infertility following synthetic progestational agents. *JAMA* 1966; 195: 160.
2 Shearman RP. Amenorrhea after treatment with oral contraceptives. *Lancet* 1966; 2: 1110.
3 Golditch IM. Postcontraceptive amenorrhea. *Obstet Gynecol* 1972; 39: 903.
4 Archer DF, Thomas RL. The fallacy of the postpill amenorrhea syndrome. *Clin Obstet Gynecol* 1981; 24: 943.
5 Mishell DR, Kletzky OA, Brenner PF, Roy S, Nicoloff J. The effect of contraceptive steroids on hypothalamic-pituitary function. *Am J Obstet Gynecol* 1976; 128: 60.

Part III
Anatomic abnormalities of the genital tract

15

The DES-exposed uterus

SIMON KIPERSZTOK & ROBERT J. STILLMAN

OVERVIEW

Estimates show that between the late 1940s and 1971, approximately 2–3 million women were prescribed diethylstilbestrol (DES) during their pregnancies. The nonsteroidal estrogen had been synthesized in 1938 by Dodds and colleagues, had a structural similarity to estradiol (Fig. 15.1), and was believed to be beneficial in treating a wide variety of pregnancy disorders such as threatened or habitual abortions, toxemia, premature delivery, postmaturity, and stillbirth [1,2]. As early as 1953 controlled clinical trials failed to demonstrate the utility of DES as definitive or prophylactic therapy for pregnancy complications [3]. However, it was not until 1971, following reports of eight women who developed clear cell adenocarcinoma of the vagina after *in utero* exposure to DES, that its use in pregnancy was banned by the Food and Drug Administration [4].

After 1971 a number of additional adverse effects from DES use during pregnancy were added to the

Fig. 15.1 Chemical structures of the natural estrogen, estradiol 17-β, and of the synthetic estrogen, diethylstilbestrol.

known association between *in utero* exposure and vaginal cancer. A study that reassessed one of the earlier trials reporting the efficacy of DES in treating pregnancy complications demonstrated that its ingestion was actually associated with a significant increase in the frequency of abortions, premature deliveries, and stillbirths [5]. Also, as evidence of anatomic abnormalities in the genital tract of females exposed to DES *in utero* accumulated, it became apparent that the drug could also be associated with an increased frequency of infertility.

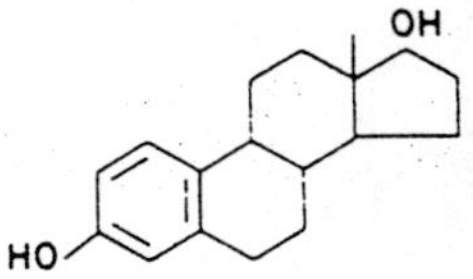

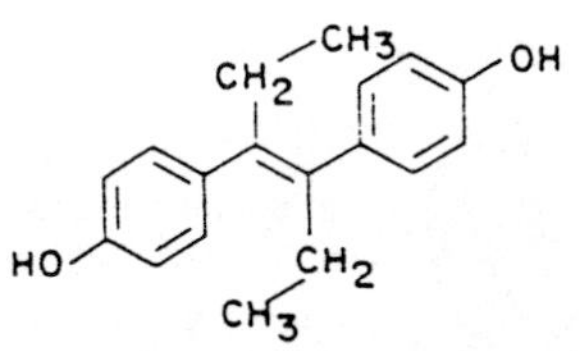

PATHOPHYSIOLOGY

During the third month of embryonic development, the uterine stroma differentiates into two distinct compartments, one of which will become the endometrial stroma, and the other the myometrium. Since there is evidence that the stroma in the female genital tract has specific inductive effects on the developments of the overlying epithelium, there is a possibility that DES may affect the stroma primarily, leading to secondary induction of abnormal epithelial changes [6]. This is more clearly conceptualized in the lower female genital tract where adenosis, ectropion, and associated squamous metaplasia are observed. Similarly, exposure to DES anywhere between the ninth gestational week through the fifth month may prevent the various mesenchymal layers of the uterus from segregating, therefore causing clinically apparent stromal hyperplasia (ridges), hypoplasia (constrictions), or abnormally contoured uterine cavities.

In 1977 Kaufman and coworkers reported, for the first time, the upper genital tract abnormalities found by hysterosalpingogram (HSG) in 40 out of 60 DES-exposed patients [7]. The abnormality most commonly encountered was a T-shaped uterus. Later, in a more comprehensive series that included 267 patients, the same workers reported that 69.3% of DES-exposed women showed evidence of upper genital tract disease by HSG [8]. The anomalies more commonly found were (in decreasing order of incidence): T-shaped uterus with a small cavity; T-shaped uterus; small uterine cavity; T-shaped uterus with a small cavity and constriction rings; T-shaped uterus with constriction; small uterine cavity with constriction and constriction rings (Fig. 15.2). These upper genital tract anomalies associated with *in utero* exposure to the synthetic hormone are part of a more widespread adverse effect in the whole female genital tract since, when epithelial changes of the vagina are observed, uterine anomalies are 5.1 times more likely to occur than in DES-exposed patients without vaginal changes. Also, in patients with structural changes of the cervix the likelihood of upper genital tract anomalies is 4.5 times higher than in unaffected DES-exposed females [9].

The fallopian tubes are usually normal both histologically and on HSG. Nevertheless, a small series reporting the findings in surgical specimens found shortened and distorted tubes with pinpoint ostia. Furthermore, the higher incidence of ectopic gestations in DES-exposed patients as compared to a non-DES-exposed population is suspicious for the presence of a functional abnormality in the tubes of the former group [10].

Despite all the evidence implicating DES as an agent which adversely affects the development of the incipient Müllerian tract, it has been difficult to establish a direct cause and effect between *in utero* DES exposure and infertility. Some data suggest a deleterious effect of DES in the fertility potential of exposed females. Menstrual irregularities and oligomenorrhea have been found to be more common in such patients; however, as these patients enter their mid 20s their menstrual regularity may become established. Also, the incidence of uterine abnormalities and of endometriosis in infertile DES-exposed females appears to be significantly higher than in nonexposed infertile controls. Notwithstanding these pathologic findings, reports on infertility rates in the exposed population as compared to that of controls remain contested. More solidly established are the significant differences in the frequency of spontaneous abortions, ectopic pregnancies, premature deliveries, perinatal deaths, and overall adverse pregnancy outcome. An increased rate of miscarriages has been consistently reported in DES daughters in both controlled and uncontrolled studies with rates ranging between 18.3 and 48.3%. The ectopic pregnancy rate has been estimated to be between 6 and 8%. Preterm delivery (defined as delivery before the 37th week of gestation or an infant weight equal to or less than 2500 g) is also found more frequently in studies of DES-exposed

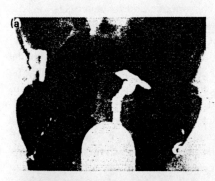
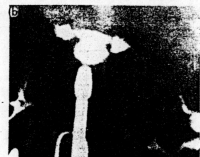
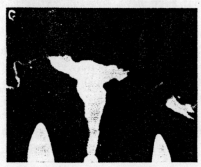
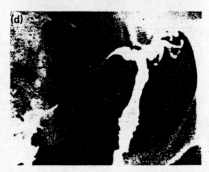

Fig. 15.2 Hysterosalpingograms of female progeny exposed *in utero* to diethylstilbestrol showing upper Müllerian tract abnormalities: (a) T-shaped uterus. (b) Constriction rings. (c) Irregularity of uterine cavity. (d) Small and irregular uterine cavity. (Reprinted with permission from [8].)

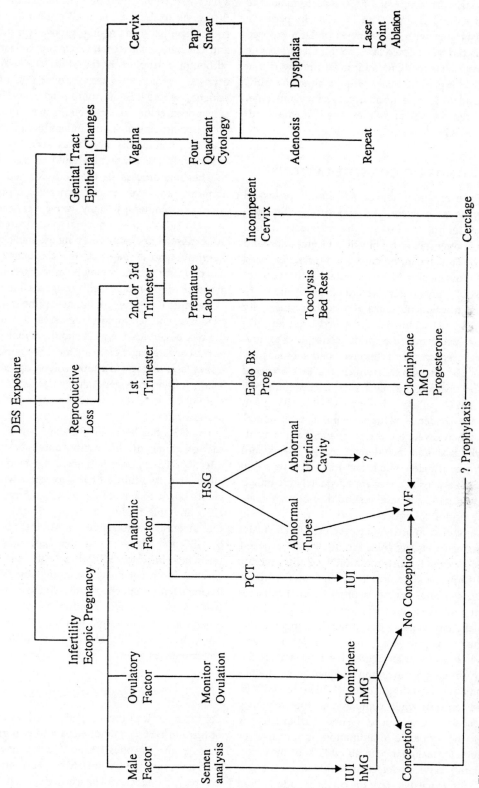

Fig. 15.3 Algorithm for the management of DES-exposure patients.

populations, with a rate of 10–30% as compared to 0–5% in control groups. The increase in perinatal death associated with pregnancies of DES-exposed females is thought to be related to the increased rate of preterm deliveries. One additional finding is that 51% of DES-exposed females with an abnormal HSG were found to have a normal pregnancy outcome, as compared to 75% of DES-exposed females with a normal HSG.

DIAGNOSTIC CONSIDERATIONS

Although every infertile couple should be asked routinely about *in utero* DES exposure in the process of an infertility work-up, the diagnosis in such patients is often made by physical examination and by HSG. The ovulatory capacity in DES-exposed infertile women should be ascertained because of the possible previously described aberrations in menstrual function. In cases of secondary infertility it should be determined if there had been any difficulty in achieving the prior conception(s) and whether a pregnancy was conceived and subsequently lost. The circumstances in which the loss occurred should be documented since such information may be useful in formulating therapy. Additionally, given the higher incidence of upper genital tract abnormalities when lower genital tract changes are present, the work-up should include a thorough assessment of the lower female genital tract in such a way that any DES-associated changes are adequately identified.

The vaginal examination should thoroughly assess the entire circumference of the vault, paying special attention to areas that may exhibit adenosis. Adenosis has been recognized in 35–90% of exposed females, is found most commonly in the anterior vaginal fornix, and is usually limited to the upper vagina. Its natural course is often spontaneous regression and, rarely, progression to an atypical and then malignant state. Appropriate cytologic evaluation involving the cervix and four fornices and observation rather than aggressive treatment is the therapy of choice since the frequency of adenocarcinoma is exceedingly low (1/1000 to 1/10 000 exposed females) when compared to the frequency of adenosis. Furthermore, when malignancy is present the cytologic examination is positive or suspicious for malignancy in about 80% of the cases.

Similarly, cervical defects should also be documented. Structural defects of the cervix include a raised ridge, usually in the anterior cervix (cockscomb), a flat rim involving part or all of the circumference of the cervix (collar), a polypoid appearance due to a circumferential constricting groove (pseudopolyp), and a diameter of less than 1.5 cm (hypoplastic cervix). Although ectropion is found in 40–60% of non-exposed females, it is seen in over 95% of exposed patients, where it is also more extensive. These areas of exposed columnar epithelium may be associated with hypermucorrhea and inflammation which may lead to inflammatory atypia, as seen on exfoliative cytology. In this context it should be recognized that the healing process in the DES-exposed female is abnormal and even minor gynecologic procedures, such as cryotherapy, may cause cervical stenosis in up to 80% of these patients, as compared to 1% of nonexposed females undergoing the same procedure. Cervical stenosis may lead to subsequent cervical–mucus factor and also may be associated with endometriosis due to increased retrograde menstruation. Since much of the columnar epithelium seen in adenosis and ectropion regresses spontaneously, the risk of cervical stenosis should be borne in mind when considering treatment for these abnormalities. Use of laser therapy to a small colposcopically defined lesion, rather than generalized pericervical therapy, should be preferred in order to minimize the area of destruction.

The HSG has been the standard test to assess the cervical canal, uterine cavity, and tubal patency in infertile DES-exposed females. As previously noted, more than two-thirds of the exposed women have been shown to have characteristic abnormalities by HSG and this finding is of significance because of the increased association of uterine abnormalities by HSG and adverse pregnancy outcomes. Magnetic resonance imaging (MRI) has been used to predict cervical incompetence in nonpregnant women and in one such prospective study DES-exposed females were found to have significantly shorter cervices when compared to normal controls [11]. We are evaluating the use of MRI in evaluation of the uterus in circumstances where HSG should be avoided.

THERAPEUTIC STEPS

For therapeutic purposes, patients who were exposed *in utero* to DES can be divided into two groups. The first group includes patients who have primary infertility, secondary infertility, and one or more ectopic pregnancies. The second group consists of patients with recurrent pregnancy loss.

In the first group a thorough infertility evaluation should include an assessment of a possible anatomic factor by means of an HSG and a postcoital test. If the HSG reveals tubal blockage or a significant tubal abnormality, the patient would benefit from *in vitro* fertilization and embryo transfer (IVF-ET). The success rate for this group of patients has been reported to be similar to other groups of patients having different infertility factors involved (24.4% pregnancy rate per cycle and 26.6% pregnancy rate per embryo transfer) [12]. If the HSG, however, reveals abnormalities within the uterine cavity then the prognosis is uncertain. Consideration may be given to IVF-ET, hoping that if conception is achieved it will not end in reproductive loss. A recent study concluded that implantation and pregnancy outcomes are impaired in DES-exposed women after IVF and a worse prognosis was seen in women who on HSG showed uterine constrictions and a combination of T-shape and constrictions [13]. Surgical correction of the uterine abnormality does not seem an option since it may further aggravate the prognosis, given the fact that the healing process in the genital tract of DES-exposed females appears impaired. With regard to embryo transfer following IVF, it should be borne in mind that in patients whose uterine anomaly decreases the intrauterine capacity, the transfer of a lesser number of embryos (e.g., two) than would have otherwise been transferred (e.g., three to four) may reduce the possibilities of pregnancy loss by reducing the frequency of multiple implantations. Of course, such action may in turn lower the pregnancy rate in that cycle.

For abnormalities consistent with a cervical factor, intrauterine inseminations (IUI) should be considered. If conception were not to occur within a reasonable period of time, then IVF can be offered. Gamete intrafallopian transfer (GIFT) is not advised because of the risk of ectopic pregnancy. If ovulation is not confirmed by biphasic basal body temperature charts and/or urinary LH surge predictors, then ovulation induction can be undertaken with the use of clomiphene citrate (CC) or human menopausal gonadotropins (hMG). If a male factor is present, as confirmed by a poor semen analysis, then consideration can be given to the performance of a hamster egg sperm penetration assay (SPA) in order to assess the functional capacity of the sperm. There have been reports linking a decrease in the infertility potential in male patients who themselves were exposed to DES. Anatomic abnormalities such as

epididymal cysts, hypoplastic testes and microphallus were reported to occur more frequently in DES-exposed than in nonexposed males. Mean sperm counts in exposed males have also been found to be significantly lower than in nonexposed random controls [10]. For abnormalities encountered in a male partner the treatment may also include IUI with hMG. When conception is not achieved within a reasonable period of time after such attempts, IVF-ET can be offered.

The group of patients that have suffered reproductive loss can be further subdivided into those who have had a first-trimester loss and those who had a second- or third-trimester loss. For those patients who had a first-trimester loss, in addition to an HSG, luteal-phase dysfunction (LPD) should be ruled out by means of a late luteal-phase endometrial biopsy. If present, LPD can be treated with CC, hMG, vaginal progesterone suppositories or injections of human chorionic gonadotropin in the luteal phase. In DES-exposed patients who have suffered reproductive loss in the second and third trimester, the etiology is often separable by presenting history to either preterm labor or cervical incompetence — both of which are more common in DES-exposed patients. If, on one hand, the primary etiology for the loss was preterm labor, then the use of tocolytics and bedrest in subsequent pregnancies can be of help. If, on the other hand, the reason for the previous pregnancy loss was cervical incompetence, then a cervical cerclage is indicated early in the second trimester. In the largest study to date, DES-exposed patients with a hypoplastic cervix or who had a previous reproductive loss had a better outcome with early cerclage than even those DES-exposed patients with a normal cervix that were followed expectantly [14]. Given these findings, there may be reasons to consider prophylactic cerclage placement in all DES-exposed patients who have achieved conception.

As previously noted, patients who have had *in utero* DES exposure are known to be at increased risk for epithelial changes in the lower genital tract. These changes may become evident at the time of evaluating the exposed patient who presents complaining of infertility. In their initial assessment, a four-quadrant cytologic evaluation of the vagina should be obtained every 6 months in addition to a cervical and endocervical smear. If adenosis of the vagina is encountered, it should be managed expectantly as the majority of these changes regress spontaneously.

CHAPTER 15

This healing process of adenosis involves squamous metaplasia. If dysplastic cytologic changes are found in this mitotically active tissue or on the cervix, then colposcopically directed biopsy would be indicated. In situations where cervical or vaginal squamous cell dysplasia is diagnosed, cryotherapy or cone biopsy should be avoided if possible to prevent cervical stenosis. Instead, colposcopically directed point ablation of the lesion with laser is preferred.

REFERENCES

1 Smith OW. Diethylstilbestrol in the prevention and treatment of complications of pregnancy. *Am J Obstet Gynecol* 1948; 56: 821.
2 Smith OW, Smith G. The influence of diethylstilbestrol on the progress and outcome of pregnancy based on a comparison of treated with untreated primigravidas. *Am J Obstet Gynecol* 1949; 58: 994.
3 Ferguson JH. Effect of stilbestrol on pregnancy compared to the effect of a placebo. *Am J Obstet Gynecol* 1953; 65: 592.
4 *Federal Register*, Vol. 36, No. 217. November 10, 1971, Washington DC.
5 Brackbold Y, Berendes HW. Dangers of diethylstilbestrol: review of a 1953 paper. *Lancet* 1978; 2: 520.
6 Cunha GR, Fujii H. Stromal parenchymal interactions in normal and abnormal development of the genital tract. In: Herbst AL, Bern HA, eds. *Developmental Effects of Diethylstilbesterol (DES) in Pregnancy*. New York: Thieme-Stratton, 1981: 179–193.
7 Kaufman RH, Binder GL, Gray PM Jr, Adam E. Upper genital tract changes associated with exposure *in utero* to diethylstilbestrol. *Am J Obstet Gynecol* 1977; 128: 51.
8 Kaufman RH, Adam E, Binder GL, Gerthoffer. Upper genital tract changes and pregnancy outcome in offspring exposed *in utero* to diethylstilbestrol. *Am J Obstet Gynecol* 1980; 137: 299.
9 Edelman DA. *Diethylstilbestrol — New Perspectives*. MTP Press, 1986: 77–78.
10 Stillman RJ, Hershlag A. Pathology of infertility and adverse pregnancy outcome after in utero exposure to diethylstilbestrol. In: Gondos B, Riddick DH, eds. *Pathology of Infertility*. New York: Thieme Medical, 1987: 41–55.
11 Hricak H, Change YCF, Cann CE *et al*. Cervical incompetence: preliminary evaluation with MR imaging. *Radiology* 1990; 174: 821–826.
12 Jones HW Jr, Jones GS, Hodgen GD (eds). *In-Vitro Fertilization — Norfolk*. Baltimore: Williams & Wilkins, 1986: 5.
13 Karande VC, Lester RG, Muasher SJ. Are implantation and pregnancy outcome impaired in diethylstilbestrol-exposed women after *in-vitro* fertilization and embryo transfer? *Fertil Steril* 1990; 54: 287.
14 Ludmir J, Landon MB, Gabbe SG *et al*. Management of the diethylstilbestrol-exposed pregnant patient: a prospective study. *Am J Obstet Gynecol* 1987; 157: 665–669.

16

Congenital absence of the vagina

THEODORE A. BARAMKI

INTRODUCTION

Congenital absence of the vagina is usually associated with congenital absence of the uterus as well. A more appropriate term would be aplasia or dysplasia of the Müllerian ducts.

The first description of this entity is attributed to Mayer in 1829. Rokitansky [1] elaborated on this condition in the *Yearbook of Medicine of the Austrian States* in 1838. Later on Küster [2] wrote an article about this entity in 1910 with a title of "Uterus bipartitus solidus rudimentarius cum vagina solida." Hauser and Schreiner [3], who reported 21 personal cases of this entity, coined the term Mayer−Rokitansky−Küster syndrome. With Hauser's prolific writing about this syndrome pointing out the high incidence of associated extragenital anomalies, this syndrome is now most commonly referred to as the Rokitansky−Küster−Hauser syndrome.

EMBRYOLOGY

The upper vagina is of Müllerian origin and arises from the caudal end of the fused and later canalized Müllerian ducts. The lower vagina arises from the urogenital sinus. If the wall between the two structures does not break down, a transverse vaginal septum is formed. The short vaginal pouch seen in some patients with the Rokitansky−Küster−Hauser syndrome is derived from the urogenital sinus, whereas the Müllerian vagina and body of the uterus are absent.

DIAGNOSIS

The usual presenting symptom is primary amenorrhea, although some patients may present with dyspareunia. The patient is a phenotypic female, normally tall, with normal secondary sex characteristics. Breast development is normal and the

pubic and axillary hair are of normal amount and distribution. Ovarian function is quite normal. The external genitalia are normal female in type. The vagina is completely absent in the majority of cases (Fig. 16.1). About 25% of patients have a short vaginal pouch, up to 4 cm in depth. The urethra opens at the proper site. Rectal examination fails to show a uterus, although small masses of rudimentary bicornuate uterus may be palpable. In obese patients,

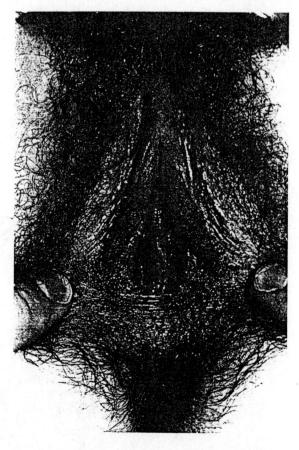

Fig. 16.1 External genitalia of a female with congenital absence of the vagina. The vagina is completely absent.

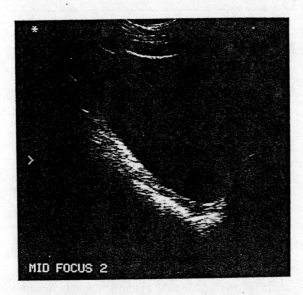

Fig. 16.2 Midline longitudinal ultrasound study showing a full bladder with no upper vagina or uterus in a female with Rokitansky's syndrome.

ultrasonography is usually helpful to demonstrate the absence of the uterus (Fig. 16.2). The chromosome analysis shows a normal female karyotype (46,XX).

As a rule, one does not have to resort to a diagnostic laparoscopy or an exploratory laparotomy to make the diagnosis. In those patients who have been explored for other reasons, the internal genitalia usually show two normal ovaries, normal or hypoplastic tubes, and two solid fibromuscular masses at the proximal ends of the tubes, suggesting a very immature bicornuate uterus (Fig. 16.3). Histologically, the masses show typical myometrium with nonfunctional basal layer of the endometrium in the substance. In rare instances one uterine horn may contain functional endometrium and the patient presents with primary amenorrhea, cyclic pelvic pain and a mass detected by rectal examination or ultrasonography. Under these circumstances, the blind uterine horn with hematometra should be excised.

Associated extragenital abnormalities include those of the urinary and skeletal systems. The renal anomalies may be in the form of congenital absence of one kidney, pelvic kidney, or crossed ectopia. Anomalies of the bones, especially the spinal column, are not uncommon. These are usually in the form of congenital fusion or absence of a vertebra.

A very unusual entity was described by Park *et al.* in 1971 [4], with two patients presenting with congenital absence of the vagina and uterus, short stature, severe bony abnormalities involving the spine, and deafness. The deafness was found to be due to bony anomalies of the small bones of the middle ear.

ETIOLOGY

The etiology of the Rokitansky—Küster—Hauser syndrome has not been satisfactorily elucidated.

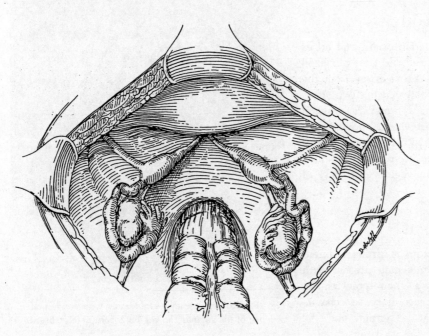

Fig. 16.3 Sketch of the internal genitalia in patients with this syndrome. The rudimentary uterine horns consist of muscle bundles and basal endometrial tissue. The tubes and ovaries are normal. (Courtesy of Dr Howard W. Jones, Jr.)

As a rule, the karyotype is 46,XX. Familial cases have been reported on occasion.

The anatomic findings suggest that the extension of the Müllerian ducts in a caudal direction during embryonic life is arrested at about 7 weeks following conception.

DIFFERENTIAL DIAGNOSIS

Imperforate hymen

After puberty, the patient with an imperforate hymen presents with a similar picture as that of congenital absence of the vagina except that she complains of cyclic pelvic pain and has a pelvic mass detected by rectal examination as well as by ultrasonography. A bulging hymen due to the hematocolpos gives the diagnosis away.

Prior to puberty, it is difficult to differentiate between patients who have imperforate hymen and those who have congenital absence of the vagina. One should resist the temptation to operate until after puberty when the diagnosis is made more easily. Rarely an imperforate hymen before puberty may present with a bulge due to accumulation of mucus in the vagina (mucocolpos). A cruciate incision of the hymen should be done.

Transverse vaginal septum

The patient with a transverse vaginal septum usually presents with cyclic pelvic pain, and a pelvic mass that is appreciated by rectal examination. Usually this septum is thick and it does not show any bulge (Fig. 16.4). Ultrasonography will demonstrate a hematocolpos and possible hematometra and hematosalpinx. Excision of the septum should be done as soon as feasible.

Testicular feminization

In this entity the patient presents as a phenotypic female complaining of primary amenorrhea, with very good breast development, scanty pubic and axillary hair, and absent or shallow vagina. The karyotype is 46,XY and the gonads are testes which may be located in the labioscrotal folds, inguinal canals or intraabdominally. Androgen and estrogen blood levels are normal for a normal male. Follicle-stimulating hormone is within normal limits, whereas lutenizing hormone is usually elevated. The latter is due to deficient androgen receptors in the pituitary and hypothalmus.

It is advisable to remove the testes as soon after

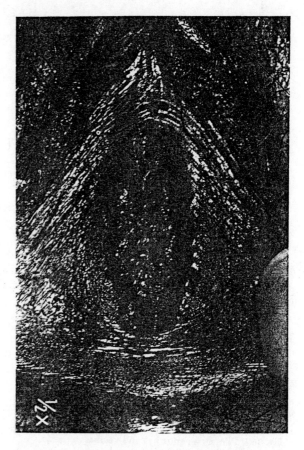

Fig. 16.4 External genitalia of a female with a low transverse vaginal septum. A large hematocolpos is producing a slight bulge.

puberty as the diagnosis is made for fear of malignant change. Estrogen replacement and a functional vagina should be addressed.

TREATMENT

Treatment of the Rokitansky–Küster–Hauser syndrome is usually centered around having a functional vagina. Vaginal dilatation (Frank's method) has been successful in patients who are highly motivated. Different types of dilators have been used. We prefer the lucite dilators of different widths which the patient can use with xylocaine 2% ointment as a lubricant and local anesthetic. The patient applies pressure for about 10 min twice daily. When sufficient depth is achieved, wider forms are used and the patient will eventually be able to have intercourse, which in itself can help complete the work that the lucite dilators started.

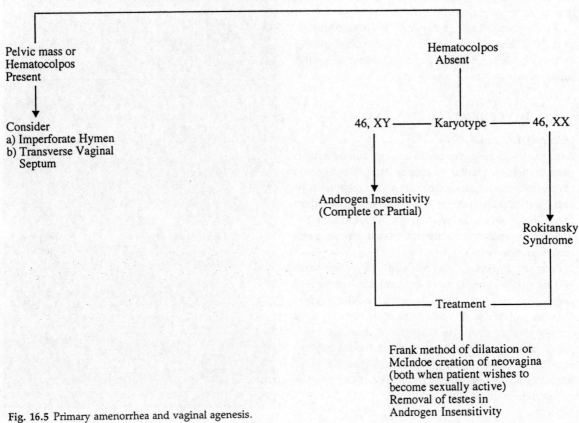

Pelvic mass or
Hematocolpos
Present

Consider
a) Imperforate Hymen
b) Transverse Vaginal
Septum

Hematocolpos
Absent

46, XY —— Karyotype —— 46, XX

Androgen Insensitivity
(Complete or Partial)

Rokitansky
Syndrome

Treatment

Frank method of dilatation or
McIndoe creation of neovagina
(both when patient wishes to
become sexually active)
Removal of testes in
Androgen Insensitivity

Fig. 16.5 Primary amenorrhea and vaginal agenesis.

Patients who are not motivated to use dilators or who have used them without success will benefit from creation of a neovagina. Our operation of choice utilizes a split-thickness skin graft (McIndoe procedure [5]) lining a newly created vagina between the bladder and rectum.

It should be stressed that vaginoplasty should not be done until the patient is desirous of becoming sexually active and responsible enough to be able to use the vaginal forms on a regular basis for several months after the surgery. Without the proper motivation and compliance, the vagina may contract due to scarring, making subsequent surgery more difficult.

REFERENCES

1 Rokitansky C. Ueber sogenannte Verdoppelung des Uterus. *Med Jb Osterreich Staates* 1838; 26: 39.
2 Küster H. Uterus bipartitus solidus rudimentarius cum vagina solida. *Z Geburtshille Gynaekol* 1910; 67: 692.
3 Hauser GA, Schreiner WE. Das Mayer—Rokitansky—Küster-Syndrom. *Schweiz Med Wochenschr* 1961; 12: 381.
4 Park IJ, Jones HW Jr, Nager GT, Chen SCA, Hussels IE. A new syndrome in two unrelated females: Klippel—Feil deformity, conductive deafness and absent vagina. In: *Birth Defects: Original Articles VIII*. New York: Alan I. Liss, 1971: 311.
5 McIndoe A. Treatment of congenital absence and obliteration conditions of the vagina. *Br J Plast Surg* 1950; 2: 254.

17

Uterovaginal anomalies

DENISE L. MURRAY & JOHN A. ROCK

The overall incidence of congenital defects of the reproductive tract is unknown. If asymptomatic at puberty, these defects may go undiscovered, presenting incidentally at the time of delivery or pelvic surgery. Most authorities estimate that from 0.1 to 0.5% of deliveries are complicated by an incidental finding of a congenital defect of the reproductive tract, with vaginal anomalies making up 10% of these.

EMBRYOLOGY

To appreciate fully the anatomy encountered in patients with vaginal anomalies, a basic understanding of the embryogenesis of the vagina is required. The uterus, fallopian tubes, and upper one-third of the vagina derives from the Müllerian ducts. The Müllerian system develops in close association with the urinary system.

The Müllerian ducts first appear as paired invaginations of the dorsal coelomic epithelium lateral to each Wolffian duct. The site of origin of the invaginations remains open and ultimately becomes the fimbriated end of the fallopian tube. At this site of origin, the Müllerian ducts each form a solid bud which later elongates and develops a lumen. The Müllerian ducts grow in a medial and caudal direction, eventually crossing the ventral aspect of the Wolffian duct. The paired Müllerian ducts then meet in the midline and become fused as part of the urogenital septum. The most cranial point of fusion is the site of the future uterine fundus. Normally, the septum separating the paired ducts disappears, leaving a single uterovaginal canal. The site of contact between the upper vagina, formed from the Müllerian-derived uterovaginal canal, and the lower vagina, developed from the urogenital sinus, is the Müllerian tubercle.

From here, a solid vaginal cord elongates caudally to meet and fuse with the bilateral endodermal

evaginations (sinovaginal bulbs) from the urogenital sinus. The point at which the upgrowths from the sinovaginal bulbs unite with the mesodermal tissue from the Müllerian tubercle is known as the vaginal plate. Canalization of these solid tissue columns results in the formation of the vagina.

Structural anomalies in the development of the vagina are clearly understood when one considers possible alterations in normal vaginal embryogenesis.

CLASSIFICATION OF UTEROVAGINAL ANOMALIES

Uterovaginal anomalies can be thought of as resulting from either disorders of vertical fusion of the sinovaginal bulbs and Müllerian tissue, or disorders of lateral fusion of the paired Müllerian ducts. Likewise, these disorders can be thought of as either obstructed or nonobstructed. This is the basis for the classification system for uterovaginal anomalies modified from the American Fertility Society Classification proposed by Rock in 1990 [1] (Table 17.1). Discussion of these anomalies will be limited to the scope of this chapter.

Table 17.1 Classification of uterovaginal anomalies. (Modified from [2])

Class	Description
Class I	Dysgenesis of the Müllerian ducts
Class II	Disorders of vertical fusion of the Müllerian ducts Transverse vaginal septum Obstructed Unobstructed Cervical agenesis or dysgenesis
Class III	Disorders of lateral fusion of the Müllerian ducts

cont.

Table 17.1 *Continued*

Class	Description

Class III	Asymmetric-obstructed disorder of uterus or vagina usually associated with ipsilateral renal agenesis
	  Unicornuate uterus with a noncommunicating rudimentary anlagen or horn
	  Unilateral obstruction of a cavity of a double uterus
	  Unilateral vaginal obstruction associated with double uterus
	Symmetric-unobstructed
	  Didelphic uterus
	    Complete longitudinal septum
	    Partial longitudinal septum
	    No longitudinal septum
	  Septate uterus
	    Complete
	      Complete longitudinal septum
	      Partial longitudinal septum
	      No longitudinal septum
	    Partial
	      Complete longitudinal septum
	      Partial longitudinal septum
	      No longitudinal septum
	  Bicornuate uterus
	    Complete
	      Complete longitudinal septum
	      Partial longitudinal septum
	      No longitudinal septum
	    Partial
	      Complete longitudinal septum
	      Partial longitudinal septum
	      No longitudinal septum
	  T-shaped uterine cavity
	  (DES drug related)
	  Unicornuate uterus
	    With a rudimentary horn
	      With endometrial cavity
	        Communicating
	        Noncommunicating
	      Without endometrial cavity
	    Without rudimentary horn

Class IV	Unusual configurations, vertical/lateral fusion defects

DES, diethylstilbestrol.

OBSTRUCTED DISORDERS OF VERTICAL FUSION

Transverse vaginal septum

The location of a transverse vaginal septum and thus the site of obstruction may occur at any point along the vaginal canal, but most frequently is found at the junction between the middle and upper thirds of the vagina. Rock and associates reported septa in the upper, middle, and lower thirds of the vagina in 46, 35, and 19% of cases, respectively [3]. A transverse vaginal septum can result from failure of union of the urogenital sinus with the Müllerian duct or from lack of canalization of the vaginal plate. A high vaginal septum is most likely to occur at the junction of the upper one-fourth and the lower three-fourths of the vagina. These tend to be substantially thicker than the septa found in the middle or lower vagina.

A transverse vaginal septum is occasionally diagnosed in infancy when a hydromucocolpos develops and results in an abdominal mass. Severe urinary tract obstruction may be associated with a large mucocolpos. More commonly, symptoms from a transverse vaginal septum begin with puberty and the onset of menses as blood and mucus accumulate and distend the vagina above the occlusion. Cyclic symptoms of pain and pressure in an adolescent girl who has not yet had menstrual blood flow is the common presentation. A delay in diagnosis of 2–3 years is not unusual and may be more frequently encountered in patients with a high transverse vaginal septum which tends to be thicker and therefore less distensible. Early diagnosis and correction are desirable in order to avoid retrograde blood flow through the uterus and fallopian tubes with subsequent development of endometriosis. Rock *et al.* [3] observed endometriosis in six of seven patients with transverse vaginal septa who underwent exploratory laparotomy. Five of these patients were noted to have a high transverse vaginal septum.

Treatment

In order to protect reproductive potential, immediate diagnosis and treatment of complete vaginal obstruction are essential. Treatment consists of excising the obstructing septum and anastomosing the upper and lower vaginal segments.

A high vaginal septum results in a smaller vaginal pouch. A long segment of atretic vagina is noted after the neovaginal space is developed. Here, the upper vagina may be located by needle aspiration of accumulated menstrual blood. However, if the distinction between the vagina and the bladder anteriorly or the rectum posteriorly is unclear, an exploratory laparotomy should be performed and a sound passed from above to identify the area for incision. The length of the obstructing septum is often difficult to assess preoperatively by physical examination and, at times, is such that anastomosis of the vaginal segments is not possible. Placement of a lucite form with an upper bulbous end and a channel for menstrual efflux is then necessary. The form should remain in place for 4–6 months to allow sufficient epithelialization with subsequent daily vaginal dilatation for another 2–4 months to prevent contracture. A graft may also be placed primarily. Alternatively, the hematocolpos may be drained sonographically, then the lower vaginal pouch dilated using the Ingram passive dilation technique [4]. Once the vaginal pouch has been dilated to sufficient length, the septum can then be resected and the vagina reanastomosed.

It should be noted that subsequent pregnancy rates have been greater in the group of patients with a vaginal septum in the lower one-third of the vagina. This may be explained by a greater vaginal capacity above the septum and thus a longer time period until development of endometriosis.

Finally, imperforate hymen will be mentioned here despite its non-Müllerian origin because of its possible confusion with the transverse vaginal septum. Because it is significantly thinner than the transverse vaginal septum, an imperforate hymen will tend to bulge out of the vagina when blood begins to accumulate behind it.

Congenital absence of the cervix
A rare Müllerian anomaly, congenital absence of the cervix is often associated with absence of all or a portion of the vagina. Because of the presence of a functioning uterine corpus, initiation of menstruation results in symptoms of cyclic lower abdominal pain without menstrual flow. Differentiation of patients with absence of the cervix from those with a normal cervix and a high transverse vaginal septum can be difficult. Magnetic resonance imaging can be helpful in the differential diagnosis. Patients with cervical dysgenesis will not have vaginal dilation from accumulation of blood above the obstruction, as is seen in the patient with a high transverse vaginal septum.

Treatment
Attempts at establishing a satisfactory outflow tract through which menstrual blood may escape have rarely been successful. Pelvic endometriosis from retrograde menstruation may develop and cause severe pain. Recurrent pelvic infections are common, at times necessitating hysterectomy and bilateral salpingo-oophorectomy. Although some controversy exists, most agree that hysterectomy with preservation of the ovaries be performed as primary therapy. In this way, severe endometriosis and infection can be avoided and ovarian function can be preserved. Reproduction with the aid of a host uterus would then remain an option.

UNOBSTRUCTED DISORDERS OF VERTICAL FUSION

Occasionally, a transverse vaginal septum is incomplete and therefore menstrual blood and mucus do not accumulate. This septum may not cause dyspareunia or reproductive compromise. The decision to correct this anomaly should therefore be individualized.

DISORDERS OF LATERAL FUSION

The third and final group in the classification of vaginal anomalies result from defects in lateral fusion of the paired Müllerian ducts. These anomalies may be obstructed or unobstructed. Unilateral obstruction is almost invariably associated with absence of the ipsilateral kidney, therefore an intravenous pyelogram is an essential diagnostic adjunct.

Obstructed uterine horn
In this group of uterine anomalies two uterine horns are present because of failure of fusion of the paired Müllerian ducts in the midline. Obstruction occurs when one uterine horn does not communicate with an outflow tract. An isolated uterine horn with only minimal connection to the unobstructed side may also result in obstructive symptoms. These patients will often present with the signs and symptoms of ectopic pregnancy. If the fallopian tube communicates with the obstructed uterine horn, retrograde menstruation and endometriosis will develop. Early diagnosis and excision of these horns provide symptomatic relief and preserve reproductive potential.

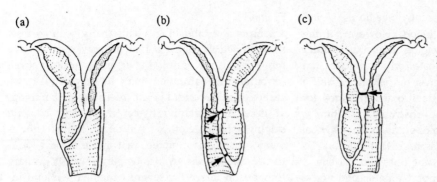

Fig. 17.1 The double uterus, complete or incomplete vaginal obstruction, and ipsilateral renal agenesis. (a) Complete vaginal obstruction. (b) Incomplete vaginal obstruction (c) Complete vaginal obstruction with a laterally communicating double uterus.

Double uterus with obstructed hemivagina and ipsilateral renal agenesis

The rare clinical syndrome of a double vagina, obstruction of the vagina, whether unilateral, partial, or complete, and ipsilateral renal agenesis presents a diagnostic challenge. According to Rock and Jones, patients can be divided into diagnostic groups depending on anatomic variations [5] (Fig. 17.1).

Group I includes patients with complete unilateral vaginal obstruction without uterine communication. Menses are regular but with severe dysmenorrhea. A paravaginal mass is palpable.

Group II patients have incomplete unilateral vaginal obstruction without uterine communication. Symptoms include severe dysmenorrhea and foul mucopurulent discharge. Intermenstrual bleeding may be present.

Group III patients have a complete vaginal obstruction with uterine communication. Menses are regular but with dysmenorrhea, and a paravaginal mass is present.

Because menses are regular in these groups of patients, suspicion of a Müllerian anomaly is low, leading to a delay in diagnosis and development of endometriosis from retrograde menstruation.

The treatment of choice for a unilateral obstructing vaginal septum communicating with a uterine horn is excision with suction and lavage of accumulated blood and mucus. Prophylactic antibiotics should be employed. Abdominal exploration is usually not necessary. Uterine reconstruction is not recommended for patients with lateral communication of uterine horns. After removal of a vaginal septum, the newly opened vagina is lined by adenomatous epithelium that is slowly replaced by metaplasia over several months.

UNOBSTRUCTED DISORDERS OF LATERAL FUSION

Unobstructed failure of lateral fusion is usually asymptomatic. Occasionally dyspareunia may require partial resection of a vaginal septum. Patients in whom a longitudinal vaginal septum is discovered should undergo hysterosalpingography as well as an intravenous pyelogram in order to document associated Müllerian and renal anomalies.

DIFFERENTIAL DIAGNOSIS

The appropriate work-up for patients with a vaginal septum is shown schematically in Figure 17.2. In general, unless discovered incidentally, patients will present with cyclic lower abdominal pain and normal secondary sexual characteristics. The menstrual history will vary. Those patients with a transverse vaginal septum or congenital absence of the cervix will report amenorrhea. Menstrual histories may be regular, however, in patients with cryptomenorrhea secondary to an obstructed hemivagina. Likewise, patients with one obstructed and one unobstructed uterine horn will report regular menses.

A careful physical examination is the initial step in the differential diagnosis of these patients. On speculum examination, visualization of a vaginal pouch would lead to the differential diagnosis of Müllerian dysgenesis versus a complete transverse vaginal septum or congenital absence of the cervix. Further differentiation with magnetic resonance imaging and pelvic ultrasound can be extremely useful. If the vagina is noted to be dilated above the point of obstruction, a diagnosis of a transverse vaginal septum is made. Alternatively, if no vaginal dilation is noted on magnetic resonance imaging (MRI) or ultrasound, a dilated rudimentary uterine

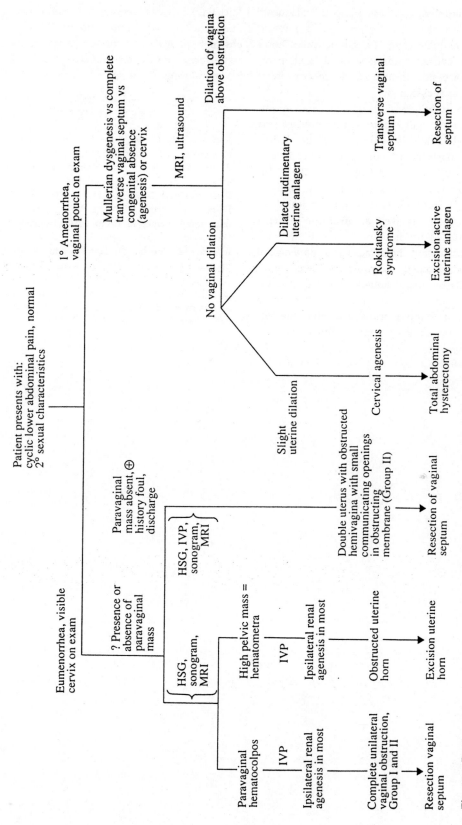

Fig. 17.2 Patient with cyclic lower abdominal pain and normal 2° sexual characteristics.

anlagen may be seen, thus assigning the diagnosis of Mayer–Rokitansky–Küster–Hauser syndrome with an active endometrium. If slight uterine dilation is noted in a patient without vaginal dilation on MRI and ultrasound, the diagnosis of congenital cervical agenesis is assigned.

If the cervix is fully visible on speculum examination, the patient will report regular menses and the differential diagnosis will include the double uterus with an obstructed hemivagina and ipsilateral renal agenesis versus an obstructed uterine horn. Bimanual examination will reveal a pelvic mass in group I and III patients with complete unilateral vaginal obstruction, as well as in those patients with an obstructed uterine horn. In patients with a group II obstructed hemivagina, a paravaginal mass may be palpated intermittently because of occasional collapse and drainage of the obstructed horn through vaginal fenestrations. In all of these patients hysterosalpingography will give the appearance of a unicornuate uterus. Ultrasound and MRI will, however, reveal the true anatomy of the double uterus with either uterine horn or vaginal obstruction. An intravenous pyelogram should also be performed in these patients in order to document ipsilateral renal agenesis.

REFERENCES

1 Rock JA. *Müllerian Anomalies in TeLinde's Operative Laparoscopy.* Lippincott, 1991 (in press).
2 American Fertility Society. Classification of Müllerian anomalies. *Fertil Steril* 1988; 49: 944.
3 Rock JA, Zacur HA, Dlugi AM, Jones HW Jr, TeLinde RW. Pregnancy success following the surgical correction of imperforate hymen as compared to the complete transverse vaginal septum. *Gynecology* 1982; 59: 448–451.
4 Ingram JM. The bicycle seat stool in the treatment of vaginal agenesis and stenosis: a preliminary report. *Am J Obstet Gynecol* 1981; 140: 867.
5 Rock JA, Jones HW Jr. The double uterus associated with an obstructed hemivagina and ipsilateral renal agenesis. *Am J Obstet Gynecol* 1980; 138: 339–342.

18

Double uterus

DOUGLAS C. DALY

The embryology of the group of congenital disorders encompassing the double uterus is actually very straightforward. The normal uterus can be viewed as having three critical steps in development: (1) the formation of the two Müllerian ducts; (2) the midline fusion of the two Müllerian ducts; and (3) absorption of the medial walls of each of the Müllerian ducts at their points of fusion. Failure of development at any one of these steps presents as a congenital abnormality. Failure of development results in uterine agenesis (Rokatansky syndrome) if bilateral or unicornuate (or unicornuate with rudimentary horn) if unilateral. These conditions are commonly associated with renal development abnormalities but are not double uterus situations. Failure of fusion results in the didelphus uterus or bicornuate uterus, characterized by external division in addition to internal division. Classically, this is associated with premature delivery and malpresentation. Failure of medial absorption leads to the complete or incomplete septum with normal external configuration. While embryologically less severe, clinically it tends to be the most important, predisposing to spontaneous abortion (Fig. 18.1).

The recognition of the double uterus as a potential pathological condition predates modern surgical technique [1]. However, the conceptual treatment has not changed. Internal division without external division leads to early loss and is relieved by correcting the internal division. External division may lead to premature loss but often requires no surgical therapy. During the proceedings of the Philadelphia Obstetrical Society in 1906 Hirsch described an effective, though by modern criteria crude, correction of the uterine septum. The cervix was dilated to admit a finger on either side of the septum. The fingers guided the incision of the septum with curved scissors. Three decades later Luikart [1] replaced the surgeon's fingers with a pair of curved stomach clamps which were left in place for 24 hours after the

septum was incised. Luikart's report also illustrated that correction of external division is not necessarily indicated. In one case a septum was incised in the cervix and lower uterus. The external division of the upper fundus (bicornuate) was left intact.

These original transvaginal approaches were replaced by the abdominal metroplasties of Jones and Tompkins in what might be called the laparotomy era of metroplasty, ushered in by improved anesthesia and antibiotics in the 1940s and closed by the advent of operative laparoscopy and hysteroscopy in the 1980s. The visualization of the septum achieved by laparotomy and hysterotomy was replaced by laparoscopic confirmation of external unity and hysteroscopic visualization of the septum for the purpose of transvaginal–transcervical incision. As technology advances the need for laparoscopic confirmation is already being replaced as transvaginal ultrasound becomes more precise in documenting anatomy. This precision is allowing the incision to be done by ultrasound guidance as well [2].

Since the principles of treatment remain unchanged, the clinician should concentrate on making the correct diagnosis. This process starts with suspicion (Fig. 18.2). The classic history of suspicion is recurrent miscarriages. The traditional definition is three consecutive spontaneous losses. In part this has been based on the relative probability of finding an abnormality of any type and in part on the consensus teaching that a uterine septum should be treated with abdominal metroplasty only after three losses has occurred. Hysteroscopic metroplasty has changed this approach [3]. Now a septum should be sought in any patient with two consecutive losses since the incidence is reasonably common and the treatment by hysteroscopy relatively benign. Further, any patient miscarrying an apparently normal pregnancy after 8 weeks should be evaluated for a uterine septum. Initially, this can be done at ultrasound during the pregnancy. The uterus will be asymmetrically

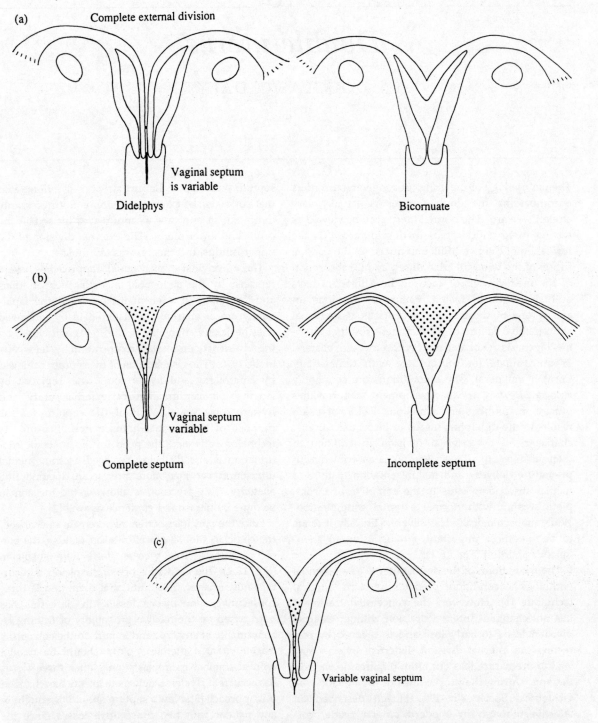

Fig. 18.1 (a) Failure of fusion: complete failure of fusion (didelphys) and incomplete failure of fusion bicornuate are not amenable to hysteroscopic correction. However, in most clinical situations correction is not necessary for successful pregnancy. (b) Failure of absorption: results when fusion is complete but midline absorption fails. The usually fibrous septum which may extend through the cervix and into the vagina can be either incised or excised with equal results (dotted area). (c) Mixed lesions occur when fusion has been incomplete and a failure of absorption has occurred as well. These are actually more common than true bicornuate uteri in the author's experience. Like a septum, these can usually be adequately treated by incision of the septal component alone (dotted area).

DOUBLE UTERUS

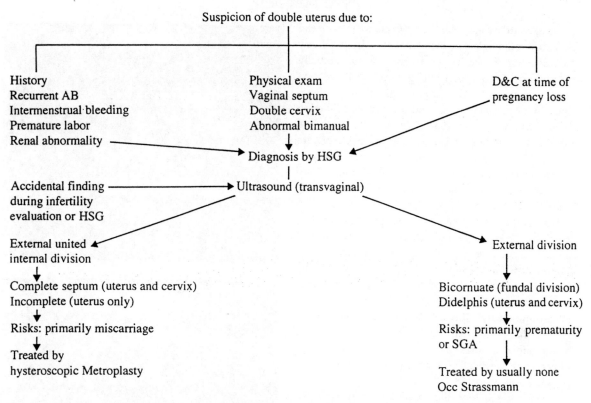

Fig. 18.2 Algorithm of diagnosis and treatment of the double uterus.

enlarged with the pregnancy in one cavity and the second cavity illuminated by the hyperechogenic endometrium. Finally, if the patient requires dilatation and curettage for retained products, careful attention should always be paid to the internal uterine contour, even at the first loss.

The other pregnancy-related event that should always trigger concern is a pregnancy loss or premature labor after 16 weeks, particularly if associated with an abnormal fetal position. While classically associated with a bicornuate uterus, a combined bicornuate–septum or septum only may present in this manner. A renal abnormality, particularly unilateral renal agensis or horseshoe kidney should trigger a concern regarding uterine structure, though these abnormalities are more commonly associated with absence of uterine development patterns. Occasionally, a patient who has not attempted pregnancy will have a uterine septum discovered during evaluation of abnormal menstrual bleeding. More commonly, a uterine anomaly will be discovered on hysterosalpingogram (HSG) performed as part of an infertility evaluation.

During the physical examination the stimuli to suspicion are quite apparent: (1) a vaginal septum; (2) a septate or double cervix; or (3) an abnormal bimanual examination. Of these the septate vagina may be the most deceptive. The vagina may only be dilated on one side and the bimanual examination does not match the speculum appearance. The non-dilated vagina can usually be found by using a sound to probe the lateral walls of the dilated vagina starting at the hymeneal ring. Almost by magic the sound will disappear behind the otherwise invisible vaginal septum into the other cavity.

Once suspicion has been aroused diagnosis is required. The standard test is the HSG. This should be done in the midfollicular phase. Careful attention should be paid to the position of the uterus. Many abnormalities have been missed by not having the uterus perpendicular to the X-ray beam or by using a cannula that occupies the uterine cavity. A single-tooth tenaculum with a Kahn's or equivalent cannula sealing the external os is ideal. Small volumes of a nonionic euosmotic dye (Conray 60-Omnipague 360), pushed slowly with a 10 ml syringe, will maximize visualization while decreasing discomfort.

Unfortunately, the traditional HSG only identifies

internal anatomy anomalies and tends to be overread by many radiologists as bicornuate [2]. In one study 55% of HSG reports were incorrect or substantially misleading. Even when the gynecologist's assessment was taken into account, 37.5% of patients referred for or seeking a second opinion for Müllerian defect has an incorrect diagnosis. Most commonly a uterine septum was misdiagnosed as a bicornuate uterus. The patients were either told no treatment was indicated at that time or abdominal metroplasty had been planned. Either of these would be inappropriate for the correct diagnosis.

The solution to this misdiagnosis problem on HSG is pelvic or transvaginal ultrasound [3]. Performed in the midluteal phase, both the external and internal anatomy can be clearly visualized (Fig. 18.3), allowing for very accurate diagnosis. With the combined approach of follicular-phase HSG and luteal-phase ultrasound, diagnostic accuracy can be improved to greater than 90% with only minor variations of the bicornuate–septum pattern being misinterpreted. This approach will allow for the proper surgery being planned and executed.

Having adequately diagnosed the anomaly, treatment should be considered. For the uterine septum hysteroscopic metroplasty is the treatment of choice and indicated for any patient with previous pregnancy loss [3,4]. It should be considered in the infertile patient when a septum is incidentally found in the evaluation, particularly when laparoscopy is to be performed as part of the evaluation/treatment. While resectoscopes, lasers, or diathermy can all be used to perform the incision or resection, these techniques have no discernible advantage over simple mechanical incision with operative scissors. Since the septal tissue is fibrous and avascular, the incised tissue tends to retract away from the cavity with little bleeding. As the incision is extended the identification of normal vasculature and less fibrous tissue is a good physiologic mark that the procedure is complete — a marker that may be missed with the other instruments. Anatomic perfection is not a necessity.

Review of patients treated by hysteroscopic metroplasty has demonstrated as good or better outcome than abdominal metroplasty, with far less morbidity. Patients with only first-trimester losses have the same prognosis in subsequent pregnancies as otherwise normal patients. However, patients with second-trimester loss or premature labor in addition to first-trimester losses remain at risk for premature delivery

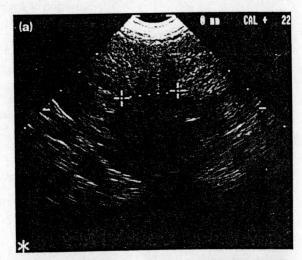

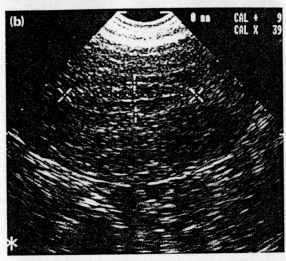

Fig. 18.3 (a) Originally diagnosed as a "bicornuate uterus" on HSG, transvaginal midluteal ultrasound reveals a unified uterus with two distinct cavities. The correct diagnosis of uterine septum was made (+----+ 22 mm septal width). (b) After hysteroscopic incision midcycle, transvaginal ultrasound reveals a normal triecho pattern in the region of the incision consistent with normal endometrial growth. This confirms both anatomic and functional correction in the previous septate region.

and should be followed aggressively in pregnancy. Septal resection had no impact on infertility [3].

At the other extreme in treatment is the true didelphus uterus with complete external division. These patients almost never require surgical intervention. While these patients are at risk for malpresentation, prematurity, and small for gestational age development, these risks are usually outweighed by the risks of scarring, infertility, and the general risks of the laparotomy performed to unify the uterus.

For the bicornuate uterus it is usually worth aggressive management of the subsequent pregnancy before considering laparotomy repair. The natural course of subsequent pregnancies is to extend longer than the initial pregnancy by an average of 4 weeks. Combined with aggressive perinatal intervention many pregnancies will progress to healthy viability before delivering. Because many patients with bicornuate patterns actually have combined bicornuate–septate patterns, careful diagnosis is warranted. If a septal component is identified, particularly in a patient who has had losses prior to 20 weeks, hysteroscopic resection of the septal component is indicated as the initial procedure. Abdominal metroplasty should only be considered if a subsequent apparently normal pregnancy is lost.

In conclusion, the physician should have a high index of suspicion, especially in the patient with pregnancy loss. Careful diagnosis by HSG and ultra-sound is necessary to differentiate the septate uterus from the didelphic/bicornuate uterus. Treatment of septate uterus should be aggressive and performed by hysteroscopic metroplasty. Treatment of bicornuate uterus by abdominal metroplasty should be with reluctance and only after conservative approaches have failed.

REFERENCES

1 Luikart R. Techniques of successful removal of the septum uteri septus and subsequent deliveries at term. *Am J Obstet Gynecol* 1936; 31: 797–803.
2 Reuter K, Daly DC, Cohen SM. Septate versus bicornuate uteri: errors in imaging diagnosis. *Radiology* 1989; 172: 749–752.
3 Daly DC, Maier D, SotoAlbors CE. Hysteroscopic metroplasty: six years experience. *Obstet Gynecol* 1989; 73: 201–205.
4 March CM, Israel R. Hysteroscopic management of recurrent abortion caused by septate uterus. *Am J Obstet Gynecol* 1987; 156: 834–842.

19

Intrauterine synechiae (Asherman's syndrome)

RAFAEL F. VALLE

Intrauterine adhesions following a delayed post-partum or postabortal curettage, resulting in the partial or complete uterine cavity occlusion, are known by the eponym Asherman's syndrome. Despite previous publications describing similar entities, it was Asherman's observations that gave this condition recognition as a pathologic entity. The original description in 1948 included only amenorrhea following curettage for postpartum hemorrhage, incomplete abortion, or missed abortion. Two years later, Asherman added to the description the partial occlusion of the uterine cavity secondary to adhesions. The term Asherman's syndrome, therefore, includes both pathologic entities [1].

This condition may result in infertility, menstrual abnormalities, particularly amenorrhea or hypomenorrhea, pregnancy aberrations such as habitual abortions, missed abortions, premature deliveries, and placental insertion abnormalities, such as placenta previa and placenta accreta (Fig. 19.1).

PATHOPHYSIOLOGY OF INTRAUTERINE ADHESIONS

The main factor associated with the development of intrauterine adhesions is trauma to the endometrium during the postpartum or postabortal period, especially at 1–4 weeks following those events. the puerperal period seems to be a vulnerable phase during which the endometrium is more susceptible to trauma with denudation of the stratum basalis and coaptation of the stratum muscularis from the opposing uterine walls. The role of acute or subacute infection in the formation of adhesions is unclear; nonetheless, it seems that infection alone, except for tuberculous endometritis, seldom will produce this pathologic condition. Pregnancy seems to be a predisposing factor to the development of adhesions in over 90% of the cases. The presenting symptomatology varies, according to the degree of uterine cavity occlusion and the severity of the adhesions. The most common symptoms are infertility (43%) and menstrual abnormalities, such as amenorrhea (37%) and hypomenorrhea (31%) [2].

Sperm migration may be impeded, and interference with the nidation of the blastocyst may occur; distortion of the uterine cavity dimensions may result in habitual abortion. Damage to the stratum basalis of the endometrium may predispose to abnormal growth of the trophoblast, resulting in pathologic placental implantations. Another mechanism of abnormal sequelae of intrauterine adhesions may be the defective vascularization of the remaining endometrium secondary to the damage of the arterial vessels; decreased pelvic vascularization may also contribute to the lack of response to estrogenic stimulus.

DIAGNOSTIC STEPS

The history of trauma by curettage in a postpartum or postabortal state is an important clue in arriving at the diagnosis. The progestin challenge test resulting in failure to withdraw bleeding may also be helpful in those patients who are amenorrheic but maintain a biphasic basal body temperature curve showing no evidence of derangement in the hypothalamic–pituitary–ovarian axis, suggesting an end-target failure. Other techniques of manipulating the intrauterine cavity with probes curettes and/or dilators may indeed occasionally suggest intrauterine adhesions by the difficulty in sounding the uterine cavity through the endocervical canal and/or the gritty sensation on passing a small currette. Nonetheless, these methods are unpredictable and dangerous and should be abandoned.

Hysterosalpingography remains the most accurate screening test in the diagnosis of intrauterine adhesions and, when the findings are abnormal or suspicious, hysteroscopy provides a definite diagnosis.

INTRAUTERINE SYNECHIAE

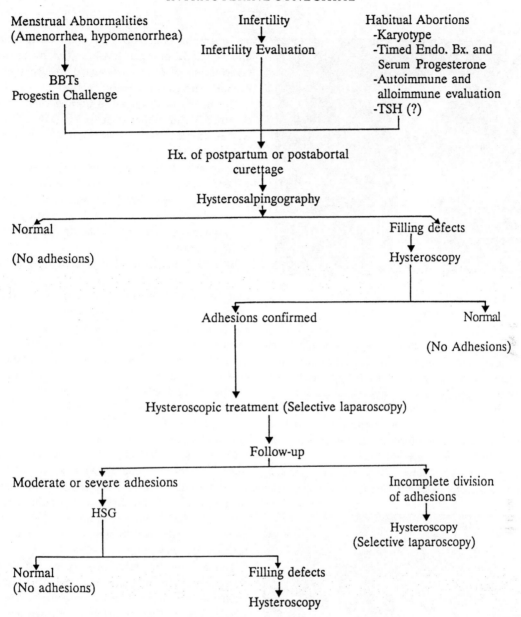

Fig. 19.1 Evaluation and treatment of intrauterine adhesions.

Routine hysterosalpingography will demonstrate intrauterine adhesions in about 1.5% of infertile patients. While hysterosalpingography will show intrauterine adhesions in about 5% of patients with a history of habitual abortions, hysterosalpingograms have shown intrauterine adhesions in about 39% of patients with a history of previous postpartum or postabortal endometrial trauma, particularly by curettage [2] (Figs 19.2 and 19.3).

TREATMENT OF INTRAUTERINE ADHESIONS

The treatment of intrauterine adhesions is surgical, by mechanical division of these adhesions. This approach is best performed by direct visualization with a hysteroscope in order selectively to divide the adhesions and reestablish the uterine cavity symmetry. Additionally, other adjunctive measures

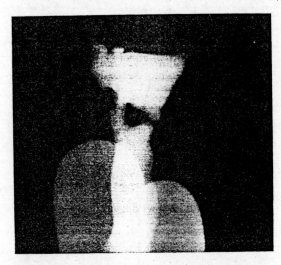

Fig. 19.2 Hysterosalpingogram showing filling defects compatible with adhesions.

are beneficial, particularly when extensive adhesions are encountered. These agents include conjugated estrogens with additional terminal progesterone, intrauterine splints, and prophylactic antibiotics.

Hysteroscopy is performed in the early proliferative phase of the menstrual cycle in those patients who are menstruating. The procedure is performed while the patient is under general anesthesia, except in those patients with filmy adhesions only partially occluding the uterine cavity. The hysteroscopes used

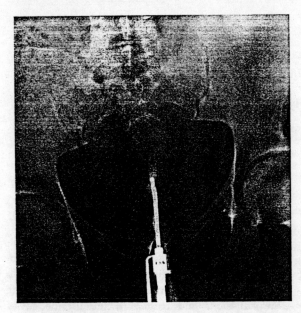

Fig. 19.3 Hysterogram shows a complete uterine cavity occlusion.

are operating endoscopes of 7 mm outer diameter and semirigid or rigid scissors. The hysteroscope-resectoscope also has been used to lyse these adhesions with electrosurgery.

The media to distend the uterine cavity are: (1) dextrose 5% in saline or in water; (2) dextran 32% w/v in dextrose 10% (Hyskon); and (3) carbon dioxide gas insufflation.

Concomitant laparoscopy is performed in those patients with extensive intrauterine adhesions on hysterosalpingography. Laparoscopy is added routinely when tubal blockage is diagnosed by hysterosalpingography, regardless of the degree and severity of intrauterine adhesions.

Visualization of the uterine cavity begins at the internal cervical os and, should adhesions extend to that area, the operation of dividing the adhesions usually begins here by systematic cutting of the adhesions and, therefore, preforming a cavity before the endoscope is advanced. As the adhesions are divided, the endoscope is advanced simultaneously. The uterine cavity is sculpted systematically until symmetry is achieved. When adhesions are focal and partially divide the uterine cavity, their division is simple and the removal of the adhesion is not attempted. Because the adhesions are divided in the middle, the remaining stumps retract and the uterine cavity distends, allowing for a better view. Both uterotubal junctions are observed and the tubal openings are examined. Once the adhesions have been divided, chromopertubation with indigo carmine is performed to assess tubal patency under laparoscopic view (Figs 19.4–19.6).

The most difficult adhesions to treat and divide are those which are marginal, particularly if they are extensive and fibromuscular or composed of connective tissue. The utmost care and gentleness are required to avoid uterine perforation. Simultaneous laparoscopic monitoring allows the laparoscopist to observe from the abdominal site the transillumination of the hysteroscopic light and alert the hysteroscopist to signs of perforation.

Following the surgical division of adhesions by hysteroscopy, other adjuvant treatments include the insertion of an intrauterine device (if available) in patients with extensive intrauterine adhesions and thick fibromuscular or connective tissue adhesions, even though the adhesions may occlude the uterine cavity only partially. If an intrauterine device is not available, a small number 8 Fr indwelling catheter inflated with 3–3.5 ml of saline solution is used; this

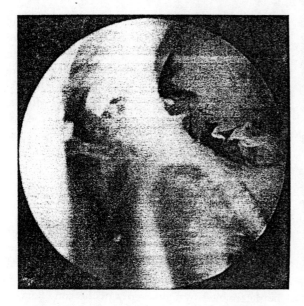

Fig. 19.4 Hysteroscopic view demonstrating an adhesion at the right uterotubal cone.

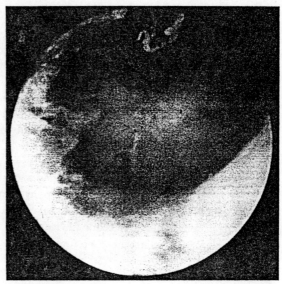

Fig. 19.6 The uterine cavity's symmetry is reestablished.

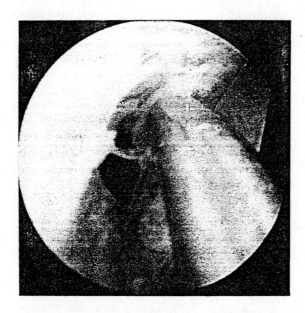

Fig. 19.5 The adhesion is divided under hysteroscopic control.

The follow-up of these patients depends on the extent and type of adhesions treated. Patients with moderate to severe adhesions may undergo a hysterosalpingography at the completion of hormonal treatment, to assess the uterine cavity symmetry. In those patients in whom adhesions were not totally divided on the first attempt, a second hysteroscopy is usually performed after the completion of the adjunctive treatment, and the remaining adhesions are divided.

CLASSIFICATION OF INTRAUTERINE ADHESIONS

To evaluate the results obtained with various treatment modalities, a uniform and standardized method of classification of this condition is important. There is a wide spectrum of adhesion formation, particularly related to uterine cavity occlusion, extension, and type of adhesions present.

It is important to observe the extent and severity of uterine cavity occlusion based on the degree of intrauterine involvement, as shown by hysterosalpingography, and the extent and type of adhesions found on hysteroscopy. Based on these factors, three stages of intrauterine adhesions are defined: mild, moderate, and severe.

Mild adhesions — filament adhesions composed of endometrial tissue producing partial or complete

is left in place for a week; the intrauterine device is left in place for 1 or 2 months, and then removed. Prophylactic antibiotics are prescribed by most physicians, and cyclic (two or three cycles) oral conjugated estrogens (Premarin) 2.5 mg b.i.d. × 30 days with terminal medroxyprogesterone acetate (Provera) 10 mg q.d. × last 10 days of the cycle are also prescribed.

uterine cavity occlusion.

Moderate adhesions — fibromuscular adhesions, characteristically thick, still covered with endometrium that bleeds upon division, and partially or totally occlude the uterine cavity.

Severe adhesions — composed of connective tissue only; lacking any endometrial lining and not likely to bleed upon division; adhesions may partially or totally occlude the uterine cavity [3].

The American Fertility Society has proposed a classification of intrauterine adhesions that is comprehensive, and includes the findings on hysterosalpingograhy and hysteroscopy; the severity of adhesions is determined by a scoring system [4].

The goals of the treatment, therefore, are: (1) to treat infertility; (2) to reestablish normal menstruation; and (3) to treat dysmenorrhea. The success in establishing normal menstruation in these patients has varied, but in collective series, a success rate of 73–92% has been achieved. The treatment of intrauterine adhesions by dilatation and curettage or blind dissection has been disappointing, with a 51% pregnancy rate after treatment, and a 55% term pregnancy rate. The type of adhesions treated, however, has not been determined by direct visualization; therefore, many of these adhesions may have been filmy adhesions or fibromuscular adhesions, excluding those formed by connective tissue. The hysteroscopic treatment of intrauterine adhesions has improved the outcome of treatment, not only in correcting menstrual abnormalities, but also in the reproductive outcome [5].

Valle and Sciarra [6] reported on 187 patients evaluated and treated by hysteroscopy over a 10-year period. The patients were classified according to the extent of uterine cavity occlusion found on hysterosalpingography and the type of intrauterine adhesions observed at hysteroscopy. Forty-three patients had mild or filmy intrauterine adhesions; 97 demonstrated moderate or fibromuscular adhesions; and 47 patients were classified as having severe connective tissue adhesions. Following hysteroscopic treatment, the restoration of normal menstruation occurred in 88.2% of patients who had menstrual abnormalities, including amenorrhea, hypomenorrhea, and dysmenorrhea. A total of 143 women achieved pregnancy, and of these, 114 (79.7%) achieved a term pregnancy and 26 women (18.1%) had a pregnancy loss. The reproductive outcome correlated with the type of adhesions and extent of uterine cavity occlusion, ranging from 81.3% term pregnancy rate

in patients with mild disease to 31.9% in patients with severe disease. Therefore, a classification of these adhesions is important in determining the prognosis for future reproductive outcome. Severe obstetric complications may occur after blind transcervical division and especially after transfundal division of intrauterine adhesions; nonetheless, following hysteroscopic division wth hysteroscopic scissors, the incidence of serious obstetric complications has generally been low.

CONCLUSIONS

The hysteroscopic treatment of intrauterine adhesions has resulted in a restoration of normal menstruation in more than 90% of patients treated. Nevertheless, the reproductive outcome seems to be determined by the severity of the condition. Of those patients who have achieved pregnancy, over 80% have carried the pregnancy to term. Although the complications related to abnormal placental implantations are markedly reduced, as compared with that following curettage or blind cervical dissection, this possibility should be kept in mind.

Despite the apparent success of the hysteroscopic approach to the treatment of intrauterine adhesions, prevention still remains the best therapy. Early diagnosis and treatment are important when adhesions are mild and filmy; in patients with severe and extensive connective tissue adhesions, even hysteroscopic division under direct view has been less than satisfactory and the reproductive outcome not very encouraging.

REFERENCES

1 Asherman JG. Traumatic intrauterine adhesions. *J Obstet Gynaecol Br Empire* 1950; 57: 892–896.
2 Schenker JG, Margalioth EJ. Intrauterine adhesions: an updated appraisal. *Fertil Steril* 1982; 37: 593–610.
3 Sugimoto O. Diagnostic and therapeutic hysteroscopy for traumatic intrauterine adhesions. *Am J Obstet Gynecol* 1978; 131: 539.
4 The American Fertility Society. The American Fertility Society classification of adnexal adhesions, distal tubal occlusion secondary to tubal ligation, tubal pregnancies, Müllerian anomalies and intrauterine adhesions. *Fertil Steril* 1988; 49: 944.
5 March CM, Israel R. Gestational outcome following hysteroscopic lysis of adhesions. *Fertil Steril* 1981; 36: 485.
6 Valle RF, Sciarra JJ. Intrauterine adhesions: hysteroscopic diagnosis, classification, treatment, and reproductive outcome. *Am J Obstet Gynecol* 1988; 158: 1459–1470.

Cervical incompetence

JOSEPH R. WAX & JOHN T. REPKE

Cervical incompetence is a diagnosis of exclusion made by a detailed history, physical examination, and laboratory evaluation of the patient. It may be defined as painless cervical dilatation associated with recurrent second-trimester pregnancy loss in the absence of genetic, endocrine, immunologic, and Müllerian abnormalities or chronic uterine infections. However, contractions may occur once the cervix has begun to dilate. The disorder is estimated to occur in 0.05–1% of all pregnancies, but may be present in up to 16% of second-trimester losses.

The etiology of incompetent cervix is unknown although several predisposing factors have been proposed. Foremost is a history of prior cervical trauma, noted in 98% of cases. Examples include forcible cervical dilatation, parturition-related lacerations, and cervical conization. Leiman et al. [1] found midtrimester losses following conization to be associated with a cone biopsy tissue volume ≥4 ml (18.2%) or biopsy height ≥2 cm (21.7%), as compared with smaller volumes (6.5%) or shorter heights (12.3%). However, a study by Buller and Jones [2] found no increased risk of second-trimester losses after conization in patients who had previously delivered successfully. Congenitally acquired incompetence, accounting for 2% of cases, should be suspected when the course of a patient's first pregnancy is consistent with incompetent cervix in the absence of prior trauma. The cause may be related to an increased ratio of smooth muscle to connective tissue or a variety of cervicouterine anomalies. Goldstein [3] has suggested a predisposition in women with *in utero* diethylstilbestrol exposure to incompetent cervix. Five of nine such patients who conceived experienced cervical incompetence, defined as painless dilatation and effacement of the cervix. All five had grossly abnormal-appearing cervices and all had term deliveries after surgical intervention.

A number of treatments for incompetent cervix are practiced, yet none have been evaluated in a randomized, prospective fashion. Placement of a vaginal pessary is felt to displace the cervix posteriorly, providing vaginal support and pressure on the internal os, while elevating the fetal head. Progestational agents in the form of 17-hydroxyprogesterone are felt to decrease cervical and isthmic diameters, and may suppress myometrial contractions. Endocervical cautery can only be performed in the nonpregnant patient and is associated with a subsequent infertility risk of up to 45%. Saling [4] has proposed a new mode of operative occlusion of the cervix for the prevention of recurrent late losses. The procedure involves hemostatic ligation of the cervix, followed by denudation of the epithelium on the portio and closure with occluding sutures. At term, the cervix is recanalized, and delivery allowed to proceed.

The mainstay of treating cervical incompetence is the cerclage — surgical placement of suture about the cervix to maintain a closed os. There are three different procedures currently in favor, each with its respective indications, advantages, and disadvantages. The most commonly performed cerclage is the McDonald technique [5] (Fig. 20.1). A purse-string suture of permanent material such as 5 mm Mersilene is placed through cervical mucosa and stroma in a circumferential fashion. Other suture material, such as 1-Prolene or 2-Tevdek, are commonly used, depending on the operator's preference and experience. It offers benefits of nonextensive surgery, low complication rate, easy removability, and a high rate of vaginal delivery. Unfortunately, the suture may dislodge, and may not be able to be placed in a very short cervix.

The Shirodkar procedure is the first described technique of cerclage. Surgical incisions are made on the cervix anteriorly and then posteriorly. The bladder is advanced off the cervix. A permanent suture is placed submucosally from the anterior incision through the posterior incision with aneurysm

(a)

(b)

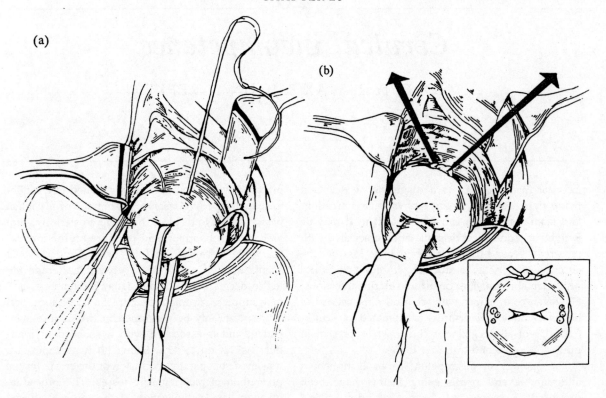

Fig. 20.1 Placement of McDonald cerclage. (a) Mersilene band being placed at level of internal os. (b) Cervix is left open to admit fingertip (knot is at 12 o'clock in this illustration).

needles, and tied posteriorly (Fig. 20.2). The mucosal incisions are then closed. This cerclage may be advantageous in patients where a pursestring suture has failed or is unable to be performed. It may be removed at term or left in permanently, but this leads to the need for elective cesarean delivery. Furthermore, the operation requires fairly extensive dissection, leading to an increased complication rate.

Finally, transabdominal cerclage entails meticulous dissection in the region of the uterine vessels and ureters for suture placement at the level of the internal os. It permits surgical occlusion of the incompetent cervix in patients with a stenosed vagina, amputated cervix, high cone biopsy, or failed vaginal cerclage with secondary damage. Unfortunately, this option requires two intraabdominal surgeries in regions close to major pelvic organs. Transabdominal cerclage is associated with the highest complication rate of the three cerclage procedures. Once a cerclage is tied, the cervix should still be able to admit the tip of the operator's small finger or similar-diameter object to allow egress of normal secretions and recognition of membrane rupture or uterine bleeding.

The preoperative evaluation serves to exclude non-surgical causes of recurrent second-trimester loss before proceeding to cerclage (Fig. 20.3). It is incomplete without a complete history and physical examination. The patient's past should be reviewed for instances of preterm labor, abruption, preterm rupture of membranes, contractions, or uterine bleeding. If the history is positive for any such events, a diagnosis other than incompetent cervix is suggested.

In the nonpregnant patient with multiple prior losses and a questionable history of incompetent cervix, any records concerning fetal anomalies, autopsies, or chromosomal studies should be obtained. Prior gynecologic surgery, *in utero* hormonal exposure, and family history of recurrent loss and congenital anomalies are documented. Laboratory evaluation includes cervical cultures for *Mycoplasma hominis* and *Ureaplasma urealyticum*. If positive, the patient is treated. Serologic studies include a test for syphilis, antinuclear antibody, anticardiolipin antibody, and lupus anticoagulant. Thyroid function tests are obtained, as well as karyotypes of each parent. Müllerian anomalies are ruled out by a hysterosalpin-

(a)

(b)

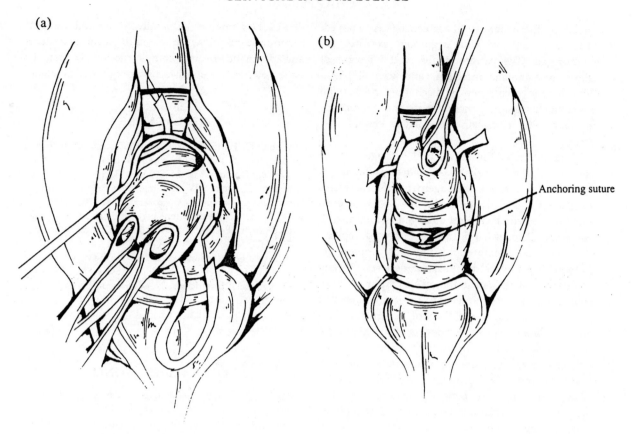

Anchoring suture

Fig. 20.2 Placement of Shirodkar cerclage. (a) Aneurysm needle guiding submucosal suture. (b) Silk sutures anchor cerclage in place prior to closing mucosal incisions.

gogram. If the patient is pregnant with a past history consistent with incompetent cervix or the current pregnancy shows signs of incompetence, ultrasound is a required examination. The study confirms fetal viability and establishes gestational age. It also rules out fetal anomalies before securing the cervix.

Not all patients with a history of incompetent cervix are candidates for a cerclage. Contraindications to the procedure include the presence of ruptured membranes, intraamniotic infection, cervical dilatation >4 cm, or persistent uterine bleeding. If the patient has entered the third trimester or has a documented fetal anomaly, cerclage generally should not be performed.

Once the diagnosis of incompetent cervix has been made, and the patient is determined to be a cerclage candidate, the procedure should be scheduled at the optimal time of 14–18 weeks' gestation. This window is beyond the period of most spontaneous abortions, before most second-trimester losses, and at a time when a detailed anatomic survey and con-

firmation of fetal viability may be performed. Some surgeons place the cerclage before pregnancy is established if the patient has a history of extensive cervical laceration or trauma. This method runs the risk of suturing in a nonviable or anomalous gestation.

Cervical cerclage is not without risk to the patient or the pregnancy. Complications may occur around the time of the procedure or remote from it. Early problems include chorioamnionitis with an incidence of 1–7.7%, dislodged McDonald cerclage (3–12%), rupture of membranes, preterm labor, hemorrhage, and those related to anesthesia. Late complications include cervical stenosis (1.4–5%), cervical laceration (2.6–13.2%), genitourinary fistula formation, and uterine rupture.

Upon completion of surgery, the patient is placed at bedrest for up to 24 hours. In the case of a McDonald or Shirodkar cerclage, surgery in the medically well patient may be performed in an outpatient setting. Light activity may then be resumed, with the exception of coitus. Nothing should be placed in the vagina by the patient until the cerclage is removed. Strenuous activity and vigorous exercise are discouraged. The patient is observed for signs of labor, intraamniotic infection, and vaginal bleeding. If none occur, she is discharged home with precautions regarding these events and instructions to contact her physician immediately should they occur.

Visualization of the cervix and cerclage may be performed every 2 weeks to ascertain any effacement, dilatation, or cerclage dislodgement. If progressive effacement and dilatation occur, the patient is evaluated for preterm labor and managed as indicated. If the suture dislodges and it is still indicated, replacement may be attempted by the most appropriate method. The suture is removed between 36 and 38 weeks' gestation, or in the case of ruptured membranes, intraamniotic infection, or vaginal bleeding of uterine origin, at the time of occurrence. Prophylactic antibiotics, tocolytics, and progestins at and beyond the time of surgery are of unproven efficacy and cannot therefore be recommended.

The success of the cerclage is difficult to assess. Most studies use the patient's own previous lost pregnancy as a control. When a cerclage was placed in the pregnancy following a loss, 75–90% of patients delivered a viable infant. However, 71–73% of those without a cerclage in the pregnancy immediately following a loss delivered a viable infant as well.

Cervical incompetence is a clinical diagnosis of exclusion, requiring meticulous patient evaluation (Fig. 20.3). Treatments are many and varied, but of uncertain value. Each awaits prospective and randomized evaluation. Operatively treated patients require careful follow-up, as outlined for procedure- and pregnancy-related complications. All patients have potential for a satisfactory pregnancy outcome.

REFERENCES

1 Leiman G, Harrison NA, Rubin A. Pregnancy following conization of the cervix: complications related to cone size. *Am J Obstet Gynecol* 1980; 136: 14–18.
2 Buller RE, Jones HW III. Pregnancy following cervical conization. *Am J Obstet Gynecol* 1982; 142: 506–512.
3 Goldstein DP. Incompetent cervix in offspring exposed to diethylstilbestrol in utero. *Obstet Gynecol* 1978; 152: 735–755.
4 Saling E. Early operative occlusion of the cervix for prevention of recurrent late abortions. Abstract No. 1, Society of Perinatal Obstetricians, New Orleans, Louisiana. Feb 1–4, 1989.
5 McDonald A. Cervical cerclage. *Clin Obstet Gynecol* 1980; 7: 461–479.

FURTHER READING

Cousins L. Cervical incompetence, 1980: a time for reappraisal. *Clin Obstet Gynecol* 1980; 23: 467–476.
Grant A. Cervical cerclage: new evidence from the Medical Research Council Royal College of Obstetricians and Gynecologists. Proceedings. *Advances in Prevention of Low Birthweight*. National Center for Education in Maternal and Child Health. Washington DC, 1988.
Harger JH. Comparison of success and morbidity in cervical cerclage procedures. *Obstet Gynecol* 1980; 56: 543–548.
Harger JH. Cervical cerclage: patient selection, morbidity, and success rates. *Clin Perinatol* 1983; 10: 321–341.

21

Uterine leiomyomas

BRADLEY S. HURST

INTRODUCTION

Leiomyomas uteri, or uterine fibroids, are the most common pelvic tumors in women. Approximately 40% of women have myomas by their 40s, and up to 50% of nulliparous women have fibroids at the age of 50. Although fibroids are quite common, most women with fibroids are asymptomatic.

CLINICAL DIAGNOSIS

History

While most women with fibroids are asymptomatic, myomas can be associated with numerous symptoms, including pelvic pain, pelvic pressure, abnormal uterine bleeding, pregnancy wastage, infertility, urinary frequency, or compressive bowel symptoms.

There is no predictable pattern of pain in women with fibroids. Pain is caused by ischemia or infarction of a myoma with growth or torsion, or due to compression of other pelvic structures. The pain generally is constant and may be quite severe with ischemia. Pain is acute and severe with torsion of the myoma, but may be constant or intermittent. Pain from myomas may be diffuse, but more commonly is focal and directly related to the fibroid causing the pain.

Pelvic pressure tends to be a constant symptom with intermittent improvement and exacerbation of symptoms. Pelvic pressure is caused by compression of pelvic and abdominal structures by the enlarging uterus.

Abnormal uterine bleeding due to fibroids usually results from mechanical distortion of the endometrial cavity. Submucous or sessile myomas directly compressing the endometrial cavity can cause bleeding at any time in the menstrual cycle. On the other hand, intramural or subserosal myomas are less likely to cause intermenstrual bleeding, but may cause menorrhagia due to mechanical enlargement of the uterine cavity. Areas of an abnormal blood supply to the endometrium due to vascular distortion from the myomas may contribute to heavy uterine bleeding.

Recurrent pregnancy wastage associated with fibroids may be caused by one of several factors [1]. First, the vascular supply to the endometrium and uterus may be abnormal, therefore interfering with implantation and growth of an early pregnancy. Second, uterine fibroids may directly alter the endometrium due to a mechanical compression. Third, uterine irritability due to myomas may interfere with implantation or cause an early miscarriage or premature labor. Additionally, submucous myomas may produce an endometrial inflammatory reaction that interferes with a developing pregnancy.

Uterine fibroids are an unusual cause of infertility. Infertility, however, may result from compression of the cornual area of the uterus by myomas. Additionally, an intracavitary myoma may result in implantation failure due to a local inflammatory reaction or mechanical alterations of the endometrium.

Urinary frequency is a result of direct compression of the urinary bladder by large intramural or submucous myomas. Constipation or diarrhea may be caused by subserous myomas that compress the sigmoid colon.

EXAMINATION

The diagnosis of uterine myomas usually is made by pelvic examination. Characteristically, pelvic examination reveals an enlarged, often irregular, firm uterus. Individual fibroids may be palpated directly on bimanual examination. On speculum examination, the cervix is drawn out of the pelvis and deviated from the midline in some patients with fibroids.

Although the diagnosis of fibroids usually is made on pelvic examination, the examination sometimes is misleading. For example, a bicornuate uterus may be mistaken for a myoma. Solid ovarian tumors may be misdiagnosed as pedunculated subserosal myomas. Additionally, uterine enlargement may be due to adenomyosis. On the other hand, patients with submucous myomas may have significant symptoms and no abnormalities detected at the time of pelvic examination.

DIAGNOSTIC EVALUATION

The diagnostic evaluation will vary considerably depending on the patient's symptoms, physical findings, and desire for uterine preservation or preservation of fertility (Fig. 21.1). However, the overall concept should be the same for any circumstances and includes the following: (1) establish the correct diagnosis; (2) rule out associated pathology; and (3) treat on the basis of symptoms, physical, and diagnostic findings, and the patient's desires for uterine preservation.

Ultrasound examination should be performed when the diagnosis of fibroids is considered, but not certain. The most common sonographic abnormalities are irregularities in uterine contour, altered areas of echogenicity, and uterine enlargement [2]. Twenty to forty percent of patients with fibroids have no sonographic abnormalities, although fibroids larger than 2 cm generally are recognized by ultrasonography.

Ultrasound also can be useful to evaluate for ureteral obstruction caused by compression from enlarging fibroids. Ureteral compression may occur as the uterus grows beyond the pelvic brim, and is seen as hydronephrosis on ultrasonography. Intravenous pyelogram (IVP) is helpful when there is a suspicion of ureteral dilatation or hydronephrosis. In addition, IVP is used to determine if the ureter is in an abnormal position due to extrinsic pressure from the fibroids.

Ultrasonography is the procedure of choice to evaluate the adnexae when enlargement of the uterus or location of myomas precludes palpation of the ovaries on bimanual examination. In general, once the adnexae are no longer palpable, usually when the uterus is 12 or more weeks' size, an ultrasound should be performed to evaluate for adnexal masses. If surgery is not performed, the adnexae should be evaluated annually by ultrasound examinations.

Magnetic resonance imaging (MRI) and computed tomography (CT) scans may be used to diagnose or confirm the diagnosis of fibroids, but both techniques have significant limitations. MRI is preferable to the

CT scan to evaluate pelvic structures because MR images are not distorted by pelvic bones and MRI provides the ability to change soft tissue contrast to enhance the image. MRI is able to demonstrate fibroids with more detail than is possible with CT scanning or ultrasound. However, MRI and CT scans are quite expensive and rarely add additional clinically relevant information than can be provided by ultrasonography. The routine clinical use of MRI or CT scans is not recommended for the diagnosis of fibroids.

A hysterosalpingogram (HSG) is advised for all patients with recurrent pregnancy wastage and infertility [3]. In addition, the HSG can provide essential information to diagnose a submucous or sessile myoma in the patient with abnormal uterine bleeding after ovulatory dysfunction, endometrial neoplasia, pregnancy, and cervical inflammation have been excluded. The HSG provides considerable information regarding size, location, and number of submucous myomas. Submucous myomas distort the normal triangular shape of the cavity and are seen as specific filling defects in the uterus. The HSG findings are more subtle with intramural myomas. Intramural myomas often cause enlargement of the uterine cavity or subtle indentations in the outline of the cavity. Fibroids may cause proximal tubal occlusion from extrinsic compression. However, the HSG is usually normal in most circumstances when intramural or subserosal myomas are present.

The HSG can only provide information if it is done properly. The uterine cavity must be parallel to the table to provide optimal anatomic detail. An early film with minimal distention of the uterus provides much more intrauterine detail of subtle defects than later films. Defects, when identified, should be evaluated with oblique views to confirm localization and shape of the myoma.

Hysteroscopy can be valuable in the diagnosis of a submucous myoma. Ideally, hysteroscopy is performed in the early follicular phase after the cessation of menses. Submucous myomas seen by hysteroscopy are smooth, firm, pale, and rounded. Fibroids can be differentiated from polyps by the lack of movement with myomas, whereas polyps will move as pressure of the distention medium varies.

Laparoscopy can be used to confirm the diagnosis of intramural or subserous myomas, but small intramural myomas and submucous myomas may not be seen with laparoscopy. Laparoscopy is advised as part of the diagnostic evaluation for a patient with

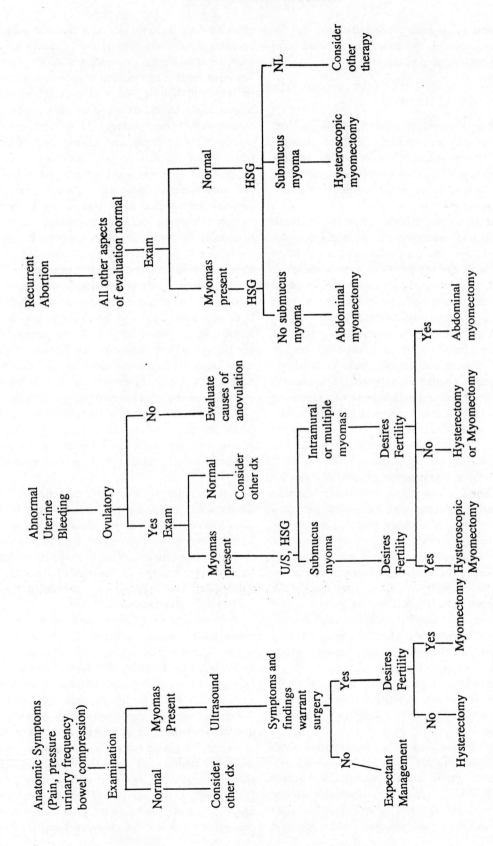

Fig. 21.1 Approach to uterine leiomyomas.

CHAPTER 21

infertility and is generally recommended at the time of a hysteroscopic myomectomy to avoid complications from uterine perforation.

THERAPY

Therapeutic options should be decided on the basis of symptoms, physical findings, and the patient's desire for future fertility. These options include expectant management, hysteroscopic myomectomy, abdominal myomectomy, vaginal hysterectomy, and abdominal hysterectomy.

Expectant management is the treatment of choice for a patient with asymptomatic or mildly symptomatic fibroids. An ultrasound evaluation is helpful to quantitate the size of the uterus for future reference. In addition, the ultrasound examination should be performed to rule out hydronephrosis and adnexal masses. Frequent follow-up pelvic examinations are essential. A pelvic examination should be performed no later than 3 months after the initial diagnosis has been made. If the uterus is growing slowly, a follow-up examination should be repeated in another 3 months. If the uterus appears to be stable, follow-up examinations at 6-month intervals are reasonable. Should the patient become symptomatic during the follow-up interval or if there is rapid enlargement of the uterus, surgery should be considered.

Although there are no approved medical therapies for uterine fibroids, gonadotropin-releasing hormone (GnRH) analog therapy provides several potential benefits. First, GnRH analogs may reduce uterine bleeding and allow for normalization of hematologic parameters in preparation for surgery in patients who are anemic. GnRH analogs decrease the uterine volume and size of fibroids, which may make them easier to remove [4]. In addition, symptomatic relief may be prolonged following GnRH analog therapy. The maximal benefit with GnRH analog therapy occurs by the third month of therapy. Further therapy usually is not warranted.

A hysteroscopic myomectomy is ideal for a patient with an isolated submucous myoma or when symptoms are attributed primarily to submucous myomas [5].

Adequate patient selection, preoperative evaluation and planning are critical to achieve optimal results with a hysteroscopic myomectomy. Patients with a submucous myoma and abnormal uterine bleeding, recurrent abortion, or infertility generally are candidates for a hysteroscopic myomectomy. If other myomas are present, their removal should be considered unnecessary to relieve symptoms, otherwise, an abdominal myomectomy should be chosen. The exact number and location of submucous myomas must be well defined prior to surgery. Thus, HSG or hysteroscopy should be done in preparation for a hysteroscopic myomectomy. The hysteroscopic myomectomy is performed in the early follicular phase after menstrual bleeding has stopped, or after endometrial suppression has been achieved with oral contraceptives, progestins, GnRH analogs, or danazol for a period of at least 3 weeks prior to surgery. However, the most important factor for a successful hysteroscopic myomectomy is for the procedure to be performed by a physician with a high level of skill at hysteroscopic surgery.

The hysteroscopic myomectomy can be performed with a modified urologic resectoscope or an Nd:YAG laser with good results. A laparoscopy may be performed at the same time to avoid complications should uterine perforation occur. Hyskon, D_5W or other nonionic fluids are used as the distending medium. A cutting current of 60 W is recommended for the hysteroscopic resectoscope, which results in a 2 mm deep burn. The cutting current is used to shave down the tumor to the base of the endometrium. A large-diameter Foley catheter can be inserted to tamponade the uterus in the event of postcautery bleeding.

Hysteroscopic myomectomy with the YAG laser deserves special comment. Although the YAG laser can be used very effectively, deaths have occurred from air embolism when carbon dioxide was used to cool the sapphire tip. Therefore, carbon dioxide should never be used as the coolant. On the other hand, fluids may be used safely. A focused sapphire contact tip is recommended.

Hysteroscopic resection of submucous and sessile myomas is carried only to the level of the endometrial lining. Uterine perforation, infection, and intra-abdominal cautery injury are risks of hysteroscopic surgery. In contrast to abdominal myomectomy, however, morbidity for this procedure is low.

Results with hysteroscopic myomectomy are good when performed by experienced hysteroscopic surgeons. Pregnancy rates of 25–33% were reported in earlier studies, but more recent studies suggest that results may be higher in well-selected patients [6]. Significant advantages of hysteroscopic myomectomy include the following: (1) it is an outpatient procedure, with a short recovery time; (2) overall, expense is much less than the expense of a major abdominal procedure; (3) blood loss usually is lower with a hysteroscopic myomectomy than an abdominal myomectomy; and (4) a cesarean section rarely is necessary following a hysteroscopic myomectomy.

Another modification of the hysteroscopic myomectomy is myomectomy combined with uterine ablation. Uterine ablation may be considered for abnormal uterine bleeding that is not controlled by medical therapy in a patient at high risk for abdominal or vaginal hysterectomy. Endometrial ablation can be accomplished at the time of hysteroscopy with a rollerball electrocautery or by contact YAG laser. Of these two options, the rollerball ablation is faster, less expensive, and more efficient.

Most patients with abnormal bleeding have significant improvement following endometrial ablation. Fifty percent of patients who have a hysteroscopic myomectomy followed by endometrial ablation will have no further uterine bleeding. Of those who experience bleeding, the bleeding is rarely severe. However, despite these encouraging results, there are no studies that evaluate the long-term safety and efficacy of endometrial ablation. There continues to be a concern that adenomyosis or cryptic endometrial adenocarcinoma may be a risk of uterine ablation.

Abdominal myomectomy is the procedure of choice for a symptomatic patient with multiple myomas or a large intramural or submucous myoma who desires preservation of fertility. Occasionally, an abdominal myomectomy may be considered for a patient who simply desires uterine preservation.

Meticulous surgical techniques are essential to provide optimal results with an abdominal myomectomy [1]. The incision chosen must provide good exposure. Exposure with a Pfannenstiel incision often is inadequate, but Maylard or vertical incisions provide excellent exposure. When doing the myomectomy, a dilute solution of vasopressin (1:20 dilution) may be injected into the myometrium to limit blood loss. The uterine incision should be made so that as many fibroids as possible may be removed through a single incision. An anterior vertical incision is not likely to result in adnexal adhesions, and is preferable. Inaccessible tumors can be removed through this incision by pushing the myomas toward the incision and removing them through a secondary myometrial incision. However, occasionally a posterior incision or multiple incisions may be required to remove multiple myomas.

The endometrial cavity should be repaired with interrupted absorbable sutures if entered during the procedure. The myometrial defect is closed with a purse-string suture at the base, then closed in layers. The serosa may be approximated with a running subserosal number 4−0 absorbable suture. However, if bleeding is persistent, figure-of-eight sutures or exposed running sutures may be necessary.

Results following myomectomy are generally good. Approximately 50% of patients with primary infertility will have a term delivery following myomectomy [7]. Recurrence of fibroids after myomectomy is common; however, only approximately 10−15% will require subsequent surgery. Cesarean section is advocated by some physicians following extensive myomectomy or entry into the uterine cavity. However, there are no well-designed studies that support the need for abdominal delivery following an extensive myomectomy. On the other hand, vaginal delivery has been successful following an extensive myomectomy [7]. Vaginal delivery should be considered following myomectomy unless the procedure was complicated by a postoperative infection or if multiple deep incisions were used during an extensive myomectomy.

Laparoscopic myomectomy has been advocated with increasing enthusiasm over the past few years. As surgical equipment has improved and surgical techniques have been refined, surgeons are attempting more aggressive laparoscopic procedures. In general, the approach and techniques used during a laparoscopic myomectomy should be comparable to those used during abdominal myomectomy [5]. As a general rule, however, most fibroids that can easily be removed with a laparoscope probably do not require surgical resection at all. The potential complications associated with laparoscopic myomectomy are serious enough that incidental or elective laparoscopic myomectomy rarely is indicated.

Hysterectomy is the recommended procedure for patients with symptomatic fibroids who have no wish for future fertility. The choice of the type of hysterectomy, abdominal or vaginal, is made depending on the size of the uterus, mobility of the uterus, vaginal compliance, and skill of the operator.

A vaginal hysterectomy should be considered when the uterus is 12 gestational weeks' size or less, although the exact uterine size that can be safely removed vaginally will depend on the pelvic anatomy and skill of the surgeon. A patient most suited for a vaginal hysterectomy will have mostly central fibroids, good uterine mobility, vaginal compliance, and good uterine descensus. Morcellation of the uterus occasionally is neccessary due to the uterine size. Morcellation should not be performed until after the uterine vascular pedicles have been secured on both sides. A patient should give consent for an abdominal hysterectomy and be emotionally prepared for the possibility of an abdominal hysterectomy, should vaginal hysterectomy prove difficult. However, vaginal hysterectomy offers the advantage of a shorter recovery time, less postoperative pain, and no visible scars compared to abdominal hysterectomy. Abdominal hysterectomy is considered the procedure of choice when hysterectomy is necessary and vaginal hysterectomy is not considered safe.

CONCLUSIONS

All too often, hysterectomy is the primary recommendation for all patients with fibroids. Although hysterectomy is an excellent approach for many, the therapy chosen must be based on symptoms, physical findings, and the patient's desire for future fertility or uterine preservation. Using these primary considerations, a rational plan may be made for the patient with symptomatic uterine myomas.

REFERENCES

1 Hurst BS, Rock JA. Uterine leiomyomata and recurrent pregnancy loss. In: Friedman AJ, ed. *Infertility and Reproductive Medicine Clinics of North America*, Vol. 2. WB Saunders, Philadelphia, 1991: 75.
2 Gross BH, Silver TM, Jaffe MH. Sonographic features of leiomyomas: analysis of 41 proven cases. *J Ultrasound Med* 1983; 2: 401.
3 Siegler AM. *Hysterosalpingography*, 2nd edn. New York; Medcom, 1974: 130.
4 Schlaff WD, Zerhouni EA, Huth JAM, Chen J, Damewood MD, Rock JA. A placebo-controlled trial of depot gonadotropin-releasing hormone analog (leuprolide) in the treatment of uterine leiomyomata. *Obstet Gynecol* 1989; 74: 856.
5 Hurst BS, Schlaff WD. Laparoscopic and hysteroscopic myomectomy. In: Azziz R, Murphy A, eds *Practical Manual of Operative Laparoscopy and Hysteroscopy*. New York: Springer-Verlag, 1992: 125–136.
6 Corson SL, Brooks PG. Resectoscopic myomectomy. *Fertil Steril* 1991; 55: 1041.
7 Babaknia A, Rock JA, Jones HW Jr. Pregnancy success following abdominal myomectomy for infertility. *Fertil Steril* 1978; 30: 644.

22

Management of the adnexal mass

BRUCE H. ALBRECHT & SANFORD M. MARKHAM

Pelvic masses in the female patient can arise from a variety of pelvic or abdominal structures. An adnexal mass may present as an unexpected finding during a routine pelvic examination or may be identified during the process of evaluating pelvic or abdominal symptomatology. In either case, the pelvic mass presents to the physician a clinical problem with a spectrum of differential diagnoses encompassing not only the wide range of benign and malignant tumors of the ovary, but also masses of nongynecologic sources.

A pelvic mass in a reproductive-age woman is most commonly felt to be physiologic by the examining physician. However, there is always an underlying concern that such a mass may represent a gynecologic cancer. Malignant disease of the ovary is the most common cause of gynecologic death in the USA. Approximately one in 70 women will develop ovarian cancer during their lifetime, and nearly 11 000 American women will die every year. In the USA 70% of ovarian cancers have metastasized by the time of diagnosis. For these reasons, early recognition of an ovarian cancer is of paramount importance, and is responsible for the anxiety physicians will commonly feel when confronted with an undiagnosed pelvic mass.

CLASSIFICATION OF ADNEXAL MASSES

Adnexal masses may be divided into two groups, those of reproductive tract origin, and those arising from surrounding or adjacent organs or tissues. These masses may be further subdivided into neoplastic and nonneoplastic lesions [1] (Table 22.1). The most common adnexal masses are either ovarian cysts or ovarian tumors, the most common of these in turn being simple or functional cysts. Nevertheless, one must always seek to exclude a more life-threatening neoplasm.

ASSESSMENT OF ADNEXAL MASSES

The key to the diagnosis and management of adnexal pathology is an accurate appreciation of the mass with regard to its size, shape, consistency, tenderness, mobility, and location. Bilaterality is important, as are other associated findings such as fever, urinary or gastrointestinal tract malfunction, ascites, or hemoperitoneum. The age of the patient is also critical in establishing an appropriate differential diagnosis. A pelvic mass in a menstruating woman may have far less significance than one in a postmenopausal or premenarchal woman. The former will much more commonly have some type of functional cyst while an adnexal mass in the latter two groups is clearly of much more concern.

Assessment of the adnexal mass begins with a careful history and thorough examination. One must always be on the alert for palpation of an unsuspected mass during routine examination because subjective complaints may not occur until a tumor is far advanced. When symptoms exist, they will usually include lower abdominal pain, pressure, or abdominal enlargement. Vague digestive disturbances or distention may also alert the physician to the possibility of a pelvic mass. Other specific complaints may relate to the location, size, and weight of the mass. A tumor expanding into the anterior pelvis can exert pressure sufficient to compromise bladder capacity or to produce outflow obstruction. Pressure at the pelvic brim may produce ureteral obstruction and secondary pyelonephritis. Compression of the rectosigmoid by an extending posterior pelvic mass may cause constipation or even intestinal obstruction. Severe pain of sudden onset, particularly when associated with nausea, low-grade fever, and leukocytosis may herald an ovarian torsion. Spontaneous torsion of a normal ovary is relatively uncommon. Rather, ovarian torsion frequently occurs in the presence of a preexisting adnexal mass such as a

Table 22.1 Classification of adnexal masses (adapted from [1])

Reproductive tract origin	Nonreproductive tract origin
Ovarian masses	*Gastrointestinal tract*
Simple cysts	Adhesions of the bowel−omentum
Physiologic cysts	Appendiceal abscess
Follicular	Diverticulosis
Corpus luteum	Endometriosis
Paraovarian cysts	Neoplastic tumors
Multiple follicle cysts (polycystic ovarian syndrome)	Stool in colon/rectum
Theca lutein cysts	
Pregnancy luteoma	*Urinary tact*
Endometriosis (endometrioma)	Bladder/ureteral stones
Surface epithelial inclusion cysts (germinal inclusion cysts)	Endometriosis
Inflammatory cysts	Neoplastic tumors
Epithelial tumors	Pelvic kidney
Sex cord-stromal tumors	Urine in bladder
Lipid cell tumors (lipoid tumors)	
Germ cell tumors	*Other pelvic masses*
Mixed germ cell and sex-cord tumors	Anterior sacral meningocele
Soft tissue tumors	Endometriosis
Unclassified tumors	Foreign body
Secondary tumors (metastatic tumors)	Hematoma
	Presacral teratoma
Nonovarian masses	Peritoneal cysts
Ectopic pregnancy	Retroperitoneal neoplasms
Endometriosis	Urachal cyst
Hydatid cysts of Morgagni	
Hydrosalpinx	
Pyosalpinx	
Congenital anomalies of the uterus/fallopian tubes	
Embryonic remnants	

benign cystic teratoma (dermoid cyst). Prompt diagnosis and surgical treatment should be initiated in such a case in order to save the ovary if at all possible. Hemorrhage into an ovarian cyst or rupture of a cyst are both causes of abdominal pain, frequently of an acute nature. These events may occur after abdominal trauma or after sexual relations. Obviously one must always exclude the possibility of an accident of pregnancy when evaluating such patients.

A careful physical and pelvic examination may be quite helpful in narrowing the differential diagnosis of a pelvic mass. For example, a cystic/solid (usually unilateral) mass in the anterior pelvis is frequently found to be a dermoid cyst. On the other hand, palpation of nodularity in the posterior pelvis, particularly along the uterosacral ligaments, may be associated with an endometrioma of the ovary as opposed to an ovarian neoplasm. A smooth regular surface suggests a benign cystic mass, whereas an irregular, nodular surface is more commonly associated with a neoplasm or malignancy. Smooth masses which may feel solid rather than cystic include leiomyomas or other solid adnexal tumors. Feces may also be a confounding finding on pelvic examination. Approximately 10% of benign tumors and 40% of malignant tumors are bilateral. The finding of a fluid wave or clinically evident ascites is clearly a very worrisome finding. Ascites is present in 25% of patients with malignant ovarian tumors and is extremely rare in patients with benign tumors.

DIFFERENTIAL DIAGNOSIS

The differential diagnosis of the pelvic mass can be subdivided into four stages of the female reproductive life cycle: prepubertal, reproductive age, pregnancy, and postmenopausal, each of which will be discussed in turn (Fig. 22.1).

ADNEXAL MASS

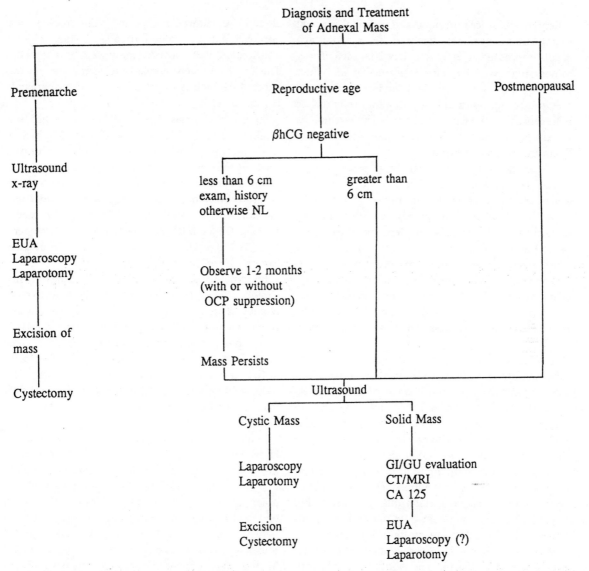

Fig. 22.1 Diagnosis and treatment of adnexal mass.

Premenarche

Because pelvic examinations are not routine in this age group, small adnexal masses are rarely detected. More commonly, a large pelvic–abdominal mass gives rise to symptoms such as distention, lethargy, or pain and is the reason for referral. While small physiologic cysts are fairly common in girls or young women, all pelvic/abdominal masses must be presumed to be either neoplasm or congenital anomaly and therefore require a careful assessment. Examination may be limited by the inability of the patient to cooperate. Abdominal/pelvic ultrasound, computed tomography (CT), or magnetic resonance imaging (MRI) may therefore be required and may be pre-

ferable to examination under anesthesia. About 60% of neoplasms in the premenarchal age group are malignant germ cell tumors such as dysgerminomas, endodermal sinus tumors, etc. Such tumors often arise in the gonads of an individual with XY gonadal dysgenesis, and therefore preoperative karyotyping to determine the presence of a Y chromosome may be advisable. If a Y chromosome is identified, it is recommended that all gonadal tissue be removed. When glycoprotein hormones are secreted by malignant germ cell tumors, they can serve as tumor markers. Therefore, human chorionic gonadotropin and α-fetoprotein should be assessed on any patient who is going to undergo surgery.

Benign germ cell tumors and gonadal stromal tumors are the next most common tumors in this age group, representing approximately 20% each. These tumors may well be hormonally active and their secretory products, estrogens and/or androgens, may produce physical findings of either isosexual or heterosexual precocious puberty. These findings should be clinically evident and lead to an accurate diagnosis in these patients.

Congenital anomalies such as a pelvic kidney should be considered. Furthermore, a pelvic mass secondary to hematometra or cryptomenorrhea can occur in a patient with primary amenorrhea and normal secondary sexual characteristics. These could be secondary to a noncommunicating uterine horn, transverse vaginal septum, or imperforate hymen. Congenital anomalies of the reproductive system are often associated with abnormalities of the urinary tract, thus an intravenous pyelogram (IVP) should be performed in a young woman with such an anomaly.

Reproductive-age group
The majority of patients with ovarian masses are in the reproductive-age group. Most of these masses occur due to cyclic hormonal stimulation, and are therefore benign and spontaneously reversible. Functional cysts are usually less than 6–8 cm in diameter. An ultrasound examination will generally show them to be simple cystic, though a persistent corpus luteum may have ultrasonographic findings consistent with blood or clot within the cyst cavity. Septations or excrescences would not be anticipated, and should generate a greater degree of concern.

When a 6–8 cm simple cyst is identified in a reproductive-age woman, she should be managed conservatively. Surgery may be indicated in the presence of persistent pain unresponsive to medical management or in the case of suspected torsion. Otherwise, the patient should be followed over the next 2–3 months, during which time the cyst is likely to resolve. Suppression of ovarian activity by use of an oral contraceptive pill should result in reduction in the size of the cyst and may also be considered, but is not necessary [2]. On the other hand, one should recognize that functional cysts rarely develop in women taking oral contraceptives so a cyst developing in a patient on oral contraceptives should be viewed with much greater concern and followed even more closely. This may be less true in women on triphasic or low-dose pills.

A patient with an adnexal cyst greater than 8 cm should be surgically explored. The conventional approach has been to perform a laparotomy with the anticipation that the cyst may well be neoplastic. The impact of new endoscopic techniques on this surgical decision is as yet unclear and further study is warranted.

Solid adnexal masses should be approached surgically due to the higher possibility of neoplasia. If there is any history of gastrointestinal or urinary tract dysfunction, preoperative evaluation should include barium enema and/or small bowel series or gastrointestinal endoscopy. An IVP would also be indicated, as would other diagnostic techniques such as CT or MRI on a selective basis. Preoperative CA-125 levels should be considered in order to facilitate careful follow-up.

Endometriosis involving uterine adnexal structures should always be considered in reproductive-age women. This diagnosis should be suspected in any reproductive-age woman presenting with noncyclic pelvic pain, dyspareunia, dysmenorrhea, or infertility. Physical findings suggestive of endometriosis include a retroflexed or fixed uterus along with posterior pelvic nodularity, adnexal masses, or indistinct masses consistent with adhesions. Ultrasound of an endometrioma will frequently show the classic appearance of a solid granite-like adnexal mass. However, the diagnosis can only be definitively made visually by laparoscopy or laparotomy. Again, the conventional approach is laparotomy with excision of the mass, resection or destruction of all endometriotic lesions, and presacral neurectomy in patients with midline abdominal pain. The potential role of endoscopic surgery continues to be uncertain. Medical management of endometriosis has included progestins, oral contraceptives, gonadotropin-releasing hormone analogs, and danazol. However, surgery should be the primary approach to women with an ovarian endometrioma in that medical management is not commonly effective.

Pregnancy
The enlarged corpus luteum in the first trimester is the most common cause of an adnexal mass and pain in pregnancy. Theca-lutein cysts are occasionally seen in normal pregnancies but are more commonly seen in patients with multiple pregnancy, diabetes, or gestational trophoblastic disease. They tend to grow rapidly and may reach 15 cm in size. They are usually multiple, giving a bilateral polycystic ovarian appearance on ultrasound examination, and regress

spontaneously when the stimulation produced by human chorionic gonadotropin is removed.

Pregnancy luteomas, though rare, may develop to a size of more than 20 cm in diameter. They are most commonly asymptomatic and are usually discovered incidentally at cesarean section or during postpartum tubal ligation. Some patients will develop masculinization during pregnancy and this should prompt consideration of a luteoma of pregnancy. Generally, the luteoma of pregnancy should be managed conservatively, like the theca-lutein cysts. Surgery is rarely indicated, and then only because of extreme size or symptoms of torsion or pain.

Small ovarian cysts (less than 5 cm in diameter) discovered in early pregnancy are usually functional and can be managed conservatively. If larger cysts persist, they are usually removed in the second trimester because of the reduced risk of complications. Mechanical complications such as torsion or rupture are managed if and when they occur, which, unfortunately, is most common in the first trimester. Only 1% of incidentally discovered cysts will undergo torsion, which is more common in pregnant than nonpregnant patients. Patients with multiple corpus luteum cysts associated with ovarian hyperstimulation syndrome are also at a significantly increased risk for torsion of the ovary.

The overriding concern of a malignant neoplasm continues to prompt consideration of surgery, even in pregnancy [3]. Approximately two-thirds of ovarian cysts measuring 5–6 cm will spontaneously resolve during pregnancy if left alone. This proportion may be even higher if a conservative policy towards surgery is implemented [4]. However, simple cysts larger than 10 cm in diameter rarely resolve and have an increased risk of both malignancy and torsion. Therefore, cysts over 10 cm should be excised.

Postmenopausal

With cessation of ovarian function at menopause, the ovaries gradually grow smaller over a period of months. In the absence of ovarian follicles, gonadotropic stimulation should be unable to produce physiologic cysts. Therefore, any mass palpated in a postmenopausal woman should be considered secondary to a neoplasm until proven otherwise. Aggressive investigation is needed as women in this age range have the highest incidence of ovarian carcinoma.

The physician should be particularly broad-minded when a pelvic mass is palpated in a postmenopausal woman. Women of this age group are particularly at risk of having a nongynecologic etiology of the pelvic mass. Specifically, diverticulitis, inflammatory bowel disease, gastrointestinal tumor, or metastatic tumor to the ovary should be carefully considered in all postmenopausal women with a pelvic mass.

ULTRASONOGRAPHIC CHARACTERISTICS

With transvaginal sonography a number of sonographic characteristics should be considered and may be predictive of diagnosis [5].

1 *Liquid phase*: intratumoral sonolucency of low-level echogenicity or completely sonolucent. A thickness of the main wall of the cystic mass greater than 4–5 mm particularly if it is irregular or shaggy in appearance, is also suspicious. Cystic masses constitute the vast majority of ovarian lesions. They may be completely sonolucent, as in follicular or functional cysts, or appear as a highly echogenic mass, as in endometrioid or dermoid cysts.

2 *Papillae*: echogenic formations protruding from the inner wall into the liquid phase, measuring from 2 mm to more than 2 cm, but not occupying more than 25% of the space of the mass. Papillary projections can be present in small (less than 5 cm) as well as large tumors. The sonograms of some benign neoplasms show papillary projections (e.g., dermoid cysts and serous cystadenomas); however, they are an ominous sign as malignancy is rarely found in cystic tumors lacking papillae.

3 *Solid lesion*: echogenic formation occupying more than 25% of the space of the mass. Solid or predominantly solid masses should always be considered true neoplasms and are generally found at surgery to be thecomas, fibromas, granulosa cell tumors, and malignant epithelial neoplasms.

4 *Daughter cysts*: circular echogenic structures protruding into the liquid phase of a larger cyst with no interstructural contingency. Most ovarian neoplasms displaying daughter cysts are benign. These include dermoid cysts and benign epithelial tumors. Occasionally, daughter cysts are also observed in serous cystadenocarcinoma.

5 *Loculation*: semicircular or circular echogenic structures protruding into the sonolucent center of the larger cyst with interstructural contingency. The sonographic implications of this finding are unclear. Many multilocular lesions are benign, including dermoid cysts, endometrioid tumors, and hemorrhagic

corpus luteum. Malignant epithelial tumors can also appear to be multilocular lesions.

6 *Septations*: structures crossing the liquid phase as echogenic bridges. Septations with a thickness of greater than 2 mm are suspicious. Septations are more common in malignant neoplasms, but they cannot be used as a certain marker for malignancy. The sonographic appearance of loculations and septations can be very difficult to differentiate. Therefore, caution should be exercised in interpreting these findings.

7 *Tumor size*: tumors greater than 10 cm in diameter are associated with a higher rate of malignancy compared to smaller ones, but there are numerous exceptions.

8 *Doppler imaging*: using flow data from color Doppler imaging, changes in the vascularity of the ovary can be detected. Given that neovascularization is an obligate event in malignant change, recognition of angiogenesis by measuring small changes in vascularity within the ovary may prove to be a highly significant advance in the use of sonography for the detection of early ovarian neoplasm.

Although ultrasonographic appearance has been used to differentiate many benign and malignant ovarian cysts preoperatively, this technique cannot be considered foolproof or firmly established. Furthermore, there is little information on the sonographic appearance of borderline tumors. Such tumors can have an echo-free internal pattern and be difficult to differentiate from benign cysts, though they more commonly have a complex appearance with internal nodules which would be rare in a simple cyst. At present, there is no accord regarding the risks or survival in patients with occult malignancies treated by laparoscopic aspiration and resection of cysts. A recent survey of gynecologic oncologists analyzed 42 ovarian malignancies identified at the time of laparoscopic cystectomy [6]. Of these, 6% were less than 8 cm, 62% cystic, 48% unilocular, and 81% unilateral. Thirteen (31%) fulfilled all four common ultrasound characteristics of benignity, while 55% satisfied at least three of four. Epithelial malignancies comprised 57% of the total and 29% were of low malignant potential.

NEW APPROACHES TO SURGICAL MANAGEMENT

Because the majority of ovarian cysts that occur during the reproductive years are functional cysts or benign neoplasms, an effective laparoscopic method of managing them may prove to be preferable to conventional laparotomy [7]. Resection of ovarian cystic masses as well as oophorectomy has been performed by laparoscopy. Laparoscopic aspiration of parovarian cysts has also been performed but is of limited therapeutic value as many cysts thus treated will quickly recur. Functional and simple ovarian cysts managed with laparoscopic or ultrasound-guided aspiration have a low recurrence rate. However, many of these may have spontaneously resolved without intervention. Fenestration and drainage of endometrioid cysts generally lead to recurrence in the majority of cases. Ablation, coagulation, or removal of the lining of endometrioid cysts reduces the rate of recurrence to 15%.

The greatest concern regarding laparoscopic treatment of ovarian masses is that the prognosis for patients with concealed malignant lesions may be adversely effected. This conclusion must be subjected to rigorous epidemiologic and statistical scrutiny.

A similar decision-making process should be entertained regarding ultrasound-guided aspiration of cysts. This may be indicated in patients who have significant pelvic pain and ultrasound characteristics suggestive of a totally benign cyst. The procedure is simple and is similar to ultrasound-guided follicle aspiration for oocytes in assisted reproductive technology procedures, It is well tolerated with minimal or no anesthesia in an office setting, and the complications are extremely rare. The decision to manage patients in this way hinges almost entirely upon the confidence one places on the ultrasonographic diagnosis, clearly demonstrated to be less than completely accurate. Ultrasound-guided aspiration of a cyst is absolutely contraindicated if there is a suspicion of malignancy, if the cyst is septate, solid, or contains papillary projections.

REFERENCES

1 Rock JA. Surgery for benign disease of the ovary. In: Rock JA, ed. *Telinde's Operative Gynecology*, 5th edn. Philadelphia: JB Lippincott, 1992.
2 Steinkampf MP, Hammond KR, Blackwell RE. Hormonal treatment of functional ovarian cysts: a randomized, prospective study. *Fertil Steril* 1990; 54 775–777.
3 Hill LM, Johnson CE, Lee RA. Ovarian surgery in pregnancy. *Am J Obstet Gynecol* 1975; 122: 565–569.
4 Hogston P, Lilford RJ. Ultrasound study of ovarian cysts in pregnancy: prevalence and significance. *Br J Obstet Gynaecol* 1986; 93: 625–628.

5 Rottem S, Timor-Tritsch IE. Ovarian pathology, In: Timor-Tritsch IE, Rottem S, eds. *Transvaginal Sonography*. New York: Elsevier, 1990: 145–173.

6 Maiman M, Seltzer V, Boyce J. Laparoscopic excision of ovarian neoplasms subsequently found to be malignant. *Obstet Gynecol* 1991; 77: 563–565.

7 Hasson HM. Laparoscopic management of ovarian cysts. *J Reprod Med* 1990; 35: 863–867.

The imperforate hymen

AMIN A. MILKI & MARY L. POLAN

The imperforate hymen is a rare congenital anomaly that most gynecologists will encounter only a few times, if at all, during the course of their practice. The incidence of this condition is estimated to be somewhere between 0.024 and 0.014% of all gynecologic admissions surveyed over several years in two major hospitals [1]. Despite the rarity of its occurrence, the diagnosis of an imperforate hymen is easy if one keeps in mind the simple fact that such an entity exists.

ANATOMY AND EMBRYOLOGY

The hymen is a thin connective tissue membrane separating the vagina from the vestibule. It is lined on both sides by stratified squamous epithelium, keratinized on the vestibular side. It has a round central opening in the majority of cases, but sometimes the opening is eccentric, or the presence of thin mucosal septa creates two or more openings.

In the fetus, the hymen is formed at about the 18th week of gestation. It is the embryologic septum between the sinovaginal bulbs above and the urogenital sinus proper below. The hymen is thus of urogenital sinus origin and is covered by endodermal epithelium. It is not derived from the Müllerian ducts [2].

PATHOPHYSIOLOGY AND SYMPTOMS

Symptoms develop secondary to the accumulation of fluid and secretions behind the imperforate hymen. Accordingly, it is not surprising that they occur at the two extremes of childhood. The presentation can be in the neonatal period if the fetal cervical glands produce a large amount of mucoid material in response to the maternal steroid hormone stimulation, leading to hydrocolpos and hydrometrocolpos. More commonly, the problem arises after puberty when the patient produces her own steroid hormones and menstruation begins. The accumulation of menstrual blood behind the hymen leads initially to hematocolpos, followed by hematometrocolpos, and possibly hematosalpinx and, rarely, hematoperitoneum.

Infantile hydrometrocolpos often presents as an abdominal mass (Fig. 23.1a) which exerts pressure on the bladder and rectum which prevents their complete emptying. Hydronephrosis is not an uncommon finding. Pelvic vein stasis can result in edema of the lower extremities and there may be respiratory distress from the decreased range of diaphragmatic motion.

The symptoms caused by an imperforate hymen in the adolescent are initially those of cyclic pelvic and abdominal discomfort without the appearance of menses (cryptomenorrhea). This is followed by continuous pain as the vagina becomes markedly distended. Pain is the most common problem that drives the patient to seek medical attention. Sometimes a noticeable suprapubic mass, with relatively little discomfort, can be the presenting symptom. Urinary complaints are not uncommon and may be manifested by dysuria, frequency, urgency, incontinence, a feeling of inadequate emptying of the bladder and, in rare instances, complete urinary retention. These findings are probably due to urethral compression, as well as bladder neck angulation caused by the vaginal fullness. Constipation can occur secondary to pressure on the rectum. Although amenorrhea is always present, it is not usually the presenting complaint, since the mean age at the onset of symptoms is in the early teens [3] when the delay in menstruation is not yet a concern.

DIAGNOSIS

The diagnosis of an imperforate hymen is typically made after the onset of puberty. The history is usually very suggestive of an obstruction to the flow of menstrual blood in a teenage girl. Secondary

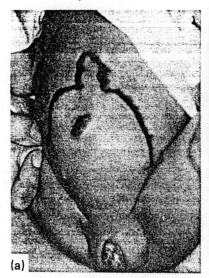 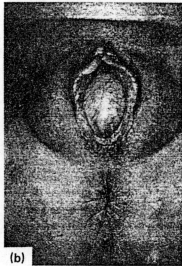 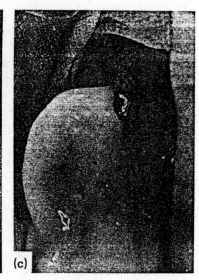

Fig. 23.1 Hydrometrocolpos in a newborn infant. (a) The abdominal mass is the vagina distended with mucus. The small mass at the top is the uterus. (b) The perineal view shows the bulging hymen. (c) Mucus draining out after the hymen was incised. (Reproduced with permission from W.B. Saunders.)

sexual characteristics are usually well developed with amenorrhea and cyclic or continuous pelvic and abdominal pain. The physical examination reveals a bulging membrane at the introitus, with a bluish discoloration if the hymen is thin enough. A fluctuant vaginal fullness of variable size can be appreciated on rectal examination and abdominal examination often reveals a suprapubic mass suggestive of a gravid uterus. The extent of the distention of the vagina and uterus depends on the delay between the onset of symptoms and the time when the diagnosis is made and therapy instituted. This delay is approximately 2 years in the series reported by Rock *et al.* describing their experience with imperforate hymen at the Johns Hopkins Hospital [3].

In the neonatal age group, it is imperative to examine the genitalia of the female with a pelvic or abdominal mass. The appearance of a bulging, tense membrane between the labia, which typically becomes more prominent with crying, strongly suggests the diagnosis (Fig. 23.1b).

The use of ultrasonography is a noninvasive technique which is very helpful in confirming the diagnosis by revealing a sonolucent mass in the vagina and possibly the uterus (Fig. 23.2). Tubal distention, if present, may also be appreciated. The amount of fluid can be estimated and the examination can serve as a baseline for future comparison to confirm the complete resolution of the condition when

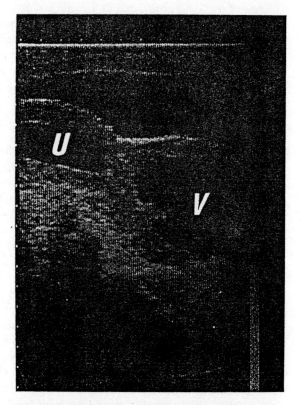

Fig. 23.2 Longitudinal scan of vagina and uterus demonstrating the sonolucent collections in the vagina (V), and uterus (U) in a patient with an imperforate hymen. (Reproduced with permission from John Wiley and Sons.)

ultrasonography is repeated after appropriate therapy. Not infrequently, the radiologist might be the one to suggest the diagnosis of imperforate hymen to the referring physician who requested an ultrasound evaluation of a pelvic mass. The actual bulging membrane itself can sometimes be seen as a septum delineating the caudal boundary of the vaginal sonolucent mass. We suggest that the kidneys be scanned as well at the time of the pelvic ultrasound to be certain there is no major anomaly. Admittedly, major renal anomalies do not seem to be present in patients with the isolated finding of an imperforate hymen. The hymen is not of Müllerian origin and its anomalies are not likely to be associated with congenital malformations of the mesonephric system. However, since the series reported in the literature lack a consistent evaluation of the urinary tract in patients with imperforate hymen, and since some patients with an isolated imperforate hymen have been shown to have a duplication of the ureter [3,4], we feel that a noninvasive ultrasonographic evaluation of the kidneys to rule out a major anomaly is probably warranted. In addition, if the hematometrocolpos is compressing the bladder and the ureters, ruling out hydronephrosis by sonographic evaluation is certainly worthwhile. We do not believe that intravenous pyelography is necessary in patients with an isolated finding of an imperforate hymen.

Differential diagnosis

The differential diagnosis in a patient with a low transverse vaginal membrane and hematocolpos includes, in addition to an imperforate hymen, a low transverse vaginal septum which can vary greatly in thickness. This condition results from the incomplete fusion of the Müllerian duct component and the urogenital sinus component of the vagina. Most of the time, a transverse septum is located in the upper half of the vagina, with only 14% occurring in the lower vagina [2]. A transverse septum can be mistaken for an imperforate hymen, although a perineal bulge is usually absent and a careful examination can reveal the presence of the hymen distal to the septum. The septum can be excised through a perineal approach with an effort to reapproximate the proximal and distal vaginal mucosa.

Another condition that should be considered in the differential diagnosis is vaginal atresia, also referred to as partial agenesis, with a small patent upper vaginal segment and a normal uterus. One could think of this as an extreme case of a transverse

vaginal septum of considerable thickness. It is compatible with future fertility if the anomaly is corrected by a procedure of the McIndoe type, and should be distinguished from vaginal agenesis where the uterine anlagen are usually vestigial and nonfunctional. With vaginal agenesis, the hymen is also absent. In less than 10% of patients with vaginal agenesis, a functional midline uterus is present and will cause cyclic menstruation with cryptomenorrhea and gradual enlargement of a lower abdominal mass. The cervix is usually absent. In these cases, as in cases where the symptoms arise from rudimentary uterine anlagen containing functional endometrial tissue, the most practical approach to therapy consists of performing a hysterectomy without unnecessary delay.

Distinguishing between these different entities

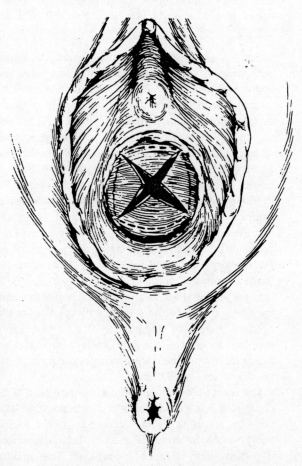

Fig. 23.3 Excision of imperforate hymen. Stellate incisions at 2, 4, 8, and 10 o'clock. The triangular flaps are then excised and the margins sutured. (Reproduced with permission from J.B. Lippincott.)

might not be possible based on the physical examination alone, and may be helped by radiologic studies, such as ultrasound and magnetic resonance imaging. Often, however, an accurate diagnosis can only be made at the time of surgery. In the rare situation where a low vaginal obstruction is discovered in an asymptomatic girl before the onset of puberty, it may be even more difficult to distinguish between an imperforate hymen, a low transverse septum, and vaginal agenesis. Rectal examination, and even a radiologic evaluation, may not distinguish a normal infantile uterus from rudimentary uterine horns. In this instance we feel that there is really no reason for immediate therapy as long as the patient is frequently monitored for any adverse symptoms of hydrocolpos or hematocolpos. A diagnosis can usually be reached more easily at the time of puberty, even if this means that a little blood is allowed to accumulate in the vagina. This is preferable to an inadvertent surgery on a prepubertal girl with vaginal agenesis, which is likely to jeopardize the success of a well-timed vaginoplasty when she is more mature.

Anomalies of the urinary tract can be present in a small percentage of patients with a transverse vaginal septum and are very significant in patients with vaginal agenesis. In this latter group, up to 40% of patients have some kind of urinary anomaly, and 15% have major renal anomalies such as agenesis of one kidney. Thus, intravenous pyelography is recommended in patients with a transverse vaginal septum and is certainly necessary in patients with any kind of vaginal agenesis.

With a high transverse septum, or vaginal agenesis with a functional uterus, the incidence of endometriosis is significantly higher, probably because less vaginal space is available, and the retrograde spillage of blood is likely to happen earlier than with an imperforate hymen.

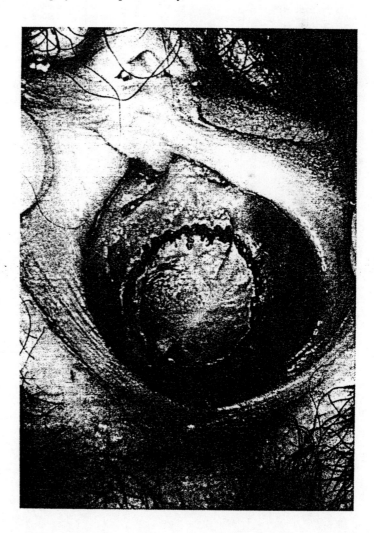

Fig. 23.4 Bulging imperforate hymen with circular incision created by CO_2 laser. (Reproduced with permission, Elsevier Science Publishing Company.)

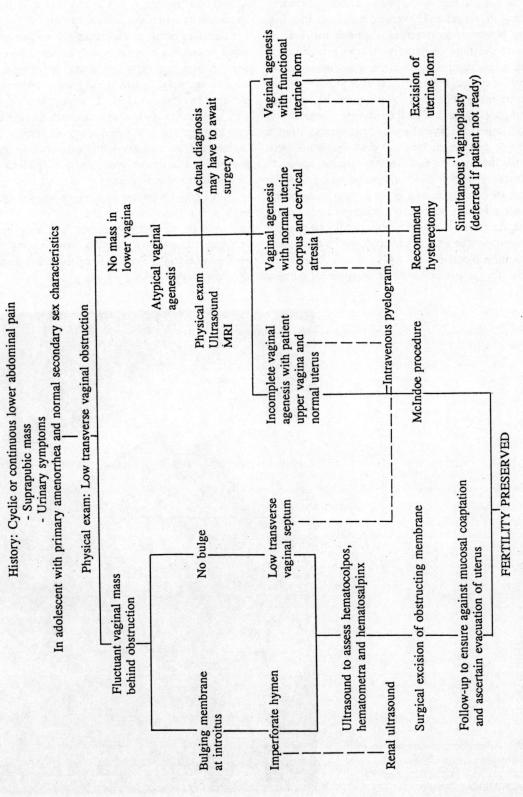

Fig. 23.5 Evaluation of the imperforate hymen.

A related condition, more commonly encountered in practice than the imperforate hymen, is the micro-perforate hymen, where a pinpoint opening allows menstruation to occur. The patient usually seeks medical attention later when she is unable to insert a tampon into the vagina, or if she experiences difficulty with sexual intercourse.

TREATMENT

The treatment of an imperforate hymen consists of the incision of the obstructing membrane. After catheterizing the bladder, the hymen is incised in a cruciate fashion at 2, 4, 8, and 10 o'clock, and then the triangular flaps created are excised (Fig. 23.3). A relatively large volume of greyish mucoid material can be observed in the newborn (Fig. 23.1c). In the prepubertal patient, the volume of blood recovered is variable, but rarely can reach several liters. The margins of the excised hymen are then reapproximated with fine nonreactive absorbable suture. Although a simple incision is likely to drain the accumulated fluid, the risk of scarring and reocclusion is too high. Even after a hymenectomy, it is recommended that the patient be checked at frequent intervals to make sure that no stenosis has occurred and that the vaginal opening remains patent. This will also allow the physician to monitor the satisfactory drainage of the hematocolpos and hematometra. The latter should clear within 2—3 weeks. If the uterine mass is still present after this interval, inspection and dilatation of the cervix should be performed to be certain that drainage from the uterus is satisfactory, At this time a follow-up ultrasound can be helpful. The presence of hematosalpinx is not an indication for the surgical drainage of the tubes, since most will spontaneously drain after the hymenectomy is performed.

General anesthesia in an operating room has been traditionally recommended for the performance of a hymenectomy in these patients. Broad-spectrum antibiotic coverage is used. However, with the recent sharp increase in office-based outpatient gynecologic surgical procedures, we believe that, in selected patients, the hymenectomy can be performed in an office setting under local anesthesia. This is particularly appropriate when there is no evidence of cervical dilatation and no hematometra on ultrasound evaluation. The laser is an elegant tool that has been used successfully in this setting [5] (Fig. 23.4). Typically, the patients have normal menstruation after the surgery. We suggest that they avoid tub bathing and swimming for two menstrual cycles. After surgical therapy, the vast majority of patients have patent tubes on hysterosalpingogram (19 of 20) [4] and the pregnancy rate in these women is quite satisfactory, with 13 of 15 women conceiving [3].

Figure 23.5 summarizes the differential diagnosis and management of the imperforate hymen.

REFERENCES

1 Warner RE, Mann RM. Hematocolpos with imperforate hymen. Report of five cases. *Obstet Gynecol* 1955; 6: 405—409.
2 Mattingly RF, Thompson JD (eds). Surgery for anomalies of the Müllerian ducts. In: *TeLinde's Operative Gynecology* 6th edn. Philadelphia: JB Lippincott, 1985: 345—380.
3 Rock JA, Zacur HA, Dlugi AM, Jones HW, TeLinde RW. Pregnancy success following surgical correction of imperforate hymen and complete transverse vaginal septum. *Obstet Gynecol* 1982; 59: 448—451.
4 Sivasamboo R. Haematocolpos. *Aust NZ J Obstet Gynecol* 1968; 8: 42—44.
5 Friedman M, Gal D, Peretz BA. Management of imperforate hymen with the carbon dioxide laser. *Obstet Gynecol* 1989; 74: 270—272.

Part IVA
Endocrinologic abnormalities: Hypothalamic–pituitary

Hyperprolactinemia and prolactin-secreting adenomas

HOWARD A. ZACUR & GIRAUD V. FOSTER

INTRODUCTION

In the presence of hyperprolactinemia, a diligent search should be made for a prolactin-secreting tumor which might be life-threatening. In most instances, however, tumors if present, are benign and should be conservatively treated whenever possible. Three errors made by physicians managing their patients with hyperprolactinemia are the failure to look for a pituitary tumor when other conditions associated with hyperprolactinemia are present, failure to reassure their patients that prolactin-secreting adenomas are rarely dangerous, and failure to stress the importance that even benign pituitary tumors require close and sometimes long-term follow-up. This chapter reviews the causes of hyperprolactinemia, how a prolactin-secreting adenoma is identified, and how the patient with hyperprolactinemia should be managed under three conditions: (1) when a large pituitary tumor or suprasellar mass is present; (2) when the patient is pregnant; and (3) when hyperprolactinemia is due to microadenomas, nonthreatening macroadenomas, other causes, or is idiopathic.

NORMAL AND ABNORMAL LEVELS OF PROLACTIN

The normal basal range of serum or plasma prolactin levels is reported to be between 0 and 25 ng/ml by most laboratories. These values, however, do not reflect the hormone's variation as affected by age, sex, pregnancy status, prandial state, state of activity, and medications. Basal prolactin concentrations are usually 0—15 ng/ml in men and 0—20 ng/ml in women. However, levels in women approximate those of men before menarche and after menopause, vary during the menstrual cycle with higher levels after ovulation, and increase during pregnancy to values between 200 and 400 ng/ml and even higher in some individuals close to term. These variations

occur because prolactin secretion is augmented by estrogen. For this reason patients on estrogen-containing contraceptives can also have increased levels of prolactin in their blood. Foods, particularly amino acids in food, stimulate prolactin secretion. Polactin levels have a diurnal pattern with values rising during sleep. Stress, too, inclusive of that produced by venipuncture in some individuals, can elevate values, since stress, by stimulating secretion of endorphins, which inhibit dopamine, the natural inhibitor of prolactin, allows prolactin to be secreted at higher than normal rates. Because of the foregoing, prolactin should be measured in the fasting state, early in the morning, preferably during the follicular period in women, and under relatively stressless conditions. Primary hypothyroidism should be ruled out by measuring thyroid-stimulating hormone (TSH) since thyrotropin-releasing hormone (TRH) is normally suppressed by thyroxine, and if it is not suppressed, it stimulates pituitary prolactin secretion.

Patients should be asked about symptoms associated with hypothyroidism and medications that promote hyperprolactinemia, inclusive of opiates, certain antihistamines, tranquilizers that have dopamine-blocking activity, and, of course, estrogen.

Finally, the physician should verify that hyperprolactinemia is present by ordering a second assay, making certain that blood is drawn under ideal conditions. Irrespective of whether or not a cause for hyperprolactinemia is found, an effort should be made to exclude a pituitary adenoma.

PROBLEMS WITH NOMENCLATURE

While an occasional patient will have a nonprolactin-secreting tumor which produces hyperprolactinemia by interfering with factors that normally inhibit prolactin secretion, most patients with tumors and elevated levels of prolactin have an excess of prolactin-secreting cells. The commonest terms used to describe the latter condition are pituitary tumor and pituitary adenoma. Unfortunately, both are semantically incorrect. A tumor is a tissue growth without physiologic function: certainly a hyperfunctioning pituitary responds to physiological stimuli. The term adenoma, on the other hand, is equally incorrect because it suggests an encapsulated cellular growth. The pituitary abnormality most commonly observed with biologically active hyperprolactinemia is nodular hyperplasia of the lactotrophs, a condition in which the hyperplastic cells are not capsulated, exhibit no cytologic or nuclear atypia, and are often geographically multifocal.

The term adenoma, however, is so well accepted that it will undoubtedly continue to be used. Adenomas are spoken of as being micro- or macroadenomas depending on their size, with microadenomas being those less than 1 cm in diameter and macroadenomas those greater than 1 cm.

RADIOLOGIC RECOGNITION OF A PITUITARY ADENOMA

A radiologic abnormality suggestive of an adenoma is observed in approximately 40% of patients with hyperprolactinemia. The best method to recognize an adenoma is by magnetic resonance imaging (MRI) of the pituitary gland. Currently, MRI scans have proven to be the imaging modality of choice. MRI has several advantages over computed tomography (CT) in that it can exquisitely display the anatomic relationships of the pituitary adenoma to adjacent structures such as the brain stem, floor of the sella turcica, and internal carotid artery within the cavernous sinus, and the optic chiasm. Looking at Figure 24.1, it is not difficult to appreciate how enlargement of the pituitary beyond its normal boundaries can compress the optic chiasm or erode into the cavernous sinus. Tumor can be readily visualized in coronal, sagittal, and axial planes. The relationship of internal carotid artery to the tumor can be easily displayed by MRI without a need for angiography. Subacute and chronic blood within the adenoma can be better recognized by MRI relative to CT scanning; however, CT is more sensitive than MRI in detecting acute hemorrhage within the tumor when pituitary apoplexy is suspected.

Microadenomas as small as 3 mm can be detected and their growth monitored by MRI. Tumors are suspected if the pituitary is enlarged, abnormally shaped, the infundibulum deviated, or density abnormally variable.

Size is determined by measuring the height of the gland through a coronal section at right angles to the diaphragm of the sella. Coronal sections generated by MRI do not require that the patient hyperextend his or her neck. Radiologists vary in their measurement of height but most consider 7–9 mm the upper limit of normal for women and 5–7 mm for men. The superior surface of the normal pituitary gland is

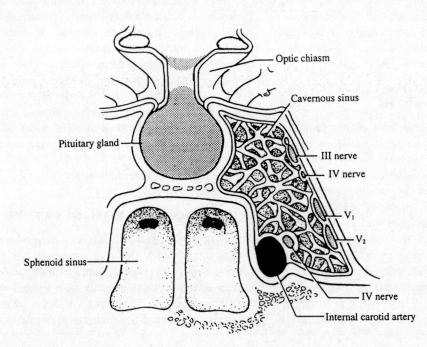

Fig. 24.1 Position of anatomic structures seen in MRI and CT scans.

usually flat or concave, whereas if an adenoma is present it is more likely to be convex. In coronal views the infundibulum should be in the midline. Deviation suggests an intrasellar mass. Various components of tumor such as calcifications or cysts can be easily detected by MRI.

TREATMENT OF HYPERPROLACTINEMIA
(Fig. 24.2)

Management of patients with large intrasellar masses

When there is significant enlargement of the pituitary or a mass near the pituitary, one has two major concerns: (1) if the mass is sufficiently large, it may impinge on the optic chiasm producing visual field detects; and (2) if it compresses the infundibulum, it may inhibit the release of dopamine, thereby provoking hyperprolactinemia.

Very rarely do pituitary lesions affect vision. This is because the optic chiasm is almost 1 cm above the superior surface of the gland itself. Therefore compression of either the chiasm or cranial nerves 3, 4, and 5 that are located in the cavernous sinuses surrounding the pituitary gland is rare unless the mass is very large. Patients with large intrasellar or superséllar tumors, on the other hand, are suspect and require an ophthalmologic examination with perimetry studies to exclude bitemporal hemianopsia caused by compression of the optic chiasm. Even more unusual are pituitary tumors large enough to produce hydrocephalus and papilledema by preventing the outflow of cerebrospinal fluid from the third ventricle. With problems of either suspected hydrocephalus or significant temporal hemianopsia, the patient should be seen and followed by a neurosurgeon.

Fortunately, most intrasellar lesions in patients

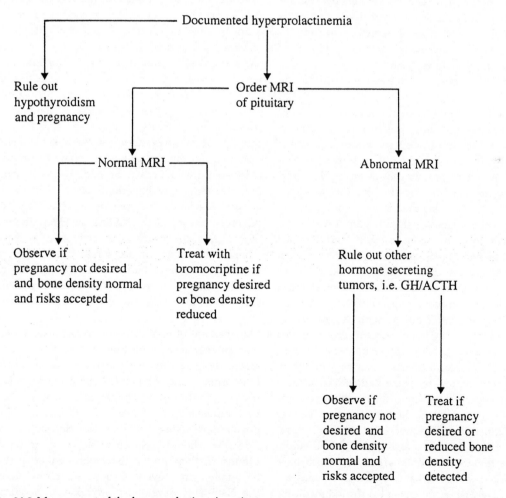

Fig. 24.2 Management of the hyperprolactinemic patient.

CHAPTER 24

with hyperprolactinemia involve only the lactotrophs. On the other hand other supersellar lesions that provoke hyperprolactinemia by interfering with dopamine production can secrete growth hormone, adrenocorticotropic hormone, gonadotropin, or thyrotropin. When large pituitary lesions are found, these hormones should be measured. Remember that growth hormone levels are measured in the fasting state and its concentration should not exceed 5 mg/l. To assess if a borderline growth hormone value is significant, a fasting plasma somatomedin C concentration should also be measured or an oral glucose tolerance test administered. If either the somatomedin C level is elevated or 75–100 g of glucose fails to suppress growth hormone levels to less than 2 mg/l after 60 min, the rate of growth hormone secretion is likely to be abnormally high.

Adrenocorticotropic hormone-producing pituitary adenomas are unlikely to be present if cortisol secretion is normal. This can be verified by demonstrating that cortisol in a 24-hour urine collection is not elevated or that 1 mg of dexamethasone, administered at 11 p.m., suppresses cortisol to 5 µg/dl or less by 8 a.m. the following day.

Until recently, much attention was paid to the secretory capacity of the pituitary when stimulated or inhibited by gonadotropin-releasing hormone, TRH, L-dopa, and insulin. The current view, however, is that these challenge tests do not distinguish between hypothalamic and pituitary disorders and need not be performed on a routine basis. However, these tests are useful in assessing pituitary hormone reserve prior to instituting medical or surgical therapy.

How to treat a patient with a large pituitary mass is a decision made by a neurosurgeon and depends on the position of the tumor, its size, and its potential for growth. The principal concern is sudden loss of vision due to a hemorrhage, which is most likely to occur in large tumors, especially those that are cystic. When the latter are present, surgery is invariably advocated. Ninety percent are removed transsphenoidally, the rest by craniotomy. Unfortunately, the long-term results of surgery are disappointing, with tumors recurring and 80% of patients becoming hyperprolactinemic again within 5 years. Nevertheless, surgery is the best way to manage nonprolactin-secreting tumors that influence prolactin secretion by compressing the infundibulum and large tumors or tumors with cysts which have the potential to hemorrhage. When adenomas are not excessively large, the patient is treated medically

with 2-brom-α-ergocryptine (bromocriptine), an ergot-derived dopamine agonist or the soon-to-be-introduced quinoline-derived dopamine agonist currently referred to as CV205–502. When shrinking of the tumor is rapid, small infarcts can occur in the pituitary; these are recognized by MRI as an increase in bright signal. Fortunately, these infarcts are not associated with adverse effects and there is no reason to stop treatment if they occur. Shrinkage of tumors occurs within weeks or months. As a result scans need not be repeated more often than every 3–6 months. If shrinkage does not occur, surgery is considered.

Management of pregnant patients with microadenomas and macroadenomas

Whenever possible, surgery is to be avoided unless there is concern for sudden loss of vision. However, in pregnant patients there is an additional cause for concern since the pituitary increases approximately 70% in size in response to increased production of estrogen, and may encroach upon the optic chiasm. In almost all instances, even when there is loss of temporal vision, changes in vision and tumor size are transient and return to normal following delivery.

There are two approaches to the management of the pregnant patient with a macroadenoma. The patient can be treated with a dopamine agonist throughout her pregnancy but the possible adverse risks of dopamine agonist therapy throughout pregnancy are not known. Second, the patient can be followed closely with periodic visual field examinations, especially during her last trimester. The latter offers the advantage of avoiding the theoretic danger of exposing the developing fetal brain to chronic stimulation by a dopamine agonist. If vision worsens, bromocriptine or surgical intervention can be considered. Most patients, however, require neither since visual defects, if they occur, are transitory.

Management of patients with prolactin-secreting microadenomas and most nonthreatening macroadenomas, hyperprolactinemia secondary to other causes, and idiopathic hyperprolactinemia

In the presence of hyperprolactinemia caused by antihistamines, antianxiety medications with dopamine-blocking activities, or cimetidine, consideration should be given to stopping these medications if they inhibit ovulation, either partially or totally, since even oligoovulation can increase the chance of developing osteoporosis because of impaired estrogen production. For the same reason patients with hyperprolactinemia secondary to prolactin-secreting adenomas should be treated with bromocriptine if ovulation is not normal and pregnancy is desired. On the other hand, if a woman has a prolactin-secreting microadenoma, nonthreatening macroadenoma, or idiopathic hyperprolactinemia and does not desire to conceive and is amenorrheic, she should be advised of the potential risks of osteoporosis and cardiovascular disease if she maintains a persistent hypoestrogenic state. She should also be told that 30% of individuals with idiopathic hyperprolactinemia may experience a spontaneous complete or partial remission without treatment and that enlargement of microadenomas without treatment is rare.

FURTHER READING

Edwards CRW, Feek CM. Prolactinoma: a question of rational treatment. *Br Med J* 1981; 283: 1561–1562.

Haney AF, McCarty KS Jr, Hammond CB. Galactorrhea-amenorrhea and hyperprolactinemia associated with pituitary tumors of growth-hormone- and adrenocorticotropic-hormone-secreting cells: a report of two cases. *J Reprod Med* 1984; 29: 883–887.

Huang HK, Aberle DR, Lufkin R, Grant EG, Hanafee WN, Kangarloo H. Advances in medical imaging. *Ann Intern Med* 1990; 112: 203–220.

Martin TL, Kim M, Malarkey WB. The natural history of idiopathic hyperprolactinemia. *J Clin Endocrinol Metab* 1985; 60: 855–858.

Melmed S. Acromegaly. *N Engl J Med* 1990; 322: 966–977.

Molitch ME. Management of prolactinomas. *Annu Rev Med* 1989; 40: 225–232.

Molitch ME, Russell EJ. The pituitary "incidentaloma". *Ann Intern Med* 1990; 112: 925–931.

Newman CB, Hurley AM, Kleinberg DL. Effect of CV 205–502 in hyperprolactinaemic patients intolerant of bromocriptine. *Clin Endocrinol* 1989; 31: 391–400.

Reincke M, Allolio B, Saeger W, Menzel J, Winkelmann W. The 'incidentaloma' of the pituitary gland. *JAMA* 1990; 263: 2772–2776.

Serri O, Radio E, Beauregard H, Hardy J, Somma M. Recurrence of hyperprolactinemia after selective transsphenoidal adennomectomy in women with prolactinoma. *N Engl J Med* 1983; 309: 280–283.

Sisam DA, Sheehan JP, Sheeler LR. The natural history of untreated microprolactinomas. *Fertil Steril* 1987; 48: 67–71.

Stein AL, Levenick MN, Kletzky OA. Computed tomography versus magnetic resonance imaging for the evaluation of suspected pituitary adenomas. *Obstet Gynecol* 1989; 73: 824–826.

Weiss MH, Teal J, Gott P et al. Natural history of microprolactinomas: six-year follow-up. *Neurosurgery* 1983; 12: 180–183.

25

Cushing's syndrome

JOHN HARRINGTON & GEORGE BETZ

Cushing's syndrome is the clinical expression of inappropriate hypercortisolism. It is most frequently encountered by the gynecologist in patients presenting with menstrual disorders, particularly when associated with central obesity, hypertension, hirsutism, muscle weakness, acne, easy bruising, purple abdominal striae, hyperglycemia, or mental disorders. In many cases, oligo- or amenorrhea may precede more overt signs and symptoms of Cushing's syndrome by months to years. This disease is much more common in women than in men, and therefore the gynecologist has a unique opportunity to identify Cushing's syndrome at an early date by the relatively simple approach to be described in this chapter. Thus, the patient may be spared years of morbidity commonly experienced before a diagnosis of Cushing's syndrome is ultimately established.

PATHOPHYSIOLOGY

Corticosteroids promote the metabolism of protein precursors to carbohydrate as well as the storage of carbohydrate as glycogen. An excess of corticosteroids therefore would result in inappropriate catabolism of proteins in plasma, muscle, and other peripheral tissue to glucose. The resultant increase in serum glucose causes an increase in insulin concentration as well, which may be related to hirsutism seen in women with Cushing's syndrome. Increased glucocorticoids also cause increased fat deposition which appears to be related to increased caloric intake rather than a primary effect of cortisol.

A number of profound effects occurs as a function of the increased cortisol. Sodium retention and potassium excretion are enhanced, resulting in electrolyte abnormalities as well as hypertension. Renal calcium excretion is increased, which may contribute to osteoporosis in Cushing's patients. Large exogenous doses of corticosteroid or high endogenous levels caused by Cushing's syndrome prevent the normal inflammatory reaction to infection or foreign substances. Inflammatory reactions are decreased, perhaps by the blockade of the action of phospholipase A_2 on arachidonic acid. Additionally, increased cortisol levels may exert an effect by interference with immune cell proliferation.

The clinical picture reflects the biologic activity of increased cortisol secretion. The onset may be gradual or quite dramatic, occurring over several days. Alterations in the menstrual cycle are frequently the first symptom in women, though obviously not a very specific one. Weight gain is common, but also a nonspecific finding. More worrisome symptoms include loss of muscle strength, emotional disturbances, and bone pain which may reflect osteoporosis.

The physical examination also may reflect a number of effects of hypercortisolism. Fullness of the face associated with central obesity reflects increased fat deposition in these areas. Atrophic skin with increased transparency and capillary fragility may reflect diminished connective tissue strength as well as poor healing. Hirsutism and masculinization may also occur. In the face of menstrual disturbances, increasing hirsutism, and a number of these other symptoms, an evaluation for Cushing's syndrome should be considered.

DIAGNOSTIC SCREENING

In order to diagnose Cushing's syndrome, the first step is to establish hypercortisolism. Once confirmed, the diagnostic process will be directed at establishing the pathophysiologic origin of the abnormality. While the excess cortisol is always secreted from the adrenal gland, the origin from the abnormality can be at the level of the adrenal gland itself or, rather, due to excess adrenocorticotropic hormone (ACTH) production at the level of the pituitary gland or from an ectopic source of ACTH. Therefore, the diagnostic discrimination will be accomplished by assessing ACTH levels as well as the suppressibility of cortisol secretion.

Screening for Cushing's syndrome should be performed in women whose symptoms as previously described make the clinician suspicious of hypercortisolism. The ideal screening test requires that it be easy to perform, have a very low false-negative rate, and be relatively inexpensive. The commonly described overnight dexamethasone suppression test fulfills these requirements. The test is performed by giving 1 mg of dexamethasone orally at 11 p.m. and obtaining a plasma cortisol at 8 a.m. the following morning. In the normal patient, morning cortisol will be suppressed to 5 μg/dl or less. There are no significant side-effects of the overnight dexamethasone suppression test, and it is well tolerated by virtually all patients. However, there will be a number of false-positive tests among patients who are obese, alcoholic, chronically ill, depressed, or suffering from a variety of emotional problems such as anorexia nervosa. In addition, treatment with some medications may cause false-positive results as well. Anticonvulsants such as phenytoin, phenobarbital, and primidone may alter dexamethasone metabolism and produce a false-positive result. Estrogen treatment may also produce false-positive values due to estrogen-induced changes in binding proteins. If a patient has a normal dexamethasone suppression test but clinical suspicion of Cushing's syndrome persists, or if the clinician is concerned that the manifestations of Cushing's syndrome are intermittent in expression, a repeat dexamethasone suppression test could be considered.

An alternative to the overnight dexamethasone suppression test is measurement of 24-hour urinary free cortisol. This test is a bit more cumbersome than the overnight dexamethasone suppression test, but may be the best discriminator of Cushing's syndrome. Normal 24-hour urinary free cortisol is less than 100 μg. Values higher than 100 μg are highly suspicious for Cushing's syndrome. There are very few reasons for false positives using this test. The additional assessment of 17-hydroxycorticoids or 17-ketosteroids along with the urinary free cortisol is not likely to be of significant benefit in the diagnosis of Cushing's syndrome.

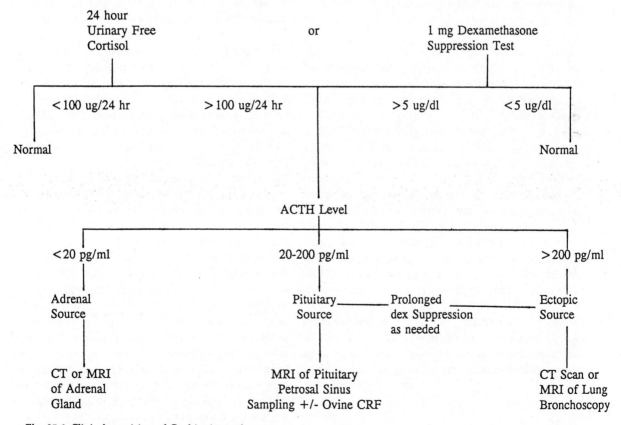

Fig. 25.1 Clinical suspicion of Cushing's syndrome.

CHAPTER 25

ETIOLOGY OF CUSHING'S SYNDROME

Once the diagnosis of Cushing's syndrome has been established, the underlying cause must be determined. Cushing's disease, or excess pituitary ACTH secretion, is responsible for 68% of cases of Cushing's syndrome. Excess ACTH from a pituitary adenoma is responsible for 40% of cases while pituitary hyperplasia due to increased hypothalamic corticotropin-releasing factor (CRF) production is responsible for the other 28%. The female to male ratio is 8:1. In general, hypercortisolism due to Cushing's disease is partially suppressible. Therefore, higher, more prolonged doses of dexamethasone than the simple 1 mg overnight suppression may well be useful in the diagnostic schema which follows.

Cushing's syndrome is a result of excess secretion of cortisol independently from the adrenal gland in 17% of cases. An adrenal adenoma is the cause of approximately 9% of cases while adrenal carcinomas are the etiology of Cushing's syndrome of approximately 8% of cases. Macro- or micronodular adenomatous hyperplasia of the adrenal glands represents an extremely rare cause of Cushing's syndrome. Adrenal tumors may produce other active hormones and therefore may be associated with virilization or, rarely, feminization, though adrenal carcinomas are less likely to be endocrinologically active than adenomas. Patients with Cushing's syndrome from an adrenal source would present with suppressed levels of ACTH.

Excess cortisol secretion from the adrenal gland due to ectopic ACTH production is the cause of approximately 15% of cases of Cushing's syndrome. Nonendocrine neoplasms are the most common source of ectopic ACTH and include oat cell carcinoma of the lung, thymoma, islet cell tumors of the pancreas, carcinoid tumors, medullary carcinoma of the thyroid gland, bronchial adenomas, and pheochromocytoma. Patients with ectopic sources of ACTH will usually have a high level of ACTH in association with hypercortisolism. Patients with ectopic ACTH production frequently present with debilitating illness rather than the other more common symptoms of Cushing's disease. This is likely due to the preeminent nature of their underlying tumor rather than the manifestations of hypercortisolism.

DIAGNOSTIC STRATEGY

The first step in determining which of the previously described etiologies is causing the observed hypercortisolism is determination of serum ACTH. Values less than 20 pg/ml would suggest that hypercortisolism is secondary to adrenal disease. Because ACTH has a relatively short half-life and is secreted episodically, several samples may be required to feel confident as to the ACTH level. It is important to check with the clinical laboratory prior to drawing an ACTH level because the radioimmunoassay is difficult and may be subject to temperature and type of collection tube, among other factors. Values between 20 and 200 pg/ml are more commonly associated with Cushing's disease, while patients with ectopic ACTH syndrome will have values greater than 200 pg/ml in 60–70% of cases. However, there is commonly some degree of overlap, particularly between patients with ectopic production of ACTH and those with Cushing's disease.

When the source of hypercortisolism appears to be the adrenal gland, the next diagnostic step should be a computed tomography (CT) scan or magnetic resonance imaging (MRI) of the adrenals. The presence of an adrenal mass virtually confirms the diagnosis of an adrenal source. Furthermore, the scan is likely able to differentiate hyperplasia from an adrenal tumor, though does not easily distinguish an adenoma from the rare carcinoma. Generally, levels of adrenal androgens such as dehydroepiandrosterone sulfate are normal or low in the case of adenomas, and are more likely to be elevated in patients with carcinoma.

The first step in attempting to distinguish Cushing's disease from the ectopic ACTH syndrome may well be a pituitary MRI, which is preferable to a CT scan. If a pituitary adenoma is identified, the diagnosis of Cushing's disease is established. However, absence of an identifiable mass on MRI does not exclude the possibility of Cushing's disease. Alternative methods to try to differentiate Cushing's disease from ectopic ACTH production include the prolonged dexamethasone suppression test, petrosal sinus sampling, or ovine corticotropin stimulation. Patients with Cushing's disease will generally have partially suppressible ACTH with prolonged dexamethasone suppression. Dexamethasone 2.0 mg is administered orally every 6 hours for 48 hours. Plasma cortisol is obtained at the end of 2 days and will be suppressed to 10 µg/dl or less in most patients with Cushing's disease but is less likely to be suppressed in patients with ectopic ACTH production. Urine 24-hour free cortisol is also likely to be suppressed, but the values most suggestive of Cushing's disease are not well established. Bilateral petrosal sinus blood sampling can also be performed in difficult cases to distinguish these two entities. This procedure should only be performed by a highly skilled invasive radiologist. The petrosal sinuses should be sampled simultaneously for ACTH levels. A gradient associated with high levels of ACTH suggests both a pituitary source of ACTH as well as the likely side affected. Ovine CRF can also be administered after the baseline ACTH sampling. Patients with Cushing's disease will likely respond significantly to CRF administration, while patients with ectopic ACTH production generally exhibit only a limited response.

Should the initial studies suggest an ectopic ACTH source, a thorough evaluation to identify the tumor should be initiated. The first step would likely be a CT scan or MRI of the mediastinum and lungs. Bronchoscopy may also be indicated. If no tumor is found, one should begin to search for other potential ectopic sources, as described earlier in this chapter.

CONCLUSIONS

Cushing's syndrome is characterized by excessive production of cortisol from the adrenal gland. The first step in diagnosis is clinical suspicion. The diagnostic strategy is first to establish the presence of hypercortisolism and then to pinpoint the origin of the problem. While it is highly advisable to coordinate the diagnostic testing with a medical endocrinologist, it is incumbent on the gynecologist to understand the decision and to initiate the process in an efficient and thoughtful manner.

FURTHER READING

Aron DC, Findling JW, Tyrrell JB. Cushing's syndrome. *Endocrinol Metab Clin* 1987; 16: 705–731.

Crapo L. Cushing's syndrome: a review of diagnostic tests. *Metaboism* 1979; 28: 955–977.

Dunlap NE, Gizzle WE, Siegel AL. Cushing's syndrome. *Arch Pathol Lab Med* 1985; 222–229.

Findling JW. Eutopic or ectopic adrenocorticotropic hormone-dependent Cushing's syndrome? A diagnostic dilemma. *Mayo Clin Proc* 1990; 65: 1377–1380.

Fuhrman S. Appropriate laboratory testing in the screening and work-up of Cushing's syndrome. *Am J Clin Pathol* 1988; 90: 345–350.

Gold EM. The Cushing's syndrome: changing views of diagnosis and treatment. *Ann Intern Med* 1979; 90: 825–844.

Schteingart DE. Cushing's syndrome. *Endocrinol Metab Clin* 1969; 18: 311–337.

26

Primary hypopituitarism

JULIA V. JOHNSON & DANIEL RIDDICK

OVERVIEW

Primary hypopituitarism results from the loss of pituicytes and decreased secretion of one or more of the trophic hormones produced by the pituitary gland (Table 26.1). Hypopituitarism is an uncommon disorder, but the practitioner should be familiar with its diagnosis and treatment. Because several causes of pituitary insufficiency are associated with pregnancy, the gynecologist has the opportunity to diagnose the disorder early in its course. Also, the patient with hypopituitarism may present with amenorrhea as the initial complaint, since the loss of gonadotropin secretion typically precedes the loss of thyroid-stimulating hormone (TSH) and adrenocorticotropic hormone (ACTH).

Unfortunately, the diagnosis of pituitary insufficiency can be difficult. The clinical presentation of hypopituitarism is variable, depending on the extent of damage to each cell type (Table 26.1). The onset of symptoms is often insidious, with the diagnosis occurring years after the precipitating event. It also may be difficult to differentiate primary pituitary disease and secondary hypopituitarism caused by the loss of hypothalamic regulation. It is the purpose of this chapter to facilitate the care of the patient with

hypopituitarism by reviewing the etiologies (Table 26.2), discussing possible clinical presentations, and outlining methods of diagnosis and treatment.

PATHOPHYSIOLOGY

Pituitary tumors

The most frequent cause of pituitary insufficiency, accounting for more than 50% of cases, is pituitary neoplasms. The most common tumor is the benign adenoma, although metastatic lesions or extrasellar neoplasms may also affect pituitary function. Because pituitary metastases from the breast, lung, or gastrointestinal tract occur in up to 25% of patients with these primary tumors, it is important to monitor

Table 26.1 Trophic hormones produced by the pituitary gland

Target organ	Pituitary cell type	Pituitary hormone
Ovary	Gonadotropes	Luteinizing hormone follicle-stimulating hormone
Thyroid	Thyrotropes	Thyrotropin
Adrenal	Corticotropes	Corticotropin
Breast	Lactotropes	Prolactin
—	Somatotropes	Growth hormone

Table 26.2 Etiologies of hypopituitarism

Pituitary tumors
  Compression of pituitary or stalk
  Apoplexy (bleeding into the tumor)

Vascular disorders/ischemic necrosis
  Sheehan's syndrome
  Diabetes mellitus
  Other systemic diseases (temporal arteritis, sickle cell disease, arteriosclerosis)

Immunologic (lymphocytic hypophysitis)

Infectious
  Syphilis
  Tuberculosis
  Fungal

Infiltrative
  Sarcoidosis
  Granulomatous hypophysitis
  Hemochromatosis
  Histiocytosis X

Iatrogenic
  Surgical removal or damage to stalk
  Irradiation to nasopharynx or sella

these patients for signs of hypopituitarism [1]. Suprasellar tumors, such as craniopharyngioma, meningioma, or dysgerminoma, cause secondary hypopituitarism by destroying the mediobasal hypothalamus, median eminence, or the pituitary stalk. Benign adenomas cause hypopituitarism by direct compression of pituicytes or by suprasellar extension with compression of the hypothalamus or stalk.

Hypopituitarism in patients with benign lesions usually has a slow onset, with laboratory evidence of hormone deficiency preceding clinical features by several years. Up to 75% of macroadenomas (>10 mm) are associated with an impairment in hormone production [1]. Fortunately, reduction of tumor mass may relieve pressure on the stalk and the pituicytes and result in resumption of pituitary function.

In contrast, an acute loss of function occurs with bleeding into the pituitary adenoma, a condition called pituitary apoplexy. Pituitary adenomas are five times more likely to have bleeding than other central nervous system (CNS) tumors. Typically, apoplexy occurs in macroadenomas; however, it is reported in microadenomas and nontumorous glands. Predisposing factors for pituitary apoplexy include pregnancy, increased intracranial pressure, trauma, coagulation disorders, upper respiratory tract infections (coughing), and radiation therapy of tumors [2].

Vascular abnormalities

Ischemic necrosis of the pituitary can occur during the puerperium, and accounts for approximately 25% of adult-onset hypopituitarism. Sheehan postulated that obstetric hemorrhage and shock may lead to arteriolar spasm with stasis of capillary blood and eventual venous thrombosis causing necrosis of the pituitary [3]. It is known that the pituicytes hypertrophy during pregnancy, making the gland more vulnerable to ischemic damage. Sheehan's syndrome is classically described in women with severe postpartum bleeding, but can occur following a normal delivery. In patients with severe hemorrhage, 3.4% will develop pituitary insufficiency with an occurrence of one in 10 000 pregnancies. As with other causes of hypopituitarism, Sheehan's syndrome has a slow onset, with diagnosis occurring up to 15 years after the pregnancy.

Ischemia and subsequent hypopituitarism may also occur in other situations. Patients with diabetes mellitus, temporal arteritis, sickle cell disease, and arteriosclerosis are at risk for ischemic necrosis and loss of pituitary function.

Immunologic and infectious diseases

Lymphocytic hypophysitis is a rare case of pituitary insufficiency with only 22 cases confirmed by biopsy or autopsy. However, this disorder occurs almost exclusively during pregnancy or the immediate postpartum period, making it of interest to the gynecologist. As with other autoimmune disorders, the gland is infiltrated by lymphocytes and plasma cells with interstitial fibrosis. Antipituitary antibodies have been identified in some cases, but are not consistent. Other autoimmune diseases may be associated, most commonly Hashimoto's thyroiditis.

Infectious diseases may rarely cause the destruction of the pituitary. The most commonly associated infections include syphilis, tuberculosis, malaria, fungal diseases, and CNS abscesses or meningitis.

Infiltrative disorders

Although sarcoidosis is a rare cause of hypopituitarism, up to one-third of women with extrapulmonary disease will have hypothalamic or pituitary involvement. The posterior pituitary is commonly involved, unlike other causes of primary hypopituitarism. Granulomatous hypophysitis, in which the gland is infiltrated by giant cells and plasma cells, is another cause of hypopituitarism. As with lymphocytic hypophysitis, this disorder occurs almost exclusively in women. Hemochromatosis, an iron storage disease which is autosomal recessive, can cause abnormalities in gonadotropin secretion in up to 25% of patients with this disorder. Finally, histiocytosis X (Hand−Schüller−Christian disease) is a granulomatous disease which can cause damage to both the hypothalamus and pituitary.

Iatrogenic causes

Although it is useful for the clinician to be aware of unusual causes of hypopituitarism, such as immunologic and infiltrative disorders, surgery and radiotherapy are more common causes of hypopituitarism. Surgical removal of pituitary macroadenomas results in loss of one or more of the trophic hormones in 10−30% of the cases. Diabetes insipidus occurs in approximately 15% of patients immediately following surgery, but rarely persists for more than 6 months. Hypopituitarism is even more common after radiation therapy, occurring in 55% of those without previous surgery and up to 67% of patients with both surgical and radiation therapy.

CHAPTER 26

CLINICAL PRESENTATION

Acute loss of pituitary function

Pituitary apoplexy commonly presents with CNS symptoms and acute pituitary insufficiency. The typical history is a sudden, severe retroorbital headache followed by nausea and vomiting and decreased visual acuity. Visual field cuts, extraocular ophthalmoplegia, meningeal signs, and loss of consciousness may follow. Upward extension of the bleed can compress the hypothalamus causing hypotension, abnormal temperature regulation, and abnormal respirations, and compression of the internal carotid artery can result in seizures or hemiplegia. Impingement on the fifth cranial nerve can cause facial pain and sensory loss, and damage to the trigeminal nerve can cause Horner's syndrome (unilateral ptosis, miosis, and anhidrosis). Up to 69% of patients will have resulting hypopituitarism. An acute loss of adrenal function can cause electrolyte imbalances, hypotension, and shock.

This condition mimics other CNS disorders, including meningitis or abscess, subarachnoid or intracerebral bleeding, or cerebrovascular accident. The diagnosis can usually be made by computed tomography (CT) scan or magnetic resonance imaging (MRI); however, immediate treatment with hydrocortisone (100 mg intravenously every 8 hours) may be life-saving. Transsphenoidal decompression has recently been recommended to prevent further extension of the bleed and increase the chance for restoration of pituitary function.

Subacute loss of pituitary function

With most conditions causing hypopituitarism, the onset of symptoms is insidious. Even with pituitary apoplexy, the patient may present long after the event with nonspecific complaints. Constitutional symptoms such as fatigue, weight loss, depression, and general malaise are frequent complaints. Because the clinical presentation varies with the specific trophic hormones lost, it is valuable to consider each deficiency as a separate entity.

Gonadotropins

Clinical symptoms of gonadotropin deficiency may be the first sign of pituitary failure. Women commonly present with secondary amenorrhea. Breast and genital atrophy may also be present if hypoestrogenism has been prolonged. Loss of libido is commonly reported. These patients do not have bleeding after progestins and have low or undetectable levels of luteinizing hormone (LH) and follicle-stimulating hormone (FSH).

Corticotropin

Patients with ACTH deficiency have symptoms which are similar to Addison's disease, including weakness, lethargy, postural hypotension, and anorexia. However, unlike Addison's they are depigmented due to a lack of melanotropin. Loss of adrenal androgens results in the loss of pubic and axillary hair. Aldosterone secretion by the renin–angiotensin mechanism decreases the risk of Addisonian-type crisis in these patients. However, severe illness or stress can precipitate an adrenal crisis, which if unrecognized may be fatal. Serum levels of both cortisol and ACTH are low in these patients.

Thyrotropin

TSH deficiency results in the same symptoms as primary thyroid disease. Patients will have cold intolerance, dry skin and hair, pallor, bradycardia, mental slowing, hoarseness, weakness, and constipation. Myxedema is rare. The reflexes are slowed and the thyroid is usually atrophic. Thiodothyronine (T_3), thyroxine (T_4), and TSH levels are low.

Prolactin

Deficiency of prolactin is clinically evident only in the postpartum period, when failure to lactate may be an early sign of pituitary necrosis. In some cases, however, prolactin levels may be elevated. When the pituitary stalk is compressed, dopamine is not transported by the portal system, and hyperprolactinemia and galactorrhea may occur. Prolactin-secreting adenomas are the most common hormone-producing tumors. With large prolactinomas, prolactin may be secreted in large amounts, while compression of the pituitary causes deficiencies in trophic hormones.

Growth hormone

Although a deficiency of growth hormone in children is typically the first clinical sign of pituitary failure, there are few symptoms of growth hormone deficiency in the adult. Fasting hypoglycemia, which is worsened in the case of concomitant ACTH deficiency, may suggest a lack of growth hormone secretion.

Antidiuretic hormone (vasopressin)

Loss of posterior pituitary function is uncommon for

most etiologies of primary hypopituitarism. However, diabetes insipidus has been reported in rare cases of Sheehan's syndrome and occurs following extensive surgery or radiation therapy. The symptoms of polydipsia, polyuria, and dehydration indicate antidiuretic hormone deficiency.

LABORATORY EVALUATION

In primary hypopituitarism, low levels of trophic hormones, with the exception of prolactin, are expected. The gynecologist who evaluates a patient for secondary amenorrhea may first suspect hypopituitarism or hypothalamic dysfunction in a patient with low levels of FSH and LH (Fig. 26.1). Unfortunately, these low values overlap with normal basal levels and a single low value may simply reflect a nadir between normal pulses. For this reason, provocative testing is required to evaluate pituitary function [4].

To evaluate for more than one hormone deficiency, a sequential testing method may be advantageous [5]. This type of testing allows the clinician to evaluate the secretion of several hormones during a single series of blood draws. Because hormone deficiencies may precede clinical symptoms, complete testing of pituitary function is reasonable in all patients with suspected hypopituitarism. A method for sequential testing, as well as procedures to evaluate individual hormone secretion, is described below.

Gonadotropin-releasing hormone (GnRH) stimulation test
This test evaluates the response of LH and FSH to

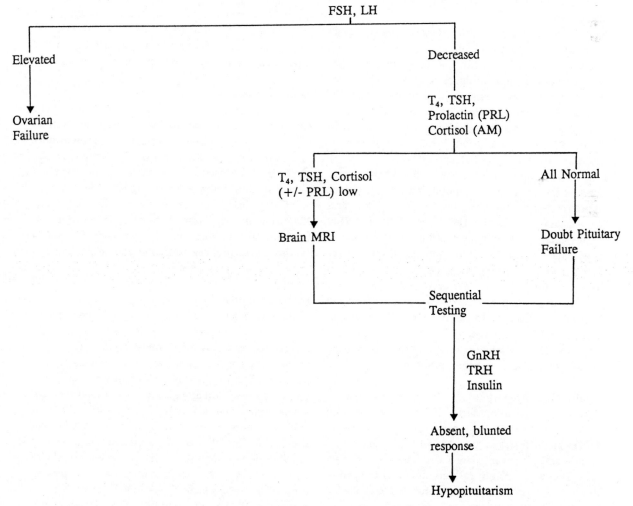

Fig. 26.1 Evaluation of primary hypopituitarism (secondary amenorrhea).

GnRH. GnRH 100 µg is administered intravenously and blood is obtained at 0, 30, 60, 90, and 120 min. In normal women during the proliferative phase the basal LH level will double at 30 min and FSH will increase 1.5 times at 60 min. During the luteal phase, there is a more pronounced response with an increase in LH and four to eight times the baseline, while FSH levels double. In patients with pituitary insufficiency there is no response of LH and FSH. Secondary hypopituitarism, caused by hypothalamic disease, results in blunted or absent response of LH and FSH. Further testing may aid in the differentiation of primary and secondary hypopituitarism. Repeat or pulsatile administration of GnRH will cause an elevation in gonadotropins in patients with hypothalamic disease, while women with pituitary disease will show no response.

Thyrotropin-releasing hormone (TRH) stimulation test

Low levels of (T$_4$) and TSH suggest hypothalamic or pituitary disease. Newer assays for TSH have increased sensitivity in the low range of the assay which improves its usefulness for diagnosing pituitary failure. These results can then be confirmed with a TSH stimulation test. TRH 500 µg is administered intravenously, and TSH levels are drawn at 0, 30, 60, 90, 120, and 180 min. When there is normal pituitary function, the TSH value will increase by 5 µu/ml to a value of 30 µu/ml by the 30-min blood draw. If there is primary hypopituitarism (secondary hypothyroidism), the basal level of TSH is low and there is no response to TRH. The additional TSH values, after the 30-min level, aid in the diagnosis of hypothalamic disease. In hypothalamic secondary hypothyroidism, the response to TRH is delayed to 60 or 120 min, with a slow return to basal levels.

Prolactin production can also be assessed with the TRH stimulation test. In response to TRH, prolactin levels should double within 30 min. Low basal prolactin values and a failure to respond to TRH indicate the loss of prolactin-secreting pituicytes.

Insulin challenge test

Corticotropin-releasing factor (CRF) has been used successfully to evaluate the decreased response of ACTH and cortisol in patients with primary hypopituitarism. However, ovine CRF is not widely available. Therefore, insulin or metyrapone is utilized to stimulate cortisol production. In the insulin challenge test, 0.1–0.2 u/kg of regular insulin is given intra-venously following an overnight fast, and cortisol levels are drawn at 0, 30, 45, 60, 90, and 120 min. The insulin-induced hypoglycemia stimulates ACTH release and an increase in cortisol of at least 10 µg/dl with a peak value of more than 20 µg/dl. If there is no increase in cortisol and a serum ACTH level of less than 10 ng/l, then pituitary or hypothalamic disease (secondary adrenal failure) is confirmed. Some authors have suggested that a low morning cortisol level, accompanied by a decreased ACTH value, is sufficient to diagnosis secondary adrenal failure.

The insulin challenge test also evaluates the production of growth hormone by the pituitary. Basal growth hormone levels are low in adults, and a challenge test using insulin, exercise, arginine, or L-dopa is required to evaluate secretion of growth hormone. To optimize this test, a decrease in serum glucose of 50% or a value <40 mg/dl should be documented. The normal response of growth hormone is an increase to >7 ng/ml at 60 min, while patients with hypopituitarism will have no response. Growth hormone-releasing hormone also been used experimentally to test growth hormone secretion.

Sequential testing

If panhypopituitarism is suspected, these three stimulation tests can be combined. Baseline levels of FSH, LH, TSH, prolactin, cortisol, and growth hormone are drawn at the onset of the testing. Hypoglycemia is induced with 0.2 U/kg of intravenous regular insulin, followed in 2 hours by 150 µg GnRH and 500 ug TRH. Blood is obtained at 20, 30, 60, and 120 min after each phase of the stimulation protocol. Utilizing this protocol in women with Sheehan's syndrome, all pituitary hormones can be evaluated in this single sequential test [5].

Posterior pituitary

Abnormal secretion of antidiuretic hormone is evaluated by water deprivation. This test is potentially dangerous, and 2 µg of desmopressin (DDAVP) is given at the conclusion of the test to prevent further fluid loss. During the 8-hour test no water is given, and the body weight and plasma and urine osmolality are monitored at 4, 6, 7, and 8 hours. A loss of weight >3% indicates excessive dehydration and the test should be discontinued. In a patient with normal antidiuretic hormone secretion, the urine osmolality should increase to >600 mosmol/kg, but plasma osmolality will remain below 300 mosmol/kg. In patients with diabetes insipidus the plasma osmo-

Table 26.3 Replacement dosages for pituitary hormones

Drug	Dosage schedule
Adrenal replacement	
Hydrocortisone	20 mg in a.m.; 10 mg in p.m.
Prednisone	25 mg in a.m.; 12.5 mg in p.m.
Fluorohydrocortisone	0.05−0.1 mg daily
Thyroid replacement	
L-thyroxine	0.10−0.20 mg daily
Gonadal replacement	
Conjugated estrogens	0.625−1.25 mg/day, 25 days/month
Medroxyprogesterone acetate	10 mg/day, 12 days/month
Posterior pituitary	
Desmopressin (DDAVP)	0.1−0.4 ml/b.i.d.

lality is >300 mosmol/kg and the urine osmolality remains dilute at <270 mosmol/kg.

Radiologic evaluation

When pituitary or hypothalamic disorder is suspected, the sellar and parasellar region should be examined by CT scan or MRI. These studies allow detailed evaluation of the pituitary and can aid in the diagnosis of tumors and apoplexy. Although CT scanning, utilizing narrow sections, provides excellent visualization of the pituitary, MRI may be superior for evaluation of the parasellar area. The choice between CT scan and MRI may depend on the experience of the radiologist with each technique.

TREATMENT

As with the clinical presentation and the diagnostic testing, the treatment of primary hypopituitarism depends on the extent of pituitary injury and the specific hormone deficiencies. The usual replacement dosages for pituitary hormones are listed in Table 26.3.

In some situations, hypopituitarism may be reversible. When the pituitary is compressed by a pituitary tumor, surgical removal results in a return of thyroid function in 57%, adrenal function in 38%, and gonadal function 32%. Prolactin-secreting macroadenomas may be successfully treated with bromocriptine alone. The patient should be placed on bromocriptine gradually, as it commonly causes postural hypotension, headache, and nausea. A dose of 2.5 mg is usually given at bedtime initially, starting a second 2.5 mg dose in the morning only after the evening dose is tolerated. Prolactin levels are used to gauge the success of bromocriptine, and if the patient remains hyperprolactinemic, the dose can be increased slowly until euprolactinemia is achieved.

If pregnancy is desired, ovulation induction can usually be accomplished with human menopausal gonadotropin (hMG) and human chorionic gonadotropin (hCG). Ovulation with hMG typically begins early in the cycle (cycle day 2 or 3), with the patient receiving 150 U/day intramuscularly. Follicular growth is monitored by ultrasound and estradiol levels, and the dosage of hMG is adjusted accordingly. When one or more follicles are between 16−18 mm in size, hCG is given to induce ovulation.

CONCLUSIONS

Primary hypopituitarism is a rare disorder which has multiple etiologies. The clinical presentation is variable and may be insidious, with patients presenting up to 15 years following the precipitating event. However, by utilizing the proper diagnostic procedures, the gynecologist can identify women with this disorder early during the course of the disease. With proper treatment, these patients can return to their former state of health, including normal ovulation and pregnancy.

REFERENCES

1 Kannan CR. *The Pituitary Gland*. New York: Plenum Medical, 1987; 423−442.
2 Reid RL, Quigley ME, Yen SSC. Pituitary apoplexy: a review. *Arch Neurol* 1985; 42: 712.
3 Sheehan HL. The pathogenesis of postpartum necrosis of

the anterior lobe of the pituitary gland. *Acta Endocrinol* 1961; 37: 479.

4 Schlaff WD. Dynamic testing in reproductive endocrinology. *Fertil Steril* 1986; 45: 589.

5 DiZerega G, Kletsky OA, Mishell DR. Diagnosis of Sheehan's syndrome using a sequential pituitary stimulation test. *Am J Obstet Gynecol* 1978; 132: 348.

Kallmann's syndrome

DANIEL KENIGSBERG

INTRODUCTION

Kallmann's syndrome has both a general and specific connotation in describing general conditions of gonadotropin-releasing hormone (GnRH) deficiency or a particular cluster of anomalies associated with primary eunuchoidism described by Kallmann and colleagues in 1944 [1].

The familial occurrence of (hypogonadotropic) hypogonadism associated with anosmia, color blindness, synkinesia, and mental defect is the classic Kallmann syndrome. Interestingly, anosmia, or lack of smell, was not found in the absence of gonadal deficiency in the original study of this disorder. This disorder was found in both sexes, but the male to female ratio was 11:1, and Kallmann's syndrome is more often listed under disorders of male hypogonadism for this reason.

Hypogonadotropic hypogonadism, or the lack of function of the testis or ovary secondary to the lack of pituitary and or hypothalamic trophic hormones, is also sometimes generally termed Kallmann's syndrome. Whether such deficiencies arise from an inborn error of hypothalamic organization and pituitary connection or damage to the hypothalamic pituitary system in prepubertal life, the manifestations of a eunuchoid or apubertal individual with potentially competent pituitary and gonadal function will result. Beyond the achievement of puberty, a similar situation can be recreated by the administration of a long-acting GnRH analog or by conditions of secondary hypothalamic dysfunction such as anorexia nervosa where shutdown of GnRH and its resultant effects cause cessation of gonadal function and even a regression of secondary sexual characteristics. Technically, these conditions are not Kallmann's syndrome but one must recognize the similarities.

PATHOPHYSIOLOGY

Gross anatomy has shown disorders of the olfactory bulbs associated with Kallmann's syndrome and Schwanzel-Eukada and coworkers have demonstrated a failure of GnRH-containing cells to migrate from the olfactory placode to the hypothalamus and preoptic area [2].

Various patterns of inheritance have been described for this obvious familial condition, and kindreds have been described with autosomal dominant, autosomal resessive, and X-linked forms of inheritance [3]. A specific deletion of the X-chromosome (Xp22.3) has been located in some cases. However, father-to-son transmission is also described.

Aside from a deficiency of GnRH, normal anterior pituitary function [4] and posterior pituitary function [5], have been demonstrated in these patients.

LABORATORY AND CLINICAL FINDINGS

The incidence of Kallmann's syndrome is one in 10 000 male births. In the absence of other obvious congenital anomalies, the presentation may be at the age of puberty — which is absent. Secondary to a lack of epiphyseal closure of the long bones, the patient's stature tends toward increased limb length relative to trunk size and the classic tall eunuchoid appearance. Variable associated findings include color blindness, deafness, cleft lip and palate, cerebellar seizures, and cardiac anomalies. Resultant associations can be cryptorchidism and an identical gonadal histology to a 7-month-old fetus. Blood levels of sex steroids, testosterone, or estradiol as well as gonadotropins, follicle-stimulating hormone (FSH), and luteinizing hormone (LH), are all extremely low.

The diagnosis can be assured by the demonstration of olfactory defect, but in the presence of olfaction

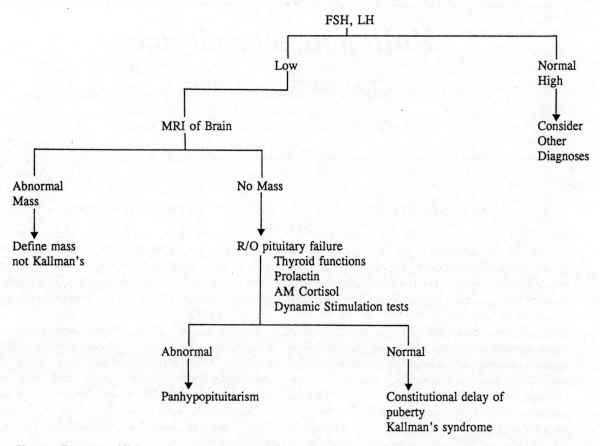

CHAPTER 27

Fig. 27.1 Diagnosis of Kallmann's syndrome (primary amenorrhea).

the diagnosis of isolated gonadotropin deficiency (IGD) is still possible.

In the absence of gross congenital anomalies, the major differential diagnosis for Kallmann's syndrome is that of delayed puberty. The lack of secondary sexual characteristics by the age of 16 in a female or

18 in a male is certainly a cause for investigation. Various strategies may be adopted for the elucidation of such cases:

1 *Nocturnal gonadotropins*. In normal puberty, even when it is delayed, if there is to be secretion of FSH and LH it will first occur in the late evening as

Table 27.1 Hypothalamic/anterior pituitary function tests* [6]

Hypothalamic releaser (i.r.)	Pituitary response	
GnRH (100 µg)	LH	13.9 ± 1.9 mIU/ml (at 30 min)
	FSH	3.0 ± 0.2 mIU/ml
CRH (1 µg/kg)	ACTH	40 ± 6.6 pg/ml (at 60 min)
GHRH (1 µg/kg)	GH	55 ± 20 ng/ml (at 60 min)
TRH (200 µg)	TSH	15 ± 2.1 µU/ml (at 30 min)
	Prolactin	92 ± 15 ng/ml (at 15 min)

GnRH, Gonadotropin-releasing hormone; LH, luteinizing hormone; FSH, follicle-stimulating hormone; CRH, corticotropin-releasing hormone; ACTH, adrenocorticotropic hormone; GHRH, growth hormone-releasing hormone; GH, growth hormone; TRH, thyrotropin-releasing hormone; TSH, thyroid-stimulating hormone.
Note that the minimum FSH rise to GnRH was obtained with combination injection.
* Values in women.

opposed to during the day. The measurement of FSH and LH at multiple times throughout the night may detect the onset of pubertal process, whereas extremely low levels of FSH and LH, even late at night, suggest an intrinsic deficiency of these hormones.

2 *Thyrotropin-releasing hormone (TRH) tests in the female.* In the absence of previous estrogen exposure, there will not be a brisk prolactin response with the administration of TRH (Table 27.1).

3 *GnRH tests.* Administration of GnRH in a one-shot bolus will provoke LH and FSH release in a primed or potentially near pubertal individual, whereas in the individual with true hypogonadotropism, an initial exposure to GnRH will not provoke an FSH and LH response (Table 27.1).

CORRELATES FOR FEMALE REPRODUCTIVE ENDOCRINOLOGY AND TREATMENT

True cases of Kallmann's syndrome are rare and predominantly occur in males. However, there are important lessons to be learned for the practice of reproductive endocrinology and infertility.

Syndromes of anovulation and resultant amenorrhea can be classified into general categories which for the purposes of discussion we will term hypothalamic and peripheral. Peripheral ovulatory disorders in the current state of knowledge can be pituitary, adrenal, or ovarian in origin, and most classically and commonly are exemplified by the polycystic ovarian syndrome. This is well discussed in other sections of the text. Hypothalamic anovulation and amenorrhea result from a hypogonadotropic state, FSH and LH deficiency, associated with disorders in GnRH secretion.

Hypothalamic disorders can be characterized by stress, such as exercise-induced amenorrhea or starvation as characterized by anorexia nervosa. There appears to be an entire spectrum ranging from total absence or regression of puberty to more subtle postpubertal disorders of low FSH and LH without other obvious abnormalities and metabolic function or body proportion. The final common pathway results in a low estrogenic state which for the purposes of skeletal well-being must, at a minimum, be supplemented with estrogens. Ovulation induction agents are necessary for the purposes of reproduction. Since there are no long-lasting stimulatory effects

beyond their given month of use, ovulation induction agents should be reserved for those cases in which fertility is desired. Antiestrogens, such as clomiphene citrate or tamoxifen, are not effective in the absence of endogenous estrogens, and therefore are not effective in these states. This leaves the alternatives of pituitary or hypothalamic replacement hormones; respectively human menopausal gonadotropins or pulsatile GnRH pump.

The use of human menopausal gonadotropins is described elsewhere in this book and is classically very effective in patients with hypothalamic disorders or even true Kallmann's syndrome. More recently, GnRH therapy has become available, but rather than requiring daily injections for perhaps 1–2 weeks per month, as is the case with human menopausal gonadotropin, GnRH administration requires a continuous pulsatile infusion pump administered either subcutaneously or intravenously for several months. GnRH therapy can take 6–12 months for full sexual development when starting from a point of total pubertal absence, but may take a shorter period of time in less absolute cases or where there has been some previous priming.

General prognosis for fertility is excellent in patients whose only fertility problem is hypothalamic amenorrhea or even total Kallmann's syndrome.

REFERENCES

1 Kallmann FJ, Schoenfeld WA, Barrera SE. Genetic aspects of primary eunuchoidism. *Am J Ment Defic* 1944; XLVIII: 203–235.
2 Schwanzel-Fukuda M, Bick D, Pfaff DW. Luteinizing hormone (LHRH)–expressing cells do not migrate normally in an inherited hypogonadal (Kallmann) syndrome. *Brain Res* 1989; 6: 311–326.
3 Bardin CW. Pituitary-testicular axis. In: Yen SCC, Jaffe RB, eds. *Reproductive Endocrinology Physiology, Pathophysiology and Clinical Management.* Philadelphia: WB Saunders, 1978.
4 Yea J, Rebar RW, Liu JH, Yen SS. Pituitary function in isolated gonadatropin deficiency. *Clin Endocrinol* 1989; 31: 375–387.
5 Thompson CJ, White MC, Baylis PH. Osmoregulation of thirst of vasopressin secretion in Kallmann's syndrome. *Clin Endocrinol* 1989; 30: 539–547.
6 Sheldon WR, DeBold CR, Evans WS *et al.* Sequential intravenous administration of four hypothalamic releasing hormones as a combined anterior pituitary function test in normal subjects. *Endocrinol Metab* 1985; 60: 623–630.

28

Sheehan's syndrome

OSCAR A. KLETZKY

Pituitary necrosis secondary to severe postpartum hypotension and shock due to hemorrhage is known as Sheehan's syndrome [1]. This cause of hypopituitarism is a rare complication of modern obstetrics (one in every 10 000 deliveries); however, it still is an important obstetric complication in developing countries [2,3]. Depending on the degree of vascular insult and extension of pituitary cell damage a variable degree of hypopituitary function can be seen, varying from a single hormone abnormality to complete panhypopituitarism [4,5].

PATHOGENESIS

The main blood supply to the anterior pituitary comes from the superior hypophyseal arteries which are branches of the internal carotids. The superior hypophyseal arteries anastomose at the upper portion of the pituitary stalk where they branch into elongated and coiled capillary loops, draining into the portal veins which empty into sinusoids of the anterior lobe. Although there is arterial communication between the anterior and posterior lobe, most of the posterior lobe blood supply comes from the inferior hypophyseal arteries. Both the anterior and posterior lobes drain into the cavernous sinus [6,7]. During pregnancy there is a significant hypertrophy and hyperplasia of the lactotropes due to the stimulatory effect of increasing levels of estrogen. Consequently, the anterior pituitary gland doubles in size during the course of pregnancy, thus increasing the need for high oxygen consumption and blood supply [8]. Under these circumstances the enlarged pituitary gland appears vulnerable to vasoconstriction and sudden ischemia which results from postpartum hemorrhage, hypotension, and shock. It is possible that severe disturbances or alterations of the clotting mechanism resulting in diffused intravascular coagulation of the portal vessels are also contributory factors in the development of the ischemic necrosis

[9]. The end-result is pituitary destruction with fibrosis developing later. Depending on the extent of tissue damage, these patients may also present with symptoms of posterior lobe damage. Post-mortem examinations have revealed a very frequent incidence of posterior pituitary lobe involvement as well as marked atrophy of mainly the supraoptic nuclei of the hypothalamus [10,11].

CLINICAL PICTURE

In the immediate postpartum period, patients may complain of failure to lactate, profound fatigue, tiredness, dizziness, and may also have hypotension. It is very important to establish the correct diagnosis of acute hypopituitarism and institute appropriate treatment, including intravenous crystalloid fluid resuscitation and hydrocortisone as life-saving measures [5]. More commonly, the syndrome develops slowly and it is not uncommon to make the diagnosis 10–15 years after the original obstetric accident. It is therefore essential to take an appropriate history, asking about possible hemorrhage, hypotension, shock, and blood transfusion occurring after a prior delivery. Almost invariably these patients will give a history of failure to lactate in the postpartum, failure to resume normal menstrual bleeding, failure of pubic hair to grow back, and then loss of all body hair. In severe acute cases, they look pale and lethargic and are at risk for stupor and death in the course of relatively minor infections or stress due to secondary adrenocortical failure [12]. Neurologic symptoms are nonspecific and vary from none to frank psychosis, which is usually completely reversible following treatment [13]. Most patients with Sheehan's syndrome show human growth hormone (hGH) and prolactin (PRL) deficiency followed in frequency of occurrence by deficient gonadotropins, thyroidstimulating hormone (TSH), and lastly by adrenocorticotropic hormone (ACTH) release [4,14–16].

Physical examination generally will demonstrate a smooth, pale, and dry skin with fine wrinkling of the face, hypopigmentation, absence of body hair, fragile nails, atrophy of the genitalia and decreased breast tissue. Some patients may also have hypotension, anemia, hypoglycemia, polyuria, polydipsia, or nocturia [12].

DIAGNOSIS

It is important to remember to ask about a past obstetric accident when taking the history. This is an essential point since many times the diagnosis is made only several years after the original accident. Final diagnosis of Sheehan's syndrome is made with laboratory tests (Fig. 28.1). Depending on the degree of pituitary necrosis, several hormones may be affected. The most commonly affected hormones are PRL and hGH [15–17]. Not only is their baseline suppressed but the PRL response to the administration of thyrotropin-releasing hormone (TRH) and the hGH response to insulin-induced hypoglycemia is either minimal or absent [16–18]. In patients with amenorrhea it is necessary to test the pituitary gonadotropin reserve with a gonadotropin-releasing hormone (GnRH) test. Measurement of free urinary cortisol in a 24-hour urine collection is adequate to test the adequacy of the pituitary–adrenal axis. Thyroid function is best determined by measuring thyroxin, free thyroxine, and triiodothyronine. Measurement of TSH is not adequate for the diagnosis of secondary hypothyroidism.

The estrogen status can be determined by either measuring serum estradiol (E_2) or by administering 100 mg of progesterone in oil intramuscularly or oral medroxyprogesterone acetate, 20 mg daily for 5 days, to induce uterine bleeding. A serum E_2 value of >40 pg/ml or the positive vaginal bleeding response to progesterone is indicative of adequate estrogen status [19]. A complete anterior pituitary function evaluation can be easily performed by combining the insulin-induced hypoglycemia, TRH and GnRH test. For that purpose the patient is admitted after an overnight fast and receives an intravenous injection of 0.15 u/kg insulin mixed with 150 µg of GnRH and 500 µg TRH. After obtaining a baseline plasma specimen the mixture is slowly given intravenously and blood samples are obtained 30, 60, and 120 min later. The concentration of glucose, cortisol, hGH, PRL, TSH, luteinizing hormone (LH), and follicle-stimulating hormone (FSH) should be measured in all samples. The amount of insulin administered should decrease plasma glucose 30 min later to at least 50% below the baseline in order to obtain an adequate hypothalamic stress response. Independent of the estrogen baseline, a significant increment in plasma hGH and cortisol should be expected unless there are impairments within the hypothalamic–pituitary axis. For hGH the minimal normal increase should be 18 ng/ml and for cortisol 6 µg%, 60–120 min after the injection of insulin [16]. Although maximal hormone response occurs at different times, all hormones should be measured in all specimens because in many instances there is a delayed maximal increase.

Animal and human experimentation have suggested that insulin-induced hypoglycemia stimulates the serotonin pathway in the hypothalamus in order to produce a pituitary response [20–22]. In patients with Sheehan's syndrome the pituitary necrosis and fibrosis will preclude any normal response. In addition, PRL should respond with a minimum of 200% above the baseline 30 min after administration of TRH. In the majority of patients with Sheehan's syndrome, the PRL increase in response to TRH is markedly diminished, if not completely absent. The completion of the pituitary function evaluation requires the measurement of TSH, LH, and FSH. Depending on the degree of pituitary necrosis, varying degrees of hormone abnormality may be demonstrated.

Patients should be given a meal rich in carbohydrates before leaving the hospital. It is recommended that a physician be present throughout this test because severe hypoglycemia with shock may occur. Although some patients have frank diabetes insipidus, abnormalities in water metabolism can be detected in many patients with less than complete Sheehan's syndrome [23,24]. In these patients a diminished ability to concentrate urine can be demonstrated by testing the vasopressin secretory capacity. It is generally accepted that water restriction followed by the administration of vasopressin is the best diagnostic method [12]. Water intake is restricted until the patient has had three consecutive hourly urine specimens with similar osmolarity. Usually this is accomplished in 12–16 hours. Therefore, it is practical to request the patients to avoid taking any food or water from 7 p.m. the evening before the test. After admission at 8 p.m. the urinary flow, urinary osmolality, and serum osmolality are measured every hour until three consecutive samples show no

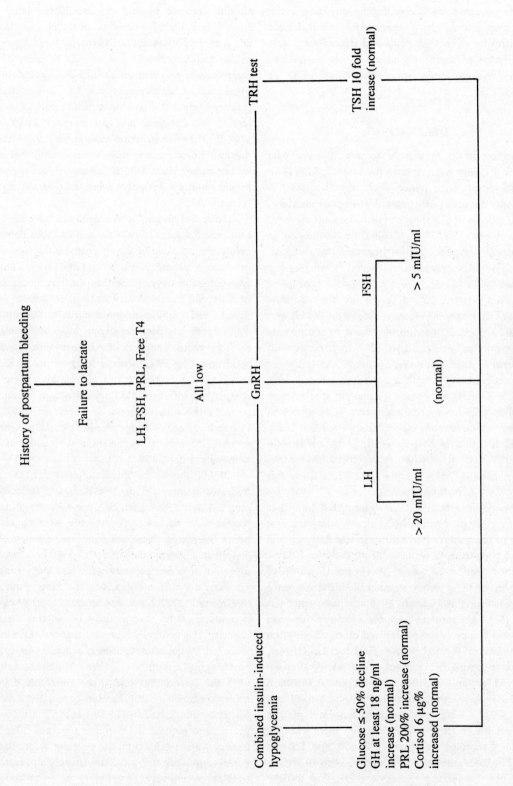

Fig. 28.1 Diagnosis of Sheehan's syndrome.

change, then again with the same frequency after receiving 5 u of aqueous vasopressin given subcutaneously. Patients with diabetes insipidus will significantly increase the urinary osmolality following the administration of vasopressin, indicating a defective endogenous secretory system. This test needs to be performed under supervision to insure that the patient does not take any water, as well as to prevent rapid dehydration and hypotension.

Case reports have been published of patients with Sheehan's syndrome and isolated abnormalities such as ACTH deficiency, psychosis, hyperlipidemia, or hypomagnesemia and polymorphous ventricular tachycardia [25–27]. Computed tomographic studies of the sella turcica in patients with Sheehan's syndrome have demonstrated the sellar volume to be significantly smaller than in control patients [28]. However, subsequent studies have instead reported an empty sella in an otherwise normal sella turcica [29,30]. Since magnetic resonance imaging is the method of choice to demonstrate an intrasellar subarachnoid herniation (empty sella), its use may have diagnostic value.

DIFFERENTIAL DIAGNOSIS

The differential diagnosis of Sheehan's syndrome includes anorexia nervosa and lymphocytic hypophysitis [31]. Patients with anorexia nervosa do not have the obstetric history, are markedly wasted, usually retain the axillary and pubic hair, and have normal serum levels of hGH and PRL. In addition, patients with anorexia nervosa have a very strong psychologic component. Patients with Sheehan's syndrome usually have lost their body hair, have low plasma levels of cortisol, hGH, and PRL, and may have evidence of hypothyroidism. Lymphocytic hypophysitis may occur in relation to pregnancy or during the postpartum period. In fact, the first case reported was a woman who died of circulatory collapse a few hours after having an appendectomy. In the chronic form the symptoms are amenorrhea, headache, lethargy, weight loss, and collapse. These patients were found to have a lymphocytic infiltration of the pituitary in postmortem studies. Some of the patients have the same infiltration in the thyroid, and thus an immunologic or autoimmune disease process has been suggested. This disease is potentially life-threatening, but it is treatable with hydrocortisone. This diagnosis should be considered in women in the reproductive age presenting with symptoms of hypopituitarism, even in the absence of significant bleeding and hypotension during labor.

TREATMENT

The determination of the ACTH reserve in patients with Sheehan's hypopituitarism is of clinical importance because of possible life-threatening situations, and treatment with hydrocortisone 10 mg twice a day should be instituted. Some patients may require 20 mg in the morning followed by 10 mg in the afternoon. Since death due to adrenal insufficiency has been reported in patients with postpartum hypopituitarism, it appears that the benefit of cortisone therapy outweighs its hazards in patients with demonstrated deficient ACTH reserve. Use of thyroid replacement will depend upon the levels of free thyroxine and not on the TSH response to TRH administration. The need for estrogen replacement will depend on the estrogen status. Patients who do not bleed to the administration of progesterone or with serum levels of less than 40 pg/ml of estradiol are severely hypoestrogenized and should receive estrogen replacement therapy.

In general the medical management of these patients consists of careful hormone replacement therapy when an indication of such deficiencies has been demonstrated [12]. Mineralocorticoids are usually not needed. Those patients with diabetes insipidus are treated with an analog of vasopressin, 1-deamino-8,D-arginine vasopressin (DDAVP). Fertility can be achieved with human menopausal gonadotropin and human chorionic gonadotropin therapy in patients with hypogonadism. Patients with preserved gonadotropin function can ovulate and become pregnant spontaneously. There have been isolated reports of partial spontaneous recovery in some patients with subsequent pregnancy. With appropriate replacement therapy the prognosis of a normal life span in these patients is good.

REFERENCES

1 Sheehan HL. Postpartum necrosis of the anterior pituitary. *Pathol Bacteriol* 1937; 45: 189.
2 Sheehan HL, Murdock R. Postpartum necrosis of the anterior pituitary. Pathological and clinical aspects. *Br J Obstet Gynaecol* 1938; 45: 456.
3 Cenac A, Develoux M, Souman I *et al*. Le syndrome de Sheehan en republique de Niger: dix-neuf observations *Med Trop* 1987; 47: 17.
4 DiZerega G, Kletzky OA, Mishell DR Jr. Diagnosis of

Sheehan's syndrome using a sequential pituitary stimulation test. *Am J Obstet Gynecol* 1978; 132: 348.

5 Rusnak RA. Adrenal and pituitary emergencies. *Emerg Med Clin North Am* 1989; 7: 903.

6 Doniach D. Histopathology of the anterior pituitary. *J Clin Endocrinol Metab* 1977; 6: 21.

7 Bergland RM, Page RB. Can the pituitary secrete directly to the brain? (affirmative anatomical evidence). *Endocrinology* 1978; 102: 1325.

8 Goluboff LG, Ezrin C. Effect of pregnancy on the somatotroph and the prolactin cell of the human adenohypophysis. *J Clin Endocrinol Metab* 1969; 29: 1553.

9 Kovacs K. Necrosis of anterior pituitary in humans. *Neuroendocrinology* 1969; 4: 170.

10 Sheehan HL, Whitehead R. The neurohypophysis in postpartum hypopituitarism. *J Pathol* 1963; 85: 145.

11 Whitehead R. The hypothalamus in postpartum hypopituitarism. *J Pathol* 1963; 86: 55.

12 Christy NP, Warren MP. Disease syndromes of the hypothalamus and anterior pituitary. In: De Groot LJ et al., eds. *Endocrinology*, vol 1. New York: Grune & Stratton, 1979: 225–229.

13 Thomas MJ, Igbal ASM. Sheehan's syndrome with psychosis. *J Assoc Physicians India* 1985; 33: 175.

14 Aons TJ, Mingawat, Kinugasa O et al. Response of pituitary LH and FSH to synthetic LH releasing hormone in normal subjects and in patients with Sheehan's syndrome. *Am J Obstet Gynecol* 1973; 117: 1046.

15 Imura H. *Hypopituitarism in the Pituitary Gland*. New York: Raven Press, 1985: 501.

16 Morenti C, Kletzky OA. Pituitary response to insulin-induced hypoglycemia in patients with amenorrhea of different etiologies. *Am J Obstet Gynecol* 1984; 148: 375.

17 Jialal J, Naidoo C, Norman RJ et al. Pituitary function in Sheehan's syndrome. *Obstet Gynecol* 1984; 63: 15.

18 Jialal J, Desai R, Rajput MC et al. Prolactin secretion in Sheehan's syndrome. *J Reprod Med* 1986; 31: 487.

19 Kletzky OA, Davajan V, Nakamura RM et al. Clinical categorization of patients with secondary amenorrhea using progesterone induced uterine bleeding and measurements of serum gonadotropin levels. *Am J Obstet Gynecol* 1975; 121: 695.

20 Gordon AE, Meldrum DS. Effect of insulin on brain 5-hydroxytryptamine and 5-hydroxy-indoleacetic acid of rat. *Biochem Pharmacol* 1970; 19: 3042.

21 Bivens CH, Lebovitz HE, Feldman JM. Inhibition of hypoglycemia induced growth hormone secretion by the serotonin antagonist cyproheptadine and methysergide. *N Engl J Med* 1973; 289: 236.

22 Plonk, JW, Bivens CH, Feldman JM. Inhibition of hypoglycemia induced cortisol secretion by the serotonin antagonist cyproheptadine. *J Clin Endocrinol Metab* 1974; 38: 836.

23 Jialal J, Desai RK, Rajput MC. An assessment of posterior pituitary function in patients with Sheehan's syndrome. *Clin Endocrinol* 1987; 27: 91.

24 Bakiri F, Benmiloud M, Vallotton MB. Arginine-vasopressin in postpartum panhypopituitarism: urinary excretion and kidney response to osmolar load. *J Clin Endocrinol Metab* 1984; 58: 511.

25 Giustina G, Zuccato F, Slavi A, Candrina R. Pregnancy in Sheehan's syndrome corrected by adrenal replacement therapy. Case report. *Br J Obstet Gynaecol* 1985; 92: 1061.

26 Ishibashi S, Murase T, Yamada N et al. Hyperlipidemia in patients with hypopituitarism. *Acta Endocrinol* 1985; 110: 456.

27 Nunoda S, Ueda K, Kameda S, Nakabayashi H. Sheehan's syndrome with hypomagnesemia and polymorphous ventricular tachycardia. *Jpn Heart J* 1989; 30: 251.

28 Sherif I, Vanderley CM, Beshyah S, Bosairi S. Sella size and contents in Sheehan's syndrome. *Clin Endocrinol* 1989; 30: 613.

29 Knobel B, Ben-Yosef S, Rosman P. Sheehan's syndrome and empty sella turcica. *Isr J Med Sci* 1984; 20: 232.

30 Fleckman AM, Schubart U, Danziger A, Fleisher N. Empty sella of normal size in Sheehan's syndrome. *Am J Med* 1983; 75: 585.

31 Nader S. Pituitary disorders and pregnancy. *Semin Perinatol* 1990; 14: 24.

29

Evaluation and treatment of pituitary sellar lesions

ANN MORRILL & GARY S. WAND

INTRODUCTION

Pituitary adenomas are the most common parasellar masses, comprising about 90% of all sellar lesions and 10% of all intracranial neoplasms. Tumors are classified as macroadenomas if their diameter is greater than 1.0 cm and as microadenomas if they are smaller. Prolactin (PRL)-secreting tumors, discussed elsewhere in this book, are the most common adenoma. Nonfunctioning adenomas, which do not secrete functional hormones, are the second most common adenoma. Although called nonfunctional, these tumors actually synthesize and secrete biologically inactive glycoprotein subunits, including the β-subunit of luteinizing hormone (LH), β-subunit of follicle-stimulating hormone (FSH), the α-subunit common to LH, FSH, and thyroid-stimulating hormone (TSH) and low concentrations of biologically active prolactin and growth hormone (GH). Next in order of frequency of occurrence are GH-secreting, mixed PRL- and GH-secreting, and adrenocorticotropin hormone (ACTH)-secreting tumors. Tumors which exclusively secrete intact LH, FSH, and TSH are rare.

Other mass lesions that can involve the sellar region include brain neoplasms, such as craniopharyngiomas, meningiomas, and glioblastomas (Table 29.1). Craniopharyngiomas are the most common. These are squamous cell tumors thought to be derived from Rathke's pouch remnants. They usually arise in the upper portion of the pituitary stalk and can extend into the sella and the hypothalamus. Metastases to the pituitary are uncommon and most often occur with breast, lung, and thyroid cancer as well as lymphoma and melanoma. Rare sellar lesions include fibromas, hemangiomas, cholesteatomas, hamartomas, teratomas, and abscesses.

In the female, the most common infiltrative disorder of the pituitary is lymphocytic hypophysitis. Enlargement of the pituitary occurs secondary to

Table 29.1 Causes of enlarged sella

Pituitary tumors
Craniopharyngiomas
Primary brain tumors (e.g., meningiomas)
Metastatic tumors
Fibromas, hemangiomas, cholesteatomas, hamartomas, teratomas
Abscesses
Lymphocytic hypophysitis
Granulomatous disease (e.g., sarcoidosis)
Primary end-organ failure (e.g., primary hypothyroidism)
Pituitary cysts
Aneurysms
Empty sella syndrome

---

inflammatory infiltration which generally progresses to pituitary fibrosis. This condition is thought to be autoimmune in nature and predominantly affects young women in late pregnancy or postpartum. Other infiltrative processes that can affect the pituitary include sarcoidosis, histiocytosis, tuberculosis, or giant cell granulomas. On occasion these states can enlarge the pituitary, causing mass effect, and result in hypopituitarism.

There are assorted states which can mimic pituitary tumors, both by clinical presentation and radiographically. These pseudotumors include pituitary hyperplasia from endocrine end-organ failure (e.g., primary hypothyroidism or primary gonadal failure) and can result in sellar enlargement. They are differentiated from tumors by appropriate hormone studies. Pituitary cysts (e.g., Rathke's pouch cysts) and aneurysms can also mimic pituitary adenomas.

The empty sella syndrome occurs most often in obese, hypertensive women. This is an enlargement of the sella thought to arise from a small arachnoid diverticulum which passes through the diaphragmatic sella with the pituitary stalk and allows cerebrospinal fluid to enter the sella. This pressure expands the sella and compresses the pituitary. Hypopituitarism is rare but can occur. A sella lesion must be differentiated from the empty sella syndrome where surgery or radiotherapy is contraindicated.

ANATOMIC–CLINICAL CORRELATIONS

The pituitary lies within a bony fossa referred to as the sella turcica (Fig. 29.1). The diaphragmatic sella is a stretched piece of dura which separates the pituitary from cerebrospinal fluid and the central nervous system. Superior to the pituitary gland and diaphragmatic sellae is the optic chiasm and the hypothalamus. The cavernous sinuses are situated laterally and on either side of the thickened walls of the sella turcica. Traversing the cavernous sinuses are cranial nerves III, IV, and VI, which regulate extraocular eye movements, and the first and second division of the trigeminal nerve. On the surface of cranial nerve III are parasympathetic fibers which regulate pupillary constriction. Most lateral in the sinus is the carotid artery. Inferior to the bony sella floor is the sphenoid sinus which communicates with the nasal cavities.

The clinical signs and symptoms which occur in patients with pituitary tumors are related to: (1) the mass effect of the lesion on the pituitary; (2) the mass effect on surrounding central nervous system structures; and (3) hypersecretion of pituitary hormones from secretory adenomas. Occasionally a pituitary tumor is incidentally discovered radiographically. Rarely, pituitary adenomas can be part of the familial multiple endocrine neoplasia syndrome type I, and thus may be associated with pancreatic islet cell tumors and hyperparathyroidism.

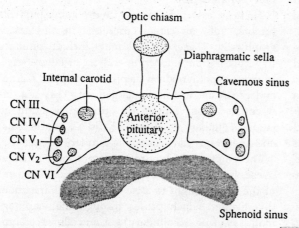

Fig. 29.1 Anatomic relationship of sella turcica.

Compression of surrounding structures

Intrasellar lesions, like all expanding masses, take the path of least resistance. In the case of the sella turcica, this is in the superior direction. Dull frontal headaches are common, resulting from the stretching of the diaphragmatic sellae, the thin piece of dura which covers the superior portion of the sella and which contains sensory nerves. With continued expansion in the superior direction, compression of the optic chiasm results in visual impairment. The first visual field loss is usually the superior temporal field due to compression of the inferior portion of the optic chiasm. Without intervention, this may progress to bitemporal hemianopsia, optic atrophy, and loss of visual acuity. Rarely, extension of tumor affects the hypothalamus resulting in disturbed consciousness, hyperphagia, and abnormal temperature regulation. Obstruction of the third ventricle and cerebrospinal fluid drainage can result in hydrocephalus. Lateral extension into the cavernous sinus often injures cranial nerves. This may result in extraocular motor palsies (e.g., compression of cranial nerve III, IV, or V), ophthalmoplegia, dilatation of the pupil (e.g., compression of the parasympathetic fibers on cranial nerve III), and facial numbness (e.g., compression of cranial nerve V). Expansion of tumor in the inferior direction can produce cerebrospinal fluid rhinorrhea and epistaxis.

Compression of the pituitary

During enlargement of a sellar lesion, the pituitary is the most vulnerable structure. Injury to the gonadotrophs (e.g., LH- and FSH-secreting cells) can cause central hypogonadism, arrested puberty, menstrual irregularities, amenorrhea, infertility, and decreased libido. Diminished PRL secretion can result in inability to lactate appropriately postpartum.

Injury to the corticotrophs (e.g., ACTH-secreting cells) will cause central adrenal insufficiency. Symptoms include arthralgias, myalgias, weight loss, anorexia, weakness, nausea, vomiting, hypoglycemia, hypotension, and circulatory collapse. In women, decreased androgens from lack of ACTH can result in decreased axillary and pubic hair. Since the mineralocorticoid axis is not dependent upon ACTH, profound volume depletion and hyperkalemia are rare. Hyponatremia, however, can result from impaired free water clearance.

Central hypothyroidism from lack of TSH (e.g., injury to thyrotrophs) can result in decreased energy, cold intolerance, dry skin, constipation, menstrual irregularities, weight gain, and diminished intellect. Myxedema is rare but has been reported. GH deficiency can result in impaired skeletal growth if the epiphyses have not yet fused. In adults, decreased muscle strength, hypoglycemia, and hyperlipidemia can occur. Should the neurohypophysis be involved, diabetes insipidus can result.

Hyperprolactinemia is not always the result of a tumor which synthesizes and secretes excess prolactin (e.g., prolactinoma). Any parasellar lesion which interferes with the synthesis (e.g., hypothalamic sarcoidosis) and/or transport of dopamine in the hypothalamus or pituitary stalk (e.g., nonfunctional tumor or craniopharyngioma) will interfere with physiologic inhibition of prolactin secretion. Dopamine is the major prolactin inhibitor. Hyperprolactinemia in this setting is from impairment of negative feedback and is always less than 200 ng/ml. Therefore, in the presence of a pituitary tumor greater than 1.0 cm in size, a prolactin level less than 200 ng/ml is strong evidence against a prolactinoma. The nonfunctional lesion associated with a mild elevation in prolactin will not shrink during the administration of bromocriptine. Dopamine agonist therapy should be used in this setting *only* to normalize the prolactin level and not in attempts to reduce tumor volume. Any etiology for hyperprolactinemia can cause amenorrhea, infertility, decreased libido, and galactorrhea. Similar to the prolactinoma, sustained hyperprolactinemia suppresses gonadotrophin release, decreases serum estrogens, and results in a higher risk for osteoporosis.

Spontaneous hemorrhage within a pituitary adenoma has been estimated to be present in about 5–20% of tumors. About one-third of these instances are recognizable as the clinical syndrome of pituitary apoplexy. This syndrome is characterized by sudden, severe headache; loss of vision (i.e., compression of the optic chiasm); diplopia and ptosis and pupillary abnormalities (compression of cranial nerves in the cavernous sinus); nausea, and vomiting, as well as the rapid development of hypopituitarism. If necrotic tissue and blood enter the cerebrospinal fluid, meningismus, hyperpyrexia, coma and death can ensue. Pituitary apoplexy must be differentiated from a subarachnoid hemorrhage or meningitis.

HYPERSECRETORY SYNDROMES

GH-secreting tumors and acromegaly

These tumors cause gigantism if the epiphyses have not yet fused, and acromegaly if the epiphyses have fused. Symptoms and signs can include: enlargement of hands, feet, and head; thickening of lips, tongue, and skin; and hyperhidrosis. Rarely, galactorrhea occurs secondary to the intrinsic lactogenic properties of GH. These patients are at increased risk of developing arthritis, hypercalciuria, carpal tunnel syndrome, osteoporosis, hypertension, early cardiovascular disease, and glucose intolerance. By the time this tumor is discovered it is frequently greater than 1.0 cm and may have resulted in significant mass effect. If a pituitary tumor is not identified radiographically, hypothalamic production of GH-releasing hormone (GHRH), or ectopic tumor production of GHRH, though rare, must be considered. Up to 40% of acromegalic tumors will secrete prolactin in addition to GH.

ACTH-secreting adenomas and Cushing's disease

ACTH-secreting adenomas result in Cushing's disease. This more often affects women in their childbearing years. The signs and symptoms are related to glucocorticoid excess. They may include proximal muscle strength weakness, truncal obesity weight gain, moon facies, hirsutism, easy bruising, purple striae, osteoporosis, psychiatric disturbances, amenorrhea, and infertility. These tumors are frequently less than 0.5 cm at the time of discovery.

TSH-secreting tumors

These tumors may, but not always, result in hyperthyroidism. These adenomas are extremely rare. Hyperthyroid symptoms may include weight loss, anxiety, sweats, tremor, palpitations, heat intolerance, hair loss, hyperdefecation, and amenorrhea. The elevated TSH and possible pituitary enlargement of primary hypothyroidism is differentiated from TSH-secreting adenomas by the clinical presentation of thyrotoxicosis and by elevated thyroid hormone levels in the patients with the adenomas. Rarely, there can be pituitary resistance to thyroid hormone. In this situation TSH and thyroxine levels are elevated but there is no evidence of a tumor or thyrotoxicosis. About one-third of these TSH-secreting tumors will also produce other hormones, most often PRL or GH.

As mentioned previously, although it is common for a pituitary adenoma to secrete biologically inactive subunits of LH and FSH, adenomas which secrete biologically active gonadotrophs are extremely uncommon. These tumors can have substantial mass by the time of discovery. Since they are so rare, there is little known about the effects on female reproduction from the hypersecretory state.

EVALUATION

Radiologic imaging is important to diagnose the presence of a pituitary tumor, define tumor limits, and to provide insight into the type of tumor. For instance, a craniopharyngioma can often be predicted by its degree of calcification and suprasellar position. The most sensitive imaging scan is a cranial magnetic resonance imaging (MRI) study with gadolinium enhancement. An alternative would be a cranial computed tomographic (CT) scan with contrast. Negative studies do not rule out the existence of a small tumor. If imaging studies show a macroadenoma, formal visual field testing should be done to evaluate optic nerve pathway impingement.

Evaluation of hormone deficiency

Hormonal evaluation is critical, to evaluate for both pituitary hormone insufficiency and excess. Static and dynamic testing should be done to assess for hypopituitarism (Table 29.2). In suspected adrenal insufficiency, a basal morning cortisol is not a very useful screen unless the value is high. Normal persons can occasionally have low values. In the setting of chronic adrenal insufficiency, the rapid ACTH stimulation test will identify pituitary–adrenal axis dysfunction. The test is performed by measuring the serum cortisol level before and 1 hour after the administration of 250 μg of cortrosyn (ACTH(1−24)). A normal test is a rise in serum cortisol of at least 7 μg/dl, with a final stimulated value of 20 μg/dl or greater. If the ACTH deficiency is more acute (e.g., less than 2 weeks old), the adrenal glands have not undergone physiologic atrophy and the rapid ACTH stimulation test is not accurate in this setting. To evaluate more accurately for secondary adrenal insufficiency, metyrapone 30 mg/kg p.o. can be administered as an overnight test to inhibit cortisol secretion. Metyrapone diminishes serum cortisol by blocking the 11 β-hydroxylase enzyme, which is responsible for catalyzing the last step in the biosynthesis of cortisol. The normal pituitary response to the ensuing inhibition of serum cortisol is to secrete ACTH and thus increase plasma 11-deoxycortisol levels, the immediate precursor to cortisol. The cortisol level the morning following metyrapone should be <5 mg/dl (e.g., indicating adequate adrenal blockade and an adequate provocation for ACTH release), and the 11-deoxycortisol level should be >7.5 μg/dl (indicating an appropriate ACTH response to hypocortisolism). If the 11-deoxycortisol level is less than 7.5 μg/dl, this indicates a suboptimal ACTH response to hypocortisolism, and thus makes the diagnosis of secondary adrenal insufficiency.

To evaluate for central hypothyroidism TSH, T_4 radioimmunoassay (T_4RIA), and T_3 resin uptake (T_3RU) can be measured. The T_4RIA and thyroid index would be expected to be low in the face of a normal or minimally elevated TSH. Though the TSH level is not usually very low, it is biologically less active than the TSH produced in a normal state.

The gonadotroph axes can be evaluated by obtaining an estradiol, LH, and FSH levels. If the FSH and

Table 29.2 Provocative tests

Test	Dose	Hormone(s) sampled	Sampling interval	Normal response
ACTH stimulation	250 μg	Cortisol	1 hour	Rise >7 μg/dl with final value ≥20 μg/dl
Metyrapone	30 mg/kg at 12 p.m.	Cortisol 11-deoxycortisol	8 a.m. next day	Cortisol 5 μg/dl 11-DOC >7.5 μg/dl
Glucose suppression	50−100 g	Growth hormone	1−2 hours	<5 ng/ml
Low-dose dexamethasone	0.5 mg q 6 hours for 48 hours	UFC	Over 24 hours	<25 μg
High-dose dexamethasone	2.0 mg q 6 hours for 48 hours	UFC	Over 24 hours	<50% baseline

ACTH, adrenocorticotropic hormone; DOC, deoxycorticosterone; UFC, urine free cortisol.

LH are inappropriately low for a decreased concentration of sex steroid, this indicates central deficiency which may or may not be secondary to a pituitary tumor. Normal LH and FSH levels in a postmenopausal patient also indicate gonadotroph damage.

Deficiency of GH in an adult is not currently considered essential to replace for relatively normal health and thus is usually not evaluated.

Diabetes insipidus, though rare with pituitary adenomas, is not unusual with other tumors such as craniopharyngiomas, and can develop after pituitary surgery. Urinary output greater than 4 liters over a 24-hour period should be evaluated with a serum sodium, serum osmolality, and a water deprivation test.

Evaluation of hormone excess

Evaluation of a patient suspected of having acromegaly should include a glucose suppression test (GST). Normally, glucose 50–100 g p.o. in solution will suppress GH levels to less than 5 ng/ml. In acromegalics after a GST, there can be: (1) a paradoxical rise in GH; (2) no glucose-induced GH suppression; or (3) a subnormal suppression (e.g., GH value greater than 5 ng/ml). Measurement of somatomedin-C level can also be diagnostic. Somatomedin-C is synthesized in the liver and is believed to be a major mediator of GH action. Rarely young, normal adults can have a falsely elevated somatomedin-C level. Isolated GH levels are not very sensitive or specific for acromegaly.

Cushing's syndrome is suspected biochemically when the patient has elevated 24-hour urine free cortisol (UFC; >100 µg). A UFC value greater than 300 µg/24 hours confirms the diagnosis of Cushing's syndrome, whereas a UFC value less than 100 µg/24 hours makes the diagnosis less likely. A UFC value between 100 and 300 µg/24 hours necessitates the low-dose dexamethasone suppression test — dexamethasone 0.5 mg every 6 hours for 48 hours (Fig. 29.2). Failure of the hypothalamic–pituitary–adrenal axis to suppress during the low-dose dexamethasone suppression test (UFC less than 25 µg/24 hours) indicates the presence of hypercortisolism or Cushing's syndrome. Once the diagnosis of Cushing's syndrome is made, the etiology of the hypercortisolism is established. Cushing's disease (hypercortisolism secondary to excess ACTH secretion from a pituitary adenoma) must be differentiated from other glucocorticoid-excess states such as functioning adrenal adenomas, ectopic tumor ACTH production, and exogenous glucocorticoid intake. The cornerstone in establishing the etiology of Cushing's syndrome is the high-dose dexamethasone sup-

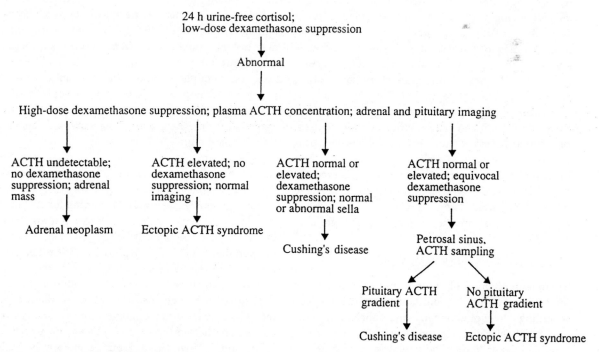

Fig. 29.2 Cushing's syndrome suspected.

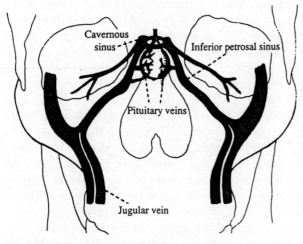

Fig. 29.3 Inferior petrosal sinus sampling.

pression test. This study takes into account that ACTH-secreting pituitary adenomas participate in glucocorticoid negative feedback, albeit at a higher set point. Therefore, during a high-dose dexamethasone suppression test (dexamethasone 2 mg every 6 hours for 48 hours) most ACTH-producing pituitary adenomas will suppress UFC levels by 50%. Ectopic and adrenal tumors generally do not have glucocorticoid receptors and therefore do not suppress during high-dose dexamethasone administration. Head imaging with CT or MRI will identify only about 30% of these small pituitary adenomas. Therefore, the diagnosis of Cushing disease is biochemic and not radiologic. When the cause of the hypercortisolism is in doubt, inferior petrosal sinus sampling should be performed (Fig. 29.3). In this study, catheters are placed in both jugular veins and then into the left and right inferior petrosal sinuses. Blood is collected simultaneously from each sinus and peripheral vein; plasma ACTH levels are then determined. Presence of an unilateral ACTH gradient from either petrosal sinus indicates Cushing's disease whereas suppressed ACTH levels in the venous effluent indicate nonpituitary Cushing's syndrome.

THERAPY

Treatment of nonprolactinoma pituitary tumors is aimed at reversing the consequences of mass effect, including hypopituitarism, and abolishing any abnormally elevated hormone levels. Therapy can be modified depending on individual patient needs and circumstances but in general, surgery is the first-line

treatment, followed by radiotherapy and medical management. Surgical resection of a pituitary lesion is a safe and effective procedure for most lesions. The transsphenoidal route — through the nasal cavity and sphenoid sinus — is preferred. The operative mortality is less than 1%. A frontal craniotomy approach is rarely indicated unless there is a very large tumor. Surgery is not indicated in empty sella syndrome.

The major advantages of surgery are the following. Immediate results are seen. This is especially important if the patient has pituitary apoplexy, rapid visual impairment, or an aggressive hypersecretory state. Surgery also allows a histologic diagnosis. Tumors such as craniopharyngiomas which are relatively radioresistant can be treated. Surgery has a low mortality and morbidity. Damage to normal structures such as the frontal lobe, optic nerves, or pituitary can occur. Rarely hemorrhage, infection, or cerebrospinal fluid rhinorrhea happens.

If surgical intervention is planned, glucocorticoid coverage is given routinely perioperatively because of the possibility of normal corticotroph damage intraoperatively. Hydrocortisone 50 mg i.v. every 6 hours or its glucocorticoid equivalent the day of surgery provides adequate coverage, and the dosage is rapidly tapered within days after surgery. Diabetes insipidus is not uncommon after pituitary surgery due to truama to the pituitary stalk. This is usually transient but if it persists beyond 4 days, it may be permanent. In some patients a brief recovery period may occur, thought to be from vasopressin release from damaged posterior pituitary cells. Fluid balance must be carefully monitored and should diabetes insipidus develop acutely, aqueous vasopressin 5 U i.m. may be given as necessary. For chronic diabetes insipidus, the long-acting vasopressin analog, DDAVP, is the preferred treatment.

Radiotherapy can avoid some surgical complications but disadvantages include: nonresponsiveness of radioresistant tumors; slow response to therapy generally, taking 6–24 months for an initial benefit to be seen, with progressive improvement over 2–5 years; significant risk of radiation-induced hypopituitarism (30–50% within 5 years of therapy); rarely, acute swelling or hemorrhage of the tumor occurs, nor is there a noteworthy incidence of damage to surrounding neural tissue. Radiotherapy modalities include conventional ionizing and heavy particle irradiation (e.g., proton beam, or α-particle irradiation). Conventional ionizing therapy is available at most institutions and requires 25 treatments

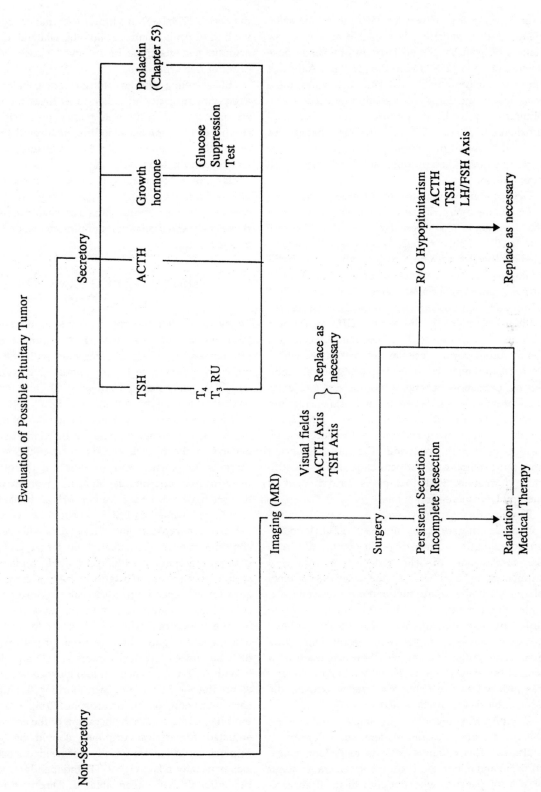

Fig. 29.4 Approach to the diagnosis of pituitary tumor.

over 5 weeks for delivery of 4500 rad to the sella. Heavy particle radiation is available at only a few centers but can be administered in one single dose delivering up to 12 000 rad to the pituitary. Although cure rates are comparable with both techniques, there is a lower incidence of radiation-induced hypopituitarism with heavy particle therapy (e.g., approximately 15% over 5 years). Radiation therapy can be used as an adjunct to surgery to prevent tumor regrowth. Radiotherapy does not preclude surgical intervention.

GH-secreting tumors are first treated with transsphenoidal surgery. If the tumor is less than 1.0 cm the cure rate is 75%; if greater than 1.0 cm the cure rate is 50%. If surgery fails to normalize GH levels, medical therapy with bromocriptine or somatostatin analog can be tried. In approximately 30% of acromegalic patients, bromocriptine in doses of 20–40 mg/day decreases but rarely normalizes GH levels. Without normalizing the serum GH level, most patients have progression of acromegalic changes. Rarely, bromocriptine use has been associated with a decrease in tumor size. The long-acting somatostatin analog, octreotide, is better at normalizing GH levels than bromocriptine. However, it is expensive and must be given by subcutaneous injection three times per day. There is some evidence that tumor size may be decreased with octreotide. The most significant long-term complication of octreotide therapy is gallstone formation. Radiotherapy is used if medical therapy is unsuccessful.

First-line therapy in Cushing's disease is transsphenoidal surgery (cure rate − 70–80%). If this is unsuccessful in normalizing glucocorticoid levels, the combination of sella radiation and medical adrenalectomy with one of the following adrenal blockers can be tried: metyrapone, ketoconazole, aminoglutethemide, trilostane, or mitotane. These drugs interfere with adrenal glucocorticoid synthesis but are usually not completely successful in inhibiting excess glucocorticoid secretion. These agents are often limited by adverse effects. If and when radiotherapy has induced a cure (50% cure rate in adults), the adrenal blocker is discontinued.

If pituitary surgery, radiotherapy, and medical therapy are unsuccessful, bilateral adrenalectomy is indicated. This commits patients to lifelong glucocorticoid and mineralocorticoid replacement. In about 5–10% of patients who undergo bilateral adrenalectomy, Nelson's syndrome or progressive enlargement of the pituitary tumor with hyperpigmentation

may occur. The Nelson's tumor is extremely aggressive and difficult to cure. Following bilateral adrenalectomy, patients must be followed closely for the onset of this syndrome.

TSH-secreting pituitary tumors are usually managed with surgery and radiation. If these modalities are unsuccessful, antithyroid management with antithyroid drugs, radioactive iodine, or surgical ablation of the thyroid can be utilized. Rarely these tumors will respond to bromocriptine.

LH- and FSH-secreting tumors are treated similarly to nonfunctioning tumors. They are so uncommon, medical therapy has not been proven but there have been case reports of tumors responding to bromocriptine.

POSTTHERAPY HORMONAL EVALUATION

To evaluate after therapy for hypopituitarism, the following course is suggested. Assessment of the pituitary–adrenal axis is completed with the overnight metyrapone test. Exogenous glucocorticoids should be held prior to this testing. Thyroid function is easily assessed by obtaining a T_4RIA and T_3RU 3–4 weeks after surgery. Since the half-life of thyroxine is about a week, it could be that long before a decrease in the thyroxine level is seen. In this setting, there is no practical purpose for the thyrotropin-releasing hormone stimulation test. In women, unless menses have resumed, estradiol, LH, and FSH levels should be obtained. A PRL level should be obtained.

Hormone replacement therapy is dictated by clinical response as mediated by target endocrine organ hormones. For deficient TSH, replacement would be thyroxine 0.8 µg/lb of body weight, with adjustment depending on clinical response and calculated thyroid index or free thyroxine serum levels. Since estrogen can be a growth factor for prolactinomas, estrogen should not be used for patients who have had mixed secretory tumors secreting prolactin.

With ACTH deficiency, an oral glucocorticoid such as prednisone 5.0 mg p.o. each morning, 2.5 mg p.o. each afternoon, or hydrocortisone 20 mg p.o. each morning, 10 mg p.o. each afternoon, or the equivalent, adjusted for clinical response should be given. Mineralocorticoids are usually not needed since this axis is usually relatively ACTH independent, unless the adrenals have been ablated. During times of stress, patients should be instructed to increase, either parenterally or orally, their usual dose of glucocorticoid 3–5 times. A medic alert device should be worn.

Women not desiring fertility who are LH and FSH deficient could be placed on conjugated estrogen 0.625 mg p.o. each day on days 1–25, and medroxy-progesterone acetate 10 mg p.o. each day on days 16–25. If they lacked a uterus then the estrogen could be continuous and the medroxyprogesterone acetate not given. To restore libido, a low dose of testosterone enanthate, e.g., 50 mg i.m., may be administered every 1–2 months.

To restore fertility in patients who are LH and FSH deficient from gonadotrophin damage, the following is recommended. Treatment with FSH injections to achieve an estrogen level of 1200 ng/ml, followed by human chorionic gonadotrophin, to mimic LH action, can result in successful ovulation. Hyperstimulated ovaries and multiple births are a risk of this therapy.

Hyperprolactinemia from hypothalamic or pituitary stalk damage can be treated with bromocriptine. If pregnancy occurs on bromocriptine, the drug can then be stopped. There is no evidence of any adverse gestational or teratogenic effect of bromocriptine in pregnancy.

FURTHER READING

Black PM et al. (eds). Secretory Tumors of the Pituitary Gland. Raven Press, 1984.

DeGroot L et al. (eds). Endocrinology. WB Saunders, 1989.

Felig P et al. (eds). Endocrinology and Metabolism. McGraw-Hill, 1987.

Molitch M (ed.). Endocrinology and Metabolism Clinics of North America, vol 16. WB Saunders, 1987.

Wand G, Identifying Cushing's syndrome and defining its cause. Grand Rounds 1989; 2: 47–56.

Weight loss amenorrhea and eating disorders

PETER R. CASSON & SANDRA A. CARSON

In our society, ingrained cultural values emphasize slimness. This bias with respect to the female form appears to be increasing, as evidenced by the decreasing measurements and weights of *Playboy* centerfolds and Miss America winners over the last 25 years [1]. Such values impose tremendous pressures among certain predisposed individuals to lose weight excessively, with a lack of regard for the adverse health consequences, which include amenorrhea.

Simple weight loss amenorrhea resolves rapidly with weight gain, and represents an attenuated form of self-inflicted hypothalamic dysfunction. In contrast to weight loss amenorrhea, the most extreme manifestations of societal pressure to lose weight are the eating disorders, such as anorexia nervosa and bulimia, which are increasing in prevalence [2], and are associated with amenorrhea in the majority of cases [3]. Amenorrhea from these eating disorders often persists even when weight normalizes [4], indicating global hypothalamic dysfunction, of which reproductive aberration is just one facet.

WEIGHT LOSS AMENORRHEA

The observation that weight loss can result in amenorrhea has long been noted, but the first systemic analysis of the phenomenon was published by Frisch and McArthur in 1974 [5]. On the basis of a longitudinal study of 181 girls, they concluded that: (1) the percentage of body fat increases through puberty in females; (2) 22% body fat is the minimum required for the restoration and maintenance of the menses; and (3) 17% body fat is the minimum amount required for the onset of menarche. Although Frisch and McArthur also used a relatively inaccurate method of determining percentage body fat (based on a calculation derived from height and weight), the concept that a certain minimal amount of stored energy reserve is necessary prior to the onset of

fertility and reproduction is teleologically appealing, and remains a useful construct. More recently, Wentz has postulated that amenorrhea results from a relative weight loss from ideal body weight of greater than 15% (30% loss of body fat) rather than an absolute weight value [6]. Subsequent studies have shown that underweight amenorrheic ballet dancers regain menstrual function with cessation of training, with no change in body weight [7]. In addition, anorexia nervosa patients will develop amenorrhea in a significant percentage of cases, prior to weight loss [8]. These findings indicate that stress and exercise levels are intimately intertwined with percentage body fat in the patient with weight loss amenorrhea, and that no one factor can be considered in isolation.

Etiology

Amenorrheic athletes who have ceased training first develop time-related luteinizing hormone (LH) secretory activity prior to their first menses, mimicking premenarchal pituitary awakening [9]. Thus, the amenorrhea associated with weight loss likely resembles the prepubertal state and may be due in part to increased hypothalamic endogenous opiate tone [10]. However, administration of naloxone (an opiate antagonist) to patients with weight loss amenorrhea yielded disappointing results [11]. This reflects an inability to correct concomitant alterations in other hypothalamic neuroendocrine modulators such as catecholestrogens, epinephrine, norepinephrine, dopamine, and serotonin. As the hypothalamic dysfunction becomes more profound, patients with weight loss amenorrhea may experience abnormalities in thermoregulation, vasopressin secretion, and thyroid and adrenal function. In any case, weight loss amenorrhea is solely a hypothalamic dysfunction; after priming, the pituitary is responsive to exogenous gonadotropin-releasing hormone (GnRH) in patients with this disorder [12]. Likewise, the ovaries are responsive to exogenous gonadotropins.

Complications

The consequences of weight loss amenorrhea are related to anovulation and hypoestrogenemia. As hypothalamic amenorrhea ensues, women develop ovulatory dysfunction, ranging from inadequate luteal phase [13] to anovulation [5,6], thus leading to infertility. When ovarian function wanes to the point of hypoestrogenemia, women with weight loss amenorrhea may experience menopausal symptoms such as hot flashes, atrophic vaginitis, and even osteoporosis [14]. Also contributing to the development of osteoporosis in these patients are dietary calcium deficiency, relative hypercortisolism, and low adrenal androgen levels. The increased physical activity seen in amenorrheic athletes does not adequately protect against osteoporosis and bone loss can still be demonstrated [15,16]. The same is probably true in weight loss amenorrhea patients. Exogenous estrogens will stabilize bone loss, but it is not known whether reversal of the process will occur with estrogens or the resumption of regular menses. Also, of concern in this group of patients are the implications of long-term estrogen deficiency on cardiovascular risk, a well-demonstrated phenomenon in postmenopausal women [17].

Medical history

Underlying diseases, such as hypothyroidism, hyperprolactinemia, or other endocrinopathies must be excluded in patients with weight loss amenorrhea. A careful chronologic history of dietary habits, exercise patterns, and weight fluctuations, and the relation of these to menstrual function is necessary. The age at which menarche and the development of secondary sexual characteristics occurred should be elicited. Inquiry about postprandial vomiting, and cathartic, diuretic, or laxative abuse is informative. During the routine medical history, particular attention should be paid to emotional and social stresses, family dynamics, and personality traits.

Physical examination

Careful measurement of height and weight can be applied to charts (Fig. 30.1) for calculation of body fat percentage. Examination of the head and neck should attempt to elicit anosmia, bitemporal hemianopsia, and an enlarged thyroid, if present. The breasts are staged according to Tanner and examined for galactorrhea. Cardiorespiratory exam may reveal bradycardia, associated with anorexia nervosa or thyroid hypofunction. A scaphoid abdomen is present. An intact, patent reproductive tract is demonstrated during pelvic examination by the presence of a uterus and cervix, and the degree of estrogenization is determined by the amount of vaginal rugation and cervical secretion present.

Laboratory and ancillary tests (Fig. 30.2)

Laboratory examination of patients in whom functional hypothalamic amenorrhea from weight loss is suspected includes a complete blood count, serum LH, follicle-stimulating hormone (FSH), thyroid-stimulating hormone (TSH), thyroxine (T_4), and prolactin (PRL) concentrations (Table 30.1). Pregnancy must be ruled out, regardless of the sexual history. Although serum carotene may be elevated in patients eating vegetable-rich diets or in hypothyroidism, the clinical utility of this assay remains questionable. If there is evidence of pituitary hypofunction, such as lack of response to first-line therapies, provocative testing is indicated to determine the degree of pituitary impairment. Insulin, thyrotropin-releasing hormone (TRH), and GnRH are administered intravenously, and serial measurements of growth hormone (GH), cortisol, TSH, LH, and FSH are measured.

A pituitary or hypothalamic lesion is ruled out with a radiologic examination of the sella turcica in patients with persistent amenorrhea, with a coned-down view, a computed tomography (CT) scan, or magnetic resonance imaging (MRI) scan. Long-standing amenorrhea necessitates baseline and follow-up radiologic investigations to evaluate bone mass with an axial skeletal CT scan.

After pregnancy has been ruled out, 10 mg of medroxyprogesterone acetate is given for 7 days to assess the presence of endogenous estrogen. If the

Table 30.1 Diagnostic tests in weight loss amenorrhea

Essential
  Height, weight, body mass index
  CBC, LH, FSH, prolactin, hCG
  Radiologic evaluation of the sella turcica (CT, NMR)
  Radiologic evaluation of bone mass (DPA, CT)
  Progestin withdrawal test

Useful
  Serum carotene
  Provocative pituitary testing

CBC, complete blood count; LH, luteinizing hormone; FSH, follicle-stimulating hormone; hCG, human chorionic gonadotropin; CT, computed tomography, NMR, nuclear magnetic resonance; DPA, dual photon absorptiometry.

CHAPTER 30

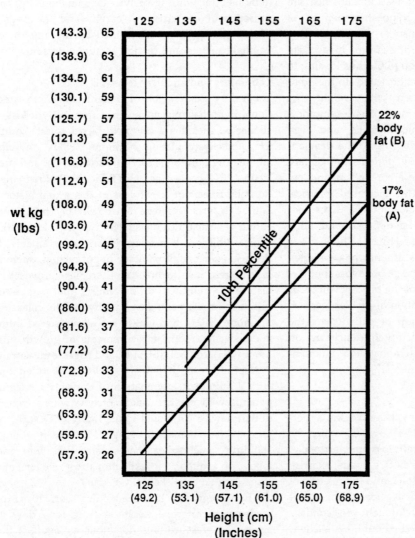

Fig. 30.1 Nomogram for the minimal weight for height for onset of menarche (A) and restoration of menses (B). (Adapted from Frisch *et al.* [51] with permission.)

patient bleeds, she has estrogenization adequate to protect bone mass and requires cyclic progestin withdrawal to reduce the risk of endometrial cancer. Patients with secondary amenorrhea who do not bleed after a progestin challenge require estrogen replacement until the cause of their amenorrhea is reversed. Patients with primary amenorrhea who do not bleed after a progestin challenge require 3 weeks of estrogen treatment prior to another progestin challenge to confirm the presence of normal anatomy.

Treatment

The treatment of weight loss amenorrhea begins with the identification and treatment of any underlying eating disorder. In many cases, simple weight gain or

cessation of exercise will result in resumption of normal menses, but many patients do not wish to change their lifestyle. Treatment then depends on the fertility aspirations of the patient. If fertility is not an issue, and a negative progestin withdrawal test reveals low levels of endogenous estrogen, low-dose oral contraceptive medications provide estrogen, cyclic menses, and reliable contraception. Alternately, any other established estrogen replacement therapy regimens can be used. Whatever therapy is instituted, calcium supplementation (1000 mg/day, or four glasses of milk) is recommended. Withdrawal bleeding after a progestin challenge implies adequate estrogenization, and cyclic progestin withdrawal is necessary. It must be emphasized that occasional

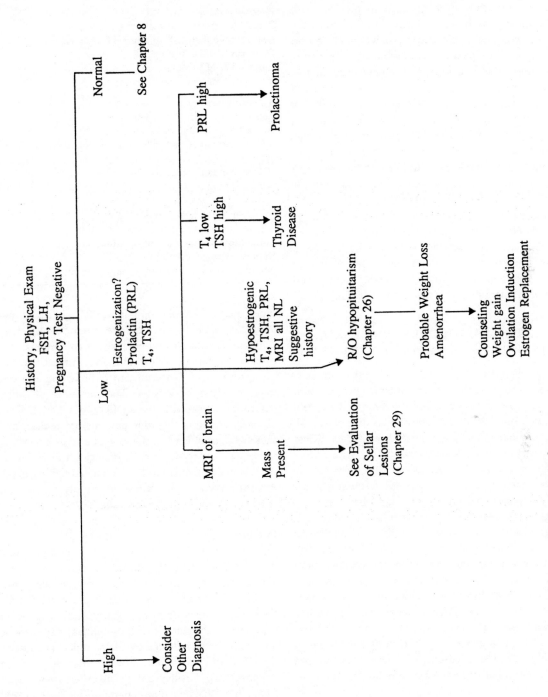

Fig. 30.2 Approach to weight loss amenorrhea.

ovulation may occur and contraception is required if the patient is sexually active.

Patients desiring fertility may be treated with ovulation induction. The decision to proceed with ovulation induction is sometimes difficult, given the asthenic body habitus and compulsive nature found in many of these patients. A psychiatrist or psychologist may be able to provide valuable input at this point. A reasonable initial approach, particularly if the progestin withdrawal test is positive, is to try clomiphene citrate 50 mg on days 5–9 after an induced menstrual period. The monthly doses may be increased in a monthly fashion to a maximum of 150 mg/day. Clomiphene is unlikely to be successful in the presence of hypoestrogenemia, as is often the case in these patients. Patients failing to ovulate with clomiphene citrate are best referred to a reproductive endocrinologist for exogenous GnRH or human menopausal gonadotropin (hMG) administration. GnRH therapy is more physiologic, resulting in a lower incidence of ovarian hyperstimulation and multiple gestation, and is also less costly [18].

EATING DISORDERS: ANOREXIA NERVOSA AND BULIMIA NERVOSA

Eating disorders are subdivided into anorexia nervosa and bulimia nervosa. Bulimics exhibit food-hoarding behaviors, binge-eating followed by self-induced vomiting, and emetic and laxative abuse [4]. They are older, more extroverted, and have a less distorted body image than anorexics [19], with greater insight into their disease. Often, despite a normal weight, menstrual disturbances still frequently occur [4]. Anorexics, on the other hand, have extreme weight loss, fear obesity, have marked body self-image distortion and lack of insight as to the disease process present [20]. Weight loss occurs through dietary restriction and variably increased degrees of physical activity. The distinction between anorexia and bulimia is blurred somewhat by frequent occurrence of bulimic behavior in anorexics [21] (bulimic anorexia nervosa — a poor prognostic sign). Similarly, one-third of bulimics have a history suggestive of anorexia [22]. Useful criteria for diagnosis of anorexia nervosa and bulimia nervosa are delineated in Table 30.2.

Epidemiology

In 1976, the prevalence of severe anorexia nervosa was 1% in women over 16 years old in a British independent school population [23]. Other populations have a higher prevalence, around 5–10% [24]. Bulimia nervosa is somewhat more common, affecting 1.3% of female college students in the USA [25]. The prevalence of intermittent bulimic and anorexic behaviors may be greater. The incidence of eating disorders increased between 1960 and 1976 [26]. In all, 90% of eating disorder patients are female, and there appear, at least in the case of anorexia nervosa, to be two age-related peaks of incidence: at age 13 (perimenarche), and age 17–18 (late adolescence) [4]. Anorexic patients are more commonly white, and from upper socioeconomic strata [27].

Etiology

The etiology of the eating disorders is multifactorial. As noted above, sociocultural pressures may play a role. Unhappy family dynamics have also been implicated. Families of anorexic patients are characterized by overprotection, rigidity, and suppressed conflict [4]. Psychiatric vulnerabilities may also be important, as is indicated by the significant incidence (20–50%) of concomitant affective disorder in these patients [28]. Finally, eating disorders may result from a hypothalamic neurochemical dysfunction [29]. Hypothalamic amenorrhea is a hallmark of these diseases. Anorexics have high cerebrospinal fluid levels of β-endorphins [30]. Other indications of global hypothalamic dysfunction include elevated

Table 30.2 Criteria for the diagnosis of anorexia nervosa and bulimia

Anorexia nervosa
Refusal to maintain normal body weight
Loss of more than 25% of original body weight
Disturbance of body image
Intense fear of becoming fat
No known medical illness leading to weight loss

Bulimia nervosa
Recurrent episodes of binge eating
At least three of the following:
  Consumption of high-calorie, easily ingested foods in a binge;
  Termination of binge by abdominal pain, sleep, or vomiting;
  Inconspicuous eating during a binge;
  Repeated attempts to lose weight;
  Frequent weight fluctuations of more than 4.5 kg
Awareness of abnormal eating pattern and fear
Depressed mood after binge
Not due to anorexia nervosa or any physical disorder

GH levels [8], and incoordinate vasopressin secretion [31], which in a minority of patients results in various degrees of diabetes insipidus. Thermoregulation, another hypothalamic function, is also impaired, with a lack of shivering noted in response to cold [12].

Complications

Anorexia nervosa may result in renal calculi, azotemia from dehydration, anemia, thrombocytopenia, diarrhea, and electrolyte abnormalities from diuretic and laxative abuse, cardiac muscle atrophy, and arrhythmias [4] (the most common cause of death in this condition). Bulimia may be complicated by acute gastric dilatation and rupture, dental erosions, parotid enlargement, esophagitis, Mallory—Weiss tears, esophageal rupture, aspiration pneumonia, and ipecac poisoning [4].

Mortality from anorexia nervosa ranges from 2 [32] to 9% [33]. It is important to note that even in the patients in whom therapeutic success is obtained, amenorrhea may still be a problem, despite attainment of normal weight.

Physical examination

The clinical features of anorexia nervosa are those of inanition. Hypothermia, bradycardia, and hypotension may be present in florid cases. Vellus hair is prominent; scalp hair may be thin. The skin is dry and in extreme cases petechiae and bruising may be present, from vitamin K deficiency and thrombocytopenia. Abdominal distention (from intestinal stasis) and peripheral edema may variably be present. Hypoestrogenemia results in breast and vaginal mucosal atrophy.

Laboratory examination

Thyroid and cortisol abnormalities are consistently seen in anorexia nervosa. While TSH remains normal, triiodothyroxine (T_3) is decreased [34,35] because thyroxine (T_4) is preferentially converted to reverse triiodothyroxine (rT_3) [36]. This "euthyroid sick state" is a nonspecific homeostatic response to starvation, resulting in a lower metabolic rate, and decreased energy expenditure. Plasma cortisol is also increased, despite normal adrenocorticotropic hormone levels [37]. In anorexia, the half-life of cortisol is increased, and the metabolic clearance is decreased [38]. These changes may be secondary to the altered thyroid status. The patient remains clinically eucorticoid, perhaps reflecting reduced tissue levels of glucocorticoid receptors [39].

Treatment

Treatment of anorexia nervosa, particularly in florid cases, is beyond the purview of the gynecologist. Historically, many therapies have been tried, from prefrontal lobotomy to hypnosis [40]. Treatment success is reduced by patient noncompliance, denial, and evasion. Once this disease is suspected diagnosis and care rest primarily with an integrated team of psychiatrists, psychologists, social workers, and internists. Weight loss greater than 30% in 3 months, metabolic disturbances, psychosis, family crisis, suicidal ideation, or severe binging and purging require hospital admission [4]. Privileges while in hospital, such as mail, visitors, and activity are linked to caloric intake and weight gain. Such behavior modification therapy [40] can be continued as an outpatient but hospital admission is necessary to initiate therapy and separate the patient from possibly unhealthy family dynamics. Continuous psychotherapy with one primary therapist is desirable [41]. In severe cases, patients require hospital admission for treatment of malnutrition, which may include tube feeding, or in the extreme, total parenteral nutrition [42]. Pharmacologic adjuvants include tricyclic antidepressants, monoamine oxidase inhibitors and serotonin antagonists, but at this time there is no clear indication for adjuvant pharmacotherapy [4]. Whatever the therapy, response rates are only moderate. A long-term follow-up study of anorexics indicates that at 4—8 years 50% resolve with therapy, 30% have an intermediate response, and 20% respond poorly [32].

Amenorrhea may persist even after successful treatment of other facets of anorexia nervosa [43]. Treatment modalities are basically the same as for the amenorrhea associated with weight loss, which have been outlined above.

CONCLUSIONS

Gynecologists are commonly presented with amenorrhea or ovulatory dysfunction of lesser degrees with a hypothalamic basis. Weight loss is an increasingly common cause, as are the more severe eating disorders. Investigation must diagnose any underlying chronic diseases or endocrinopathies. The high incidence of concomitant eating disorders makes an index of suspicion for these conditions essential. In simple weight loss amenorrhea, restoration of weight is often all that is required to restore normal reproductive function. However, if this is unsuccessful, the patient must be actively treated to protect her from the consequences of hypoestrogenemia, or of unopposed estrogen, and to allow fertility, if so desired.

REFERENCES

1 Garner DM, Garfinkel PE, Schwartz D, Thompson M. Cultural expectations of thinness in women. *Psychol Rep* 1980; 47: 483–491.

2 Willi J, Grassmann S. Epidemiology of anorexia nervosa in a defined region of Switzerland. *Am J Psychiatry* 1983; 140: 564–567.

3 Warren MP, Vande Weile RL. Clinical and metabolic features of anorexia nervosa. *Am J Obstet Gynecol* 1973; 117: 435–449.

4 Herzog DB, Copeland PM. Eating disorders. *N Engl J Med* 1985; 313: 295–303.

5 Frisch RE, McArthur JW. Menstrual cycles: fatness as a determinant of minimum weight for height necessary for their maintenance or onset. *Science* 1974; 185: 949–951.

6 Wentz AC. Body weight and amenorrhea. *Obstet Gynecol* 1980; 56: 482–487.

7 Abraham SF, Beumont PJV, Fraser IS, Llewellyn-Jones D. Body weight, exercise and menstrual status among ballet dancers in training. *Br J Obstet Gynaecol* 1982; 89: 507–510.

8 Newman MM, Halmi KA. The endocrinology of anorexia nervosa and bulimia nervosa. *Endocrinol Metab Clin North Am* 1988; 17: 195–212.

9 Yen SSC, Jaffe RB. *Reproductive Endocrinology, Physiology, Pathophysiology, and Clinical Management*, 2nd edn. Philadelphia: WB Saunders, 1986: 552.

10 Quigley ME, Sheehan KL, Casper RF, Yen SSC. Evidence for increased dopaminergic and opioid activity in patients with hypothalamic hypogonadotropic amenorrhea. *J Clin Endocrinol Metab* 1980; 50: 949–954.

11 Giusti M, Torre R, Traverso L, Cavagnaro P, Attanasio R, Giordano G. Endogenous opioid blockade and gonadotropin secretion: role of pulsatile luteinizing hormone-releasing hormone administration in anorexia nervosa and weight loss amenorrhea. *Fertil Steril* 1988; 49: 797–801.

12 Vigersky RA, Andersen AE, Thompson RH, Loriaux DL. Hypothalamic dysfunction in secondary amenorrhea associated with simple weight loss. *N Engl J Med* 1977; 24: 1141–1145.

13 Ellison PT, Lager C. Moderate recreational running is associated with lowered salivary progesterone profiles in women. *Am J Obstet Gynecol* 1986; 154: 1000.

14 Rigotti NA, Nussbaum SR, Herzog DB, Neer RM. Osteoporosis in women with anorexia nervosa. *N Engl J Med* 1984; 311: 1601–1606.

15 Marcus R, Cann C, Madvig P *et al*. Menstrual function and bone mass in elite women distance runners. *Ann Intern Med* 1985; 102: 158–163.

16 Drinkwater BL, Nilson K, Chesnut CH III, Bremner WJ, Shainholtz S, Southworth MB. Bone mineral content of amenorrheic and eumenorrheic athletes. *N Engl J Med* 1984; 311: 277–281.

17 Stampfer MJ, Willett WC, Coldite GA, Rosner B, Speizer FE, Henekens CM. A prospective study of postmenopausal estrogen therapy and coronary heart disease. *N Engl J Med* 1985; 313: 1044.

18 Wong PC, Asch RH. Induction of follicular development with luteinizing hormone-releasing hormone. *Semin Reprod Endocrinol* 1987; 5: 399–409.

19 Casper RC, Eckert ED, Halmi KA, Goldberg SC, Davis JM. Bulimia: its incidence and clinical importance in patients with anorexia nervosa. *Arch Gen Psychiatry* 1980; 37: 1030–1035.

20 Mansfield MJ, Emans SJ. Anorexia nervosa, athletics, and amenorrhea. *Pediatr Clin North Am* 1989; 36: 533–549.

21 Garfinkel PE, Moldofsky H, Garner D. The heterogeneity of anorexia nervosa. *Arch Gen Psychiatry* 1980; 37: 1036–1040.

22 Fairburn C, Cooper PJ. The clinical features of bulimia nervosa. *Br J Psychiatry* 1984; 144: 238.

23 Crisp AH, Palmer RL, Kalucy RS. How common is anorexia nervosa? A prevalence study. *Br J Psychiatry* 1976; 128: 549–554.

24 Pope HG, Hudson JI, Yurgelun-Todd D, Hudson MS. Prevalence of anorexia nervosa and bulimia in three student populations. *Int J Eat Disord* 1984; 3: 45–51.

25 Schotte DE, Stunkard AJ. Bulimia vs bulimic behaviors on a college campus. *JAMA* 1987; 258: 1213–1215.

26 Jones DJ, Fox MM, Babigan HM, Hutton HE. Epidemiology of anorexia nervosa in Monroe County, New York. *Psychosom Med* 1980; 42: 551–558.

27 Speroff L, Glass RH, Kase NG. *Clinical Gynecologic Endocrinology and Infertility*, 4th edn. Baltimore: Williams & Wilkins, 1989: 197.

28 Herzog DB. Are anorexic and bulimic patients depressed? *Am J Psychiatry* 1984; 141: 1594–1597.

29 Mecklenburg RS, Loriaux DL, Thompson RH, Andersen AE, Lipsett MB. Hypothalamic dysfunction in patients with anorexia nervosa. *Medicine* 1974; 53: 147–159.

30 Kage WH, Pickar D, Naber D, Ebert MM. Cerebrospinal fluid opiate activity in anorexia nervosa. *Am J Psychiatry* 1982; 139: 643.

31 Gold PW, Walter K, Robertson GL, Ebert M. Abnormalities in plasma and cerebrospinal-fluid arginine vasopressin in patients with anorexia nervosa. *N Engl J Med* 1983; 308: 1117–1123.

32 Hsu LK, Crisp AH, Harding B. Outcome of anorexia nervosa. *Lancet* 1979; i: 61–65.

33 Seidensticker JF, Tzagournis M. Anorexia nervosa — clinical features and long term follow-up. *J Chronic Dis* 1968; 21: 361–367.

34 Miyai K, Yamamoto T, Azukizawa M, Ishibashi K, Kumahara Y. Serum thyroid hormones and thyrotropin in anorexia nervosa. *J Clin Endocrinol Metab* 1975; 40: 334–338.

35 Moshang T Jr, Parks JS, Baker L *et al*. Low serum tri-

iodothyronine in patients with anorexia nervosa. *J Clin Endocrinol Metab* 1975; 40: 470–473.

36 Vagenakis AG, Burger A, Portnay GI *et al*. Diversion of peripheral thyroxine metabolism from activating to inactivating pathways during complete fasting. *J Clin Endocrinol Metab* 1975; 41: 191–194.

37 Takahara J, Hosogi M, Hashimoto K *et al*. Hypothalamic pituitary adrenal function in patients with anorexia nervosa. *Endocrinol Jpn* 1976; 23: 451.

38 Boyar RM, Hellman LD, Roffwarg H *et al*. Cortisol secretion and metabolism in anorexia nervosa. *N Engl J Med* 1977; 296: 190–193.

39 Kontula K, Andersson LC, Huttunen M, Pelkonen R. Reduced level of cellular glucocorticoid receptors in patients with anorexia nervosa. *Horm Metab Res* 1982; 14: 619–620.

40 Halmi KA, Powers P, Cunningham S. Treatment of anorexia nervosa with behavior modification. *Arch Gen Psychiatry* 1975; 32: 93–96.

41 Lucas AR, Duncan JW, Piens V. The treatment of anorexia nervosa. *Am J Psychiatry* 1976; 133: 1034–1038.

42 Pertschuk MJ, Forster J, Buzby G, Mullen JL. The treatment of anorexia nervosa with total parenteral nutrition. *Biol Psychiatry* 1981; 16: 539–550.

43 Kohmura H, Miyake A, Aono T, Tanizawa O. Recovery of reproductive function in patients with anorexia nervosa: a 10-year follow-up study. *Eur J Obstet Gynecol Reprod Biol* 1986; 22: 293–296.

44 Frisch RE. Body fat, menarche, and reproductive ability. *Semin Reprod Endocrinol* 1985; 3: 45–54.

31

Abnormal gonadotropins

ELI RESHEF & ROBERT A. WILD

INTRODUCTION

Disorders of gonadotropin (GT) secretion (abnormal levels or abnormal secretion patterns of luteinizing hormone (LH) and/or follicle-stimulating hormone (FSH)) often pose a diagnostic challenge. Because numerous etiologies to these disorders are possible, a systematic approach is needed to avoid unnecessary expense, patient discomfort, and delay of diagnosis. GTs have changing dynamics during various phases of life. What might be considered normal in one phase (e.g., elevated FSH and LH in the post-menopausal years) may be abnormal when applied to another phase (e.g., during the reproductive period). The pulsatile nature of GT secretion, as well as the presence of a midcycle surge just prior to ovulation, should be taken into consideration when abnormal GTs are encountered.

Disorders of GT secretion may be the sequelae of serious and sometimes life-threatening pathology (Tables 31.1 and 31.2). The first responsibility of the health care professional, therefore, is to rule out such etiologies while arriving at the correct diagnosis in as logical and economical fashion as possible. In this chapter, following a short description of normal GT physiology, a practical approach to the diagnosis of GT abnormalities based on their most common clinical presentations will be offered. Since the majority of GT disorders in the reproductive years in the female are manifested as menstrual aberrations, the reader should refer to related chapters in this book which specifically outline the work-up and treatment of menstrual disorders. The goal of this chapter is to guide the reader to situations in which LH and FSH tests are warranted, and to aid in pursuing logical diagnostic and therapeutic alternatives once GT abnormalities are detected.

Table 31.1 Etiologies of elevated gonadotropins (GTs) by clinical presentation

Physiologic

Midcycle surge
Menopause

Pathologic

Ambiguous genitalia
   Partial androgen insensitivity

Precocious puberty (central)
   Idiopathic
   Cerebral
   Ectopic GT

Delayed puberty or primary amenorrhea
   Congenital gonadal failure
      Pure gonadal dysgenesis
      Chromosomal aberrations (Turner's, Klinefelter's)
      Defects in androgen synthesis
      Defects in androgen receptors (testicular feminization)
      Polymalformation syndromes
   Acquired gonadal failure
      Gonadal surgery
      Chemo-, radiotherapy
      Trauma
      Infection
      Autoimmune
   Polycystic ovary syndrome

Secondary amenorrhea
   Congenital gonadal failure (rare)
   Chromosomal aberrations (Turner's mosaic)
   Polycystic ovary syndrome
   Acquired gonadal failure
      Gonadal surgery
      Chemo-, radiotherapy
      Trauma
      Infection
      Autoimmune
   Idiopathic
      Premature menopause

Table 31.2 Etiologies of decreased gonadotropins (GTs) by clinical presentation

---

Physiologic

Childhood
  Pregnancy
  Exogenous hormones

Pathologic

Primary amenorrhea
  Congenital
    Isolated GT deficiency
    Kallmann's syndrome (anosmia)
    Polymalformation syndromes
    Congenital adrenal hyperplasia
  Acquired
    Eating disorders (anorexia nervosa, bulimia)
    Exercise-related
    Intracranial tumors
    Intracranial trauma

Secondary amenorrhea
  Acquired pituitary or hypothalamic failure
    Eating disorders
    Exercise-related
    Intracranial tumors
    Intracranial trauma, surgery
    Intracranial infection/inflammation
    Pituitary apoplexy (Sheehan's syndrome)
    Systemic illness
  Peripheral steroid hormone excess
    Androgen or estrogen-producing neoplasms
    Obesity
    Liver, renal disease

NORMAL GONADOTROPIN PHYSIOLOGY

The gonadotropins FSH and LH are glycoproteins composed of two subunits, α and β. The α-subunits of FSH and LH, as well as that of thyroid-stimulating hormone (TSH) and human chorionic gonadotropin (hCG) are virtually identical, whereas the β-subunits differ. FSH and LH are secreted in a pulsatile fashion from the anterior pituitary under the influence of pulsatile gonadotropin-releasing hormone (GnRH) from the medial basal hypothalamus. The GTs in turn influence gonadal activity, namely follicular development, ovulation, and corpus luteum function in the ovary. These events occur in part due to stimulation of gonadal steroid production by FSH and LH.

Negative and positive feedback mechanisms exist whereby the gonadal steroids estrogen and progesterone, as well as other substances (e.g., inhibin, androgens, progestins) influence hypothalamic secretion of GnRH or pituitary GT secretion. The complex interrelationship between the central nervous system (CNS), hypothalamus, pituitary, gonads, and end-organs changes throughout life. These changes must be considered when an abnormality of GTs is suspected.

During the first 4 months after birth, a temporary rise in FSH and LH represents the escape of the newborn pituitary from negative feedback by high levels of placental estrogen and progesterone. LH and FSH secretion is suppressed between the end of the first year of life and the onset of puberty. FSH begins to rise after age 8, whereas LH rise occurs at age 10–12 years. Episodic LH pulses occur at early puberty, first during sleep, then, as pulsatile GnRH secretion occurs, LH and FSH patterns during the day resemble that of the adult and menses occur. During the normal menstrual cycle, FSH and LH rise in the preovulatory phase in a rapid manner. The rapid midcycle rise in LH (LH surge), thought to be triggered by positive feedback from rising estrogen and progesterone, helps to initiate ovulation and corpus luteum function.

Negative feedback by estrogen and/or progesterone on the pituitary and hypothalamus causes decrease in GTs during the midfollicular and midluteal phases of the cycle. During the perimenopausal period, as follicular function and estrogen and progesterone production decline, FSH and LH begin to rise, with the former dominating. FSH and LH peak approximately 1–3 years after menopause, then decline slightly but remain elevated. This peri- and postmenopausal rise in GTs is a response to declining ovarian function.

PATHOLOGY

Abnormalities of GT secretion may result from disturbances in any of the major stations in the hypothalamic–pituitary–gonadal axis. In childhood, GT disorders are very uncommon or nonapparent due to the absence of menstrual periods. The most common presentation of abnormal GTs in the newborn period and infancy in females is ambiguous genitalia, which is most commonly due to adrenal enzyme deficiency in the female, but can also be due to partial androgen insensitivity in the male. In childhood, the most common clinical presentations of abnormal GTs are precocius (premature) puberty and chromosomal abnormalities (e.g., Turner's syndrome) with their unique physical features.

During adolescence, GT abnormalities are most commonly manifested as delayed puberty and primary amenorrhea. During the reproductive years, the most common manifestations of abnormal GT pattern are expressed as menstrual aberrations or signs and symptoms of estrogen deficiency. The etiologies of primary amenorrhea differ from those of secondary amenorrhea (Tables 31.1 and 31.2). This fact may influence the choice of diagnostic procedures.

Generally, decreased or absent ovarian function, whether congenital or acquired, will result in a compensatory elevation of FSH and LH (hypergonadotropic hypogonadism). Only rarely will hypergonadotropic hypergonadism be due to primary pituitary or hypothalamic lesions such as functional GT tumors. Factors causing hypothalamic deficiency will cause decrease in GTs as well as ovarian hormones (hypogonadotropic hypogonadism). Primary pituitary insufficiency, a rare disorder, is also characterized by low GTs and low ovarian hormones (hypogonadotropic hypogonadism).

In certain endocrine disorders, such as polycystic ovary syndrome or androgen insensitivity, serum GT levels will be normal or near normal, but the secretion pattern and/or ratio of LH to FSH will be altered. Normal GT levels in the presence of reduced ovarian activity often is indicative of impaired hypothalamic function, since the intact hypothalamus–pituitary axis is expected to respond with a compensatory elevation of FSH and LH when ovarian function is impaired. Therefore, "normal" GT levels do not always imply normal hypothalamic function.

DIAGNOSIS

The history and physical examination are the cornerstone of the diagnosis. The major issue to be addressed is whether the disorder is of central, hypothalamic, pituitary, or gonadal origin. If a menstrual dysfunction exists, its nature should be thoroughly examined since primary amenorrhea has different etiologies than secondary amenorrhea. A summary of pertinent historic details which might be elicited during an interview when an abnormality in gonadotropins is suspected is presented in Table 31.3.

The physical examination may give important clues

Table 31.3 History and physical examination when disorders of gonadotropins are suspected

History
General
  Energy, weight change
Skin
  Hair pattern, pigmentation changes
HEENT
  Headaches, visual symptoms, head trauma, CNS infection, smell
Thyroid
  Cold/heat intolerance, hair changes, GI changes
Breasts
  Discharge
Abdomen
  Pain, bowel habits, history of irradiation, surgery, chemotherapy,
Gynecologic
  Surgeries, infections, hormonal therapy, vaginal dryness, hot flushes, sexual function
Menses
  Primary versus secondary amenorrhea, menarche, puberty and development, characteristics of flow, cyclic pelvic or abdominal pain
Other
  Collagen–vascular disease, anemia, arthritis, myasthenia gravis, diabetes, eating disorders, stress
Family history
  Congenital malformations, endocrine disorders, collagen–vascular diseases, premature menopause, delayed puberty, hirsutism

Physical examination
General
  Stigmata of Turner's, Klinefelter's, Cushing's, polymalformation syndromes, hypothyroidism, hypopituitarism, adrenal dysfunction
Skin
  Hirsutism, lack of hair, vitiligo, striae
HEENT
  Smell, visual fields
Thyroid
  Enlargement, nodules
Breasts
  Galactorrhea, Tanner's stage
Abdomen
  Scars, masses, tenderness
Pelvic
  External genitalia ambiguity, escutcheon, Tanner's stage, vulvar atrophy, patency of lower genital tract, uterus present or absent, adnexal masses

HEENT, head, eyes, ears, nose, throat.

regarding uncommon etiologies. Stigmata of Turner's and Klinefelter's syndromes are readily discerned. Ambiguous genitalia, signs of precocious puberty, and the absence of vagina are easy to recognize. Pertinent areas on which to focus during the physical examination are summarized in Table 31.3.

The presence or absence of secondary sexual characteristics may direct the clinician toward the correct diagnosis. The presence of breasts reassures the clinician that the gonads are present and functional, and that the etiology of the menstrual dysfunction is from either abnormal genital tract development or CNS—pituitary factors. The presence or absence of the uterus, diagnosed by pelvic examination and/or ultrasound, should be determined early. Absent uterus and/or vagina is most commonly the result of Müllerian dysgenesis in the female or androgen insensitivity in the male.

Once the physician has classified the initial clinical presentation into the six clinical categories which warrant determination of GT levels (Table 31.4), he or she should next refer to Figure 31.1 for the recommended initial laboratory tests. Since a detailed description of the work-up and treatment of each GT disorder is beyond the scope of this chapter, and since each of the six clinical categories is covered separately elsewhere in this book, the reader is referred to the corresponding chapters for a more detailed description of the appropriate diagnostic tests and treatment.

When elevated levels of GT are encountered, and normal physiologic states which are associated with elevated GT are ruled out, gonadal failure is overwhelmingly the most likely diagnosis. Etiologies of gonadal failure should then be vigorously pursued, since some may be life-threatening (Table 31.1). Decreased levels of GTs are less frequently encountered and often do not pinpoint where in the CNS—hypothalamus—pituitary the defect exists. In these situations, the clinician has to rely on characteristic clinical clues (e.g., signs and symptoms of stress, dietary alterations, athletic activity, etc.) and additional diagnostic procedures. As in situations where GT levels are elevated, serious and life-threatening underlying etiologies of decreased GTs must be ruled out first (Table 31.2).

TREATMENT

Numerous etiologies for GT disorders exist. The reader is advised to refer to corresponding chapters in this book (Fig. 31.1) for specific treatments. The primary responsibility is to rule out and treat (or refer) a life-threatening disorder, such as intracranial, adrenal, or adnexal tumors, pituitary or adrenal insufficiency, or anorexia nervosa. The next priority is to diagnose and treat conditions which are not life-threatening but are readily amenable to treatment, such as idiopathic central precocious puberty. Another objective is to prevent long-term adverse sequelae of GT disorders, such as osteoporosis in long-standing hypogonadal disorders or short stature and social maladjustment in precocious puberty.

The first priority when encountering the problem of ambiguous genitalia is to provide gluco- and/or mineralocorticoids in those affected by salt-losing forms of congenital adrenal hyperplasia (see Chapter 4); and perform gonadectomy in those phenotypic females with XY chromosomes in which the gonads are likely to develop neoplastic changes. Significant masculinization of female external genitalia may warrant corrective surgery. In the case of precocious puberty, treatment of the underlying disorder (tumor, infection, etc.) is required. Where the underlying etiology cannot be found or completely treated (e.g., idiopathic central precocity), the treatment objective should be to suppress the prematurely activated central—pituitary—gonadal axis so that the final attained stature will not be compromised and to avoid psychologic trauma associated with the condition (Chapter 1).

Hypogonadal states, both hyper- and hypogonadotropic, should be treated with estrogen and progestin replacement to prevent osteoporosis, vulvovaginal atrophy, and adverse cardiovascular sequelae. Hyperandrogenic and hyperestrogenic conditions in which GT secretion patterns may be abnormal (e.g., polycystic ovary syndrome) should be treated with exogenous progestins (low-dose combination oral contraceptives or progestins alone) in order to induce

Table 31.4 Clinical situations in which gonadotropin levels should be obtained

---

Ambiguous genitalia
Precocious (premature) puberty
Delayed puberty
Primary amenorrhea
Secondary amenorrhea — only if pregnancy has been
  ruled out
Menopausal symptoms

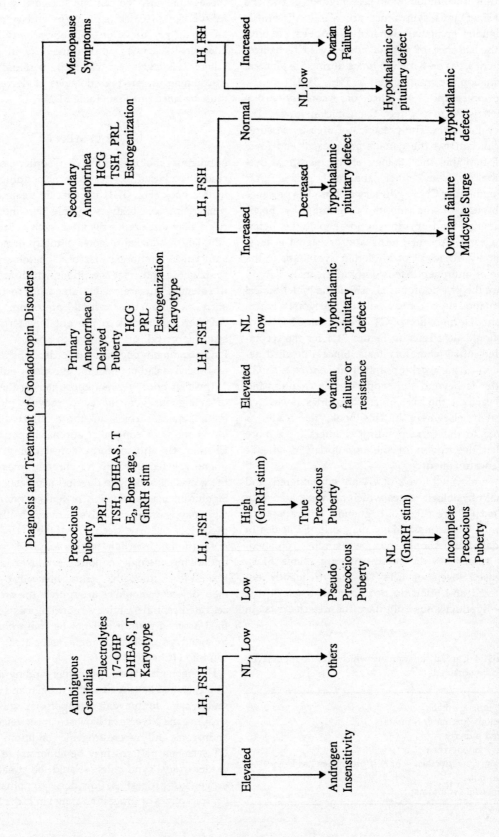

Fig. 31.1 Algorithm for the diagnosis and treatment of gonadotropin disorders. 17-OHP, 17-hydroxyprogesterone; DHEAS, dihidroepiandrosterone sulfate; T, testosterone; E₂, estradiol; GnRH stim, GnRH stimulation test; TSH, thyroid stimulating hormone; HCG, human chorionic gonadotropin.

endometrial sloughing, thus preventing endometrial hyperplasia and cancer, and reduce hirsutism. Ovulation induction (e.g., with clomiphene citrate) may be indicated if fertility is desired (Chapter 74).

FURTHER READING

Bourguingnon JP, Franchimont P. The gonadotropins: clinical disorders of LH and FSH in males and females — their investigation and management. In: DeGroot L, ed. *Endocrinology*, 2nd edn. Philadelphia: WB Saunders, 1989: 296–317.

Mishell DR Jr, Davajan V, eds. *Infertility, Contraception and Reproductive Endocrinology*, 3rd edn. Oradell: Medical Economics, 1991.

Speroff L, Glass RH, Kase NG. *Clinical Gynecologic Endocrinology and Infertility*, 4th edn. Baltimore: Williams & Wilkins, 1990.

Yen SSC, Jaffe RB, eds. *Reproductive Endocrinology*, 3rd edn. Philadelphia: WB Saunders, 1991.

Endocrinologic abnormalities: Thyroid gland

Thyroid-stimulating hormone

YOMNA T. MONLA

BIOSYNTHESIS

When extracted from the pituitary, thyroid-stimulating hormone (TSH) is in the form of a glycoprotein with a molecular weight of 30 000 Da. It is composed of two noncovalently bound subunits (α and β). It has a tertiary structure similar to the other glycoproteins, namely luteinizing hormone (LH), follicle-stimulating hormone (FSH), and human chorionic gonadotropin (hCG) and has ~15% carbohydrate content. The α-subunit is common to all glycoprotein hormones and it is the β-subunit which confers the biologic specificity to each hormone.

Recent advances in molecular biology techniques enabled researchers to study the TSH biosynthesis at the genomic level. The synthesis of each subunit appears to be dependent on a separate gene and occurs by way of ribosomal translation of a separate messenger RNA. The transcribed peptide is then cleaved in the rough endoplasmic reticulum and its glycosylation occurs in the Golgi apparatus. The β-subunit synthesis appears to be the rate-limiting step in TSH synthesis since the α-subunit is produced in excess with a molar ratio of 2.7. The integrity of the structure of the α-subunit is important to both subunit–subunit interaction and expression of biologic activity. The high carbohydrate content of TSH is required for the protection of TSH from degradation, for the facilitation of TSH binding to its receptor, and for the coupling of the TSH-receptor complex to alterations in cellular functions.

METABOLISM

The normal TSH production and degradation is 40–150 mU/day. It is metabolized by the liver and the kidney. Its half-life is 54 min and its normal mean basal concentration is 0.5–5.5 mU/ml. In hypothyroidism, its metabolism is decreased and its production rate is increased (>4000 mU/day), leading to an increased TSH level. In hyperthyroidism, the reverse occurs, leading to a suppressed TSH level. In chronic liver and kidney disease, its degradation is decreased, leading to an elevated TSH level.

REGULATION OF TSH SECRETION

The hypothalamus determines the set-point of the pituitary–thyroid feedback control and mediates environmentally influenced changes related to stress, temperature, and circadian rhythm. In normal subjects, there is a small circadian variation in serum basal TSH concentration. The nadir/peak values range from 50 to 200% of the 24-hour mean value. Peak TSH levels occur between 8 p.m. and 12 midnight just before the onset of sleep; nadir values are found between 10 a.m. and 12 noon. Early-onset sleep blunts the evening rise; the rise is greater when sleep is delayed. This circadian variation is absent in patients with pituitary TSH tumors.

TSH secretion from the pituitary is regulated by the hypothalamus and midbrain, the thyroid gland, and by TSH itself. TSH is under dual control from the hypothalamus, i.e., tonic stimulation by thyrotropin-releasing hormone (TRH) (a neuropeptide secreted by the tuberoinfundibular system) and tonic inhibition by somatostatin (secreted by the paraventricular and median eminence — part of the third ventricle) and dopamine (secreted by the arcuate nucleus). It seems that TRH pulsation is responsible for the circadian rhythm of TSH. TRH stimulates TSH synthesis via cyclic adenosine monophosphate — an effect counteracted by dopamine. TRH appears to regulate also the TSH β-subunit transcription and the terminal processing of the carbohydrate chain during TSH biosynthesis (an event very important for the biologic activity of TSH, which may be reduced in some cases of tertiary hypothyroidism — see below).

There are certain hormones and drugs which

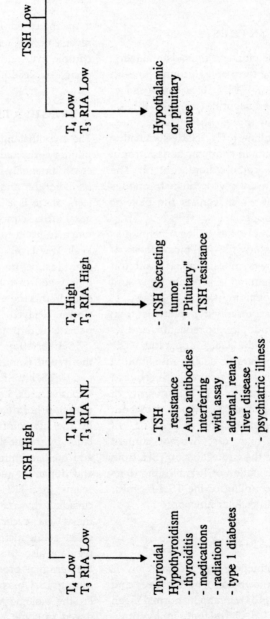

Fig. 32.1 Approach to abnormal thyroid stimulating hormone.

TSH Low

T₄ NL
T₃ RIA NL
→ - Nonthyroidal illness
- Pregnancy

T₄ Low
T₃ RIA Low
→ Hypothalamic or pituitary cause

TSH High

T₄ High
T₃ RIA High
→ - TSH Secreting tumor
- "Pituitary" TSH resistance

T₄ NL
T₃ RIA NL
→ - TSH resistance
- Auto antibodies interfering with assay
- adrenal, renal, liver disease
- psychiatric illness

T₄ Low
T₃ RIA Low
→ Thyroidal Hypothyroidism
- thyroiditis
- medications
- radiation
- type 1 diabetes

modulate TSH secretion at the hypothalamic level. Examples of these are: cortisol (via decreased pituitary responsiveness to TRH); growth hormone; cholecystokinin; gastrin; calcitonin; and vasopressin, all of which decrease TSH synthesis. Dopamine agonists (dopamine receptors are present on thyrotrophs and dopamine causes tonic inhibition of prolactin and TSH), morphine, and valium (via α-aminobutyric acid — GABA) also decrease TSH synthesis.

It is also very important to note that any situation where the pituitary stalk is sectioned or compressed (e.g., pituitary tumors, empty sella, etc.) results in a decreased TSH level since TRH reaches the anterior pituitary via the hypophyseal portal system which runs in the pituitary stalk. In addition, stress, altitude, starvation, psychiatric illness (unipolar depression and anorexia nervosa), and Parkinson's disease can cause a decreased TSH synthesis via a decreased TRH secretion.

On the contrary, an increase in TSH secretion is produced by estrogen (which sensitizes the pituitary to TRH via an increase in the number of TRH receptors and a decrease in the inhibition of thyroid hormone on TSH — see below), amphetamine, and dopamine antagonists.

TSH synthesis is also under sympathetic influence from the midbrain: norepinephrine and epinephrine stimulate (via α_2-receptor) and inhibit (via α_1-receptor) TSH synthesis at the pituitary and hypothalamic levels. Histamine appears to increase TSH synthesis, while endorphins and GABA decrease it.

Finally, the thyroid hormone secreted by the thyroid gland causes a negative feedback inhibition on TSH secretion at both the hypothalamic and pituitary levels, with the major effect being at the pituitary level. The hypothalamic effect is through decreased TRH secretion, while the pituitary effect is through decreased TRH receptors on the thyrotrophs. There is also evidence that the thyroid hormone may regulate TSH synthesis at its β-subunit level by modulation of its transcription and/or its messenger RNA metabolism.

Triiodothyronine (T_3) is the predominant effector of thyroid hormone action within the thyrotrophs. T_3 binds more tightly than thyroxine (T_4) to pituitary cells, causing a greater TSH suppression on a molar basis. The degree and time course of TSH suppression varies with the type and the concentration of thyroid hormone (e.g., a sudden treatment with 0.1 mg of T_4/day, causes a decrease in TSH 4–6 weeks later; however, a sudden treatment with T_3 50–75 µg t.i.d. causes a decrease in TSH 4–10 days later!). Pituitary T_3 is derived 50% from the peripheral circulation and 50% from monodeiodination of T_4 inside the pituitary cells (via T_4-5'deiodinase type II). This type II T_4-5'deiodinase activity is regulated depending on the disease state: in primary hypothyroidism, its activity is decreased both in the periphery and the pituitary, causing a decreased intrapituitary T_3 level and an increased TSH level. In starvation and nonthyroidal illness its activity is decreased in the periphery but not in the pituitary, leaving an intrapituitary T_3 level high enough to maintain a decreased TSH level. Other intrinsic changes that may occur in nonthyroidal illness or sick euthyroid disease state include either a decrease in TRH secretion or an increase in inhibitory hormones like somatostatin, dopamine, and glucocorticoid. All these changes lead to decreased TSH production in face of decreased T_3 and T_4 peripheral levels — a mechanism seen in severely ill patients in an attempt to dampen wasteful metabolic processes and conserve body stores.

There is recent evidence of the existence of an "ultrashort loop" type of TSH-negative feedback regulation at the pituitary level, whereby TSH increases the number of dopamine receptors present on the thyrotrophs, thereby enhancing the functional tonic inhibition of its release by dopamine.

MECHANISM OF ACTION OF TSH

TSH regulates the thyroid gland function by a process that involves the initial interaction of TSH with its specific receptor on the plasma membrane of thyroid cells.

TSH receptor

The recent cloning of the TSH receptor revealed that it is a glycoprotein with an oligomeric structure and a molecular weight of 84 501 Da. The protein component contains 743 amino acids and is divided into three parts: the first part is extracellular, water-soluble, and includes 394 amino acids. It has a binding site for TSH and TSH-like molecules (e.g., thyroid-stimulating immunoglobulin or TSI; hCG). The second part is intracellular and includes 83 amino acids. This part interacts with a regulatory G protein and an adenylate cyclase system. The third transmembrane connecting part includes 266 amino acids and is composed of seven segments (I–VII). A high degree of homology exists (in segments II, III, VI, VII) between the TSH receptor and the LH, hCG, and FSH receptors, which makes this TSH receptor a member of the G protein-coupled subfamily of receptors, all of which work via adenylate cyclase activation.

Regulation of thyroid function and growth

Upon binding of TSH to its receptor on the thyroid cells, a cascade of events occurs whereby regulation of thyroid cell function and modulation occurs. In this process cyclic adenosine monophosphate is generated, a protein kinase is activated and many nuclear proteins are phosphorylated inside the thyroid cells. This cascade of events leads to increased iodide transport into the thyroid cells, increased colloid resorption, and hormone secretion. TSH action is supported, modulated, and counteracted by a variety of signaling factors, the most important being prostaglandins and catecholamines.

Alterations in the TSH receptor coupling to adenylate cyclase may explain TSH refractoriness in certain TSH-resistant states.

LABORATORY TESTS

The ideal laboratory test for the thyroid status would be to measure the thyroid hormone actions directly at the tissue level. Among many thyroid function tests currently available for clinical use, measurement of TSH concentration comes closest to such an ideal test for two reasons: TSH from the pituitary works like a signal from a thermostat. When the hypothalamic–pituitary axis is intact, serum TSH reflects thyroid hormone action, assuming that thyroid hormone actions in other organs parallel those in the pituitary. The negative feedback of the thyroid hormone on TSH amplifies the TSH response (e.g., a minor change in the thyroid hormone level elicits a 10 times larger inverse change in pituitary TSH release).

TSH ASSAYS

Since TSH action is mediated via cyclic adenosine monophosphate, this reaction has been used as a bioassay endpoint for TSH quantitation in the past. It has been shown over the years that this TSH bioassay technique was useful to assay TSH levels in pituitary tissue (with enough TSH concentration)

but was neither sensitive enough to detect TSH levels in serum, nor specific enough to differentiate between TSH and TSI.

Two other more sensitive bioassay tests were developed later on, namely the cytochemical TSH bioassay and the radioreceptor TSH bioassay. The first assay is based on the ability of TSH to increase the permeability of the thyroid cell lysosomes. The second assay is based on the ability of unlabeled TSH to inhibit the binding of I^{125} radiolabeled TSH to TSH receptors on the plasma thyroid membrane, an activity called TSH displacement activity. Both tests measured the bioactivity of TSH, but had a limited specificity because of cross-reactivity with TSI. At present, the use of these bioassay techniques is restricted to the measurement of TSI and to the detection of an altered TSH bioactivity.

Later, the TSH-radioimmunoassay (TSH-RIA) was introduced. This assay is based on a competitive binding technique, whereby TSH from the patient's sample competes with I^{125} radiolabeled TSH for a limited amount of TSH antibody. Separation of bound from unbound radioactivity is by anti-TSH antirabbit immunoglobulin G technique. The more the unlabeled TSH is present, the less the labeled TSH binds to the antibody and vice versa. TSH standards and controls are used, and TSH values are plotted against the radioactivity measured, and the patient's TSH value is computed by extrapolation from a standard curve. The rabbit anti-TSH antibody is directed primarily at the β-subunit of TSH in order to provide reasonable specificity toward TSH alone. However, many anti-TSH sera still react to some degree with the α-subunit of TSH and of other glycoproteins like FSH, LH, and hCG. Such antisera must be absorbed first with a source of α-subunit, such as hCG, before being used in the assay. Most TSH-RIAs are sensitive to detect levels as low as 0.5–1 mU/ml of TSH; some may detect levels as low as 0.1 mU/ml of serum.

A highly sensitive assay was introduced in the early 1980s — the new sTSH-IMA assay or supersensitive TSH by immunoradiometric technique. This technique is based on the use of two monoclonal antibodies, each directed against a different part of the TSH molecule, with at least one of them against the β-subunit of TSH. Usually one of the antibodies is immobilized on a solid phase to which the patient's serum is added. After separation of the solid phase, a second labeled antibody is used to quantify the bound TSH sandwiched in between the two antibodies. This sTSH-IMA has two advantages over TSH-RIA: It is 10−100 times more sensitive in detecting the suppressed levels of TSH in hyperthyroidism (normal range for TSH level by this method is <0.4−4.5 mU/ml), and it is more specific and has less cross-reactivity with LH, FSH, and hCG.

It also helps in the early detection of minor thyroid abnormalities (e.g., subclinical hyperthyroidism), facilitates the fine tuning of thyroid hormone replacement therapy, and allows better monitoring of thyroid-suppressive treatment (e.g., an incomplete replacement treatment results in only partial restoration of TSH levels to normal).

A fourth test, used by many endocrinologists to assess the TSH pituitary reserve, is the TRH stimulation test. An intravenous bolus injection of 100−400 μg of TRH is given and blood for TSH levels is sampled at 15, 30, 60, 90, 120, and 160 min. A normal response is indicated by a peak TSH level at 20−40 min of ~16 mU/ml or a five times increase from basal. It helps to detect subclinical hyper- and hypothyroidism and to differentiate between the various causes of decreased or elevated TSH levels.

CAUSES OF ELEVATED TSH LEVELS

Thyroid/pituitary diseases

TSH levels are elevated in subclinical or clinical primary hypothyroidism. In subclinical hypothyroidism, metabolism is normal, free T4 is normal, and TSH is elevated. In clinical primary hypothyroidism, hypometabolism is present, free T4 level is low, and TSH is elevated. Subclinical and clinical hypothyroidism may be encountered in patients with endemic goitre, autoimmune, or postpartum thyroiditis, with the intake of dietary goitrogens (soybean, cabbage, etc) or drugs (antithyroid medications, amiodarone, lithium) and after radiation therapy to the head and neck region. Subclinical or clinical hypothyroidism may also be seen in any female patient with a history of menorrhagia, galactorrhea, and/or infertility (TSH, LH, and prolactin levels are elevated because of an underlying increased hypothalamic dopamine turnover). In all these cases the TRH stimulation test may be hyperreactive.

A rare situation in which an elevated TSH level is seen with eumetabolism or hypothyroidism and goiter is diffuse TSH resistance. This is associated with an abnormal TSH molecule with decreased biologic activity.

An elevated TSH level with clinical hyperthyroidism (elevated free T_3 and T_4 levels) is also rare and can present with evidence of a goiter, galactorrhea, and/or hyperprolactinemia. Examples are TSH resistant states at the pituitary level and TSH secreting pituitary tumors. In the TSH-resistant state, the pituitary is resistant to TSH suppression by T_3 secondary to pituitary T_3 receptor function abnormalities. To suspect a pituitary tumor, a patient should have symptoms of increased intracranial pressure, bitemporal hemianopsia, and an elevated TSH level >600 μU/ml (versus an elevated TSH level of only 2−3 μU/ml in resistant TSH states!). An even better screening index is an α-subunit : TSH ratio of >1, because of the greater α-subunit secretion than TSH secretion in pituitary tumors.

The TRH stimulation test is hyperreactive in a TSH-resistant state and blunted in the case of a pituitary tumor.

No evidence of thyroid/pituitary disease

TSH levels may be spuriously elevated in some patients who harbor antimouse immunoglobulin G antibodies that may interfere with RIA or TSH-IMA assays. These antibodies may be induced by vaccination with material contaminated with animal serum or endogenous TSH antibodies.

TSH levels may also be elevated in the recovery phase of sick euthyroid disease (up to 30 mU/l) − a situation to keep in mind in a patient recovering from a severe debilitating disease.

Other causes of elevated TSH levels, with neither thyroid nor pituitary disease, are: chronic renal failure; chronic liver disease; Addison's disease and cortisol deficiency; psychiatric illness; premenstrual syndrome; and drug use like dopamine antagonists (metoclopramide, haloperidol), cholestyramine, sulfonamides, and furosemide. Transient TSH elevations are also seen with propranolol, amiodarone, and intravenous contrast solutions.

The TRH stimulation test is normal in nonthyroidal illness, blunted in psychiatric illness, and hyperreactive in the follicular phase of the menstrual cycle and with the intake of the above-mentioned drugs.

CAUSES OF DECREASED TSH LEVELS

Thyroid/pituitary diseases

Decreased TSH levels and subclinical or clinical hyperthyroidism should be sought in any patient with thyroid disease (multinodular goiter, autoimmune, or post partum thyroiditis). Also, look for these decreased levels in any pregnant patient who has a goiter (hyperthyroidism may be mediated by hCG in cases of hydatidiform mole or chorio-carcinoma — see elevated hCG, T_3, T_4 levels and decreased TSH level) or in any female patient with pelvic problems but no goiter (hyperthyroidism may be mediated by extrathyroidal secretion of thyroid hormone, as in the case of struma ovarii — see elevated free T_4 and decreased TSH level). In all these cases the TRH stim test is blunted.

In cases of decreased TSH levels and clinical hypo-thyroidism, an underlying hypothalamic (e.g., tertiary hypothyroidism due to TRH deficiency or insensitivity or both) or pituitary disease (e.g., secondary hypothyroidism due to TSH deficiency, as in empty sella or pituitary tumors) should be ruled out.

The TRH stimulation test is normal or delayed in tertiary hypothyroidism, hyperreactive in empty sella syndrome, and blunted in secondary hypothyroidism.

No evidence of thyroid/pituitary disease
No evidence of thyroid or pituitary disease is found in 17% of cases with decreased TSH.

In the first trimester of pregnancy, the TSH level may be low because of the weak effect of the thyroid-stimulating action of a large amount of hCG produced by the placenta at that time. (hCG has 1/1000th of TSH activity).

The TRH stimulation test is contraindicated in

pregnancy because of its questionable safety (the injected TRH may cross the placenta and affect the fetal pituitary—thyroid axis).

The TSH level may be low in a patient with non-thyroid illness (e.g. diabetes mellitus, infection, malignancy) without evidence of thyroid disease. The thyroid is a component of a very complex system, and defects at other levels may affect the thyroid status. In a patient on some drugs (e.g. dopamine, dopamine agonists such as bromocriptine, gluco-corticoids, phenytoin), the TSH level may also be low and the TRH stimulation test may be normal or blunted.

FURTHER READING

Bergman DA. Thyroid physiology and immunology. *Oto-laryngol Clin North Am* 1990; 23: 231–249.

Misrahi M, Loosfelt H, Atger M, Sar S, Guiochon-Mantel A, Melgrom E. Cloning, sequencing and expression of human TSH receptor. *Biochem Biophys Res Commun* 1990; 166: 394–403.

Pierce JG, Magner JA, Weintraub BD, Field JB, Utiger RD. Thyrotropin. In: Ingbar SH, Braverman LE, eds. *Werner's The Thyroid: A Fundamental and Clinical Text*, 5th edn. Philadelphia: JB Lippincott, 1986: 267.

Refetoff S. Thyroid function tests and effects of drugs on thyroid function. In: Degroot LJ, ed. *Endocrinology*, 2nd edn, vol 1. Philadelphia: WB Saunders, 1989: 590.

Sarne DH, Degroot LJ. Hypothalamic and neuroendocrine regulation of thyroid hormone. In: Degroot LJ, ed. *Endocrinology*, 2nd edn, vol 1. Philadelphia: WB Saunders, 1989: 574.

33

Hypothyroidism

RONALD C. STRICKLER

Dietary iodine is trapped by the thyroid gland where, stimulated by pituitary thyroid-stimulating hormone (TSH), enzymatic reactions synthesize thyroid hormones. Thyroxine (T_4) is produced only in the thyroid gland. Triiodothyronine (T_3) is produced in the gland (20%) and formed from T_4 by extrathyroid deiodination (80%). The biologically inactive reverse-T_3 (rT_3) is 97.5% formed by extrathyroid deiodination. The plasma half-lives are T_4, 6−7 days and T_3, 24−30 hours.

Hypothalamic thyrotropin-releasing hormone (TRH) stimulates the anterior pituitary gland to secrete TSH. Prolactin and growth hormone are also stimulated by TRH. Thyroid hormone feeds back to the pituitary gland with less compelling evidence for regulation in the hypothalamus. Although T_3, the more biologically active hormone, is capable of entering the pituitary gland from plasma, deiodination of T_4 to form T_3 in the adenohypophysis is the primary regulatory mechanism.

Primary hypothyroidism, in 95% of cases, describes thyroid gland failure. Plasma T_4 and T_3 levels are low and TSH measures very high. Pituitary thyrotroph (and to a lesser extent, lactotroph) hypertrophy and hyperplasia can enlarge the pituitary gland, cause local pressure symptoms, affect adjacent tropic-cell functions, and expand the pituitary fossa to mimic pituitary tumor on imaging studies. Hyperprolactinemia is frequently found with primary hypothyroidism. Secondary hypothyroidism, in 5% of cases, results from inadequate TSH or TRH stimulation. All hormones in the thyroid axis are present in low levels. Peripheral thyroid hormone resistance is a very rare third explanation for hypothyroidism: elevated blood T_3 and T_4 concentrations can give near-normal tissue effects of thyroid hormone despite this probably postreceptor defect (Table 33.1).

FREQUENCY

The prevalence of previously undiagnosed, non-treatment-related, clinical hypothyroidism has been estimated from community-based studies worldwide at 2−4/1000 population. If cases of prior surgery and radiotherapy treatments are included, the prevalence approximates 1/100. Addition of subclinical cases (elevated TSH with normal thyroid gland hormone levels) enriches the prevalence to 5/100 population. The annual incidence of hypothyroidism is 1−2/1000 women, which is 10 times more common for women than for men.

CLINICAL FEATURES

Thyroid hormone is needed for normal function in most organs, and the clinical presentation varies according to the magnitude and duration of thyroid hormone deficiency, and the degree of slowing in different systems. The spectrum ranges from asymptomatic through overt hypothyroidism to myxedema coma.

1 *Subjective*: lethargy, weakness, fatigues easily, and inability to continue usual mental and physical activities at the expected levels of performance. Cold intolerance, even in warm environments.

Table 33.1 Causes of hypothyroidism

Goiter	No goiter
Hashimoto's thyroiditis	
Iodine deficiency	Idiopathic
Drugs (iodine, lithium, propylthiouracil, sulfonylureas)	^{131}Iodine surgery
Infiltration of the thyroid (lymphoma, amyloid, sarcoid)	Thyroid dysgenesis
Impaired peripheral sensitivity to thyroid hormone	Hypothalamic−pituitary insufficiency

CHAPTER 33

2 *Thyroid*: normal, enlarged by goiter, or withered by autoimmune cytotoxicity.

3 *Skin*: dry, scaly, pale, cool skin. Decreased sweating. Coarse hair which falls out easily. Thinning of the outer third of the eyebrows. Nonpitting facial and peripheral edema causing weight gain.

4 *Nervous system*: mental slowness, diminished alertness, sleepiness. Paresthesias, ataxia. Carpal tunnel syndrome. Psychosis or depression.

5 *Cardiovascular*: bradycardia, cardiomegaly, heart failure, pericardial effusion.

6 *Ear, nose, and throat*: hoarse voice. Thick, enlarged tongue. Diminished hearing. Nasal congestion.

7 *Respiratory*: slow respirations. Pleural effusion. Hypercarbia.

8 *Gastrointestinal*: nausea, constipation, abdominal distention. Delayed gastric emptying, slow bowel transit time, paralytic ileus, megacolon.

9 *Musculoskeletal*: myalgia, cramps, muscle stiffness. Arthralgia, joint stiffness, and effusion.

HYPOTHYROIDISM SCREENING

Thyroid hormone testing is recommended for:
1 All newborn babies.
2 Children with precocious puberty or short stature.
3 Teenagers with dysfunctional bleeding.
4 Women with galactorrhea.
5 Postpartum patients with any suggestive symptom.
6 Elderly women with any suggestive symptom.
7 Women with autoimmune diseases (Schmidt's syndrome is the combination of immune hypothyroidism and immune Addison's disease).

PRESENTATIONS IN REPRODUCTION

Newborn
Hypothyroidism affects 1/4000 liveborn babies and is not clinically apparent. Routine screening for an elevated blood TSH is necessary to begin treatment before age 3 months and thereby avoid mental retardation. Congenital hypothyroidism does have a family tendency, can be diagnosed before birth by amniotic fluid iodothyronine levels, and the baby can be treated *in utero* with intraamniotic T$_4$.

Short stature
Endocrine causes are uncommon etiologies. Hypothyroidism, hypopituitarism, and hypercortisolism are most probable. Hypothyroidism is usually congenital and less commonly of juvenile onset.

Sexual precocity
Most true precocity in girls (breast development, estrogenized vaginal mucosa, vaginal bleeding) is idiopathic; central nervous system tumors and polyostotic fibrous dysplasia (Albright's syndrome) are uncommon. In a small number of patients with clinically obvious hypothyroidism, true sexual precocity has been described. Short stature, delay in bone age, and galactorrhea may be associated features. Sellar enlargement which remodels with T$_4$ therapy can be confused with pituitary tumor. The precocious sexual development reverses with thyroid hormone treatment.

Hirsutism
Juvenile hypothyroid patients may experience mild hirsutism.

Dysfunctional bleeding
Dysfunctional bleeding describes the result of many pathologies: hypothalamic–pituitary–ovarian hormonal dysfunction; uterine and ovarian diseases; pregnancy complications; and systemic illness. When thyroid hormone levels are low, estriol is formed in excess and anovulation, probably due to altered neurotransmitter and releasing hormone dynamics in the pituitary gland, is common.

In a Toronto study, 3/70 women undergoing hysterectomy for menorrhagia had hypothyroidism and 15/67 had an exaggerated TSH response to TRH stimulation testing [1].

In women, especially teenagers, whose severe dysfunctional uterine hemorrhage (flooding) is unresponsive to intravenous estrogen therapy, thyroid function should be evaluated.

Amenorrhea
In overt hypothyroidism, usually after months of irregular, heavy menstrual bleeding, secondary amenorrhea does occur. As thyroid disease presentations are less typical in teenagers, primary and secondary amenorrhea in this group will be explained occasionally by thyroid hormone studies.

Galactorrhea
Drugs, prolactinomas, and idiopathic dysfunction are common causes for nonpuerperal lactation, and hypothyroidism explains 3% of presentations. The serum prolactin level is <100 ng/ml. Because thyroid therapy is so straightforward and rewarding, TSH should be routinely measured in women with hyperprolactinemia.

208

Infertility

Thyroid dysfunction, by contribution to anovulation, luteal-phase defect, or hyperprolactinemia, may be associated with infertility. Although thyroid hormone profiles are recommended studies in women with unexplained infertility, the tests are unrewarding.

Hypothyroidism explains an occasional male with oligospermia, but again, testing in the absence of clinical symptoms or signs is unproductive.

The empiric administration of thyroid hormones to euthyroid men or women to promote fertility is a myth which is condemned.

Recurrent abortion

The rate of abortion in women with untreated hypothyroidism is double that of euthyroid peers. Within every paradigm to evaluate women with habitual abortion is a recommendation to measure thyroid hormones. In the absence of clinical symptoms or signs, hypothyroidism is an unlikely finding.

Pregnancy

Hypothyroidism rarely complicates pregnancy because most untreated women have ovulatory/menstrual disturbances and reduced libido. Although myxedematous women have delivered normal babies, hypothyroid women are anemic (31%), develop preeclampsia (44%), and experience placental abruption (19%), and postpartum hemorrhage (19%) more often than euthyroid pregnant women. The babies also fare less well: low birth weight (31%) and fetal death (12%) are reported.

Women who become pregnant on thyroid replacement therapy may experience increased T_4 requirements, as reflected by an increase in serum TSH concentrations. Although deleterious effects of modest hypothyroidism in pregnancy are unclear, it seems prudent to measure serum TSH levels each trimester and adjust the T_4 dose to maintain a normal range value.

The fetal hypothalamic—pituitary—thyroid axis is autonomous and the unborn does not depend on thyroid hormone from mother for development. Nonetheless, the rate of congenital anomalies in babies of untreated hypothyroid women is triple that of the general population. This increased risk for anomalies may continue even if replacement therapy is being given.

Postpartum thyroiditis

Autoimmune thyroiditis occurs in 5% of parturients. The clinical course is silent inflammation of the thyroid gland which stimulates transient hyperthyroidism 2—4 months postpartum, followed by hypothyroidism. The hypothyroid symptoms are often attributed to lactation and nocturnal feeding schedules, new mothering responsibilities, or resolution of pregnancy changes. There is a strong association with antithyroid antibodies.

When T_4 therapy is required, it can be withdrawn after 6—12 months as >80% of women will undergo spontaneous recovery. However, there is a strong likelihood of recurrence after subsequent gestations. Lifelong follow-up is a wise precaution as it is unknown how many of these women will experience future thyroid failure.

The differential diagnosis of postpartum hypothyroidism must include Sheehan's postpartum pituitary necrosis. Failure to lactate is the early clinical clue. The blood TSH and T_4 levels are low: the TRH-stimulated rise in both TSH and prolactin is blunted.

LABORATORY DIAGNOSIS

Serum TSH is the most valuable measurement in patients suspect for hypothyroidism (Fig. 33.1). The level is markedly elevated in primary hypothyroidism; slightly elevated in compensated or subclinical hypothyroidism; and normal/decreased in secondary hypothyroidism. Current TSH assays can clearly separate the normal range from both the elevated and suppressed levels of disease states. Further, there is new precision as the lower end of the scale allows titration of replacement therapy without risk of overdosage and iatrogenic hyperthyroid effects (Table 33.2).

Serum total and free T_4 levels are low. Total T_4, but not free T_4, concentrations are spuriously low when T_4-binding globulin levels are low or drugs compete with T_4 for its protein carrier.

Serum T_3, despite its biological importance, is a poor measure of hypothyroidism. The enzyme activity, type II T_4 5'-deiodinase, which forms T_3 in peripheral tissues, rapidly increases with a reduction in T_4. This likely explains the observation of low T_4 and normal T_3 plasma levels in symptomatic hypothyroid patients.

TRH stimulates TSH secretion, which peaks in 20—30 min. Blood samples are drawn shortly before bolus intravenous injection of 200—400 µg TRH, and after 30 min. A normal response approximates a two- to fivefold increased TSH level. An exaggerated response implies inadequate thyroid hormone feedback on to the pituitary gland and a blunted response implies absent endogenous TRH or diseased pituitary thyrotrophs.

Antibodies against thyroglobulin and thyroid microsomes indicate autoimmune thyroiditis, but provide no information about thyroid function. Antithyroid antibodies may be present at low levels in up to 15% of elderly subjects. High levels indicate disease in all ages, and low levels are significant in children and adolescents.

LABORATORY ALTERATIONS

Laboratory alterations include the following: mild anemia; low serum levels of sodium, glucose, angiotensin-converting enzyme, and thyroglobulin; reduced electrocardiogram voltage: reduced basal metabolic rate; and prolonged Achilles' reflex half-relaxation time.

There are elevated serum concentrations of cholesterol, triglycerides, creatine phosphokinase, aminotransferases, lactate dehydrogenase, and partial pressure of carbon dioxide. Prolactin secretion is increased.

SICK EUTHYROID SYNDROME

Clinically euthyroid patients who are ill with nonthyroid disease can show abnormal thyroid function tests. The most common plasma hormone pattern is low T_3, low to low-normal T_4, and normal TSH. The hallmark of this syndrome is a shift in T_4 metabolism from T_3 to rT_3 and the circulating level of this biologically inactive T_4 metabolite is elevated.

Surgery, epidural and general anesthesia, psychosis, myocardial infarction, renal failure, cirrhosis, uncontrolled diabetes mellitus, and systemic infection have all been associated with sick euthyroid syndrome. The changes from systemic illness are also compounded by aging (T_3 formation decreases with age), poor nutrition (decreased binding protein), and drug effects (corticosteroids, amiodarone, propanolol, heparin, dopamine, contrast dyes) on thyroid gland and hormone metabolism.

TREATMENT

T_4 is the best treatment for hypothyroidism. A single daily dose of T_4 provides a long-lived pool of hormone for peripheral formation of the biologically important T_3. Since this conversion is regulated by a variety of nutritional and metabolic factors unrelated to the thyroid gland itself, and since local formation of T_3 in tissues such as the pituitary gland is more important than levels available in plasma, it is not logical to bypass these controls with exogenous T_3.

The usual adult daily dose of T_4 is 100 µg. Young patients can be given this dose immediately. Elderly patients or those at risk for cardiovascular symptoms such as angina, congestive failure, or arrhythmia should begin with 25 or 50 µg with increases after 4–6 weeks. Adequacy of dosage is judged primarily by the resolution of symptoms and signs of hypothyroidism. A TSH level within the normal range is the best biochemical monitor of correct dosage.

The association between hypothyroidism and hypoadrenalism must always be considered. Pituitary insufficiency requires that corticosteroid replacement precede T_4 replacement. Autoimmune hypothyroidism should suggest primary adrenal insufficiency. Since it is impractical to evaluate adrenocorticotropic hormone reserve in many patients, consider glucocorticoid therapy when underreplaced hypothyroid patients face significant stress.

Most patients will require lifelong thyroid replacement therapy. There is no test to identify the continuing need for exogenous thyroxine while receiving therapy. To decide if continuing therapy is necessary, T_4 replacement must be discontinued. Euthyroid patients may experience transient clinical and biochemical hypothyroidism, but normal function will be restored within 1 month. In contrast, hypothyroid subjects will experience increasing symptoms and signs, which will be a florid syndrome by 1 month.

Myxedema coma is a medical emergency. Immediate, rapid T_4 replacement therapy is started with concurrent corticosteroid coverage. Careful monitoring and support of ventilation, fluid and electrolyte balance, temperature regulation, and cardiovascular dynamics are imperative.

Table 33.2 Laboratory profiles

	TSH	Free T_4	rT_3
Hyperthyroid	Low	High	High
Hypothyroid	High	Low	Normal
Compensated	High	Normal	Normal
Pregnancy	Normal	Normal	Normal
Sick euthyroid	Normal	Low/normal/high	High

TSH, thyroid-stimulating hormone; T_4, thyroxine; rT_3, reverse-triiodothyronine.

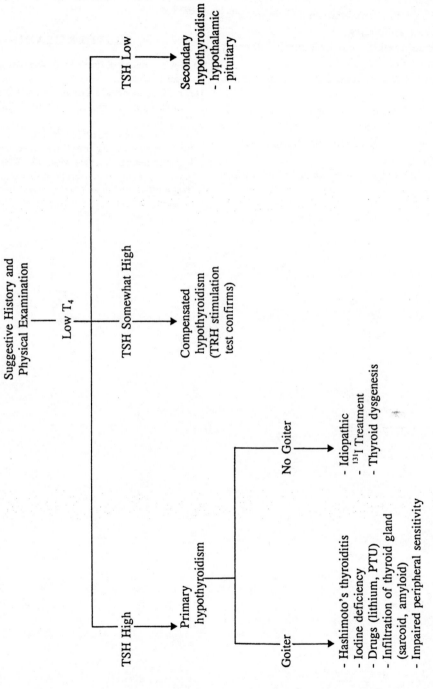

Fig. 33.1 Approach to hypothyroidism.

TRANSIENT HYPOTHYROIDISM

Temporary biochemical and sometimes clinical hypothyroidism occurs:

1 In newborns with maternal-transmitted thyrotropin-receptor blocking antibodies.

2 After subtotal thyroidectomy or iodine-I^{131} therapy for hyperthyroidism.

3 Postpartum in women with autoimmune thyroid disease.

4 Postpartum in women with isolated pituitary TSH deficiency.

5 Following withdrawal of chronic thyroid replacement therapy.

T_4 treatment is often unnecessary or can be withdrawn after 3–12 months.

REFERENCE

1 Wilansky DL, Greisman B. Early hypothyroidism in patients with menorrhagia. *Am J Obstet Gynecol* 1989; 160: 673–677.

FURTHER READING

Bailliere's Clinical Endocrinology and Metabolism, Vol. 2, August, 1988.

Davis LE, Leveno KJ, Cunningham FG. Hypothyroidism complicating pregnancy. *Obstet Gynecol* 1988; 72: 108–112.

Mandel SJ, Larsen PR, Seely EW, Brent GA. Increased need for thyroxine during pregnancy in women with primary hypothyroidism. *N Engl J Med* 1990; 323: 91–96.

Thomas R, Reid RL. Thyroid disease and reproductive dysfunction: a review. *Obstet Gynecol* 1987; 70: 789–798.

34

Hyperthyroidism

JAN M. BRUDER & MARGARET E. WIERMAN

Hyperthyroidism is a clinical syndrome that results when peripheral tissues are exposed to an excess of thyroid hormone. The syndrome is characterized by a constellation of signs and symptoms related to the thyroid hormone excess and confirmed by specific thyroid function tests. The underlying etiology of the hyperthyroidism can then be established by the performance of a radioactive iodine uptake (RAIU) and scan (Fig. 34.1).

The clinical features of hyperthyroidism include nervousness, anxiety, emotional lability, weight loss, heat intolerance, perspiration, palpitations, hyperdefecation, and menstrual irregularity. Hyperthyroidism is also in the differential diagnosis of the infertile patient, usually associated with an inadequate luteal phase or oligomenorrhea.

On physical examination, clinical findings include: tachycardia, systolic hypertension, multiple eye findings including lid lag, a stare, ocular irritation with chemosis, and periorbital swelling. Exophthalmos, proptosis, and extraocular muscle paresis are ocular signs characteristic of Graves

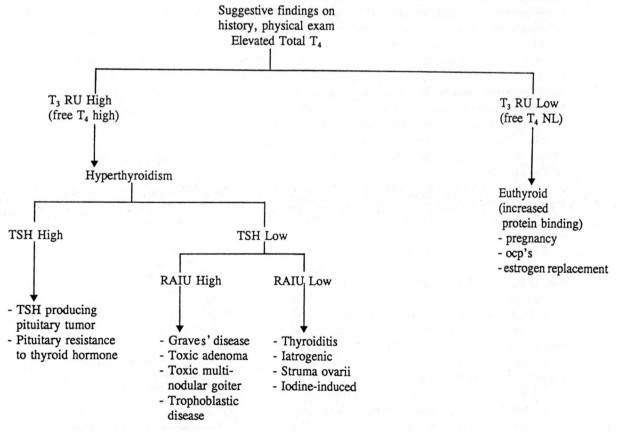

Fig. 34.1 Approach to hyperthyroidism.

disease. In addition, the patient has smooth skin, a tremor, excess perspiration and onycholysis. On neck examination, a goiter, or enlarged thyroid gland, is almost always present. In the elderly, the classic signs and symptoms of hyperthyroidism may not be apparent and the disorder has been described as apathetic hyperthyroidism.

In a patient with these clinical symptoms and signs, the diagnosis can be confirmed with appropriate laboratory tests. The laboratory work-up includes assessment of a total thyroxine (T_4) and triiodothyronine resin uptake (T_3RU). A T_4 level of greater than 12 (nl 5–12) µg/dl and T_3RU greater than 35% (nl 25–35) suggests the diagnosis of hyperthyroidism. A suppressed thyroid-stimulating hormone (TSH) level in a sensitive immunoradiometric assay (IRMA) assay of less than 0.01 µU confirms the diagnosis. A total T_3 level by radioimmunoassay is elevated to a greater extent than the total T_4 in some disorders, but because of cost is usually not obtained.

To interpret the thyroid tests, it is important to remember that T_4 is the major hormone secreted from the thyroid gland. It circulates bound to proteins including thyroid-binding globulin (TBG), albumin, and prealbumin. Also, a smaller percentage (0.03%) circulates in the unbound or free state. The free hormone is the physiologic, active hormone. The total T_4 assay measures both bound and unbound T_4. Free T_4 levels can also be measured but the assay is expensive and cumbersome. An indirect measurement of the free T_4, however, is the T_3RU. In this test, a small amount of radioactive labeled T_3 is added to a mixture of the patient's serum and a resin that binds T_3. The number of binding sites in the resin is fixed. The number of binding sites in the patient's serum depends on the amount of protein in that serum sample and the fraction of sites already occupied by circulating thyroid hormone. The labelled T_3 distributes equally between the resin and the patient's serum-binding proteins. The serum is then separated from the resin and the resin counted to determine the amount of radioactive T_3 bound to the resin. This percentage indicates how many binding sites are unoccupied. If few sites are available in the serum sample, the resin will bind most of the radiolabeled T_3. If many sites are available in the serum, the radiolabeled T_3 will bind to the patient's serum; thus, little will be bound to the resin. Therefore, a high T_3RU value indicates few unoccupied serum-binding sites.

In hyperthyroidism, both total T_4 and the T_3RU are elevated; in conditions that result in hyper-

thyroxinemia but not hyperthyroidism, an elevated T_4 but low or normal T_3RU reflects states of TBG excess. This pattern of thyroid function tests is seen in pregnancy with oral contraceptives or with estrogen replacement therapy in the menopause. In addition, a similar pattern is observed in acute and chronic active hepatitis. The advent of the supersensitive TSH assay allows one to differentiate between these disorders. A suppressed TSH level makes the diagnosis of hyperthyroidism. A normal TSH level excludes the diagnosis.

Hyperthyroidism may be due to one of many different disorders (Table 34.1). The three most common causes of hyperthyroidism in the general population as well as the obstetric population are: (1) Graves disease (~85%); (2) thyroiditis (~15%); and (3) excessive exogenous thyroid hormone replacement (<3%). Once the diagnosis of hyperthyroidism has been made, RAIU is useful to classify the underlining pathophysiology and to determine the appropriate treatment options. The differential diagnosis can be broadly subdivided into two major categories: (1) disorders that are associated with an increased RAIU; and (2) disorders that result in a decreased RAIU (Table 34.2). Conditions that increase the RAIU stimulate thyroid hormone synthesis as well as release. Conditions that decrease the RAIU do not affect thyroid hormone synthesis, but instead result in destruction of the parenchymal tissue of the thyroid with subsequent release of excessive

Table 34.1 Causes of hyperthyroidism

Graves' disease
Toxic adenoma
Toxic multinodular goiter
Thyroiditis
  Subacute
  Lymphocytic
  Postradiation
Drug-induced
  Factitious
  Iatrogenic
  Iodine-induced
Ectopic
  TSH-producing pituitary tumor
  Trophoblastic tumor
    Choriocarcinoma
    Hydatidiform mole
  Struma ovarii

TSH, thyroid-stimulating hormone.

Table 34.2 Hyperthyroidism: elevated T_4, elevated T_3RU

Elevated RAIU		Decreased RAIU
Elevated TSH	Decreased TSH	Decreased TSH
TSH-producing pituitary tumor	Graves' disease	Subacute thyroiditis
Pituitary resistance to thyroid hormone	Toxic adenoma	Lymphocytic thyroiditis
	Toxic multinodular goiter	Iatrogenic
	Trophoblastic disease	Struma ovarii
		Iodine-induced

T_4, thyroxine; T_3RU, triiodothyronine resin uptake; RAIU, radioactive iodine uptake; TSH, thyroid-stimulating hormone.

thyroid hormone. In addition, a suppressed RAIU can also be due to an excessive iodine load resulting in an increased precursor pool for thyroid hormone synthesis.

Graves' disease occurs in 0.5% of the population and is also the most common cause of hyperthyroidism in pregnancy. The hallmark features include a diffuse, homogeneous goiter with or without exophthalmos, proptosis, and other ocular symptoms. Additionally, a dermopathy termed pretibial myxedema may be observed. Graves' disease is an autoimmune disease characterized by circulating immunoglobulins that stimulate the thyroid gland, resulting in overproduction and release of T_4. The eye findings are due to retrobulbar inflammation and infiltration of the extraocular muscles. The diagnosis is made with the clinical picture and an elevated T_4, elevated T_3RU and suppressed TSH level. In the nonpregnant state, RAI scan and uptake demonstrates a homogeneous, diffuse increase in the uptake of the thyroid gland. The amount of RAIU and the size of the gland can be used to calculate the dose of radioactive iodine to treat the patient. Other options include the administration of antithyroid drugs and β-blockers or rarely surgery.

Making the diagnosis of hyperthyroidism in pregnancy is occasionally difficult because of the hyperdynamic status of the pregnant patient. The prevalence of hyperthyroidism in pregnancy is 0.2%. It may present as hyperemesis gravidarum. Because of the increasing estrogen levels in pregnancy, TBG levels are increased. Therefore, the diagnosis of hyperthyroidism is usually made with a T_4 value of greater than 15 μg/dl, a T_3RU in the normal or elevated range, and a suppressed TSH level. Since a radioactive iodine scan is contraindicated in pregnancy, the etiology of the hyperthyroidism must be made on clinical grounds alone.

The intensity of the thyrotoxicosis due to Graves' disease fluctuates during pregnancy. Patients tend to have remissions during the second and third trimesters and exacerbations during the postpartum period. These fluctuations are thought to be due to changes in the immunologic milieu during pregnancy. Although radioactive iodine ablation is the most common treatment for Graves' disease, it is contraindicated in pregnancy and the patient is treated with the antithyroid drug, propylthiouracil (PTU) and β-blockers.

The second most common etiology of hyperthyroidism is thyroiditis. Thyroiditis accounts for about 5–20% of all newly diagnosed cases of thyrotoxicosis. There are two major types: (1) subacute or painful thyroiditis following a viral syndrome; and (2) lymphocytic thyroiditis, often occurring in the postpartum period. Thyroiditis is due to an inflammatory process of the thyroid resulting in destruction of the thyroid gland and release of T_4. The disease usually proceeds through four phases of thyroid function: initially, hyperthyroidism followed by a period of euthyroidism; then hypothyroidism, and finally a return to a euthyroid state. In some patients, treatment with thyroid replacement is necessary for a short period of time for hypothyroid symptoms. If thyroid autoantibodies are present and remain in significant titers, however, the patient may require long-term thyroid hormone replacement.

Subacute thyroiditis is also known as painful, granulomatous, de Quervain's, or giant cell thyroiditis. Classically, patients complain of a painful, diffuse, small goiter following a viral illness and have an elevated sedimentation rate. Because of the inflammatory destruction of the thyroid, there is excessive release of T_4 and T_3 into the peripheral circulation to cause the hyperthyroxinemia. To distinguish thyroiditis from Graves' disease, there are no associated eye findings and the RAIU is very low rather than increased. Treatment options include temporary use of β-blockers and nonsteroidal anti-inflammatory agents for local symptoms.

Lymphocytic thyroiditis resembles subacute thyroiditis in that the RAIU is also low when the patient is in the hyperthyroid state. Unlike subacute thyroiditis, the thyroid gland is nontender and the disease does not follow a viral illness. The pathology reflects a lymphocytic infiltration. Some 5–9% of pregnancies result in thyroiditis in the postpartum period. In addition, the disease may recur with subsequent pregnancies. Treatment includes the use of β-blockers for symptomatic relief of the hyperthyroid symptoms. Occasionally, a patient requires thyroid hormone replacement for a short period of time. The medication can be discontinued at 6–12 months to assess whether the patient needs longer term thyroid hormone replacement.

Factitious or iatrogenic thyrotoxicosis results from exogenous thyroid hormone ingestion or overzealous hormone replacement. It should be suspected when the T_4 and T_3RU are elevated, the TSH is suppressed but no goiter is palpated. The RAIU is also suppressed. When exogenous thyroid medication is discontinued, the pituitary–thyroid axis returns to normal within 6 weeks. β-Blockers may be administered for symptomatic relief but usually are not required.

Other causes of hyperthyroidism include a single toxic adenoma and toxic multinodular goiter. These are benign growths of the thyroid that function autonomously from the remaining thyroid. The thyroid scan reveals an increased RAIU in the area of the nodule with little tracer activity in the remaining gland, as normal tissue is suppressed. A toxic multinodular goiter has multiple areas of autonomy which suppress the normal gland. These disorders can be treated with radioactive iodine, antithyroid drugs, or surgery.

Rarely, excessive iodine ingestion or an iodine load from contrast dye can result in thyrotoxicosis, termed the jodbasedow effect. Since iodine is a substrate for thyroid hormone synthesis, excessive iodine can cause hyperthyroidism in a patient with an underlying multinodular goiter. Other rare causes of thyrotoxicosis include oversecretion of TSH by a pituitary adenoma, struma ovarii, due to an ovarian teratoma which contains hyperfunctioning thyroid tissue, trophoblastic tumors such as hydatidiform mole or choriocarcinoma in which high levels of chorionic gonadotropin cross-react with the TSH, and pituitary resistance to thyroid hormone.

Treatment options in thyrotoxic disorders depend on the underlying etiology. Disorders associated with an increased RAIU such as Graves' disease, toxic multinodular goiter, or solitary toxic nodules are usually treated with radioactive iodine as a primary mode of therapy. Alternative options include antithyroid drugs as well as β-blockers for symptomatic relief. Surgery is rarely indicated in these disorders. Hyperthyroidism due to thyroiditis is a self-limiting disease and usually treated symptomatically.

Radioactive iodine (I^{131}) ablates the thyroid gland by its β-emission and produces follicular cell necrosis and later fibrosis. The usual treatment dose of radioactive iodine is in the range of 5–15 mCi. Higher doses may be needed to treat a toxic adenoma or multinodular goiters. Subsequent 10-year follow-up of patients receiving radioactive iodine indicates an incidence of hypothyroidism of 40–70%. However, the natural history of the Graves' disease suggests an ultimate progression to hypothyroidism. Thus, the risk of hypothyroidism is discussed with each patient and is an expected consequence of radioactive iodine therapy. If hypothyroidism occurs, the patient can be placed on a physiologic dose of thyroid hormone replacement.

Radioactive iodine therapy is contraindicated in pregnancy. Thus, a negative β-human chorionic gonadotropin is mandatory prior to treating women in the child-bearing age. In pregnancy, treatment of hyperthyroidism is with antithyroid drugs and β-blockers. The goal of treatment is to use the lowest dose of drugs to optimize the T_4 levels in the upper limits of the normal range, avoiding the hypothyroid state and its effects on the fetus, and discontinuing β-blockers at the time of labor and delivery.

If antithyroid drugs are utilized, there are two drugs currently available: (1) PTU; and (2) methimazole (Tapazole). Both of these drugs block the formation of thyroid hormone by inhibiting tyrosine iodination and coupling. PTU, unlike methimazole, also blocks the peripheral conversion of T_4 to T_3. PTU requires administration at 6–8-hour intervals, while methimazole can be administered once a day. Although both drugs cross the placenta,

PTU is the drug of choice in the pregnant patient because methimazole has been associated with aplasia cutis (a minor scalp defect seen in children of mothers who took methimazole during pregnancy). The initial dose of PTU is 300 mg/day and methimazole is 30 mg/day. In severe thyrotoxicosis, larger doses up to 600–1200 mg of PTU daily or 60–80 mg methimazole may be needed. The drug dose should be reduced to the smallest amount to maintain the euthyroid state once the thyrotoxicosis is controlled. Serum thyroid function tests must be measured very frequently to adjust the dose and the patient must be monitored carefully for side-effects. Minor side-effects include fever, rash, arthralgias, arthritis, and leukopenia. Major reactions include cholestatic jaundice with methimazole, toxic hepatitis with PTU, and agranulocytosis with both drugs. Patients should be instructed to seek medical attention if a sore throat or fever develops in order to prevent potentially fatal agranulocytosis.

β-Blockers are useful adjuncts in the treatment of thyrotoxicosis. They do not alter the underlying course of the disease but alleviate the symptoms of tachycardia, tremor, anxiety, and hyperactive behavior. Theoretically, they also block T_4 to T_3 conversion. Propranolol doses can range from 40 to 160 mg/day. The usual starting dose is 10–20 mg every 8 hours and the dose is titrated to control the tachycardia. Rarely, iodides have been used to treat thyrotoxicosis but are usually reserved for the treatment of thyroid storm or to prepare a patient for emergency surgery. Iodides initially block organification of iodine within the gland in an action termed the Wolff–Chaikoff effect. Iodide also blocks the release of thyroid hormone into the circulation; however, escape can occur.

In summary, hyperthyroidism is a clinical syndrome manifested by classic symptoms and signs of excess thyroid hormone in the peripheral circulation. The clinical signs and symptoms together with pertinent thyroid function tests and RAIU and scan allow the physician to make the correct diagnosis and select the appropriate treatment for the individual patient.

FURTHER READING

Becker DV. Choice of therapy for Graves' hyperthyroidism. N Engl J Med 1984; 311: 464–466.

Borst GC, Eil C, Burman KD. Euthyroid hyperthyroxemia. Ann Intern Med 1983; 98: 366–378.

Burrow GN. Management of thyrotoxicosis in pregnancy. N Engl J Med 1985; 313: 562–565.

Cooper DS. Antithyroid drugs. N Engl J Med 1984; 311: 1353–1362.

DeGroot LJ, Larsen PR, Rifetoff S, Stanbury JB. The Thyroid and its Disease, 5th edn. 1984.

Hamburger JI. The various presentations of thyroiditis. Ann Intern Med 1986; 104: 219–224.

Kaplan MM, Larson PR. Thyroid disease. Med Clin North Am 1985; 69: 937–973.

Williams RH. In: Wilson JD, Foster DW, eds. Textbook of Endocrinology, 7th edn. Philadelphia: 1985: 743–775.

35

Thyroid mass

DEAN M. MOUTOS

INTRODUCTION

Abnormalities of the thyroid gland are among the most commonly encountered endocrinologic problems. Virtually any type of thyroid disorder can present as a thyroid mass. Because most thyroid disorders are more common in women, it is likely that the gynecologist will encounter a thyroid mass at some time in his or her practice. This chapter will review the diagnostic tools available for the evaluation of a thyroid mass and a management scheme will be presented.

HISTORY AND PHYSICAL EXAMINATION

The initial evaluation of a thyroid mass begins with a thorough history. Several benign thyroid conditions including Graves disease and Hashimoto's thyroiditis have familial tendencies. A family history of malignant thyroid disease, especially medullary thyroid carcinoma, should raise the suspicion of cancer. Previous head and neck irradiation is associated with an increased incidence of both benign and malignant thyroid nodules. External radiation to the head and neck was used in the past for a variety of benign conditions including tonsillitis, thymic enlargement, and various dermatologic conditions. Older patients should be carefully questioned about a childhood history of such radiation exposure. Persons exposed to nuclear fallout are also at increased risk, as are patients with a previous head or neck malignancy treated with radiation.

Palpable thyroid abnormalities occur in 20–30% of patients exposed to head and neck radiation, compared to an incidence of 4% in the general population [1]. Rapid enlargement of a new or preexisting thyroid nodule should alert the physician to a possible malignancy, although hemorrhage within a benign nodule can also be associated with rapid growth. Cervical adenopathy, dyspnea, dysphagia, and hoarseness should raise the suspicion of cancer, but they can also be seen with benign conditions. A thyroid nodule that has been present for many years should not automatically be considered benign. Thyroid cancer usually grows slowly and cancer has been found in nodules that have been present for many years. All thyroid nodules, regardless of their duration, should be carefully evaluated.

Numerous drugs, including propylthiouracil, methimazole, and lithium carbonate can be associated with thyroid enlargement. Large doses of iodide may result in iodide-induced hypothyroidism (Wolff–Chaikoff effect) and subsequent goiter formation in susceptible individuals. Iodine-containing drugs such as the antiarrhythmic amiodarone and X-ray contrast media should be noted as they too can precipitate thyroid dysfunction.

Physical examination of the thyroid should be performed with an understanding of basic thyroid anatomy. The normal thyroid gland weighs approximately 20 g and consists of two lobes lying anterolaterally to the trachea with the right lobe often slightly larger than the left. The two lobes are united in the midline by an isthmus situated between the second and third tracheal cartilages. Each lateral lobe extends upward to the midportion of the thyroid cartilage and downward to the fourth tracheal ring. One-third of patients have a narrow projection of thyroid tissue extending upward from the isthmus to the thyroid cartilage, usually to the left of the midline. This projection is known as the pyramidal lobe and when prominent may be mistaken for a thyroid mass. Agenesis of a thyroid lobe can result in a more prominent contralateral lobe which can also be mistaken for a mass.

The neck should be carefully inspected. The normal thyroid is usually visible only at the isthmus. Palpation of the thyroid requires relaxation of the neck muscles which can be accomplished by flexing the neck and turning the chin slightly to the side. The normal thyroid is soft to palpation and rises with swallowing. Fixation of the gland to surrounding neck structures is abnormal. The presence or absence of nodules is one of the most important physical findings. Nodules as small as 0.5 cm can usually be palpated. Auscultation of an enlarged thyroid should be performed. A to-and-fro bruit is suggestive of a toxic goiter. Systemic manifestations of hypothyroidism or hyperthyroidism should be noted.

The distinction between a single nodule and multinodular or diffuse goiter is important because there is a higher incidence of malignancy in solitary nodules. Approximately 10% of solitary nodules harbor a malignancy. The presence of a diffuse or multinodular goiter is generally considered a sign of a benign process, but thyroid malignancies are occasionally found in diffuse or multinodular goiters. Furthermore, clinical assessment of thyroid nodularity is often inaccurate and on further investigation 25% of clinically solitary nodules will actually be more prominent nodules in a multinodular gland. Nevertheless, categorizing thyroid masses as either uninodular or multinodular is a useful starting point in the diagnostic evaluation.

DIFFUSE AND MULTINODULAR GOITER

Thyroid function studies, including a total thyroxine, triiodothyronine (T_3) resin uptake (T_3RU) and an ultrasensitive thyroid-stimulating hormone (TSH) assay, should be obtained. Clinical and laboratory parameters are used to classify patients as hyperthyroid, hypothyroid, or euthyroid.

The most common cause of a diffuse goiter with hyperthyroidism is Graves disease (toxic diffuse goiter). In addition to hyperthyroidism and a diffuse goiter, Graves disease is characterized by ophthalmopathy, the presence of thyroid-stimulating immunoglobulins, and occasionally dermopathy. The diagnosis of hyperthyroidism is not necessarily synonymous with Graves disease and every effort should be made to determine the exact etiology of the hyperthyroidism.

Subacute thyroiditis typically presents as an enlarged, painful gland. It is a self-limiting disease which is most likely viral in etiology and is often preceded by an upper respiratory tract infection. Laboratory findings include an elevated erythrocyte sedimentation rate and a low TSH. Radionuclide scanning will show a decreased uptake of isotope by the gland, although scanning is not necessary to make the diagnosis. Subacute thyroiditis is often associated with mild hyperthyroidism, but transient hypothyroidism may be seen. Salicylates are sometimes required for symptomatic relief, but further treatment is not usually needed.

Multinodular goiter is characterized by a long history of a slowly enlarging gland. Any chronic, low-grade stimulus to thyroid growth can cause multinodular goiter. Physical examination reveals an enlarged, multinodular thyroid gland. Thyrotoxicosis often develops insidiously in long-standing multinodular goiter, and when present the condition is termed toxic multinodular goiter. Ophthalmopathy and dermopathy are absent. Clinical hyperthyroidism is usually mild, but radioactive iodine or surgery may be required in extreme cases. If thyrotoxicosis is absent, the condition is termed nontoxic multinodular goiter. Treatment of nontoxic multinodular goiter is not required unless cosmetic problems develop. Thyroxine-suppressive therapy can be tried, but it is of questionable benefit. Radioactive iodine or surgery is occasionally required in severe cases.

Colloid goiter describes a gland filled with uniformly distended follicles. The gland is symmetrically enlarged and feels spongy on examination. This condition occurs almost exclusively in young women and thyroid function tests are usually normal. Colloid goiter may resolve or it may persist. Persistent colloid goiter may be a precursor or multinodular goiter. Treatment is not required unless the goiter causes cosmetic problems. Thyroxine-suppressive therapy can be tried for mild enlargements, but surgery may be necessary in extreme cases.

The patient presenting with firm, lobular thyroid enlargement and hypothyroidism most likely has Hashimoto's thyroiditis. Microsomal and thyroglobulin antibodies are present in 95 and 60%, respectively, of patients with this disorder. An increased incidence of thyroid lymphoma is seen in Hashimoto's thyroiditis, therefore an enlarging or suspicious nodule should undergo fine-needle aspiration (FNA).

Iodine deficiency is a rare cause of goiter in developed countries, but it is the most common cause of thyroid enlargement worldwide. Genetic defects in thyroid hormone synthesis can result in hypothyroidism and goiter, but these disorders are extremely rare. Pituitary tumors secreting TSH are an uncommon cause of goiter and other pituitary abnormalities are usually present in addition to the hyperthyroidism.

CHAPTER 35

If a thyrotoxic patient does not clearly have Graves disease then radionuclide scanning should be performed to help establish the cause of the hyperthyroidism. Scanning, however, provides little additional information in the euthyroid or hypothyroid patient with a goiter.

THE SOLITARY THYROID NODULE

Evaluation of the solitary thyroid nodule is controversial. While thyroid nodules are common, thyroid cancer is uncommon. There are approximately 40 cases of thyroid cancer per million persons, but there are 40 000 cases of thyroid nodules per million persons. Most thyroid cancers, with the exception of anaplastic tumors, are indolent compared to other malignancies and only about 1000 people die each year in the USA of thyroid cancer. Thyroid nodules are uncommon in the young, but become more prevalent with advancing age. Autopsy studies have shown that approximately one-half of clinically normal thyroid glands have one or more nodules.

Thyroid cancer most commonly presents as a solitary nodule in a euthyroid patient. It is very uncommon for a malignant thyroid tumor to cause thyrotoxicosis. Thyroid function tests may be obtained but are frequently not helpful as the vast majority of solitary nodules, benign and malignant, are associated with normal results. With the exception of elevated calcitonin levels in medullary carcinoma, there are no reliable serum markers for thyroid cancer. Elevated thyroglobulin levels, antimicrosomal antibodies, and antithyroglobulin antibodies can be found in benign and malignant conditions and are not useful in the evaluation of the solitary nodule. Optimal evaluation of the solitary nodule should minimize the number of patients with benign disease who undergo surgery and correctly identify the 5–10% of patients with a malignancy who require surgery.

Radionuclide imaging has been the primary diagnostic tool in the evaluation of solitary nodules. Currently, however, many experts recommend FNA as the initial diagnostic procedure. This procedure is simple and inexpensive to perform. Anesthesia is not required and morbidity is low. A 22-gauge 1.5-inch (4 cm) needle is attached to a 10 ml syringe and inserted into the nodule. Aspiration is performed as the needle is moved back and forth inside the nodule. The aspirated material is placed on a slide and cytologic analysis performed. If a cyst is aspirated

the fluid should be sent for cytologic analysis as the presence of a cyst does not eliminate the possiblity of cancer. After a cyst is aspirated, any remaining solid component should also be aspirated.

The cytology is reported as benign, malignant, or suspicious. Malignant and suspicious lesions should undergo surgical excision. One of the limitations of FNA is in the evaluation of follicular thyroid neoplasms. Cytologic analysis cannot usually differentiate benign from malignant follicular neoplasms and the cytology will often be reported as suspicious, thus necessitating surgical excision.

Patients with benign cytology by FNA should be placed on thyroxine-suppressive therapy (0.1–0.3 mg levothyroxine/day), although the efficacy of this management has been questioned [2]. An ultrasensitive TSH assay should be performed while on thyroxine therapy to ensure that TSH suppression is complete. Nodules that persist or enlarge on suppressive therapy should undergo repeat FNA. Cysts should be followed clinically and repeat FNA performed if the cyst recurs.

The false-negative rate of FNA is generally reported to be less than 10% with some studies reporting rates as low as 2%. False-positive rates range from 2 to 5%. Approximately 10% of FNA will be nondiagnostic and require repeat aspiration. Large or cutting needle biopsy has been proposed as a method to avoid some of the inadequacies of FNA, but large-needle biopsy is associated with increased morbidity and requires greater skill to perform. It does not offer any significant advantages over FNA and should not be routinely used. Use of FNA has resulted in a 50% reduction in the number of patients requiring surgery and has doubled the incidence of cancer found in those patients who have surgery. A prerequisite for the use of FNA is the availability of a pathologist skilled in the interpretation of aspiration cytology. If such a person is not available, then radionuclide imaging should be the initial diagnostic step performed.

Radionuclide imaging with radioiodine (^{123}I) or technetium 99 m is recommended by some authorities as the initial diagnostic procedure. ^{123}I is preferred over ^{131}I because it delivers only 1% of the radiation of ^{131}I and has a shorter half-life — 13 hours versus 8 days [3]. Nodules are classified according to their ability to concentrate the isotope. A cold nodule is nonfunctioning or hypofunctioning and either does not take up the isotope or concentrates it to a lesser degree than the surrounding tissue. Uptake by a warm nodule is similar to that of the surrounding

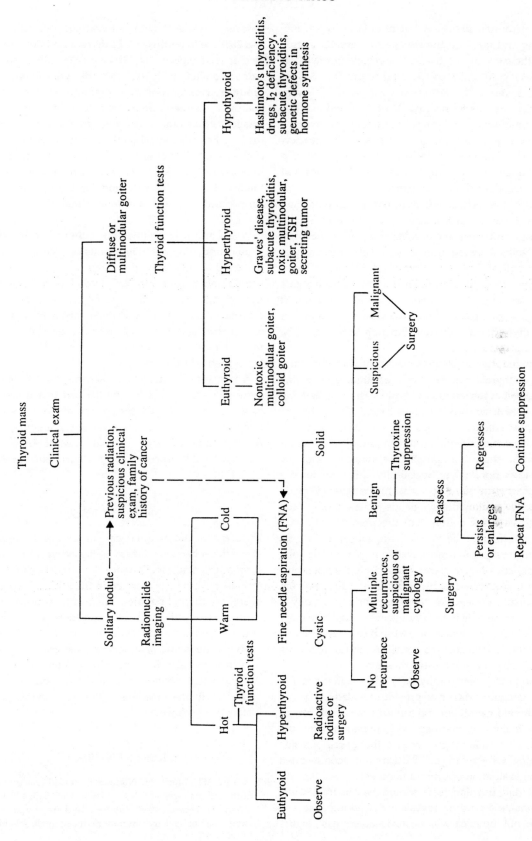

Fig. 35.1 Work-up of a thyroid mass.

normal thyroid tissue. A hot nodule is hyperfunc-tioning and takes up the isotope to a greater degree than the surrounding tissue. In a review of the litera-ture, Ashcraft and Van Herle [4] found that 84% of nodules were cold, 10.5% were warm, and 5.5% were hot. Cancer was found in 16% of cold nodules, 9% of warm nodules, and 4% of hot nodules. Although a cold nodule carries the greatest risk of malignancy, most cold nodules are benign. The presence of a hot nodule significantly decreases, but does not eliminate, the risk of malignancy.

One of the main criticisms of radionuclide imaging is that it cannot distinguish benign from malignant nodules and since most solitary nodules are cold, FNA will still be required. It is for these reasons that many authorities now recommend FNA over radio-nuclide imaging. Although radionuclide imaging gives an overall indication of thyroid activity, it should not be used to diagnose the hyperthyroid or hypothyroid state. Thyroid function tests should be used for this purpose.

Sonography has also been advocated in the evalu-ation of thyroid nodules. High-resolution sonography can detect cystic lesions as small as 1 mm in diameter and solid lesions as small as 3 mm. Up to 40% of clinically solitary nodules are found to be multi-nodular on sonographic examination [5]. The signifi-cance of these sonographically detected multiple nodules is not known. Specifically, it is not known if they carry the same low risk of malignancy as do clinically multinodular glands. Sonography can identify a cystic nodule, but the presence of a cyst does not rule out the possibility of cancer. Pure cysts are uncommon and most cysts will have some solid component on sonogram. There are no sonographic criteria that can reliably distinguish benign from malignant nodules. For these reasons sonography is not recommended in the routine evaluation of solitary thyroid nodules. It may be useful in selected cases for localizing small nodules for FNA or for following nodule size on suppressive therapy.

Computed tomography (CT) and magnetic reson-ance imaging (MRI) can provide detailed images of the thyroid gland, but still cannot distinguish benign from malignant nodules. The radiation exposure with CT scanning is greater than that of radionuclide imaging. CT scanning and MRI are not recommended in the evaluation of thyroid nodules.

Thyroid function tests should be obtained when radionuclide imaging reveals a hot nodule. Most of these hot nodules will be toxic adenomas. Eighty

percent of patients with hot nodules are euthyroid and 20% are hyperthyroid. Euthyroid nodules should be managed expectantly. Of the expectantly managed euthyroid hot nodules, 10–20% will eventually produce symptoms of hyperthyroidism. This occurs mainly in nodules 3 cm in diameter or greater, while smaller nodules rarely become symptomatic. Hyper-thyroid hot nodules should be treated with either radioactive iodine or surgery. The risk of permanent hypothyroidism is low with radioactive iodine therapy because the extranodular thyroid tissue is suppressed and will not concentrate much of the isotope.

Warm and cold nodules on radionuclide imaging should undergo FNA. The results of FNA should be managed as previously described.

Metastatic disease to the thyroid is uncommon. Lymphoma, renal cell carcinoma, and adenocar-cinomas of the breast, lung, and ovary may occasion-ally metastasize to the thyroid. A patient with a thyroid mass and a history of one of these malig-nancies should undergo FNA.

A suggested management scheme is outlined in Figure 35.1. It should be emphasized that if signifi-cant risk factors for cancer are present such as pre-vious radiation, suspicious clinical examination, or a positive family history of thyroid cancer, FNA should be performed irrespective of other hormonal or radio-logic findings.

CONCLUSIONS

Diffuse and multinodular goiters are usually associ-ated with a benign process. Solitary thyroid nodules carry a 10% risk of malignancy. Radionuclide imaging or FNA should be performed in the initial evaluation of solitary thyroid nodules. There is no consensus as to which one is the best, although there is a growing body of evidence supporting the use of FNA.

Hypofunctioning or otherwise suspicious nodules in a multinodular gland should be subject to FNA. All persistent solitary nodules must be resolved and most of the time this will require cytologic or histologic specimens.

REFERENCES

1 Rojeski MT, Gharib H. Nodular thyroid disease, evalu-ation and management. *N Engl J Med* 1985; 313: 428–436.
2 Gharib H, James M *et al.* Suppressive therapy with levo-thyroxine for solitary thyroid nodules: a double-blind

controlled clinical study. *N Engl J Med* 1987; 317: 70–75.

3 Griffin JE. Southwestern internal medicine conference: management of thyroid nodules. *Am J Med Sci* 1988; 296: 336–347.

4 Ashcraft MW, Van Herle AJ. Management of thyroid nodules. II: scanning techniques, thyroid suppressive therapy and fine needle aspiration. *Head Neck Surg* 1981; 3: 297–322.

5 Mazzaferri EL, de los Santos ET, Rofagha-Keyhani S. Solitary thyroid nodule: diagnosis and management. *Med Clin North Am* 1988; 72: 1177–1211.

Part IVC

Endocrinologic abnormalities: Ovary and adrenal gland

Abnormal androstenedione

CRAIG A. WINKEL

INTRODUCTION

Androgens are defined as substances that stimulate the male reproductive tract. These compounds are, for the most part, steroid hormones that promote the development of masculine secondary sexual characteristics and lead to nitrogen retention. Since androgens are defined biologically rather than chemically, it is necessary to understand the differences in their relative potencies. In the human, androgens that are present in the circulation in any significant quantities include: dihydrotestosterone (DHT), testosterone (T), androstenedione (A_4), and dehydroepiandrosterone (DHEA) [1]. DHT is the most potent naturally occurring androgen in the human, but the concentration of DHT is low in plasma under normal circumstances. T is the second most potent androgenic steroid, and the principal androgen secreted by the male gonad. In the normal female, approximately 25% of T is secreted by the adrenal gland, 25% secreted by the ovary, and 50% arises by conversion in peripheral sites from precursors secreted by both the ovary and the adrenal (Fig. 36.1). DHEA, which circulates usually as the sulfate (DHEAS), is the least potent androgenic steroid hormone and a principal secretory product of the adrenal gland. A_4, with an androgenic potency between T and DHEA, is unique in the sense that it plays a major role as a precursor of not only the potent androgen, T, but also of the estrogen, estrone.

PHYSIOLOGY

The distribution of the production of A_4 between the ovary and the adrenal gland varies according to the phase of the ovarian cycle and the time of day. The mature graafian follicle synthesizes and secretes an increasing amount of A_4 as the time of ovulation approaches — a phenomenon that is reflected in the rising concentrations of A_4 in plasma near midcycle. This increase in circulating level is maintained during the luteal phase of the cycle by the action of the corpus luteum.

On the other hand, the contribution of the adrenal gland to the circulating concentration of A_4 is responsive to the action of adrenocorticotropic hormone (ACTH) and this is reflected in the diurnal variation in plasma concentrations of A_4 observable during the early portion of the follicular phase of the ovarian cycle. In the morning, adrenal secretion may account for nearly 80% of the A_4 in the circulation whereas in the evening a substantial reduction in the adrenal component is observed [2]. These facts become of obvious importance when assessments are made for suspected abnormalities in the production or metabolism of A_4 since timing of blood sampling may become critical to the correct interpretation of assay results.

PATHOPHYSIOLOGY

Abnormalities of the production or metabolism or A_4 androstenedione may result in signs and symptoms attributable to the actions of the potent metabolites of A_4—T, and estrone, but usually not the actions of

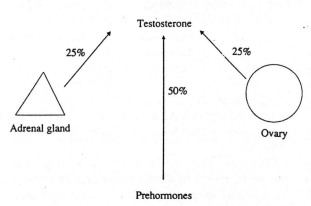

Fig. 36.1 The origins of testosterone in the human female.

A_4 *per se*. For the most part, the complaints attributable to abnormal production of A_4 are the result of overproduction and result in symptoms associated with excessive androgen action, excessive estrogen action, or occasionally both. While patients with reduced biosynthesis of A_4 may well have a variety of disease states, the complaints associated with adrenal hypofunction or anovulation tend to result from abnormalities other than the fact of reduced formation of A_4.

EXCESSIVE ESTROGEN FORMATION

Of the four endogenously produced estrogen precursors (T, DHEA, DHEAS, and A_4), MacDonald *et al*. demonstrated that A_4 is converted to estrogen in peripheral tissues to a greater extent than the other three [3]. Indeed, A_4 is converted to estrogen in the female five times more efficiently than the other three precursor steroids. The estrogen derived from circulating A_4 is solely estrone. The quantity of estrone formed from endogenously produced circulating A_4 depends ultimately not only upon the extent of conversion of A_4 to estrone, but also on the quantity of A_4 available for this process. In the normal female, production rates of A_4 have been estimated at 3.4 mg/day. Since the normal female has the capacity to convert 1.3% (range 1.0–1.7%) of her circulating A_4 to estrone, it can be calculated that 44 µg of estrone could be expected to be formed daily in a normal female.

Under a variety of pathophysiologic conditions, the extraglandular formation of estrogen (which occurs primarily in muscle cells, adipocytes, hair follicles, and skin fibroblasts) may be excessive and result in a state of relatively constant, elevated estrogen action. Unopposed, excessive estrogen action has been associated in the human female with endometrial hyperplasia, abnormal uterine bleeding, and the development of endometrial carcinoma. In addition, it has been suggested that such an estrogenic state may also play a significant role in the development of cystic changes in the breasts as well as breast carcinoma.

Acyclic extraglandular estrogen formation can develop under conditions associated with excessive production of the precursor A_4-androstenedione. It is estimated that 60% of the A_4 in circulating plasma is of adrenal origin and 40% of ovarian origin [4] (Fig. 36.2). Conditions associated with excessive adrenal steroidogenesis may result in overproduc-

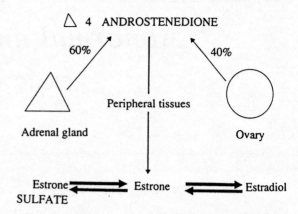

Fig. 36.2 The origins of androstenedione and estrogen in the human female.

tion and secretion of A_4. Females with adrenal 21-hydroxylase deficiency have reduced capacity for the formation of cortisol by the adrenal gland. Secretion of ACTH from the pituitary gland is uninhibited. As a result, plasma 17-hydroxyprogesterone levels rise and A_4 as well as T is formed in excess. If the patient is obese, excessive estrone and estradiol may be formed in adipose tissue by way of the extraglandular aromatase enzyme system. Alternately, in females with polycystic ovarian disease, ovarian thecal hyperplasia "overproduces" A_4. The A_4 thus formed may be converted into estrone in peripheral tissues. Interestingly, among women under the age of 35 years found to have endometrial carcinoma, associated history of polycystic ovarian disease was identified in the vast majority.

Obesity *per se* is associated with exaggerated capacity for aromatase activity that appears to be the result of an absolute increase in numbers of adipocytes. Aging has been shown also to be associated with a two- to fourfold increase in the formation of estrone from A_4. This appears, however, to be secondary to age-related increases in the aromatase enzyme activity in aging adipocytes and not an increase in cell numbers. The importance of this phenomenon is augmented by the fact that in the aging female, the ovary continues to produce significant quantities of A_4, even in the postmenopausal state when ovarian estrogen formation essentially ceases.

Under all conditions in which excessive production of A_4 results in acyclic extraglandular estrogen formation, therapy, in addition to attempting to reduce the daily production of A_4, should be aimed at reducing the impact on the estrogen target organs, breast, and uterus. It has been demonstrated by a number of investigators that the consequences of unopposed estrogen action on the endometrium can be obviated by treatment, in a cyclic fashion, with oral progestogens. For these reasons, it is recommended that the anovulatory female with an acyclic, endogenous source of estrogen, be it estrone or estradiol, should be treated for a minimum of 10–12 days per month to prevent endometrial hyperplasia. While still somewhat controversial, there are little data to support any specific therapy to reduce the impact of prolonged unopposed estrogen action upon the breast.

EXCESSIVE ANDROGEN FORMATION

A_4 is the major plasma precursor of T and, as stated in the introduction, 50% of the plasma concentration of T is derived from A_4. On the other hand, 2% of plasma A_4 is converted into the very potent androgen, DHT. DHT is 1.5–3 times more potent than T and approximately 15% of the total daily production of DHT (75 µg) arises from T (about 10 µg). Since the normal female produces about 3300 µg of A_4 per day, it can be calculated that 66 µg of DHT (about 80% of the daily production) arises from A_4. It is no wonder that excessive production of A_4 is associated with overproduction of potent androgens that result in the signs and symptoms of androgen excess — hirsutism, acne, and virilization.

The conditions associated with excessive androgen production as a result of abnormal formation of A_4 may be divided into those associated with an ovarian source of excessive A_4, those associated with an adrenal source, or those in which both ovary and adrenal might be involved. The major difficulty often lies in distinguishing which exists so that proper therapy can be instituted.

A significant elevation of essentially all of the androgenic steroid hormones and their precursors has been observed in patients with polycystic ovarian disease. In addition to the persistently elevated levels of estrone derived from the extraglandular conversion of A_4, augmented formation of T and DHT, also derived from A_4, is observed. Despite the diversity of symptoms associated with polycystic ovarian disease, acne, hirsutism, obesity, and menstrual dysfunction are the most frequent. Acne and hirsutism could be the result of either excessive androgen production or of increased androgen action. It has been demonstrated, however, that the obesity

seems to play a critical role in the manifestations of this disease [5]. Simple weight reduction has been shown to result in reduced plasma concentrations of A_4 and other androgens as well as reduced extraglandular estrogen formation and the restoration of cyclic ovarian estrogen production.

Although hyperandrogenemia in the patient with polycystic ovarian disease is well established, the issue of whether the adrenal gland is involved or not remains to be elucidated. Indeed, only 50% of patients with polycystic ovarian disease have elevated plasma concentrations of adrenal androgen, namely, DHEAS. It appears that suppression with oral dexamethasone (0.5 mg nightly) of plasma concentration of DHEAS is readily achievable, whereas suppression of plasma concentrations of A_4 and T by similar treatment is unlikely, reflecting the ovarian contribution to circulating androgens in patients with this abnormality. Nonetheless, it is clear that the polycystic ovarian syndrome represents two subtypes: those with an adrenal androgen component and those without.

Pure adrenal sources of excessive A_4 production tend to be unusual or relatively rare conditions. For the most part, patients with complaints referable to mild or moderate elevations in A_4 production are most likely to have an ovarian source to their problems, likely associated with polycystic ovarian disease. On the other hand, patients with evidence of severe elevations in androgen production are more commonly found to have adrenal disease, androgen-producing tumors of the adrenal gland, Cushing's disease, or adrenal hyperplasia secondary to a congenital enzyme deficiency, to name a few.

When confronted by the patient with evidence of excessive androgen production, it is important to rule out a potentially life-threatening disease such as a tumor. This can be accomplished usually by quantification of plasma androgen concentrations. It has been reported, for example, that it is unlikely that a tumor exists if the plasma T concentration is less than 200 ng/dl. Plasma concentrations of A_4 that might point toward a tumor have not been defined.

A useful approach to the problem of defining the source of the excessive androgen production so that therapy may be directed specifically is as follows: plasma samples may be obtained and quantification of T, DHEAS, and A_4 should be ordered. If DHEAS and T are elevated but A_4 is normal, it is likely that there is an adrenal source; if T and A_4 are elevated but DHEAS is normal, then an ovarian source is likely; if

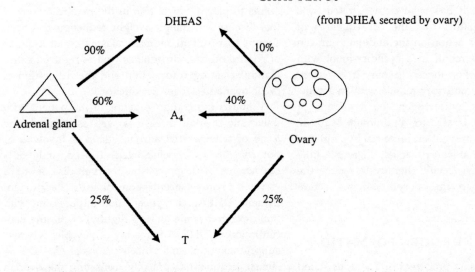

Fig. 36.3 The origins of potent and weak androgens in the human female. Clinical utilization of circulating levels for diagnostic purposes.

DHEAS and A_4 are elevated, then a combined adrenal and ovarian source is likely (Fig. 36.3). While the method of interpreting the results is not foolproof, it has been found to be a rather simple, relatively quick way of defining the source of androgen excess short of complex and time-consuming suppression/stimulation tests. These latter tests still retain their value in more intense investigations of the patient with excessive androgen production, however, and cannot be replaced by simply quantitating T, DHEAS, and A_4.

TREATMENT

The treatment of the patient with a complaint referable to abnormal production of A_4-androstenedione must be directed primarily at the source of the excessive hormone production. Clearly, if a tumor is involved, extirpation is the only proper mode of therapy. On the other hand, if the possibility of a tumor can be eliminated, then medical therapy may be pursued. Medical therapy might be subdivided according to the expected origin of the excessive androgen production. If the adrenal gland is involved, then suppression of pituitary ACTH production (and thus stimulation of the adrenal gland) can be accomplished by replacement of insufficient cortisol with exogenous glucocorticoid hormone. If the ovary is involved, then suppression of pituitary luteinizing hormone production can be accomplished, which will result in decreased ovarian thecal stimulation. This can be accomplished by the use of oral contraceptives or by treatment with gonadotropin-releasing hormone analogs.

REFERENCES

1 Kirschner MA, Bardin CW. Androgen production and metabolism in normal and virilized women. *Metabolism* 1972; 21: 667.
2 Yen SSC, Jaffe RB. *Reproductive Endocrinology, Physiology, Pathophysiology, and Clinical Management*. Philadelphia: WB Saunders, 1986; 446–448.
3 MacDonald PC, Rombaut RP, Siiteri PK. Plasma precursors of estrogen, I. Extent of conversion of plasma androstenedione to estrone in normal males and nonpregnant females. *J Clin Endocrinol Metab* 1967; 27: 1103.
4 MacDonald PC, Chapelaine A, Gonzalez O, Gurpide E, VandeWiele RL, Lieberman S. Studies on secretion and interconversion of the androgens, III. Results obtained after the injection of several radioactive C_{19} steroids, singly or as mixtures. *J Clin Endocrinol Metab* 1965; 25: 1557.
5 Bates GW, Whitworth NS. Effect of body weight reduction on plasma androgens in obese infertile women. *Fertil Steril* 1982; 38: 406.

Abnormal testosterone

M. YUSOFF DAWOOD

To understand abnormal testosterone levels in women, it is essential that the practitioner has a basic understanding of the sources contributing to testosterone levels in normal women. This chapter will therefore address first the sources of testosterone in normal women and then the causes of and further work-up of women with abnormal testosterone levels.

SOURCE OF TESTOSTERONE IN NORMAL WOMEN

Testosterone is secreted directly by the ovaries and the adrenals and also contributed from peripheral metabolism of prehormones, mainly androstenedione and to a lesser extent dehydroepiandrosterone (DHEA) [1]. Based on measurements of blood level gradients of testosterone in ovarian and adrenal veins, it has been suggested that 25% of the daily testosterone production comes directly from adrenal secretion, 25% directly from ovarian secretion, and the remaining 50% from extragonadal or peripheral metabolism of prehormones [2]. Androstenedione is secreted by both the adrenals and ovaries in about approximately equal amounts. The DHEA is largely of adrenal origin. Therefore, about half to two-thirds of

peripheral levels of testosterone are ovarian in origin while the remainder comes from the adrenals. The daily production rate of testosterone is $230 \pm 30\,\mu g$ with insignificant variation throughout the menstrual cycle.

During the menstrual cycle, circulating levels of plasma or serum testosterone as measured by radioimmunoassay showed slight fluctuations with an increase during the preovulatory period that has been thought to give rise to increased sexual activity [3,4]. Serum testosterone levels are slightly but not significantly higher during the luteal phase than in the follicular phase. The normal ranges of plasma concentration of testosterone, androstenedione, DHEA, and dehydroepiandrosterone sulfate (DHEAS) are summarized in Table 37.1.

Testosterone is carried in the circulation in a form tightly bound to sex hormone-binding globulin (SHBG; 85%) and loosely bound to albumin (10–13%) with only 1–2% existing in the free form, not bound to any protein. About 10–15% of the circulating testosterone is biologically active and available from the albumin-bound and the free fractions. Serum testosterone measurements reflect the non-SHBG-bound form while serum free testosterone levels

Table 37.1 Serum androgen levels in women

Condition	Testosterone (ng/ml)	Androstenedione (ng/ml)	Dehydroepi-androsterone (ng/ml)	Dehydroepi-androsterone sulfate (ng/ml)	17-Hydroxy-progesterone (ng/ml)
Menstrual cycle					
Follicular phase	0.2–0.8	1.4–2.2	2.2–8.4	1250–1950	0.15–0.70
Midcycle peak	0.2–0.8	1.4–2.2	2.2–8.4	1250–1950	0.15–0.70
Luteal phase	0.2–0.8	1.4–2.2	2.2–8.4	1250–1950	0.4–3.0
Postmenopausal women	0.1–0.4			230–370	0.2–0.7
Children (female)	0.1–0.4				0.3–0.90

Normal ranges may vary from laboratory to laboratory, with the assay kits employed, and with the specificity of the antisera used.

which can also be determined reflect the 1−2% of circulating testosterone which is in the free form.

Testosterone is metabolized mainly in the liver and peripherally in target tissues such as the skin and hair follicle. In the liver, testosterone is mainly metabolized to androstenedione and then excreted as androstenedione and etiocholanolone, both of which are 17-ketosteroids. A small amount of testosterone is metabolized to testosterone glucuronide and excreted in the urine. Thus, only a portion of circulating testosterone is detected when urinary 17-ketosteroids are measured since testosterone itself is not a 17-ketosteroid. At the biologic target sites such as the skin and hair follicle, testosterone is metabolized to dihydrotestosterone (DHT) under the enzymatic action of 5α-reductase [5]. Peripheral circulating levels of DHT are about 2−5% of testosterone [3]; because DHT is not produced from the ovaries or the adrenals, changes in DHT levels reflect almost entirely testosterone metabolism at androgen target sites. Locally produced DHT is further metabolized to androstanediol (5α-androstane-3α,17β-diol), which is also present in the conjugated form as androstanediol glucuronide [6]. All three metabolites — DHT, androstanediol, and androstanediol glucuronide — have potent androgenic properties. It should be further noted that 5α-reductase activity at the androgen target tissues also converts DHEA, DHEAS, and androstenedione to DHT and androstanediol. Both DHT and androstanediol reflect peripheral androgenic activity at target tissues such as the skin and hair follicle better than testosterone levels. Since androstanediol is a stable metabolite after further local metabolism of DHT, the latter is therefore only partially excreted into the circulation while blood levels of androstanediol are a better index of peripheral androgen metabolism and androgenic activity.

ABNORMAL TESTOSTERONE LEVELS

Abnormal testosterone levels may be due to the use of exogenous testosterone agents or endogenous overproduction of testosterone. The possibility of exogenous agents such as testosterone cream, androgen-related anabolic agents, and androgens can all give rise to elevated plasma levels of testosterone. If such a possibility has been ruled out by careful history, elevated levels of serum testosterone are usually due to endogenous overproduction. The causes of endogenous overproduction of testosterone are summarized in the algorithm in Figure 37.1. Elevated serum testosterone from overproduction is due to either a tumor or a nontumor cause and both can arise from either the ovary or the adrenal. In clinical practice, serum testosterone is usually measured to rule out androgen-producing ovarian or adrenal tumors rather than necessarily confirming hypertestosteronemia when the presenting complaint is obvious hirsutism and/or virilism. If the serum testosterone level is more than 2 ng/ml, an androgen-producing tumor should be ruled out unless clinically the patient is typical for testicular feminization syndrome (see below). Therefore, further diagnostic work-up to rule out an adrenal or ovarian tumor producing testosterone should be undertaken, using such modalities as computed tomography scan, magnetic resonance imaging, and selective catheterization of ovarian and/or adrenal vessels [7] for measurement of androgen levels, as deemed appropriate.

With prolonged elevation of serum testosterone levels characteristic of androgen-producing tumors, virilization is usually present. Symptoms of virilization include change in voice (more hoarse or deep), loss of frontal scalp hair, increased libido, and increase in aggression or aggressive behavior. Signs of virilization include clitoromegaly, frontal baldness or male-type receding frontal hairline, increased muscle mass, and sometimes acanthosis nigricans (best looked for in the antecubital fossa, axilla, and nape of the neck).

Marked elevation of serum testosterone can be associated with and due to some types of abnormal gonad development presenting with androgen insensitivity. These patients usually have primary amenorrhea or external sexual ambiguity present, together with a Y chromosome detectable in blood or in gonadal tissues.

Dexamethasone suppression test

A rapid overnight dexamethasone suppression test using a low dose of dexamethasone is able to evaluate the suppressibility of cortisol secretion. A baseline serum testosterone, DHEAS, and cortisol are taken at 8 p.m., 0.5 mg dexamethasone is ingested and repeat serum testosterone, DHEAS, and cortisol are taken at 8 a.m. the following day. If a nontumor, adrenal hyperactivity is responsible for the elevated androgen, the hormone levels measured are suppressible the following morning after taking dexamethasone. The rapid overnight dexamethasone suppression test is, however, not very satisfactory for evaluating suppression of adrenal androgen secretion due to

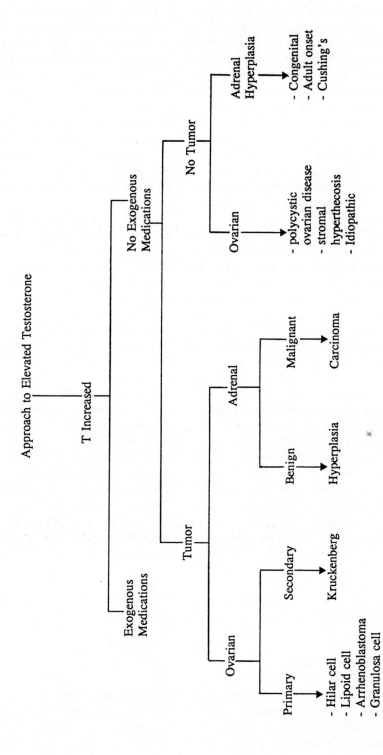

Fig. 37.1 Diagnosis of elevated testosterone levels in nonpregnant women.

probably the longer half-life of DHEAS. Usually at least 5 days of adrenal suppression with 3 mg of dexamethasone are required to evaluate suppression of adrenal androgen. Plasma levels of DHEAS, DHEA, testosterone, and androstenedione are then repeated at days 5 and 6 and should permit evaluation of the adrenal contribution for the elevated testosterone and other androgens determined. Results should be interpreted in relation to the menstrual cycle as cyclic variations may persist.

Androgen-producing tumors

Androgen-producing tumors may be benign or malignant. Benign androgen-secreting adrenal adenomas are rare but they respond to human chorionic gonadotropin stimulation and are suppressed by exogenous estrogens. More often, benign and malignant adrenal tumors present with elevated cortisol levels and are uncovered during work-up for possible Cushing's syndrome. Levels of other androgens, including DHEA, DHEAS, and androstenedione, are also elevated.

Androgen-secreting ovarian tumors are usually arrhenoblastomas, hilar cell tumors, lipoid cell tumors, and sometimes Krukenberg tumors (metastatic). Less frequently, granulosa cell tumors may produce increased testosterone levels from the stromal cells stimulated by some factor produced by the granulosa cell tumor. Luteomas of pregnancy are another testosterone- or androgen-producing tumor of the ovary but more likely to present during pregnancy. With testosterone-secreting ovarian tumors, DHEA and DHEAS levels are within normal limits but androstenedione may be elevated.

Although testosterone-producing tumors may rarely present with serum testosterone of 2 ng/ml or less, such levels are more likely to reflect nontumor causes. With such a laboratory finding of serum testosterone, it is essential to identify whether the adrenal or the ovary is the principal cause of the elevated testosterone so that the correct treatment can be given.

Androgen insensitivity syndrome

With the complete form of testicular feminization syndrome or other forms of androgen insensitivity, the patients have primary amenorrhea, normal female external genitalia with a short vagina (sometimes absent), normal breast development, scanty pubic and axillary hair, presence of testicular tissue, and absent uterus and tubes (Müllerian agenesis).

Testosterone levels in such patients range from 4 to 15 ng/ml but they fail to convert testosterone at peripheral target tissues due to absence of the enzyme 5α-reductase, absence of androgen receptors, or defective androgen receptors. Thus, the high circulating levels of testosterone do not express androgenic effects while the low levels of estrogen from both glandular and extraglandular sources allow breast development. Chromosome karyotype should be done and DHT levels are normal for a female. The abnormal gonads need to be localized, identified, and removed after puberty is established due to the high incidence of malignant transformation of such gonads, usually after the age of 20 years.

Polycystic ovary syndrome (PCOS)

With PCOS, there is chronic anovulation as reflected by oligoamenorrhea but ovulation may continue in 10–15% of patients. Hirsutism is present in about two-thirds of patients with PCOS and serum testosterone is elevated but usually below the 2 ng/ml range. However, in some PCOS patients with marked hirsutism, serum testosterone can be more than 2 ng/ml and virilism is also present. Obesity, if present, further compounds the hypertestosteronemia by increasing free testosterone levels secondary to a decrease in SHBG which is inversely related to obesity. In some instances, there may be an adrenal component to the PCOS and this is reflected by elevated serum DHEAS or DHEA levels. While serum luteinizing hormone (LH) levels may be increased, this determination is not clinically crucial to the diagnosis of PCOS; a serum LH : FSH (follicle-stimulating hormone) ratio of more than 2 may be helpful in the diagnosis but is not invariably found. The testosterone levels and the polycystic ovaries are readily suppressed with birth control pills or gonadotropin-releasing hormone agonists (such as nafarelin, leuprolide acetate, or buserelin). Less frequently needed and practiced today is ovarian wedge resection which will result in a significant lowering of serum testosterone but lasting an average of about 14–16 months, after which the levels are often up again.

Idiopathic hirsutism

Hirsutism may be found in women whose serum testosterone and other androgen levels are not elevated. While this condition was referred to as idiopathic or constitutional hirsutism, it is now clear that many of these patients have increased 5α-reductase activity that converts testosterone to DHT and androstanediol. Since DHT is also further metabolized in the peripheral tissues to androstanediol, the latter is increased in the blood and in the urine. Therefore, serum androstanediol glucuronide or 24-hour urinary excretion of androstanediol glucoronide can be expected to be elevated while serum testosterone may or may not be elevated in such patients. Antiandrogens such as spironolactone, cimetidine, and cyproterone acetate that block peripheral action of testosterone or inhibit 5α-reductase activity are effective for treatment of this condition. Nevertheless, in the evaluation of serum testosterone in patients with hirsutism, it is often necessary to determine whether the increased levels are due to an adrenal or ovarian source and baseline serum DHEAS and androstenedione levels can be useful. Thus, elevated serum T and DHEAS would suggest an adrenal source while elevated serum T and androstenedione suggest an ovarian origin. Further definition of the source can be delineated through the dexamethasone suppression test (see above). This test is not always clear and differential catheterization of the ovarian and adrenal vein (which can be tricky) can be performed to determine testosterone levels and therefore the source of any elevation.

Adult-onset congenital adrenal hyperplasia

Patients with adult-onset congenital adrenal hyperplasia (CAH) have elevated testosterone levels. CAH due to either 21-hydroxylase or 11β-hydroxylase deficiency causes decreased cortisol biosynthesis, giving rise to increased ACTH secretion that in turn stimulates the adrenals further to produce more cortisol precursors, including both 17-hydroxypregnenolone and 17-hydroxyprogesterone. These steroids are converted to DHEA and androstenedione because of the enzyme block and further peripherally converted to testosterone to produce elevated testosterone levels. Incomplete forms of the enzyme block or defects usually may not produce symptoms or signs of increased androgen production until after puberty [8]. Adult-onset CAH may be a commoner cause of elevated testosterone levels than hitherto recognized and many may be erroneously diagnosed as PCOS. Menstrual irregularity is the usual early presentation for the incomplete forms of the enzyme defect in the adult-onset CAH. At a later stage, hirsutism, oligoamenorrhea, and amenorrhea occur. The increased testosterone levels further lower the SHBG levels and lead to increased free estrogen levels,

causing stimulation of toxic LH release which further drives ovarian androgen production. A family history of postpubertal onset of hirsutism, mild evidence of virilization, and DHEAS levels of more than 5 μg/ml is indicative of CAH. The diagnosis can be confirmed with plasma 17-hydroxyprogesterone levels that are elevated (usually more than 8 ng/ml). If 17-hydroxyprogesterone levels are between 3 and 8 ng/ml, an ACTH stimulation test is carried out after an overnight dexamethasone 1 mg suppression is performed. A baseline 17-hydroxyprogesterone level is drawn the morning after dexamethasone is given, 25 IU of synthetic ACTH is given as a bolus dose and the 17-hydroxyprogesterone level is repeated 1 hour later. A post-ACTH 17-hydroxyprogesterone of 20 ng/ml or more confirms the diagnosis. Treatment is with continuing glucorticoids.

Hyperthyroidism

In patients with hyperthyroidism, plasma testosterone levels are markedly increased secondary to increased SHBG capacity. Thus, the free testosterone fraction is decreased but the concentration is normal and the metabolic clearance rate of testosterone is decreased. The blood production rate of testosterone remains normal.

REFERENCES

1 Abraham GE. Ovarian and adrenal contribution to peripheral androgens during the menstrual cycle. *J Clin Endocrinol Metab* 1974; 39: 340–346.
2 Kirschner MA, Bardin CW. Androgen production and metabolism in normal and virilized women. *J Clin Endocrinol Metab* 1972; 21: 667–687.
3 Dawood MY, Saxena BB. Plasma testosterone and dihydrotestosterone in ovulatory and anovulatory cycles. *Am J Obstet Gynecol* 1976; 126: 430–435.
4 Morris NM, Udry JR, Khan-Dawood FS, Dawood MY. Marital sex frequency and midcycle female testosterone. *Arch Sex Behav* 1987; 16: 27–37.
5 Ito T, Horton R. The source of plasma dihydrotestosterone in man. *J Clin Invest* 1971; 50: 1621–1627.
6 Horton R, Lobo RA. Peripheral androgens and the role of androstanediol glucuronide. *Clin Endocrinol Metab* 1986; 15: 293.
7 Kirschner MA, Jacobs JB. Combined ovarian and adrenal vein catheterization to determine the site(s) of androgen overproduction in hirsute women. *J Clin Endocrinol Metab* 1971; 33: 199–209.
8 Lobo R, Goebelsmann U. Adult manifestation of congenital adrenal hyperplasia due to incomplete 21-hydroxylase deficiency mimicking polycystic ovarian disease. *Am J Obstet Gynecol* 1980; 138: 720–726.

38

Elevated DHEAS

JOUKO K. HALME

Dehydroepiandrosterone sulfate (DHEAS) is the most abundant circulating steroid in both women and men. Essentially all of this hormone is produced and secreted by the adrenal glands. Interestingly, the fetal adrenal produces 10 times more than the adult one, due to the presence of the so-called fetal zone that will regress after birth. In adults DHEAS is converted to DHEA by slow continuous enzymatic hydrolysis although the majority of DHEA also arises from adrenal secretion. The physiologic function(s) of DHEAS is (are) not well established but changing levels during childhood and adult life have been clearly demonstrated. This hormone has also proven to be a useful indicator of abnormal adrenal function in some patients with signs of hirsutism or virilization.

PHYSIOLOGIC LEVELS IN CHILDREN

Several studies have demonstrated a progressive increase of DHEA and DHEAS in boys and girls by the age of 7 or 8 that continues to 13–15 years of age. During this time the levels increase approximately 20-fold. This increase in adrenal activity occurs approximately 2 years prior to the increase in gonadotropins and gonadal sex steroid secretion. This so-called adrenarche is associated with a rise in several adrenal enzyme activities that appears to promote the increase in adrenal androgen production. The control of this production is not yet fully understood but it is believed that the pituitary has a dual control mechanism separate from the pituitary–ovarian axis. Both adrenocorticotropic hormone (ACTH) and an insufficiently characterized pituitary cortical androgen-stimulating hormone (CASH) are apparently required. This hypothesis is borne out by observations that patients with premature adrenarche who have elevated levels of DHEA and DHEAS enter puberty and experience menarche within the normal age range. Moreover, prepubertal children who have congenital adrenal insufficiency with deficient or absent adrenal androgens usually have a normal onset and progression of puberty when on gluco- and mineralocorticoid replacement. Thus, early activation of adrenal androgen secretion does not commonly lead to precocious puberty, nor is deficient adrenal androgen output usually associated with delayed puberty, suggesting separate controls for adrenal androgen, cortisol, and ovarian steroids.

PHYSIOLOGIC LEVELS IN ADULTS

In adult life the levels of DHEAS peak between the ages of 15 and 25 years and start decreasing steadily after age 30 in both sexes, leading to almost undetectable levels after the age of 70. This is in contrast to cortisol secretion which remains relatively constant throughout life. It has been, therefore, proposed that DHEAS levels may serve as a specific marker for aging. Menopause is associated with an acceleration in the decline of DHEAS levels but estrogen replacement does not appear to influence that change.

The cause for the age-related decline in DHEAS levels remains unknown, but several possibilities can be considered. Aging may be associated with decreased pituitary production of the presumptive CASH or aging may lead to preferential utilization by the adrenal zone of the $\Delta 5$ pregnenolone precursor for cortisol. A third possibility is that aging may be associated with a decrease of cells in the androgen-producing zona reticularis (in contrast to adrenarche, when the cell mass increases).

METABOLISM OF DHEAS

The metabolic clearance rate for DHEAS is only 15 l/day, meaning that 1 liter of blood needs to go through the liver 100 times before all DHEAS is removed from it (given that all clearance, in the liver and hepatic blood flow, is 1500 l/day). DHEAS appears to be undergoing slow, continuous hydrolysis, thus contributing to the pool of free DHEA. The

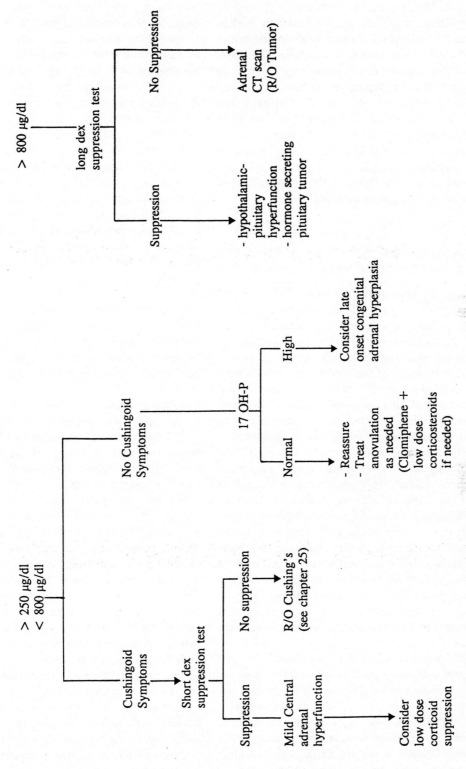

Fig. 38.1 Approach to elevated DHEAS (>250 µg/dl).

CHAPTER 38

slow clearance rate is reflected in the fact that in contrast to DHEA which has a diurnal variation, no such variation or menstrual cycle variation exist in DHEAS levels. DHEAS is a very weak androgen and only 5% of it is converted to testosterone. Therefore, modest elevations of this hormone will not lead to significant clinical androgenization. In fact, increased DHEAS levels have been reported with hyperprolactinemia without signs of hirsutism and the levels return to normal with suppression by bromocriptine. The cause for elevated DHEAS may be secondary to the persistent anovulatory state induced by the increased prolactin, although a direct prolactin effect on the adrenal cannot be excluded.

ELEVATED DHEAS IN EVALUATION OF HIRSUTISM OR VIRILIZATION

Clinically, the ease of measurement of DHEAS and the absence of short-term fluctuations have made it a reliable guide in evaluation of abnormal adrenal secretion and help in the differential diagnosis of chronic hyperfunction of the adrenal glands. Serum DHEAS measurement has largely replaced 24-hour urine determination of 17-ketosteroids as an initial evaluation of adrenal androgen secretion. A random sample is adequate, needing no correlation for body weight, creatinine excretion, or random variation.

Most laboratories report normal values of DHEAS up to 250 μg/dl, although higher normal ranges are sometimes quoted. In evaluation of hirsutism or virilization with or without chronic anovulation, when DHEAS is within the normal range, an adrenal abnormality is very unlikely. In this case excess androgen production by the ovaries is the most likely explanation. However, if serum testosterone is *markedly* elevated one should still be entertaining the rare possibility of an adrenal tumor secreting testosterone. An adrenal computed tomography (CT) scan should in this case be obtained to rule out such a tumor.

Slight elevations above the upper limit of normal are quite commonly seen in anovulatory patients with polycystic ovarian disease and it does not appear productive to pursue adrenal evaluation in these patients if their basal 17-OH-progesterone is normal. In patients with late-onset adrenal hyperplasia DHEAS levels are not usually elevated, consequently they are not useful in screening for such disorder — unlike the 17-OH-progesterone level.

Short dexamethasone suppression test

In patients with signs and symptoms of cortisol excess such as centripetal obesity and purple striae, an overnight dexamethasone test is a simple way to rule out Cushing's syndrome by giving 1 mg dexamethasone (2 mg if really obese) at 11 p.m. and checking the serum cortisol at 8 a.m. next morning. If it is less than 5 μg/dl, one can rule out Cushing's.

When anovulatory patients have slightly elevated DHEAS levels it is often beneficial to use mild adrenal suppression with oral low-dose corticosteroids (either 0.5 mg dexamethasone daily late p.m. or 5 mg prednisone p.m. and 2.5 mg a.m.) in order to improve their response to ovulation induction by clomiphene citrate or human menopausal gonadotropins. Serum DHEAS levels provide a useful guide in such therapy. Adequate suppression is usually reached when DHEAS returns to the high-normal range in these patients.

Long dexamethasone suppression test

Elevations of DHEAS more than two to three times the upper normal limit suggest significant adrenal hyperfunction and adrenal suppression with dexamethasone is in order to exclude an adrenal tumor as the source. To this end a longer, more complete hypothalamic suppression will be needed to suppress the adrenal glands adequately. Dexamethasone 2 mg q.i.d. is given for 5 days and serum DHEAS obtained before and after treatment. A suppressed DHEAS level suggests hypothalamic–pituitary hyperfunction or a hormone-secreting pituitary tumor.

The diagnosis of a virilizing adrenal tumor is made on the basis of clinical signs along with markedly elevated DHEAS that is not suppressed. This lack of adrenal suppression indicates the presence of an autonomously (not dependent on ACTH or CASH) functioning adrenal tumor. In Cushing's syndrome, where signs of cortisol excess are sometimes accompanied by signs of virilization, especially when caused by an adrenal carcinoma, the DHEAS may be grossly elevated and would not suppress with dexamethasone. In these cases a CT scan of the adrenals is by far the most helpful diagnostic tool for localization of such a tumor. It can reliably detect tumors as small as 1 cm in diameter and can identify bilateral enlargement in patients with pituitary ACTH-producing tumors. CT may also differentiate between a well-demarcated adenoma and irregular, lobulated, or infiltrating carcinoma.

CONCLUSIONS

DHEAS provides important information about the contribution of the adrenal glands in patients with signs and symptoms of androgen excess. In addition to its usefulness in the diagnosis of adrenal tumors or hyperfunction it can be utilized as a guide in monitoring adrenal suppression in the context of ovulation induction.

FURTHER READING

Chang JR, Abraham GE. Effect of dexamethasone and clomiphene citrate on peripheral steroid levels and ovarian function in a hirsute amenorrheic patient. *Fertil Steril* 1976; 27: 640.

Daly DC, Walters CA, Soto-Albors CE *et al*. A randomized study of dexamethasone in ovulation induction with clomiphene citrate. *Fertil Steril* 1984; 41: 844.

Hoffman DI, Klove K, Lobo RA. The prevalence and significance of elevated dehydroepiandrosterone sulfate levels in anovulatory women. *Fertil Steril* 1984; 42: 76.

Lobo RA, Paul, WL, Goebelsmann U. Dehydroepiandrosterone sulfate as an indicator of adrenal function. *Obstet Gynecol* 1981; 57: 69.

Rittmaster RS, Loriauk DL. Hirsutism. *Ann Intern Med* 1987; 106: 95.

Speroff L, Glass RH, Kase NG. Hirsutism. In: *Clinical Gynecologic Endocrinology and Infertility*. Baltimore: Williams & Wilkins, 1989: 233–263.

Uno H. Biology of hair growth. *Semin Reprod Endocrinol* 1986; 4: 2.

Abnormal sex hormone-binding globulin

GEORGE T. KOULIANOS & IAN H. THORNEYCROFT

INTRODUCTION

Steroid hormones circulate in the blood stream either bound to plasma proteins or unbound. These binding proteins are produced by the liver and can be nonspecific or highly specific. For androgens these proteins are primarily albumin and sex hormone binding-globulin (SHBG). Various drugs, hormones, and clinical conditions can affect their blood levels.

ANDROGEN BINDING AND TRANSPORT

Of the nonspecific proteins, albumin is the most important since it is present in such high concen-

trations. Due to its high concentration (4.2 g/dl), albumin has a high binding capacity for androgens but has a low affinity ($K_D = 10^{-6}$ mol/l) [1]. Thus, androgens are loosely bound by albumin. In normal women, albumin binds 10–19% of circulating testosterone (T) and both the loosely bound albumin fraction and free fraction are biologically active.

SHBG is a β-globulin synthesized by the liver. Although present in serum in smaller concentrations (65.1 mmol/l), SHBG is the principal specific steroid-binding protein for androgens. Some 80–85% of T is bound to SHBG (Fig. 39.1). SHBG binds less hormone than albumin since it is present in smaller concentrations but its affinity ($K_D = 10^{-9}$ to 10^{-8} mol/l) for

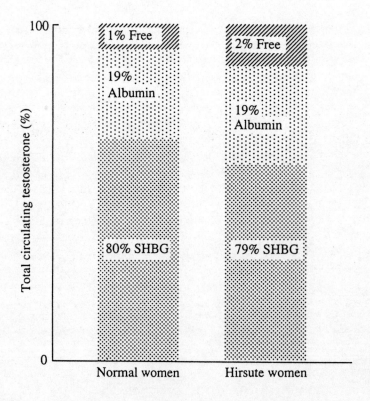

Fig. 39.1 Testosterone binding in normal and hirsute women.

androgens is much greater than that for albumin [1]. For example, the affinity of SHBG for testosterone is 10^5 times that of albumin for testosterone. Thus, steroids bind tightly to SHBG.

For androgens to bind with SHBG they must have a 17β-hydroxyl group. These would include T, 5α-dihydrotestosterone (DHT), 5α-androstane-3α-17β-diol (3α-Adiol), Δ5-androstenediol (Δ5-Adiol). Estradiol also binds to SHBG because of its 17-OH group. DHT has the highest affinity, followed by the Adiols. The androgen with the lowest affinity is T and of all steroids, estradiol possesses the weakest affinity. Only 35% of estradiol is SHBG bound [2]. The weak androgens androstenedione, dihydroepiandrosterone, and dehydroepiandrosterone sulfate do not bind to SHBG since they possess a 17β-ketone. There is no specific binding protein for these androgens and thus they only nonspecifically bind to albumin.

Binding between steroid and protein involves hydrogen and hydrostatic bonds. An equilibrium occurs between the bound and free steroid, for example:

$$T + SHBG \rightleftharpoons T \cdot SHBG$$

where T·SHBG represents bound steroid. The relative amounts of free and bound T are determined by the T and SHBG concentrations. These concentrations can be affected by a number of physiologic and pathologic conditions, which will be discussed later.

As free hormone enters the cell its concentration in the serum falls and the equilibrium reaction shifts in favor of the free hormone. Bound steroids are biologically inactive since they cannot enter the cell. Only the free fraction and the fraction loosely bound to albumin exert biologic activity. The amount of SHBG binding can also affect the metabolic clearance rate (MCR) for a particular steroid. The greater the SHBG fraction, the lower the MCR. Thus, in men, where the SHBG concentration is lower than women, the MCR for T is higher than in women. As the concentration of SHBG decreases the amount of free steroid increases, resulting in increased biologic activity. This is especially important with androgens where an increase in free T can result in hyperandrogenic sequelae, i.e., hirsutism.

Recently information suggesting a new role for SHBG has been reported [3]. In addition to the ability of free hormone to enter the cell by simple diffusion and exert its effect it also appears that SHBG binds to cell membranes and induces a second messenger.

In vitro studies suggest that SHBG increases both adenylate cyclase activity and the accumulation of cAMP. SHBG appears to be an allosteric protein with both steroid and membrane-binding sites. The membrane-binding site is masked when its steroid binding site is occupied. Thus, any specific biologic effect of SHBG on cell membranes other than its traditional transport function must occur after free SHBG binds to cell membranes. Once SHBG binds it is then able to bind steroid and activate its second messenger (Fig. 39.2). *In vitro* second messenger activity appears to depend on the steroid bound with DHT inducing the largest effect. This new second messenger role for SHBG is still poorly understood and should be considered experimental until more definitive data becomes available.

FACTORS AFFECTING SHBG CONCENTRATION

A number of factors modulate SHBG production by the liver. Of greatest clinical relevance is that androgens decrease SHBG and estrogens increase SHBG. Conditions which increase SHBG include pregnancy and hyperthyroidism. Drugs such as Dilantin, Tamoxifen, and exogenous estrogens also increase SHBG. The role of exogenous estrogen will be discussed in the treatment section. The estrogenic stimulus of pregnancy induces a profound increase in SHBG, bringing about a threefold rise in the total testosterone concentration and decreases the unbound fraction. Consequently, the MCR of T decreases. Hyperthyroidism increases SHBG by directly stimulating the liver to produce SHBG [3].

Conditions which diminish SHBG include obesity, hirsutism, insulin resistance, polycystic ovary syndrome, hypothyroidism, hyperprolactinemia, liver disease, and menopause. Drugs such as progestins, danazol, and glucocorticoids decrease SHBG. The effect of different progestational agents will be discussed in the treatment section. Lowered levels of SHBG result in an increased free T fraction. As previously discussed, the greater the free fraction, the greater the biologic activity. Thus, conditions which lower SHBG increase free T, resulting in hyperandrogenic sequelae. These conditions can occur separately or together and their effect on SHBG is primarily mediated by testosterone. Diet can also affect SHBG, a high carbohydrate diet causes a 35–40% increase in plasma SHBG.

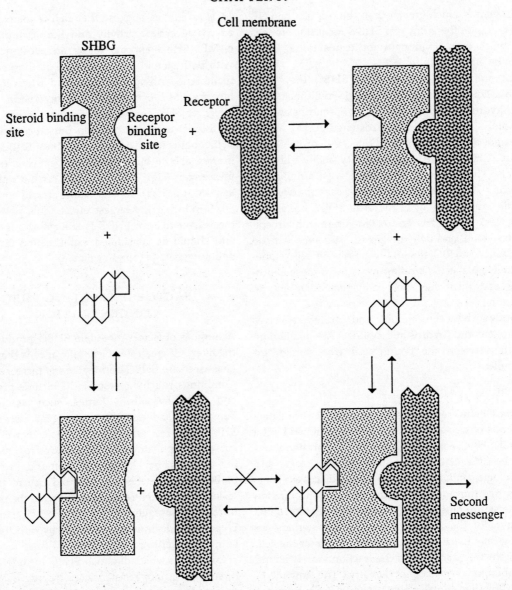

Fig. 39.2 Model for receptor SHBG steroid binding. (Adapted from [3].)

ANDROGENS AND SHBG

The most important androgen, when discussing SHBG, is T, and our subsequent discussion on the effect of androgens will primarily be limited to T. Even moderate obesity (30% above ideal body weight) can be associated with diminished SHBG and elevated free T with normal total T [4]. The mechanism causing this is poorly understood. Obese individuals are often hyperinsulinemic and insulin has been shown to lower SHBG secretion profoundly *in vitro* [3]. This may help to explain why obesity lowers SHBG. Several investigators have shown that weight loss can reverse this effect and bring both SHBG and free T back into the normal range.

Patients with polycystic ovary syndrome frequently are obese, hirsute, and hyperandrogenic. So it is not surprising that SHBG is markedly diminished (28 nmol/l) when compared to normal controls (78 nmol/l) [2]. This diminished binding capacity results in an increase in biologically active or non-SHBG-bound T and enhances the clinical features of hyperandrogenism. Since SHBG weakly binds estrogen, the non-SHBG fraction is elevated, even

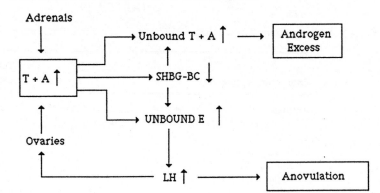

Fig. 39.3 Scheme depicting the possible role of adrenal-derived androgens (T, testosterone; A, androstenediol) in initiating androgen excess and anovulation (E, estradiol). (Adapted from [2].)

though total estrogen levels are normal, causing a hyperestrogenic state. This can affect luteinizing hormone (LH) production and lead to anovulation. The importance of SHBG binding in the development or propagation of this syndrome is illustrated in Figure 39.3.

Other conditions which diminish SHBG that are not secondary to hyperandrogenism are menopause, liver disease, hypothyroidism, and hyperprolactinemia. The most important of these is menopause. Circulating estrogen levels are profoundly reduced in menopausal women, resulting in a decrease in SHBG. Menopausal women with hot flushes have even lower estrogen and SHBG levels.

TREATMENT

Patients with diminished SHBG typically are hyperandrogenic and complain of obesity, anovulation, hirsutism, acne, and/or polycystic ovary syndrome. Since androgens and obesity lower SHBG, treatment is based on lowering androgen levels and weight loss. In obese women weight loss can return SHBG, total T, and free T concentrations to normal. For example, a 10% weight loss can return SHBG to normal in mildly obese women [5] (Table 39.1).

The primary pharmacologic agent used to increase SHBG and decrease testosterone is an oral contraceptive. Ethinylestradiol, the estrogen present in all low-dose oral contraceptives, alone can more than double SHBG concentrations. The increased SHBG results in T being more avidly bound, resulting in much lower unbound T levels. In addition oral contraceptives diminish ovarian androgen synthesis directly by suppressing LH synthesis.

Unfortunately, since the progestins in oral contraceptives are 19-nortestosterone derivatives, they

appear partially to counteract the effects of estrogen and lower SHBG. This may be a direct effect on SHBG synthesis or an indirect effect through displacement of T from SHBG. The higher the progestin potency of the pill, the lower the SHBG. When choosing an oral contraceptive, 35 µg ethinylestradiol is sufficient significantly to increase SHBG and lower T. Higher-dose pills exert a more profound increase in SHBG but they do not lower free T levels more than low-dose pills do. It appears that one can only lower T by so much by increasing SHBG.

In general one should use a low-dose birth control pill with estrogenic properties to maximize the SHBG effect. Data on the SHBG effect of various oral contraceptives are limited and to date there are no controlled randomized studies comparing the triphasic contraceptives in normal and hyperandrogenic women, but enough information is available to allow one to make an appropriate choice. Table 39.2

Table 39.1 Effect of weight loss on sex hormone-binding globulin (SHBG) and testosterone (T). (Adapted from [5])

Parameter	Value
Height (in)	64.2
Weight (lb)	
Before	228
After	203.2
Weight loss (%)	10.7
SHBG (ng/DHT bound/ml)	
Before	1.59
After	2.02
T (ng/ml)	
Before	0.89
After	0.67

DHT, dihydrotestosterone.

CHAPTER 39

Table 39.2 Effect of birth control pills on SHBG, total T, and free T in normal women. (Adapted from [6–9])

Oral contraceptive pill	SHBG change (%)	Total T change (%)	Free T change (%)
Triphasil EE 30, 40, 30 µg; L 0.05, 0.075, 0.125 mg	+92	−26	−35
Lo-ovral EE 30 µg; Nor 0.3 mg	+24	−21	−37
Ovcon EE 35 µg; NE 0.4 mg	+271	−3	−49
Ortho Novum 1/35 EE 35 µg; NE 1.0 mg	+92	−36	−
Nordette EE 30 µg; L 150 mg	+28	−16	−31

EE, ethinylestradiol; L, levonorgestrel; Nor, norgestrel; NE, norethindrone; −, not reported.

lists the effects of several birth control pills in normal women on SHBG, total T, and free T. Only pills available in the USA are discussed.

Given this information, it appears that any low-dose pill will elevate SHBG and suppress ovarian androgens. The most important gauge of the effectiveness of a particular oral contraceptive should be its ability to suppress free T since this is what is biologically active. The effect on SHBG is also important but should not be the only consideration since a marked increase in SHBG does not result in an equally marked decrease in free T. Oral contraceptives also decrease free T by decreasing total T. From Table 39.2 we can see that all of the contraceptives listed exerted a similar effect on free T. An equally profound effect can be seen in women with acne vulgaris where triphasic oral contraceptive use can decrease free T by approximately 25%, increase SHBG by over 100%, and moderately to significantly improve acne in 86.5% of patients [10]. Unfortunately, the data on hirsute women are not quite as clear-cut but it does appear that oral contraceptives will increase SHBG and lower free T [11].

MEASUREMENT OF SHBG

Commercially available kits using radioimmunoassay are available but are not frequently used. Usually a thorough history and physical examination with special emphasis on amenorrhea, oligomenorrhea, hirsutism, acne, or male hair patterns coupled with serum total and free T measurements are sufficient. Although the inverse relationship between T and SHBG is not absolute, the correlation is strong enough to defer SHBG determination on a routine basis.

CONCLUSIONS

SHBG is a steroid hormone-binding protein produced by the liver. It is affected by a number of factors, the most important of which is hormones. Estrogen increases SHBG and androgens decrease SHBG. The clinical importance of SHBG is that it is decreased by a number of hyperandrogenic conditions, resulting in an elevated free testosterone fraction and resultant increase in hyperandrogenic sequelae. The principal treatment is low-dose oral contraceptives, which increase SHBG and decrease ovarian androgen production, resulting in lower free T. All low-dose contraceptives appear to exert a similar effect on free T, although their effect on SHBG is variable.

REFERENCES

1 Clark AF. Androgen biosynthesis, production, and transport in normal and hyperandrogenic women. *Semin Reprod Endocrinol* 1986; 4: 77–87.
2 Mishell DR, Davajan V, eds. *Infertility, Contraception, & Reproductive Endocrinology*. Oradell: Medical Economics Books, 1986.
3 Rosner W. The functions of corticosteroid-binding globulin and sex hormone-binding globulin: recent advances. *Endocr Rev* 1990; 11: 80–91.
4 Wajchenberg BL, Marcondes JAM, Mathor MB *et al*. Free testosterone levels during the menstrual cycle in obese versus normal women. *Fertil Steril* 1989; 51: 535–537.

244

5 Harlass FE, Plymate SR *et al*. Weight loss is associated with correction of gonadotropin and sex steroid abnormalities in the obese female. *Fertil Steril* 1984; 42: 649–652.

6 Hammond GL, Langley MS, Robinson PA *et al*. Serum steroid binding protein concentrations, distribution of progestins, and bioavailability of testosterone during treatment with contraceptives containing desogestrel or levonorgestrel. *Fertil Steril* 1984, 42: 44–51.

7 Granger LR, Roy S, Mishell DR. Changes in unbound sex steroids and sex hormone binding globulin-binding capacity during oral and vaginal progestogen administration. *Am J Obstet Gynecol* 1982; 144: 578–584.

8 Murphy AA, Cropp CS, Smith BS *et al*. Effect of low-dose oral contraceptive on gonadotropins, androgens, and sex hormone binding globulin in nonhirsute women. *Fertil Steril* 1990; 53: 35–39.

9 Jung-Hoffmann C, Kuhl H. Divergent effects of two low dose oral contraceptives on sex hormone-binding globulin and free testosterone. *Am J Obstet Gynecol* 1987; 156: 199–203.

10 Lemay A, Dewailly SD *et al*. Attenuation of mild hyperandrogenic activity in postpubertal acne by a triphasic oral contraceptive containing low doses of ethinyl estradiol and dl-norgestrel. *J Clin Endocrinol Metab* 1990; 70: 8–14.

11 Talbert LM, Sloan C. The effect of a low-dose oral contraceptive on serum testosterone levels in polycystic ovary disease. *Obstet Gynecol* 1979; 53: 694–697.

40

Androgen excess

RICARDO AZZIZ

Disorders of androgen excess lead to the symptoms of hirsutism, acne, and oligoovulation. In this chapter the author will outline normal androgen metabolism, the symptoms, differential diagnosis, work-up, and treatment of androgen excess.

NORMAL ANDROGEN METABOLISM

Androgens are 19-carbon steroids derived from cholesterol, and secreted by the adrenal cortex and the ovaries. Androgens may also be derived (not secreted) from the conversion of other androgens by peripheral tissues (e.g., adipose tissue, muscle, skin, etc.) Principal circulating androgens include testosterone (T) and its metabolite dihydrotestosterone (DHT), androstenedione (A_4), and dehydroepiandrosterone (DHEA) and its metabolite dehydroepiandrosterone sulfate (DHEAS).

In premenopausal women T originates approximately 25% from the ovary, 25% from the adrenal, and 50% from the peripheral conversion of A_4. A_4 is produced equally from the ovary and the adrenal cortex. T and A_4 are further metabolized to the potent androgen DHT in the liver and skin, through the action of the enzyme 5α-reductase. Approximately 90% of DHEA and 99% of DHEAS are produced by the adrenal cortex. Although DHEAS is the most abundant androgen in circulation, in a circulating concentration 8000–10 000 times more than that of T, this steroid, DHEA, and A_4 are weak androgens compared to T and DHT.

T and DHT circulate tightly bound to an α-globulin produced by the liver called sex hormone-binding globulin (SHBG), while A_4 is weakly bound, and DHEA and DHEAS are not bound at all. Since androgens act through a specific cytoplasmic/nuclear receptor and only free (unbound) steroid is able to act on this receptor, the action of T and DHT is greatly influenced by the circulating SHBG level. If the SHBG level is low, the free fraction of T and DHT

is altered and their androgenic effect is also increased. Furthermore, the higher the free fraction of T and DHT, the greater their clearance from the body, since only free androgen can be metabolized and removed by the liver and peripheral tissues. Paradoxically, the circulating SHBG level is decreased by androgens and increased by estrogens. Thus, if androgens increase, the SHBG concentration subsequently decreases, possibly resulting in a normal total T circulating level in face of an elevated free fraction.

Androgen production and clearance are affected by various physiologic states. Androgen clearance and production are accelerated in obesity, although relatively normal circulating levels are maintained. In part, this is due to an obesity-related decrease in the circulating level of SHBG, which leads to higher levels of rapidly metabolizable free T and DHT. The circulating concentration of androgens is also affected by aging and, of course, by the removal of either the adrenals or the ovaries. Adrenal androgens (DHEA, DHEAS, and to a certain extent, A_4) decrease in a linear fashion, beginning about age 30. Normally the circulating concentration of A_4 in the postmenopausal woman is about one-half of that observed in premenopausal females, in part due to the decreased adrenal and ovarian secretion. Alternatively, T levels are only minimally lower in women immediately following natural menopause and decrease slowly thereafter, since the ovary continues to produce significant amounts of T. Since the amount of estradiol (E_2) produced by the postmenopausal ovary is minimal, the effective androgen : estrogen ratio is higher in the menopause, which may result in slight hirsutism in some postmenopausal women. This is more frequently noted in women whose ovaries have not been removed, and especially if they suffered from androgen excess prior to menopause. Nevertheless, evidence of mild androgen excess may also be evident in oophorectomized women as a result of continued, albeit decreasing, adrenal androgen secretion.

SIGNS AND SYMPTOMS OF ANDROGEN EXCESS

Androgen excess in women leads to a number of signs and symptoms including hirsutism, acne, oily skin, oligo- or amenorrhea, increased or decreased libido, increased appetite, weight gain, or virilization/masculinization. In the absence of androgen-producing tumors or classic congenital hyperplasia, the signs and symptoms of androgen excess generally develop slowly and insidiously.

Hirsutism

Hair follicles cover the entire body, with the exception of the soles of the feet, the palms of the hands, and the lips. While there are racial and ethnic differences in the numbers of follicle, there is no such dissimilarity between sexes within each race/ethnic group. The differences observed between men and women do not relate to the number of hair follicles, but rather to the type of hair arising from these follicles. In general there are three types of hair. Lanugo is the soft unmedullated hair covering the surface of the fetus, which is shed some time in late gestation or the early postpartum period. Vellus hairs are short (2–5 mm), soft, fine, unmedullated, and usually nonpigmented, and cover the apparently hairless areas of the body. Terminal hairs are long, coarse and medullated, composing the eyebrows, eyelashes, and scalp, pubic, and axillary hair.

A number of hormones control hair growth. Thyroid and growth hormone produce a generalized growth in hair. Hyperthyroidism yields a fine friable hair which is easily lost, while hypothyroidism produces a coarse brittle hair which is also easily shed. Androgens are the most important determinant of the type and distribution of hairs throughout the body. Progesterone has a minimal effect, while estrogens oppose the effect of androgens, most importantly by increasing SHBG and decreasing free T and DHT.

The principal circulating androgens T and A_4 are converted in the hair follicle to DHT, through the action of 5α-reductase. DHT then acts on the dermal papilla to increase the growth and thickness of terminal hairs. DHT also stimulates vellus-producing follicles to produce terminal hairs, an irreversible process. The effect of androgens on the hair follicle depends on the specific skin area. Some skin areas (e.g., eyelashes, eyebrows, lateral, and occipital aspects of the scalp) are relatively independent of the effects of androgens (nonsexual skin). Other areas are quite sensitive to the effect of even low levels of androgens, due to their high 5α-reductase activity, and include the lower pubic triangle and the axilla (ambosexual areas). These areas begin to develop terminal hair quite early in puberty, accompanying the minimal increases in adrenal androgens. Other parts of the skin contain less 5α-reductase activity and respond only to high levels of androgens, including the chest, lower abdomen, lower back, upper thighs, upper arms, chin, face, and upper pelvic triangle (sexual areas). Terminal hair growth in these areas is characteristically masculine and, if present in women, is considered hirsutism.

It is most important for the examining physician to determine whether a patient truly has hirsutism. The excessive growth of vellus hairs, producing a fuzzy appearance, is called *hypertrichosis* and should not be considered hirsutism. While a number of medical problems or medications can lead to hypertrichosis, it is more commonly familial. The excessive growth of coarse hairs *only* on the lower forearms and lower legs does not constitute hirsutism. However, a woman suffering from hirsutism may also note worsening hair growth in these areas. While hirsutism is usually obvious, it may be important to standardize the examination for future reference using a scoring system. It is important to remember that not all hyperandrogenic women demonstrate hirsutism (e.g., oriental women rarely do so), while other patients with hirsutism have normal circulating androgen levels (see the section on idiopathic hirsutism, below).

Acne

The pilosebaceous unit, in addition to the hair follicle, also may contain a sebaceous gland which produces an oily protective secretion (sebum) in response to androgen action. The excessive production of sebum leads to oily skin, clogged hair follicles, folliculitis, and subsequent acne. Although many teenagers suffer from acne, skin problems that persist into the 20s should raise the suspicion of androgen excess.

Oligo- or anovulation

Androgens are converted to estrogens in adipose tissues, and excessive levels of both these steroids disrupt the hypothalamic–pituitary–ovarian axis with the development of ovulatory problems. Furthermore, excessive androgen levels directly inhibit follicular development, leading to the formation of multiple small cysts within the ovarian cortex (the so-called polycystic ovary). The effect of androgens on ovulatory function may be very subtle, with some patients demonstrating only a shortened menstrual cycle and a luteal-phase defect. Other women demonstrate an increase in the length of their menstrual cycle, with infrequent or absent ovulation.

Virilization and/or masculinization
When androgen excess is massive and persistent, women may develop virilization, including temporal and frontal balding, clitoromegaly, reduction in breast size, and severe hirsutism. In general, virilization should raise the suspicion of an androgen-producing tumor, severe hyperthecosis, or the hyperandrogenemia—insulin resistance—acanthosis nigricans (HAIRAN) syndrome (see below). If the high levels of androgens have been present for a long period of time, especially prior to puberty (e.g., as in classic congenital hyperplasia), the patient's body habitus may undergo masculinization with an absence of breast development, an increase in muscle mass, upper body obesity, and virilization.

Polycystic ovaries
Excessive levels of circulating androgens from *any* source may disrupt follicular development with the accumulation of many small, atretic follicles in the ovarian cortex, producing a polycystic-like ovary. The appearance of polycystic ovaries, either on laparoscopy or sonography, is not exclusive or diagnostic for the so-called polycystic ovary syndrome (PCOS, see below); rather it is a sign of inadequate folliculogenesis.

DIFFERENTIAL DIAGNOSIS OF ANDROGEN EXCESS

Nonandrogenic causes

Acromegaly
Between 10 and 15% of acromegalics initially present with hirsutism. Accompanying the hirsutism will be an enlargement of the hands and feet, and a coarsening of the facial features. The diagnosis is based on a determination of excessive growth hormone secretion.

Chronic skin irritation
Chronic irritation of the skin secondary to depilating agents, environmental toxins, etc., will lead to a local increase in terminal hair growth, since teleologically hair protects the skin.

Anabolic drugs
Certain anabolic medications cause a generalized growth of many tissues, particularly hair, and include Dilantin, Nilevar, and Anavar. However, they generally lead to hypertrichosis and not hirsutism.

Androgenic causes
The diagnosis in this category is based on the finding of elevated circulating androgen levels.

Late-onset adrenal hyperplasia
Between 1 and 6% of hyperandrogenic women suffer from late-onset adrenal hyperplasia (LOAH), which generally results from a deficiency in the adrenocortical enzyme 21-hydroxylase, essential for the production of cortisol. The steroid precursors to 21-hydroxylase, 17-hydroxyprogesterone (17-HP) and A$_4$, accumulate in excess. The excessive production of A$_4$, which in part is converted to T, leads to the symptoms of androgen excess.

Patients with LOAH are clinically indistinguishable from other hyperandrogenic patients. Serum levels of the exclusive adrenal androgen, DHEAS, are not any higher than that of other hyperandrogenic women. The measurement of 17-HP in the follicular part of the menstrual cycle (or following withdrawal bleeding if the patient is amenorrheic) can be used to screen for this disorder. If the baseline 17-HP level is higher than 2 ng/ml (or 200 ng/dl), the patient should undergo an adrenocorticotropic hormone (ACTH) stimulation test. Alternatively, if the level of 17-HP is below 2 ng/ml it is very unlikely that the patient suffers from 21-hydroxylase deficient LOAH. These patients are readily treated with corticosteroid replacement. See Chapter 41 for additional discussion of LOAH.

HAIRAN syndrome
Between 1 and 5% of hyperandrogenic women suffer from this disorder. It is characterized by extremely high circulating levels of insulin (generally >80 uu/ml in the fasting state, and >300 μU/ml following an oral glucose tolerance test). The high levels of insulin are usually due to a genetic deficiency in the number of insulin receptors and/or a postreceptor defect. Rarely some of these women demonstrate circulating anti-insulin antibodies. In general, their fasting glucose levels are normal. This syndrome should not be confused with the mild degrees of insulin resistance noted among some patients with PCOS.

Patients with HAIRAN syndrome demonstrate

acanthosis nigricans, a velvety hyperpigmented change of the crease areas of the skin. These girls are usually severely hyperandrogenic, and can even be virilized or masculinized. A fasting insulin and glucose will serve to select and/or diagnose most patients with the HAIRAN syndrome. Rarely is an oral glucose tolerance test (measuring both glucose and insulin responses) required.

Cushing's syndrome
Excessive adrenocortical function, either due to adrenal carcinoma, an ectopic ACTH-producing tumor, or a pituitary tumor (Cushing's disease) can lead to excessive adrenal androgen secretion and the development of hyperandrogenic symptoms. Most of these patients present with typical Cushingoid features including yoke-like centripetal obesity, thinning and striae of the skin, muscle wasting, glucose intolerance, and osteoporosis.

The diagnosis of excessive cortisol production (Cushing's syndrome) can best be established by a 24-hour urine free cortisol. A more simple method is the measurement of a morning fasting cortisol following the oral administration of 1 mg of dexamethasone the evening before, although the false-positive rate can be as high as 15% among obese women or depressed patients, with a false-negative rate of approximately 2%.

Androgenic tumors
Androgen-producing tumors are relatively rare, and are usually of ovarian or adrenal origin. They should be suspected when the onset of androgenic symptoms is rapid and sudden, and when virilization and/or masculinization is present. Steroid-secreting neoplasms may also manifest other systemic symptoms including weight loss, anorexia, a feeling of abdominal bloating, back pain, etc., particularly if malignant. It is most important to remember that suppression and stimulation tests (including corticosteroid and/or oral contraceptive administration) can be misleading and are not encouraged for the diagnosis of these neoplasms.

Androgen-producing adrenal tumors are relatively rare. These adrenal tumors should be suspected when the DHEAS level is greater than 7000 ng/ml, or the T level is above 2 ng/ml, or when hirsutism is accompanied by other symptoms of excessive corticosteroid action. The diagnosis is usually established by a computed tomography (CT) scan of the adrenal, with images obtained at 0.5 cm intervals. Adrenal

carcinomas are usually associated with Cushingoid features, and are generally large (greater than 6 cm) and irregular on CT scan. Unfortunately, their prognosis is very poor.

Ovarian tumors are somewhat more common. They are usually palpable on pelvic examination and/or are associated with a unilateral ovarian enlargement on ultrasound or CT scan. They are generally not malignant, and include Sertoli–Leydig cell tumors and lipoid cell tumors. Ovarian tumors should be suspected when the circulating T level is consistently greater than 2 ng/ml. However, it is important to remember that approximately 20% of androgen-producing ovarian tumors may have T levels below this value, and that the majority of women with T levels over 2 ng/ml have HAIRAN syndrome, hyperthecosis, or PCOS, and not an ovarian tumor.

Hyperthecosis
These patients are usually severely androgenized and have very high levels of circulating T. The diagnosis is established pathologically after removal or wedge resection of the ovary. Islands of hyperplastic theca cells are noted between small atretic follicles. In contrast to PCOS, hyperthecotic ovaries have relatively few cortical cysts. Circulating luteinizing hormone (LH) and follicle-stimulating hormone (FSH) levels may be relatively low (4–8 mIU/ml) due to the very high circulating T levels. These patients are particularly difficult to treat, although the use of long-acting gonadotropin-releasing hormone (GnRH) agonists has been promising.

PCOS
This disorder has been commonly termed the polycystic ovarian syndrome, although it is better referred to as the hyperandrogenic chronic anovulatory syndrome. These patients comprise between 65 and 85% of all hyperandrogenic women seen. The diagnosis is one of exclusion, having eliminated other causes of hyperandrogenemia. It is established by an elevated circulating level of total and/or free T, with or without an elevated DHEAS (which is above normal in approximately 50% of these patients). Prolactin levels are usually normal or only slightly elevated (generally less than 40 ng/ml). The LH : FSH ratio is usually 3 : 1, although this is only observed in approximately 60% of these patients. Pathologically, the ovarian cortex contains multiple intermediate and atretic follicles measuring 2–5 mm in diameter, which give the ovary its polycystic appearance at sonography or

CHAPTER 40

laparoscopy. Some 40–60% of these patients are obese, 60–90% are hirsute, 50–90% are amenorrheic, 7–16% have regular menses, and 55–75% complain of infertility. These patients do not generally present with symptoms of virilization or masculinization.

Idiopathic hirsutism

The diagnosis of idiopathic hirsutism is assumed only when the circulating total and free androgen levels appear to be normal on repeated study, and the patient is obviously hirsute. Furthermore, these patients usually do not suffer from oligomenorrhea. Approximately 5–25% of hirsute women suffer from idiopathic hirsutism. However, it should be understood that many of these patients simply demonstrate degrees of androgen excess that are not detectable by routine clinical androgen assays, and in fact may more accurately reflect a deficiency in the laboratory.

In many women with idiopathic hirsutism the 5α-reductase activity in the hair follicle is excessive, leading to hirsutism in face of "normal" circulating levels of androgens. The measurement of serum 3α-androstanediol-glucuronide, a metabolite of DHT and a reflection of peripheral 5α-reductase activity, may help confirm the hyperfunction of this enzyme and monitor therapy. However, the diagnosis of idiopathic hirsutism is usually established by default, when normal circulating androgen levels are repeatedly encountered in the face of hirsutism and regular menses.

WORK-UP OF ANDROGEN EXCESS

History

Drug or medication use, skin irritants, menstrual history, onset and progression of hirsutism, change in extremity or head, change in face contour, balding and hair loss, and family history of similar disorders should be elicited. The etiology of the hirsutism can often be suspected during this part of the evaluation.

Physical examination

The type and pattern of excessive hair growth and/or acne should be noted and scored. The presence of galactorrhea, virilization, masculinization, pelvic and abdominal masses, obesity, Cushingoid features, bluntness of facial features, thyroid enlargement, or signs of systemic illness should be sought. It is most important during the physical examination to determine whether hirsutism is truly present and whether it is related to other endocrinologic features.

Laboratory assessment

For general screening purposes a total and free T, 17-HP, and DHEAS should be obtained in all patients suspected of suffering from androgen excess, optimally in the follicular phase of the menstrual cycle and in the fasting state.

While free T is the more sensitive indicator of hyperandrogenemia, total T and DHEAS serve to screen for ovarian and adrenal tumors. If the total T level is repeatedly above 2 ng/ml an ovarian ultrasound (preferably transvaginal) and an adrenal CT scan (with images at 5 mm intervals) should be obtained. A DHEAS level consistently over 7000 ng/ml also mandates an adrenal CT scan. One must keep in mind that approximately one-half of patients with PCOS demonstrate DHEAS levels that are mildly elevated.

If the basal follicular phase 17-HP level is over 2 ng/ml (200 ng/dl), the patient should undergo an acute ACTH adrenal stimulation test. In oligoovulatory patients the simultaneous measurement of progesterone can establish the validity of this basal 17-HP measurement. If the progesterone level is greater than 5 ng/ml (indicating that the patient is in the luteal phase), the 17-HP level will also be elevated and misleading. Adrenal stimulation testing is performed by administering 250 µg (1 vial) of Cortrosyn (1–24 ACTH) intravenously and measuring 17-HP 60 min after ACTH administration. If the post-stimulation 17-HP level is greater than 10 ng/ml (or 1000 ng/dl), the diagnosis of 21-hydroxylase-deficient LOAH is established. In order to rule out other rarer deficiencies of the adrenal cortex, including that of 3β-hydroxysteroid dehydrogenase and 11β-hydroxylase, the levels of 17-hydroxypregnenolone or 11-deoxycortisol, respectively, can also be measured following adrenal stimulation (see Chapter 41).

If the patient has signs or symptoms of thyroid disorder (myxedema, tachycardia, hair loss of the lateral eyebrows, goiter, heat/cold intolerance, etc.) a thyroid panel including a thyroid-stimulating hormone and free thyroxine should be obtained. If the patient is oligoovulatory an FSH, LH, prolactin, and basal body temperature chart should be obtained. If the patient has features suggestive of acromegaly, a fasting growth hormone (with the patient as relaxed as possible) should be obtained, and normally should be below 10 ng/ml. If the patient has signs suggestive of Cushing's syndrome a fasting morning cortisol following 1 mg of dexamethasone the evening before, or preferably a 24-hour urine cortisol, should be measured. The 24-hour free cortisol is normally less than 100 μg/24 hours, while the morning cortisol after overnight dexamethasone should be less than 5 μg/dl. Abnormally elevated cortisol levels require further testing, and these patients should be referred to an endocrinologist.

TREATMENT OF ANDROGEN EXCESS

In order to treat patients suffering from androgen excess properly it is important first to establish the goals of therapy. If the patient is oligoovulatory and desires fertility she should proceed with ovulation induction (see Chapter 74). It is usually not possible to treat the hirsutism or acne while ovulation induction for fertility is being pursued. Alternatively, if the patient only manifests oligo- or amenorrhea and does not require contraception, monthly progestin withdrawal (e.g., medroxyprogesterone acetate, 10 mg from days 1 to 12 of each month) can be utilized. In this fashion one will prevent the continued estrogen stimulation of the endometrium, and the development of dysfunctional uterine bleeding and/or endometrial hyperplasia.

The treatment of hirsutism should be undertaken as soon as the diagnosis is established. In young children or teenagers with hirsutism initially its degree may not be alarming. However, one must remember that these disorders are usually progressive, and the production of terminal hairs is irreversible. Hirsutism is not only disfiguring but can become a significant handicap to a young woman's social life and emotional stability.

Mechanical means of hair removal, by themselves, do little to affect the long-term course of hirsutism. However, while awaiting the full effect of hormonal therapy it is best to encourage the patient to shave (either with a blade or a machine) since this causes minimal trauma to the skin. Although shaving can lead to a blunt hair end which may feel stubble-like, it does not lead to a worsening of the hirsutism. Plucking or waxing should be discouraged since they do not kill the hair follicle, may induce folliculitis with damage to the hair shaft and the development of ingrown hairs, and stimulate the growth of surrounding follicles. Depilating agents, particularly on the face, can lead to skin irritation and worsening of hirsutism. Electrolysis is the only method available for the irreversible destruction of follicles producing terminal hairs. It use should be combined with hormonal therapy once sufficient time has elapsed. It

may not be applicable to large areas of the body, or to sensitive areas such as the periareolar region.

Hormonal therapy of hirsutism has the objective of stopping new terminal hairs from growing and may also reduce the growth rate, thickness, and pigmentation of terminal hairs already present. However, it will not reverse the androgen-induced transformation of vellus to terminal hairs. Only electrolysis can eliminate terminal hairs by destroying the follicle altogether. It is most important to emphasize to the patient that therapy may take 6 or 8 months for a positive effect to be observed.

The mainstay of treatment of androgen excess is the oral contraceptive pill (OCP) which, by suppressing the secretion of gonadotropins (LH and FSH), leads to a decrease in ovarian androgen production. Furthermore, OCPs decrease adrenal androgen production by a mechanism not yet clear. The progestin in the birth control pill can also antagonize 5α-reductase and the androgen receptor. The estrogen fraction in the OCP increases circulating SHBG, with a subsequent decrease in free T levels. Since the progestin in the OCP may alternatively decrease SHBG, it is most important to select a pill whose progestin is least androgenic (e.g., ethynodiol diacetate in Demulen). OCPs should be administered in the usual cyclic fashion. It is important periodically to monitor circulating androgen levels to insure full normalization of androgen levels, which is usually observed within the first 2 months of treatment.

Spironolactone (SPA) is an aldosterone antagonist and a mild diuretic. More importantly, it also antagonizes the androgen receptor, 5α-reductase, and the binding of T to SHBG. Furthermore, it has a suppressive effect on various enzymes involved in androgen production. Initially, a dose as high as 100–200 mg/day should be used. If the dose is slowly increased by 25 mg increments, from 25 mg a day, the patient will have minimal side-effects, which most commonly include polyuria, fatigue, headaches, and irregular menses. Hypertensive patients on a potassium-saving diuretic rarely develop hyperkalemia. SPA is extremely effective for treating hirsutism, in particular idiopathic hirsutism. Since it acts through mechanisms different from that of OCPs, it is possible to improve the overall therapeutic effectiveness by combining these medications. Furthermore, the use of OCPs with SPA eliminates the irregular bleeding associated with the sole use of SPA, while providing adequate contraception.

Dexamethasone (0.25–0.5 mg every to every other

evening) or prednisone (5–10 mg daily) can be used as adjuvants for the treatment of hirsutism, particularly in patients with significant adrenal hyperandrogenemia, or for the treatment of patients suffering from LOAH. The use of oral estrogen (with a progestin administered in a cyclic fashion when the uterus is present) has also been advocated for older females or those not tolerating the oral contraceptives. The doses of estrogen needed are usually higher than that required for regular postmenopausal hormonal therapy. Oral estrogen increases SHBG, decreases circulating LH and FSH levels, and potentially antagonizes the effect of androgens at the hair follicle level. High doses of progestin only (e.g., 20–30 mg of medroxyprogesterone acetate daily) can also be used, increasing the clearance of T by the liver and possibly decreasing circulating LH levels. However, high doses of progestins also decrease the circulating SHBG concentration which may decrease the effectiveness of this regimen. Furthermore, side-effects may be unacceptable and include breakthrough bleeding, liver dysfunction, possibly vascular changes, depression, and hot flushes.

Cyproterone acetate is a strong progestin and antiandrogen. It decreases circulating T and A$_4$ levels through a decrease in circulating LH levels. Furthermore, it antagonizes the effect of androgens at the peripheral level. Side-effects may include adrenal insufficiency and loss of libido. This drug is currently not available in the USA and it is unlikely that it will be Food and Drug Administration-approved, since SPA appears to be equally effective. Cimetidine has been proposed as an antiandrogen since it weakly competes for the androgen receptor. However, it does not change circulating levels of T, DHT, and adrenal androgens. It has no therapeutic benefit over SPA, but is more expensive and has a higher incidence of side-effects.

In the past, ovarian wedge resection has been used for the treatment of ovarian hyperandrogenism, with satisfactory results. More recently, laparoscopic wedge resections or fulguration of multiple areas of the ovarian cortex has been proposed. In general, these destructive procedures should be used as the line of last defense, since they almost invariably lead to ovarian adhesions. It is a rare patient who requires a bilateral ovarian wedge resection today, with the exception of those suspected of having an ovarian tumor, and in some hyperthecotic or HAIRAN syndrome patients. A long-acting GnRH agonist may be a better method of treating these patients since it

produces a reversible oophorectomy, without the surgical risk or possibility of adnexal adhesions. It may take 2 or 3 months of GnRH agonist suppression fully to suppress androgen levels in these extremely hyperandrogenic patients. Rarely are individuals so affected that a bilateral oophorectomy need be considered. This may be a viable alternative for women nearing the menopause and who have increasingly severe hyperandrogenic symptoms.

The treatment of hyperandrogenemia is of medical, and not only cosmetic, importance. The long-term effects of excessive androgens include lipid changes associated with an increased risk of cardiovascular disease. Furthermore, oligomenorrhea can lead to the development of endometrial hyperplasia and subsequent adenocarcinoma at a young age. It suffices to say that if an endocrinologic disorder (Cushing's, acromegaly, LOAH, etc.) is diagnosed during the evaluation, the patient should be treated and referred if necessary. Patients who suffer from hirsutism usually require long-term follow-up, counseling, and emotional support. Following menopause a worsening of the patient's hyperandrogenic symptoms may occur, since the ovary and adrenal continue to produce a significant amount of androgens while the antagonistic effects of circulating estrogens are almost eliminated.

FURTHER READING

Azziz R, Gay F. The treatment of hyperandrogenism with oral contraceptives. *Semin Reprod Endocrinol* 1989; 7: 246.

Azziz R, Zacur HA. 21-hydroxylase deficiency in female hyperandrogenism: screening and diagnosis. *J Clin Endocrinol Metab* 1989; 69: 577.

Barbieri RL, Ryan KJ. Hyperandrogenism, insulin resistance, and acanthosis nigricans syndrome: a common endocrinopathy with distinct pathophysiologic features. *Am J Obstet Gynecol* 1983; 147: 90.

Correa de Oliveria RF, Novas LP, Lima MB et al. A new treatment for hirsutism. *Ann Intern Med* 1975; 83: 817.

Cummings DC, Yang JC, Rebar RW, Yen SSC. The treatment of hirsutism with spironolactone. *JAMA* 1982; 247: 1295.

Hatch R, Rosenfield RL, Kim MH, Tredway D. Hirsutism: implications, etiology and management. *Am J Obstet Gynecol* 1981; 140: 815.

Kirschner MA, Zucker IR, Jespersen D. Idiopathic hirsutism – an ovarian abnormality. *N Engl J Med* 1976; 294: 637.

Maroulis GB. Evaluation of hirsutism and hyperandrogenemia. *Fertil Steril* 1981; 36: 273.

Mattox JH, Phelan S. The evaluation of adult females with testosterone producing neoplasms of the adrenal cortex. *Surg Obstet Gynecol* 1987; 164: 98.

Meldrum DR, Abraham GE. Peripheral and ovarian venous

concentrations of various steroid hormones in virilizing ovarian tumors. *Obstet Gynecol* 1979; 53: 36.

Pittaway DE, Maxson WS, Wentz AC. Spironolactone in combination drug therapy for unresponsive hirsutism. *Fertil Steril* 1985; 43: 878.

Rittmaster RS, Loriaux DL. Hirsutism. *Ann Intern Med* 1987; 106: 95.

Surrey ES, DeZiegler D, Gambone JC, Judd HL. Preoperative localization of androgen-secreting tumors: clinical, endocrinologic, and radiologic evaluation of ten patients. *Am J Obstet Gynecol* 1988; 158: 1313.

Uno H. Biology of hair growth. *Semin Reprod Endocrinol* 1986; 4: 2.

41

Late-onset adrenal hyperplasia

RICARDO AZZIZ

Adrenal enzyme deficiencies which lead to the appearance of hyperandrogenic symptoms at some time after birth have been alternatively called late-onset, nonclassical, postpubertal, attenuated, mild, or acquired. In this chapter the term late-onset adrenal hyperplasia (LOAH) will be used to address these disorders. Patients previously thought to suffer from the polycystic ovary syndrome (PCOS) and related hyperandrogenic disorders are now being diagnosed as having this genetic disease. By definition, LOAH is an autosomal recessive disorder which causes symptomatic hyperandrogenemia (e.g., hirsutism, acne, oligomenorrhea, etc.) peri- or postpubertally. All of these patients demonstrate a normal female external genitalia. If a girl presents with evidence of an adrenal enzyme deficiency and demonstrates virilization of the genitalia, however minor, the disorder is classified as *congenital* or classical adrenal hyperplasia (CAH), because the adrenal hyperandrogenemia was present *in utero* during genital development.

Adrenal enzyme deficiencies leading to androgen excess involve 3β-hydroxysteroid dehydrogenase (3β-HSD), 21-hydroxylase (21-OH), or 11-hydroxylase (11-OH; Fig. 41.1) [1]. In brief, these patients have a genetic defect of one of these enzymes which decreases their catalyzing activity. Since these enzymes are required for the biosynthesis of cortisol, an essential steroid, it is presupposed that this deficiency is compensated for by an increase in adrenocorticotropic hormone (ACTH) stimulation. It should be noted, however, that elevated circulating ACTH levels have not been documented in LOAH. The increased adrenocortical stimulation leads to normal circulating cortisol levels, although the production of enzymatic precursors, including adrenal androgens, is increased above normal.

A deficiency in 21-OH activity constitutes 90–95% of all cases of CAH, and it is assumed that this enzyme defect is also the most common among patients with LOAH. Following, we will discuss the pathophysiology of LOAH, its diagnosis, screening, treatment and outcome, on occasion comparing it to its more severe variant, classical CAH. We will focus primarily on 21-OH deficiency since it has been more thoroughly characterized.

21-OH-DEFICIENT LOAH

The 21-OH gene is located on the short arm of chromosome 6 in the midst of human leukocyte antigen (HLA) region. There appears to be two 21-OH genes, one active and the other a pseudogene (not active, although very similar in DNA sequence). The HLA complex encodes for a large number of leukocyte surface antigens, important in human organ transplantation. Every individual carries two HLA haplotypes, one inherited from each parent. Due to the extreme heterogeneity of the HLA antigens, it is highly unlikely (1 : 20 000) that two random individuals will have the same HLA haplotype. Because of the close linkage between the 21-OH genes and specific HLA alleles, HLA-typing has been used in family studies to ascertain the inheritance pattern of the 21-OH deficiencies. In this regard, CAH appears to be closely linked to the HLA-B47 allele, while LOAH patients exhibit a greater frequency of HLA-B14, DR1.

LOAH appears to affect between 1 and 2% of hyperandrogenic women [2], although studies of more select populations (such as those from tertiary medical centers-treated high-risk populations) may report a higher frequency in the range of 6–20% [3]. Overall, Speiser and associates estimated that LOAH was far more common than CAH (which occurs in approximately 1/8000 births) [4]. Prevalence of the disorder was particularly high among Ashkenazi Jews (3.7%), Hispanics (1.9%), Yugoslavs (1.6%), and Italians (0.3%), compared to other Caucasians (0.1% or 1/1000). They estimated that the carrier frequency

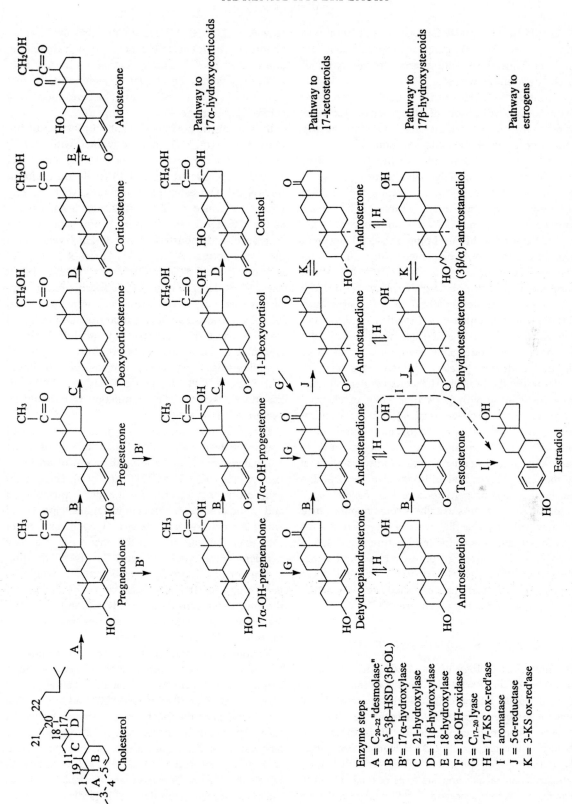

Fig. 41.1 Major pathways of steriod biosynthesis from cholesterol. The flow of hormonogenesis is usually to the right and downward. C_{17-20} lyase (enzyme step G) is also termed 17,20-desmolase. (From [1].)

Enzyme steps

A = C_{20-22} "desmolase"
B = Δ^5–3β–HSD (3β-OL)
B' = 17α-hydroxylase
C = 21-hydroxylase
D = 11β-hydroxylase
E = 18-hydroxylase
F = 18-OH-oxidase
G = C_{17-20} lyase
H = 17-KS ox-red'ase
I = aromatase
J = 5α-reductase
K = 3-KS ox-red'ase

for LOAH in the general Caucasian population was approximately 7%, compared to approximately 2% for CAH. Thus, the resulting carrier frequency for all 21-OH deficiencies was 9%.

In contrast to CAH, LOAH patients do not demonstrate any virilization of the external genitalia. Hyperandrogenic symptoms most commonly appear peri- or post-pubertally, although some children may present with premature adrenarche, the development of pubic and axillary hair before age 8 years in girls and 9 years in boys. Women with LOAH generally demonstrate mild symptoms of hyperandrogenism, if at all. DeWailly and colleagues described three clinical LOAH phenotypes [5]. Seven of their 20 patients (39%) presented with features suggesting PCOS, although a high serum luteinizing hormone : follicle-stimulating hormone (LH : FSH) ratio was not consistently found. Seven other women (39%) presented only with hirsutism and no oligomenorrhea. The remaining four women (22%) did not have hyperandrogenic symptoms in spite of elevated androgen levels and were considered to have the cryptic LOAH. The absence of symptoms in some women with LOAH, in spite of elevated androgen levels, probably relates to the weak androgenic potential of adrenal androgens, the individual variability in susceptibility to androgens (due to variations in androgen receptor affinity, peripheral 5α-reductase activity and androgen clearance), and to the duration of androgen exposure (e.g., patient's age).

Although symptoms usually become manifest near or after puberty, the diagnosis is often established only late in life, due to the mild nature of the symptoms. In males suffering from LOAH, clinical symptoms may never become apparent, although these boys may be shorter than expected with premature facial, pubic, and axillary hair growth.

DIAGNOSIS AND SCREENING

The molecular biology of the 21-OH deficiencies is becoming better characterized, and we may soon be able to screen for or diagnose the disorder using these techniques. However, currently the diagnosis is established endocrinologically. It is difficult to distinguish biochemically LOAH women from other hyperandrogenic patients. The hypothalamic–pituitary–adrenal axis appears to be normal in LOAH. Circulating testosterone and dehydroepiandrosterone sulfate levels are not different from those observed in patients with PCO, and in fact may be normal.

However, LOAH patients do not usually have an abnormally high LH : FSH ratio. Although circulating androstenedione is usually higher in LOAH than in PCO patients, the overlap is significant, so that screening for this disorder cannot be performed using solely this hormone.

In light of the obvious difficulty in differentiating the patient with PCO from the women with LOAH, an easy screening test would be most helpful. Basal 17-hydroxyprogesterone (17-HP) levels are useful in this regard. Untreated patients with CAH invariably have an elevated basal 17-HP serum level, usually above 1000 ng/dl. The majority of untreated LOAH women also demonstrate basal 17-HP levels which are above normal. A basal 17-HP level of >200 ng/dl is approximately 30% predictive for LOAH, while a basal 17-HP level of less than 200 ng/dl almost completely rules out LOAH. These measurements should be obtained in the follicular phase of the menstrual cycle, since 17-HP increases in the luteal phase. Dexamethasone should not be administrated prior to sampling since it may falsely decrease the circulating 17-HP level. If the screening 17-HP is >200 ng/dl, the more specific ACTH stimulation test should be performed.

The ACTH stimulation test is the most useful diagnostic test for LOAH. This test measures the adrenal response to the administration of an intravenous bolus of 1–24 ACTH (Cortrosyn). The general principle is that the rise in enzymatic precursor(s) and in the precursor : product ratio(s) following ACTH administration reflects the activity and amount of the enzyme in question. If the enzyme is relatively deficient or completely absent, the rise in the precursors or in the precursor : product ratio would be very high. For the diagnosis of 21-OH deficiency, the precursors considered are 17-HP and/or androstenedione (A_4), while the precursor : product ratio includes 17-HP/11-deoxycortisol.

Various interpretations of the adrenal stimulation test have been used to estimate 21-OH activity and to diagnose LOAH. The measurement of a single 17-HP serum level 30 or 60 min post-ACTH administration was found to be the most cost-effective and simplest to interpret. Furthermore, data from this and other laboratories indicate that acute adrenal stimulation with a bolus of 0.25 mg of 1–24 ACTH (the amount in which the vials of Cortrosyn are available) provides maximal adrenal stimulation, regardless of body weight [6]. The use of prestimulation dexamethasone suppression is unnecessary since the steroid levels

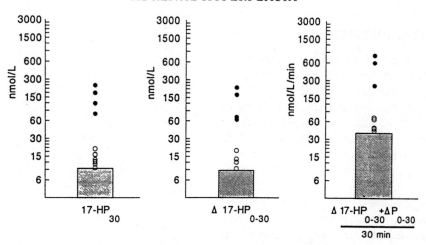

Fig. 41.2 From a population of 164 hyperandrogenic patients studied consecutively, all women with abnormal 21-OH measures after stimulation with 1-24 ACTH are plotted on a logarithmic scale. Measures include the 17-HP level 30 minutes following ACTH administration (17-HP$_{30}$), the net increment of 17-HP (Δ17-HP$_{0-30}$), and the sum of increments in 17-HP and progesterone divided by the stimulation time ([Δ 17-HP$_{0-30}$ + ΔP$_{0-30}$]/30 minutes) yielding the rate of rise of these two steroids. The boxed area represents the control response (up to the 95th percentile of normal). •, LOAH; ○, patients with a mild exaggeration in their 17-HP response to ACTH. (Reprinted with permission from [2].)

following ACTH administration do not change. For best interpretation, the test should be performed in the follicular phase of the menstrual cycle, or within 10 days of withdrawal bleed.

Individuals with LOAH are noted to have a 17-HP response to ACTH which is at least three to four times the upper normal limit. In our laboratory, the 95th percentile response of normal women is a 17-HP serum level of 320 ng/dl at 30 min and 350 ng/dl at 60 min post-1–24 ACTH. In most studies, 21-OH-deficient LOAH patients have a 17-HP response to acute ACTH stimulation of at least 1000 ng/dl [2,7]. Patients with CAH demonstrate stimulated 17-HP levels greater than 20 000 ng/dl [6]. A small number of hyperandrogenic women demonstrate a 17-HP response following adrenal stimulation that is above the normal limit but below 1000 ng/dl. These individuals do *not* have LOAH and the clinical significance of their abnormality is unclear.

Patients with LOAH and symptomatic hyperandrogenemia respond well to suppressive doses of glucocorticoids. Normally, between 20 and 25 mg/m^2 of cortisol (or hydrocortisone) is required daily. Prednisone is three- to fourfold more potent than hydrocortisone, while dexamethasone is 10- to 15-fold more potent. Thus, the average glucocorticoid replacement dose for a normal-sized woman is 30–40 mg hydrocortisone/day, 10–15 mg prednisone/day,

or 0.5–1.0 mg dexamethasone/day. However, some women may metabolize dexamethasone more slowly and will only require 0.25 mg/day, or 0.5 mg every other day, for adequate adrenal suppression. Furthermore, because of its shorter half-life prednisone may be easier to regulate. Avgerinos and colleagues [8] have demonstrated that treatment with every-other-day prednisone adequately suppresses adrenal androgen levels, without long-term suppression of the hypothalamic–pituitary–adrenal axis or impairment in cortisol response. Medications should be taken at night to maximize adrenal suppression. Addition of spironolactone may also be helpful in treating hirsutism in these patients.

Overall, prognosis for fertility in oligomenorrheic LOAH women is good. However, it is important to counsel LOAH patients with regard to their risk of producing offspring with 21-OH deficiency. Since the carrier rate in the general population for 21-OH deficiencies of all types may be as high as 9%, the risk of producing offspring with a 21-OH deficiency would be approximately 4.5%. Although the majority of affected children will suffer from LOAH, some may have CAH, since some individuals with LOAH are compound heterozygotes carrying one gene for LOAH and another for CAH. Consultation with a genetic counselor may be most helpful.

11-OH DEFICIENCY

A less common cause of adrenal hyperplasia is 11-OH deficiency, which constitutes approximately 5% of all cases of CAH. Severe deficiency in 11-OH activity leads to the accumulation of deoxycorticosterone (DOC), a potent mineralocorticoid, in addition to androgens. With the increase in DOC levels, sodium is retained and hypertension may result. However, one should note that the clinical picture in 11-OH-deficient CAH varies significantly, and is indistinguishable from that of other hyperandrogenic women. The diagnosis of 11-OH-deficient CAH can be established by measuring the basal level of 11-deoxycortisol (compound S), which usually exceeds 40 ng/ml.

The prevalence of 11-OH-deficient LOAH and its diagnostic criteria are less clear than with the better characterized 21-OH-deficient LOAH. In order to establish the prevalence of this or any other genetic disorder it is necessary to find a reliable genetic marker. The 11-OH gene has been localized to the middle of the long arm of chromosome 8. However, due to the chromosomal localization of the 11-OH gene, the congenital deficiency of 11-OH is not linked to the HLA system, and a reliable molecular marker for this disorder has yet to be elucidated.

In the absence of a reliable genetic marker, the diagnosis of 11-OH-deficient LOAH can be presumed when the 11-deoxycortisol level following ACTH stimulation exceeds a preestablished arbitrary value. Based on our experience with 21-OH-deficient LOAH, we have selected an 11-deoxycortisol response to stimulation greater than three times the 95th percentile in normal women to be consistent with 11-OH-deficient LOAH. In our laboratory, this represents a poststimulation 11-deoxycortisol serum level of greater than 25 ng/ml (Fig. 41.3). Obligate heterozygotes (carriers) for the congenital form of 11-OH adrenal hyperplasia usually demonstrate poststimulation compound S levels within normal, and always less than 12 ng/ml [9].

The prevalence of presumed 11-OH-deficient LOAH appears to be low. In our hyperandrogenic population arising from a large referral area in the eastern and southeastern USA, the prevalence of presumed 11-OH-deficient LOAH was 0.18% compared to 1.9% for 21-OH-deficient LOAH [10]. In small numbers of reported cases, clinical outcome, including fertility, appears to be good, sometimes even in the absence of treatment.

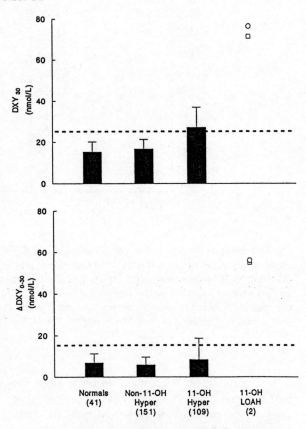

Fig. 41.3 In a population of 262 hyperandrogenic patients studied consecutively (after excluding all patients with 21-OH deficient LOAH), the increment in 11-deoxycortisol ($\blacktriangle DXY_{0-30}$) and DXY level ($DXY_{30}$) following acute 1–24 ACTH is depicted (mean ± one standard deviation) for normal women (normals), hyperandrogenic women with a normal 11-OH response (non-11-OH hyper) and hyperandrogenic patients with a mildly exaggerated DXY response (11-OH Hyper), and in two patients with presumed 11-OH deficient LOAH. The dashed line represents the upper 95th percentile of normal than control or 11-OH normal hyperandrogenic women (Adapted from [10].)

3β-HSD-DEFICIENT LOAH

The diagnosis of 3β-HSD deficiency is based on the 17-hydroxypregnenolone (17-HPREG) and/or dehydroepiandrosterone (DHEA) response to ACTH stimulation. Extremely high basal or stimulated levels of 17-HPREG (generally above 60 ng/ml) herald 3β-HSD-deficient CAH. This disorder leads primarily to the excessive production of the weak androgen, DHEA, and may actually decrease the adrenal production of the stronger androgens A_4 and testosterone. Furthermore, the enzymatic production of both

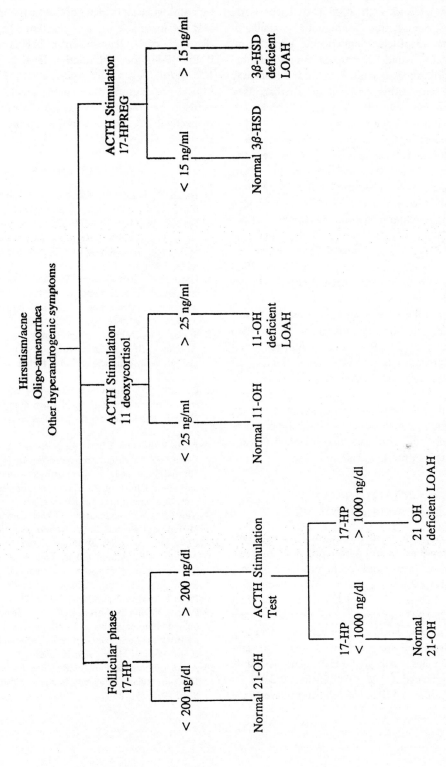

Fig. 41.4 Approach to LOAH. 17-HP, 17-hydroxyprogesterone; 17-HPREG, 17-hydroxypregnenolone; 21-OH, 21-hydroxylase; 11-OH, 11-hydroxylase; 3β-HSD, 3β-hydroxysteroid dehydrogenase; LOAH, late-onset adrenal hyperplasia.

the adrenal cortex and the gonads is affected. There appears to be considerable phenotypic heterogeneity. Thus, males affected with 3β-HSD-deficient CAH may actually demonstrate ambiguous genitalia at birth, due to insufficient androgenic stimulation. The female fetus usually demonstrates only minimal degrees of virilization, if at all. Some individuals may demonstrate salt-wasting, while others are diagnosed only later in life with the appearance of hyperandrogenic signs and symptoms.

Various reports have documented the existence of a 3β-HSD-deficient form of LOAH. However, the diagnostic criteria for this disorder are not clear. Some authors have presumed 3β-HSD-deficient LOAH simply if the stimulated 17-HPREG was above the normal limit (either mean plus 2 s.d., or the upper 95th percentile). However, if one uses the experience with 21-OH deficiency as a model, 3β-HSD-deficient individuals should demonstrate a 17-HPREG-stimulated value of at least three times the upper normal limit. Therefore, in the absence of firm diagnostic criteria, each investigator must establish normal standards. In our laboratory, the upper 95th percentile for the 17-HPREG level 60 min following ACTH administration is 5.0 ng/ml. Thus, the diagnosis of 3β-HSD-deficient LOAH is presumed if the stimulated 17-HPREG level is above 15 ng/ml. Using this criterion, we were unable to detect any such patient among 78 consecutively studied hyperandrogenic women. Thus, it appears that 3β-HSD deficiency is the most rare of the LOAHs.

CONCLUSIONS AND RECOMMENDATIONS

Among Caucasian patients presenting with hyperandrogenic symptoms, including hirsutism, androgenic oligomenorrhea, acne and premature adrenarche, approximately 1–2% will suffer from 21-OH-deficient LOAH, 0.5–1.0% from 11-OH LOAH and less than 0.5% from 3β-HSD deficiency. The prevalence may be higher among certain populations, including Ashkenazi Jews and some Italian, Yugoslavian, and Hispanic families. All hyperandrogenic patients should be screened for 21-OH-deficient LOAH by obtaining a serum 17-HP in the follicular phase of the

menstrual cycle. If this hormone is above 200 ng/dl, an acute adrenal stimulation test should be performed by administering 0.25 mg of Cortrosyn intravenously and obtaining a serum sample 30 or 60 min later. The diagnosis of 21-OH-deficient LOAH is usually made if the 17-HP post-stimulation level is greater than 1000 ng/dl. Eleven hydroxylase and 3β-HSD-deficient LOAH are presumed when the levels of 11-deoxycortisol or 17-HPREG exceed 15 and 25 ng/ml, respectively. A summary of the approach to LOAH is shown in Figure 41.4.

REFERENCES

1 Hatch, Rosenfield RL, Kim MH, Tredway D. Hirsutism: implications, etiology and management. *Am J Obstet Gynecol* 1981; 140: 815–830.
2 Azziz R, Zacur HA. 21-Hydroxylase deficiency in female androgenism; screening and diagnosis. *J Clin Endocrinol Metab* 1989; 69: 577–584.
3 Lobo RA, Goebelsmann U. Adult manifestation of congenital adrenal hyperplasia due to incomplete 21-hydroxylase deficiency mimicking polycystic ovarian disease. *Am J Obstet Gynecol* 1980; 138: 720–726.
4 Speiser PW, DuPont B, Rubinstein P, Piazza A, Kastelan A, New MI. High frequency of nonclassical steroid 21-hydroxylase deficiency. *Am J Hum Genet* 1985; 37: 650–667.
5 DeWailly D, Vantyghem-Haudiquet M-C, Sainsard C et al. Clinical and biological phenotypes in late-onset 21-hydroxylase deficiency. *J Clin Endocrinol Metab* 1986; 63: 418–423.
6 Azziz R, Bradley E Jr, Huth J, Boots LA, Parker CR Jr, Zacur HA. Acute adrenocorticotropin-(1-24) (ACTH) adrenal stimulation in amenorrheic women: reproducibility and effect of ACTH dose, subject weight and sampling time. *J Clin Endocrinol Metab* 1990; 70: 1273.
7 New MI, Lorenzen F, Lerner DJ et al. Genotyping steroid 21-hydroxylase deficiency: hormonal reference data. *J Clin Endocrinol Metab* 1983; 57: 320–326.
8 Avgerinos PC, Cutler GB Jr, Tsokos GC et al. The association between cortisol and adrenal androgen secretion in patients receiving alternate day prednisone therapy. *J Clin Endocrinol Metab* 1987; 65: 24–29.
9 Pang S, Levine LS, Lorenzen F et al. Hormonal studies in obligate heterozygotes and siblings of patients with 11β-hydroxylase deficiency congenital adrenal hyperplasia. *J Clin Endocrinol Metab* 1980; 50: 586.
10 Azziz R, Boots LR, Parker CR Jr, Bradley E Jr, Zacur HA. 11β-hydroxylase deficiency in hyperandrogenism. *Fertil Steril* 1991; 55: 733–741.

42

Hirsutism

ANNE COLSTON WENTZ

THE CHIEF COMPLAINT

The patient who complains of hirsutism is usually most worried first about her cosmetic appearance. Much less frequently she thinks about a serious problem, such as tumor, and rarely about a problem of gender identity. She notices the growth of chin and moustache hair, and sometimes shaves the hair on her lower abdomen and inner thighs so she can wear a bikini. She thinks of acne as something she should have outgrown. She decides she needs help when the problem intrudes on her life or she is convinced she has a serious problem.

The physician's first decision is whether the hirsutism needs evaluation, and next, how. The patient may present with another complaint, for example, infertility, irregular periods, or dysfunctional uterine bleeding, and she may perceive the hirsutism as incidental. The physician has to decide which problem takes precedence, whether they have a common underlying etiology, and if solving one solves all.

The patient's next decision may be difficult: choosing to treat the hirsutism may by necessity preclude conception, or pregnancy may preclude treating the hirsutism, but the treatment of both at the same time is mutually incompatible.

PATHOPHYSIOLOGY

There are three types of hairs: lanugo or fetal hairs primarily under the control of growth hormone; vellus hairs, which are fine, thin and nonpigmented, which respond to growth hormone, and which cover the body, except for the palms, soles and lips; and terminal hairs, which are coarse, curly, and pigmented, and which are transformed from the vellus hairs in sex hormone-responsive hair follicles. The sensitivity of this transformation from vellus to terminal hair depends upon the genetic or racial background, the site of the body stimulated, and the degree of andro-

genic exposure. The most sex hormone-sensitive are the axillary and pubic areas, followed in order by the upper lip, lower abdomen, chin, chest, and lower back.

Patterns of hair growth can be divided into asexual hair growth, with scalp hair, eyebrows, and eyelashes being obvious examples; ambisexual growth patterns with terminal hairs in pubic and axillary areas, stimulated by androgen regardless of sex; and sexual growth patterns, with male-pattern hair distribution involving beard, chest, abdomen, and sacral areas. In women, an ambisexual growth pattern is seen when androgen levels are within normal limits for females. Elevated androgen levels in women stimulate vellus-to-terminal transformation of hairs and promote a male distribution; once this transformation has occurred, the life cycle of the hair continues without the need for the excessive androgen stimulation required for transformation. Normal androgen levels then maintain the male-pattern hirsutism. More generalized hypertrichosis without a sexual or ambisexual pattern suggests a nonandrogen etiology.

The hair growth cycle has three phases: anagen, the phase of active growth which determines hair length; catagen, a brief but important involutional phase; and telogen, the resting phase during which hairs are shed as a result of trauma or reactivation of follicles. Hair follicles have totally different rhythms of activity, depending on their body location; scalp hair has a long anagen phase, which lasts for years. Since hormonal therapy can only be effective on the hair follicle during the catagen and telogen phases, the actively growing hair is unaffected. Due to this life cycle, a year or more of treatment may be needed before a perceptible decrease in numbers of terminal hairs may be seen in the chin and moustache area.

Most women with male-pattern hirsutism have had elevated circulated androgens, but androgen levels may be entirely normal at the time of presentation since male-pattern hirsutism will be maintained at androgen levels normal for the normal female. To change a hair follicle from terminal to vellus hair production, circulating androgen levels must be decreased or suppressed to well below normal. This explains why pursuit of fertility and pursuit of the treatment of hirsutism are mutually incompatible.

STEPS IN DIAGNOSIS

The goals of the evaluation should be established, and discussed with the patient. The first of these is to rule out serious disease, and the second to manage her chief complaint, whether hirsutism, irregular dysfunctional bleeding, or infertility.

The history of the development and progression of hirsutism is important. Whether rapid or slow gives an indication of the seriousness of the situation. Did the hirsutism come on quickly, or has it been progressive over many years? If progressive, has virilization occurred, or has the change been almost imperceptible? Has the hair growth not changed but been maintained? Are there any clues in the history? What about a family history of hirsutism? Does the patient take androgenic medications, have there been changes in menstrual cyclicity, is there evidence of androgen production from a tumor source as indicated by deepening of the voice, very rapid hair growth, balding, or increased libido? Has there been weight loss or gain? What about the onset of fatigue, skin changes, and easy bruising, nocturia, or the development of a moon facies? Is the patient athletic, perhaps "pumps iron," and likely to take anabolic steroids, which might not be volunteered in the history?

A careful physical examination should clarify the presence or absence of some of the entities suggested by the history. Does the patient have hypertension? Evaluation of nutritional status and muscle mass can be revealing. How much hair is present, and in what pattern? Terminal hair is unusual in such areas as the shoulders, chest, and upper abdomen, and indicates elevated androgen stimulation. Signs of Cushing's syndrome should be evaluated, including the presence of purple striae, buffalo hump, hypertension, central obesity, facial plethora and acne, and proximal muscle weakness. The presence of acanthosis nigricans suggests insulin resistance. A generalized increase in vellus hair may indicate drug-induced hypertrichosis as seen with minoxidil, cyclosporin, and phenytoin.

The pelvic examination should reveal the degree of hyperestrogenism; a careful bimanual examination, perhaps accompanied by ultrasonographic evaluation, should detect the presence of adnexal masses. An indication for endometrial biopsy should be considered; patients with hirsutism and long-standing amenorrhea or anovulation who have evidence of hyperestrogenism could have endometrial hyperplasia.

The decision as to what laboratory test to order for screening purposes is straightforward. Anovulatory and/or amenorrheic patients with hirsutism require an evaluation for the etiology of the anovulation. Laboratory tests to be ordered at the initial visit for anovulatory patients include: serum gonadotropins, follicle-stimulating hormone (FSH) and luteinizing hormone (LH); serum testosterone; serum dehydroepiandrosterone sulfate (DHEAS); and serum prolactin, serum gonadotropins, FSH and LH. Thyroid function tests should be ordered if the patient has profuse lanugo hair or hypertrichosis to diagnose hypothyroidism. Patients with anorexia nervosa may have increased lanugo hair on the basis of increased growth hormone stimulation, but it is not necessary to measure growth hormone levels unless acromegaly is suspected.

Ovulatory patients should have their hormonal evaluation limited to the assessment of serum testosterone and DHEAS, and perhaps a prolactin level. Other hormone levels, including free testosterone, androstenedione, sex hormone-binding capacity, 3α-androstanediol glucuronide, and 17α-hydroxyprogesterone (discussed below) are not useful in clinical diagnosis. Having ordered tests at the initial visit, the physician must decide if further evaluation would be useful before the initial screening test results are available. Three diagnoses, which require additional testing, should be considered.

If Cushing's disease is suspected on the basis of hypertension, thin skin with bruising, buffalo hump, central obesity, facial plethora and purple striae, then an overnight dexamethasone suppression test should be done. Dexamethasone 1.0 mg is given at 11 p.m., and serum cortisol is measured at 8 a.m. the next morning. Serum cortisol less than 5 µg/dl is a normal response and virtually rules out Cushing's disease. Normal women who do not have Cushing's disease but do have severe psychologic depression may fail to have normal suppression, and thus have a false-positive overnight dexamethasone suppression test. Morning cortisol greater than 10 µg/dl should be followed up with a measure of urinary free cortisol and other testing as indicated.

If an androgen-producing tumor is suspected on the basis of the rapid progression of hirsutism and the presence of virilization, then the site of androgen production must be actively sought. A serum testosterone level of 2.5 times the upper limits of normal for the assay used is further indication of a serious underlying disease process; an elevated DHEAS level might suggest adrenal involvement, but is not diagnostic. Ruling out the presence of an adrenal tumor is easier than diagnosing an ovarian tumor, and the radiologist should be consulted as soon as a tumor is suspected. A computed tomographic (CT) scan, or magnetic resonance imaging (MRI) of the adrenal gland diagnose a tumor with accuracy; previously used modalities such as intravenous pyelography (IVP), adrenal ultrasonography, and adrenal vein catheterization are less useful. If an adrenal tumor has been eliminated, then ovarian ultrasonography, or an MRI, may be helpful. Ovarian tumors which produce androgens may be quite small; laparoscopy will not be useful in eliminating a suspected ovarian tumor, as bivalving of the ovaries may be the only way to locate a small lipoid cell androgen-producing ovarian tumor. Importantly, dynamic tests of adrenal suppression with dexamethasone or stimulation with adrenocorticotropin hormone (ACTH), or ovarian suppression with oral contraceptives and gonadotropin-releasing hormone (GnRH) analogs, or stimulation with human chorionic gonadotropin (hCG), are not useful in diagnosing tumors or even in delineating the differential site of excessive androgen production. Testosterone-producing adrenal tumors have been found in the presence of normal DHEAS levels and may respond to hCG stimulation. The unreliability of these determinations makes reliance upon radiologic procedures essential.

If congenital adrenal hyperplasia is suspected, Cortrosyn stimulation is necessary for diagnosis. Because the various forms of congenital adrenal hyperplasia mimic polycystic ovary syndrome (PCOS), it has been recommended that all patients with hirsutism be screened for congenital hyperplasia. The measurement of baseline 17α-hydroxyprogesterone is imperfect; it is only reliable in the follicular phase of a patient with ovulatory menstrual cycles, and may be normal in patients with cryptic or heterozygotic congenital adrenal hyperplasia. If the baseline 17α-hydroxyprogesterone level is greater than 5.0 ng/ml, the diagnosis is likely, and Cortrosyn testing unnecessary (if the patient has not ovulated);

levels between 2 and 5 ng/ml are elevated, and testing is clearly indicated, while patients with levels less than 2 ng/ml are less likely to have congenital adrenal hyperplasia, and may only be identified by Cortrosyn stimulation. The stimulation test involves the intravenous administration of synthetic ACTH1-24, Cortrosyn 0.25 mg with the measurement of 17α-hydroxyprogesterone before stimulation, and after 30 and 60 min; the result is applied to a nomogram [1]. Another test, based on the rate of rise of 17α-hydroxyprogesterone, measures both progesterone and 17α-hydroxyprogesterone before and 30 min after the intravenous administration of 1.0 mg Cortrosyn; the sum of the two hormones at zero level is subtracted from the sum of the two hormones at the 30-min level, and divided by 30; greater than 6.8 ng/dl per min is the upper limit of normal and the dividing line between patients with and without congenital adrenal hyperplasia. The 30-min test is easily accomplished in the office setting, either at the first office visit, or scheduled to avoid the luteal phase in a patient with ovulatory menstrual cycles.

Hirsute women, in whom the various diagnoses of Cushing's syndrome, adrenal or ovarian androgen-producing tumor, and congenital adrenal hyperplasia have been eliminated, can probably be assigned the diagnosis of either idiopathic hirsutism or polycystic ovarian syndrome. PCOS is best described as chronic anovulation with hyperandrogenism; those women with hirsutism who are not chronically anovulatory are classified as having idiopathic hirsutism, particularly if circulating androgen levels are normal. Making the diagnosis of polycystic ovarian syndrome is neither precise nor easy, but patients who do not fit into any of the other diagnostic categories will usually fit some investigator's criteria for polycystic ovarian syndrome.

With a diagnosis of PCOS, there are some characteristic hormonal findings. An elevated LH to FSH ratio is confirmatory, but not diagnostic, and the absence of this ratio does not preclude the diagnosis. Most patients with PCOS have hyperandrogensim with elevated testosterone and/or androstenedione levels, but some do not. Most patients with PCOS have a pathognomonic history of irregular periods, occasional dysfunctional uterine bleeding, infertility, obesity, and other signs of hyperandrogenism. However, there are thin patients with polycystic ovarian syndrome, as well as patients who have polycystic ovaries on ultrasonography who appear to be ovulating regularly. Therefore, this syndrome is controversial in terms of description, definition, and diagnosis.

Idiopathic hirsutism is usually diagnosed in those patients who have hirsutism and normal circulating androgen levels. In most of these patients, a careful history will reveal that the patient was probably hyperandrogenic at some point in her life, and that the hyperandrogenism correlated with the development of the hirsutism. Total testosterone levels are normal, but the use of more sophisticated diagnostic testing may reveal the elevation of circulating free testosterone, a decrease in sex hormone-binding capacity, or another abnormality. In these patients, a serious underlying cause is unlikely (if testing has been thoroughly carried out as described above), and treatment of hirsutism is not different.

TREATMENT OF HIRSUTISM

The first rule, find and treat the etiology, is sometimes difficult in patients presenting with hirsutism; obviously detection of an ovarian or adrenal tumor dictates the management. Medication- or drug-induced hypertrichosis or hirsutism may be identified, and the treatment may be as simple as stopping the drug. The hyperandrogenism associated with obesity may be responsible for hirsutism, and weight loss may be beneficial. Patients who are anorectic with hypertrichosis and increase in lanugo hair may be improved by restoring normal body weight.

The rule that the "hair that is there" can only be managed by cosmetic approaches has a physiologic basis, in that the transformation from terminal back to vellus hair only occurs during the involutional and resting phases of growth. Hair can be removed by depilatories, creams, shaving, plucking, and other innovative means. Shaving is one of the least irritating forms of hair removal (except in black people), although perhaps the most psychologically damaging. Electrolysis, which destroys the hair follicle selectively, may cause significant damage to the epidermis and should only be accomplished by experienced operators.

Restoration of ovulation does not lower androgen levels enough to be therapeutic for hirsutism. Therefore, although the patient may become ovulatory and achieve pregnancy, her hirsutism is not likely to be improved.

Ovarian suppression using oral contraceptives may decrease androgen levels enough to exert an effect, but clinical experience suggests that a discernible change may take a year to observe. Oral contraceptives have other benefits which must be taken into consideration, including their safety, relative lack of side-effects, relative inexpense of long-term administration, induction of regular cyclic bleeding, and contraception. Ovarian suppression using GnRH analogs is an effective means of decreasing androgen levels below those in the normally cycling woman. Over time, hirsutism will be improved, but at the price of symptomatology including hot flashes, hypoestrogenism, and the potential of demineralization of bone. Further, these analogs are quite expensive, and therefore problematic for routine use in the treatment of hirsutism.

Adrenal suppression is an inadequate approach to the treatment of hirsutism, primarily because androgen levels are rarely suppressed below those encountered in the normal ovulatory cycle. The use of glucocorticoids, for example dexamethasone, is frequently associated with increased weight gain, bloating and water retention. Glucocorticoids are clearly the treatment of choice in adrenal hyperfunction, but unlikely to benefit most patients presenting with hirsutism.

The use of antiandrogens is an effective approach. Local antiandrogen application, in the form of a progesterone cream or lotion, has not been thoroughly tested, although progesterone is a potent endogenous antiandrogen. Antiandrogens, including spironolactone, cimetidine, and cyproterone acetate (not available in the USA), all exert their effect by blocking androgen receptors and effectively decrease androgen stimulation to the hair follicle. Spironolactone has not been cleared by the Food and Drug Administration for the indication of treatment of hirsutism; on the other hand, it is effective if administered in large-enough doses (150–200 µg/day), a not inexpensive regimen. Despite the high doses of spironolactone needed, very few complications are seen, although there are some precautions. Patients on long-term administration regimens should be monitored for the theoretic development of hyperkalemia. If spironolactone is administered to a woman with irregular menstrual cycles, she may develop even worse dysfunctional uterine bleeding. Further, spironolactone is contraindicated in any woman at risk for pregnancy, because a male fetus exposed to an antiandrogen risks the possibility of ambiguous development of the external genitalia. Therefore, in patients exposed to pregnancy, spironolactone should not be administered for treatment of hirsutism. A convenient and effective approach is to administer an oral contraceptive, restore cyclic bleeding, and supplement with spironolactone to induce an enhanced effect. This combined use of oral contraceptives and spironolactone has proven beneficial.

Some women with hirsutism elect no treatment. This may be problematic, as patients may ovulate sporadically and inconsistently, running the risk of unwanted pregnancy. Further, they may develop profuse abnormal uterine bleeding, and being anovulatory, run the risk of endometrial hyperplasia. Since the patient with hirsutism probably has hormonal abnormalities, no treatment would be selected if the physician decides that the patient does not have significant risk for the development of other problems.

In conclusion, the diagnosis and treatment of hirsutism involve some simple and some difficult decision making. Hirsutism may present as simply a cosmetic problem, but its underlying pathophysiology may suggest a serious disorder. Therefore, the approach to diagnosis and treatment must be thorough and specific, to rule out serious problems, and to address the patient's chief complaint.

REFERENCE

1 New MI, Dupont B, Pollack MS, Levine LS. The biochemical basis for genotyping 21-hydroxylase deficiency. *Hum Genet* 1981; 58: 123.

FURTHER READING

Azziz R, Zacur HA. 21-hydroxylase deficiency in female hyperandrogenism: screening and diagnosis. *J Clin Endocrinol Metab* 1989; 69: 577.

Ehrmann DA, Rosenfield RL. Clinical review 10. An endocrinologic approach to the patient with hirsutism. *J Clin Endocrinol Metab* 1990; 71: 1.

Rittmaster RS, Loriaux DL. Hirsutism. *Ann Intern Med* 1987; 106: 95.

Diagnosis and management of hair loss in women

ANDREW S. COOK

The female patient presenting with hair loss may have a serious emotional reaction to her condition with an underlying fear of impending baldness and its associated social embarrassment and humiliation. A systematic approach to the patient will allow for the correct diagnosis of her condition. The clinician is then in the position to institute treatment, when appropriate, and to help alleviate the patient's anxiety with an explanation of her condition and its prognosis.

PHYSIOLOGY OF HAIR GROWTH

The hair follicle is an epidermal appendage which extends into the dermis, and in some cases, into subcutaneous tissue. The hair shaft is composed of compact sulfur-rich keratin strands covered by a delicate cuticle comprised of plate-like scales. The human scalp contains approximately 100 000 hairs with a diameter of 0.08 mm and a rate of growth of 0.4 mm/day (1.2 cm/month).

Hair grows in a cyclic fashion, alternating between phases of activity and inactivity. Hair can be in the anagen, catagen, or telogen phase. Anagen hairs by definition are in the growth phase and normally account for approximately 85–90% of hair. Catagen hairs are in a phase of rapid involution which lasts 1 or 2 weeks. Telogen hairs or "club hairs" are in the end-stage and make up the remaining 10–15% of hair. The duration of the anagen phase is approximately 1000 days and the telogen phase is approximately 100 days. The basic hair types include lanugo, vellus, and terminal hair. Lanugo hair, which is present on fetuses and some newborn infants, is replaced by vellus hair, which is the fine, light-colored hair usually found on arms and legs of children, and terminal hair, which is coarse, thick and pigmented. Both sexes experience progressive hair loss beginning about age 50.

EVALUATION OF THE PATIENT WITH HAIR LOSS

A thorough history, physical examination, and screening laboratory tests provide the basis for diagnosis of the various types of alopecia. The physician should inquire into both the patient's current situation and events which occurred several months prior to the time at which the patient presents with complaints of hair loss. An acute emotional or physical stress, chronic illness, various drugs, poor nutrition, crash diets, high fever, or prolonged surgery which predate the patient's hair loss by several months may all be possible precipitating events.

A thorough examination of the scalp and use of objective techniques for evaluation of hair loss are essential for accurate diagnosis of the patient's hair loss. The various physical findings associated with the different types of alopecia are described under their individual subheadings.

The use of screening laboratory tests may aid in the diagnosis of the cause of hair loss [1]. These tests will evaluate the patient's androgen, thyroid, and nutritional status as well as screening for signs of various chronic diseases. Females as well as males may be predisposed to androgen-related (androgenetic) hair loss. This type of hair loss requires both a genetic predisposition and exposure to androgens in order for hair loss to occur. An increased androgen level may, therefore, exacerbate the hair loss experienced by the female patient. Evaluation of the androgen status is accomplished with dehydroepiandrosterone sulfate (DHEAS), testosterone, sex hormone-binding hormone, and potentially, free testosterone. Both hypothyroidism and hyperthyroidism may result in hair loss. The hypothyroid patient characteristically experiences loss of the lateral portion of the eyebrows. A thyroid-stimulating hormone (TSH), thyroxine, triiodothyronine, and free thyroxine index will provide information on the patient's thyroid status. Chronic disease arrests hair growth and subsequently results in hair loss. A screening evaluation for various chronic diseases and the patient's nutritional status is provided by obtaining a complete blood count (CBC), an unsaturated iron-binding capacity, serum iron, and antinuclear antibodies. Secondary or tertiary syphilis can result in a "moth-eaten" appearance of hair loss [2]. A VDRL will screen for the presence of this condition.

TECHNIQUES USED IN ASSESSMENT OF HAIR LOSS

Hair pull
This technique involves the removal of 50–70 hairs with a hemostat whose jaws have been covered with rubber tubing. The bulb ends of the hair are cut off and mounted on a slide with mounting medium or clear nail lacquer and covered with a glass coverslip. Assessment of the shaft diameters and the ratio of telogen to anagen hairs is determined. The telogen: anagen ratio may be helpful in determining the etiology of hair loss (Fig. 43.1).

Hair count
The patient is asked to collect all of her lost hair for 7 consecutive days. This includes all hair from her comb, brush, shower drain, etc. She brings in a record of the 7-day count and the last day's hair sample, which is mounted and evaluated in the same manner as described with the hair pull.

Density mapping
The density of scalp hair, which is rated on a scale from 1 to 10, is mapped out on a diagram of the head. This allows for objective evaluation of progression of disease over time.

Scalp biopsy
Under local anesthesia, a 4mm punch biopsy is obtained. This is essential in the evaluation of most scarring alopecias and will often help in the diagnosis of nonscarring alopecia, such as alopecia areata.

TYPES OF HAIR LOSS

Alopecia, the loss of hair from areas in which it is normally present, falls into two basic categories — scarring and nonscarring (Table 43.1). The hair follicle is destroyed in the scarring type of alopecia. Since

Table 43.1 Types of alopecia

Scarring alopcia
Physical trauma — extended traction on hair, X-rays (>1200 rad), third-degree burns
Chemical injury
Bacterial and spirochetal infection — tuberculosis, tertiary syphilis
Ringworm infections
Viral infection — herpes zoster
Neoplasms — basal cell carcinoma, squamous cell carcinoma
Psychogenic conditions — neurotic excoriation
Hereditary disorders/developmental defects — recessive X-linked ichthyosis
Destructive diseases producing scarring — scleroderma, pseudopelade of Brocq

Nonscarring alopecia
Anagen effluvium
Telogen effluvium
Androgenetic alopecia
Alopecia areata
Drugs
Bacterial and spirochetal infections — secondary syphilis
Trichotillomania
Chronic illness — systemic lupus erythematosus
Traction — rollers, hot comb
Endocrinology — hypothyroidism, hypopituitarism

neogenesis of the hair follicle does not occur in the adult this is an irreversible type of hair loss. The patient who presents to her primary care physician with scarring alopecia will usually need a referral to an appropriate specialist for further evaluation and treatment.

The hair follicle is preserved in nonscarring alopecia and the hair loss is therefore potentially reversible. The growth of cells in the follicular matrix is very sensitive to an acute stressful event, which may precede hair loss by as much as 6–8 months. The stressful event may be emotional stress, prolonged surgery, crash diets, or endocrine changes. Chronic illness due to a variety of disorders, including malignancy, diabetes, renal failure, or collagen vascular disease can result in hair loss. Poor nutrition and — particularly in women — iron deficiency is a common cause of hair loss. Hypopituitarism and thyroid dysfunction are potential causes of hair loss. Environmental factors (shampooing, sun, and blow-drying) may result in cuticular damage and hair loss. Some hereditary disorders which result in intrinsic anomalies of the cuticle result in hair loss as well. The

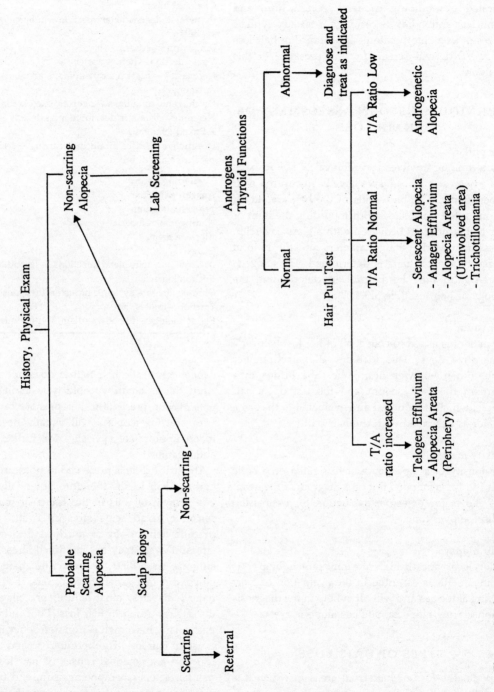

Fig. 43.1 Work-up of hair loss. T/A, telogen/anagen.

patient with nonscarring hair loss is more commonly encountered. In many cases care may be provided to the patient with nonscarring hair loss by the primary physician who has a comprehensive understanding of the various types of alopecia.

Telogen effluvium

Telogen effluvium refers to an abnormal amount of shedding of hair secondary to an excessive number of hairs in the telogen phase. The precipitating event, which prematurely converts a large number of follicles from the anagen to telogen phase, precedes the loss of hair by 2−4 months. The diagnosis requires a telogen count of >25% on the hair pull test.

Clinically, the patient notices an increase in hair loss prior to alopecia. Normally, 40−100 hairs are lost daily. The patient with telogen effluvium loses 120 to over 400 hairs daily. There is no specific treatment of telogen effluvium. The large number of telogen hairs shed are actually a result of new hair in the anagen phase pushing out the club hair. The prognosis is good if the hair loss is related to a specific precipitating event.

Potential precipitating events of telogen effluvium cover a wide range of possibilities (Table 43.2). Hair loss precipitated by a traumatic emotional stress tends to last longer and is more likely to recur than other types of telogen effluvium. Chronic illnesses such as cancer, tuberculosis, Hodgkin's disease, cirrhosis, malignant lymphoma or leukemia have been noted to cause telogen effluvium. Postpartum telogen effluvium usually begins 2−5 months after delivery with a telogen count between 24 and 46%. The patient may continue to experience hair loss up to 1 year after the birth of her child. However, normally even in prolonged cases regrowth of the patient's hair is complete. Postfebrile telogen effluvium is occasionally seen following infections with influenza, scarlet, or typhoid fever with telogen counts which may exceed 50%. Drug-induced telogen effluvium has been noted with a variety of agents (Table 43.2). Crash diets with less than 500 calories a day and weight loss of 25−35 lb may precipitate hair loss. This phenomenon is also seen following gastric bypass surgery.

Anagen effluvium

When a severe metabolic insult occurs, cellular division in the matrix is slowed and eventually arrested. As the thinned portion of the hair shaft reaches the surface of the scalp, this weak area breaks. Chemo-

Table 43.2 Causes of telogen effluvium

Acute stress — emotional shock, hemorrhage, blood donation
Chronic illness
Postpartum
Fever — influenza, pneumonia, scarlet fever
Drugs
  Allopurinol
  Amphetamines
  Anticonvulsants
  Antidepressants
  Antithyroid drugs
  Aspirin
  β-Blocking agents (Inderal)
  Carbamazepine (Tegretol)
  Cholesterol reducers
  Clofibrate (Atromid-S)
  Cocaine
  Coumarin
  Gentamicin
  Heparin
  Iodides (cough medicines)
  Isotretinoin
  Levodopa
  Lithium
  Nicotinic acid
  Oral contraceptive pill
  Penicillamine
  Propylthiouracil
  Tripanol
  Warfarin (Coumadin)
  Vitamin A excess
Poor nutrition
Crash diet — <500 calories per day
Iron deficiency
Prolonged surgery/anesthesia

therapeutic agents (alkylating agents, antimetabolites, and mitotic inhibitors), ionizing radiation, and various chemicals (arsenic, borate, lead, and mercury) are common causes of anagen effluvium. Hair loss is usually seen within the first 2 weeks following the precipitating insult. The club hairs in the telogen phase may be the only hair left following this type of hair loss. Growth of the normal follicle resumes with cessation of the insulting agent.

Alopecia areata

Alopecia areata usually presents as several well-circumscribed areas of hair loss 1−5 cm in diameter. The patches of baldness are usually found on the scalp but are occasionally present in the axilla or pubic areas. Alopecia areata is equally prevalent in males and females. It most commonly presents in the second and third decade of life. The etiology of alopecia areata is likely autoimmune and is associated with a specific mononuclear cell infiltrate at the hair bulb.

Physical examination reveals a bald patch with short broken-off hairs broken at the periphery. If removed, these loose telogen hairs may be seen to have a broad tip and narrow at the level of the scalp — thus the term "exclamation point" hair. A normal anagen : telogen ratio is seen if a biopsy is taken from a normal-appearing portion of the scalp but the loose hairs at the border of the lesion are only in the telogen phase.

The primary differential diagnosis is trichotillomania (manual removal of normal hair by the patient). In this condition the hairs found at the periphery are in the anagen phase and securely attached to the scalp. One other less common condition which can resemble alopecia areata is alopecia neoplastica. The bald patches seen with alopecia neoplastica are caused by metastatic adenocarcinoma of the breast. This can potentially be the first sign of metastatic breast cancer [3].

The natural progression of alopecia areata is hair loss over a period of 3–6 months, followed by 3–6 months of no hair growth, with return of hair growth (in >90% of patients) over the subsequent 3–6 months. Thirty to eighty percent of patients will experience recurrence within their lifetime. Rarely the patient may lose all of the hair on her scalp (alopecia totalis) or body hair (alopecia universalis), in which case the prognosis for hair regrowth is poor. Treatment of alopecia areata is varied, primarily using steroids (oral, topical, or intralesional) or topical irritants. These patients should be referred to a dermatologist for confirmation of diagnosis and appropriate treatment.

Trichotillomania

Trichotillomania is hair loss due to the patient pulling, plucking, eating, knotting, or twisting her hair. This condition is seven times more common in children than adults. Cases which are severe enough to present to a physician are often associated with a significant mental disturbance, but may infrequently present as a nervous tic comparable to nail-biting. In contrast to alopecia areata, which has a bald patch with short loose hairs at the periphery, trichotillomania has ill-defined areas of incomplete hair loss with indistinct borders. The remaining hair is of varying length and is not easily removed since these are normal hairs in the anagen phase. The areas of hair loss may be more extensive on the side of the dominant hand. Trichotillomania may be an unconscious habit on the part of the patient, or more commonly in the adult, this may represent an underlying psychologic disorder for which the patient will need referral for psychiatric treatment. Occasionally, diagnosis of this condition is difficult to make and may require referral to a dermatologist. It may be useful to shave the affected area and have the patient return in a couple of weeks. The shaved area will show uniform regrowth of hair since this is normal hair in the anagen phase. Alternatively, colloidin may be applied to the area, which will prevent patient access to hair with subsequent regrowth.

Androgenetic alopecia

Androgenetic alopecia is the term coined by Orentreich in 1960 for male-pattern baldness, but may actually been seen in both sexes. The pathophysiology in the male and female is the same, with an increased binding and metabolism of androgens, primarily dihydrotestosterone. The age of onset and the pattern of hair loss, however, are different in the female and male with androgenetic alopecia [4]. The male patient will experience hair loss, usually beginning in the third decade of life, primarily in the temporal and vertex regions with a gradual recession of an M-shaped hairline. In contrast, the female patient will experience hair loss in a more diffuse pattern in the centrofrontal region 15–20 years later than her male counterpart.

The three primary contributing factors to androgenetic alopecia in both the male and female are: (1) androgens; (2) age; and (3) familial tendency. The age of onset and severity of hair loss is less in the female as a result of lower androgen levels. Hair loss rarely progresses to the point that bald areas develop in the female patient with androgenetic alopecia. Initially it was thought that androgenetic alopecia was transmitted by an autosomal dominant gene with variable penetrance with a multigene distribution. Recent evidence suggests that the transmission of androgenetic alopecia is more likely of a polygenic inheritance pattern. The predisposition of a woman to develop androgenetic alopecia seems to be transmitted through an affected mother rather than through an affected father [2]. Occasionally, a woman presenting with androgenetic alopecia will have findings consistent with hyperandrogenism, such as hirsutism or virilization. These patients must be evaluated for excess ovarian and adrenal androgen production.

Diagnosis of androgenetic alopecia in the female patient is based upon: (1) diffuse thinning of the centrofrontal region; (2) normal to slight decrease in the anagen : telogen ratio; and (3) a variety of hair diameters which is pathognomonic of androgenetic alopecia. The hair pull test reveals a normal anagen : telogen ratio with the percentage of telogen hairs occasionally as high as 20%. With magnification, variation in the hair shaft diameter is observed. Greater than 30% of hairs have a thin diameter (0.03−0.05 mm). The remaining hairs have a normal diameter (0.08 mm).

Treatment of androgenetic alopecia has employed a variety of different agents, but has met with limited success. Because the hair loss is diffuse, use of surgical hair transplantation from unaffected areas is rarely useful in the female patient. The initial clinical results using minoxidil in the treatment of women with androgenetic hair loss are encouraging: however, the use of minoxidil in women has not been adequately studied. Spironolactone has been successful in the treatment of women with androgenetic hair loss and elevated DHEAS [5]. Topical estrogen may help to slow or arrest the progression of hair loss. Topical corticosteroid solutions may be beneficial as well.

Senescent alopecia

Nearly all individuals over the age of 50 experience progressive thinning of their scalp hair. The age at which this becomes clinically apparent varies; however, most individuals presenting with this type of hair loss are in their 60 s and 70 s. In contrast to other types of alopecia, there is a decreased density of the entire scalp. Hair loss may be pronounced in the bitemporal, centrofrontal, and vertex areas, but is present in the occipitoparietal area as well. The hair pull test reveals a normal anagen : telogen ratio. Topical estrogen can be used in an attempt to slow the hair loss; however, there is no effective treatment for this type of alopecia.

REFERENCES

1 Reid RL, Van Vugt DA. Hair loss in the female. *Obstet Gynecol Surv* 1988; 43: 135.

2 Domonkos AN, Arnold HL Jr, Odom RB. Diseases of the skin appendages. In: *Andrews' Diseases of the Skin, Clinical Dermatology*, 7th edn. Philadelphia. WB Saunders, 1982: 935.

3 Bertolino AP, Freedberg IM. Hair. In: Fitzpatrick T *et al.*, eds. *Dermatology in General Medicine: Textbook and Atlas*, 3rd edn. New York: McGraw-Hill, 1987: 627.

4 Ludwig E. Classification of the types of androgenetic alopecia (common baldness) arising in the female sex. *Br J Dermatol* 1977; 97: 249.

5 Kassick JM et al. *Adrenal androgenetic female-pattern alopecia: sex hormones and the balding woman. Cliv Clin O* 1983; 50: 111.

44

Clitoromegaly

LUTHER M. TALBERT

Development of both internal and external genital organs in male and female fetuses is identical up to about 8 weeks of gestational age. Development of the external genitalia beyond this time is controlled by secretions from the fetal gonads. In the absence of gonads the internal and external genitalia always will develop as female. Testosterone secreted by the fetal testis directs the development of the external genitalia to a male configuration. Under the stimulation of androgens, the genital tubercle in the male undergoes enlargement and elongation to form a penis, and the genital folds elongate and fuse to form the male urethra. In the absence of stimulation by androgens, the genital tubercle in the female develops into the clitoris. While testosterone is responsible for virilization of the Wolffian ducts, virilization of the external genitalia requires the peripheral conversion of testosterone to 5α-dihydrotestosterone by the enzyme 5α-reductase [1,2].

Ambiguous external genitalia may be a result of virilization of the female by excessive amounts of androgen (female pseudohermaphroditism) or may result from incomplete virilization of the male (male pseudohermaphroditism). Since male pseudohermaphrodites with less than adequate phallic development are often reared as females, this group of individuals will also be discussed in this presentation.

FEMALE PSEUDOHERMAPHRODITISM

Virilization of the external genitalia in a female neonate with a 46,XX karyotype may result from congenital adrenal hyperplasia, maternal ingestion of androgenic steroids during pregnancy, or virilizing tumors in the mother. The former is by far the most common and accounts for at least 95% of all cases of female pseudohermaphroditism. Table 44.1 is a classification scheme for female pseudohermaphroditism.

Table 44.1 Female pseudohermaphroditism

Congenital virilizing adrenal hyperplasia
Transfer of excess androgen from maternal circulation:
  Maternal ingestion of androgenic compounds
  Maternal virilizing tumor

MALE PSEUDOHERMAPHRODITISM

Incomplete virilization of the external genitalia in the male may result from either insufficient testosterone production or inadequate response to testosterone at the end-organ level.

Several enzymatic defects which reduce or eliminate testosterone biosynthesis in the testes and result in less than adequate virilization have been described (Table 44.2).

The androgen insensitivity syndromes are comprised of individuals with either reduced numbers or absence of receptors for testosterone at the end-organ level or the presence of abnormal testosterone receptors. 5α-Reductase deficiency is a rare genetically transmitted abnormality in the peripheral utilization of testosterone and causes less than adequate penile

Table 44.2 Male pseudohermaphroditism

Inborn errors of testosterone synthesis
  Cholesterol desmolase deficiency
  3β-Steroid dehydrogenase deficiency
  17α-Hydroxylase deficiency
  17–20 Lyase deficiency
  17β-Oxyreductase deficiency

Androgen insensitivity
  Complete
  Incomplete
  5α-Reductase deficiency

Dysgenetic male pseudohermaphroditism

development. Virilization and a degree of phallic enlargement may occur at puberty.

Chromosomal abnormalities in the male fetus often result in incomplete testicular development and secondarily cause inadequate virilization of the genitalia. Mosaic sex chromosome patterns are most common.

Most males with severe developmental abnormalities of the external genitalia are best raised as females, and therefore management of the phallic abnormalities in these individuals is identical to that in female pseudohermaphrodites.

CLITORAL ENLARGEMENT IN THE ADULT

Clitoral enlargement in the adult invariably occurs as a result of excess androgens, from either an endogenous or an exogenous source. While significant enlargement may occur in this group of patients, it is rarely of sufficient extent to result in any social embarrassment or disfigurement and as a general rule needs no therapy other than attempts to correct the hyperandrogenism.

Management of clitoral enlargement

Sex rearing of neonates
It is important that a final decision as to sex of rearing of the neonate be established within a few

weeks of birth. This decision is based on the etiology, the karyotype of the infant and, most importantly, the potential of the individual to achieve normal sexual function as an adult. Female pseudohermaphrodites are appropriately raised as females, although reconstructive surgery may be required to allow normal appearance of the genitalia and normal sexual function.

Male pseudohermaphrodites with severe developmental defects of the external genitalia usually are better raised as females after removal of any gonadal tissue present.

It is necessary to make a judgment as to whether the phallic enlargement will be of sufficient magnitude as to cause social embarrassment, and if so, it probably is advisable to do corrective surgery on the phallus before 2 or 3 years of age [4].

Surgical techniques for reduction of clitoral size
1 *Clitoridectomy.* Surgical removal of the clitoris was the most common approach to management of gross phallic enlargement up until relatively recent years [5]. This operation is still occasionally carried out in some parts of the world, but is no longer thought to be the optimal operation for reduction of clitoral size. If clitoridectomy is to be carried out, it is important that the corpora be completely dissected off the pubic ramus, so that no clitoral remnants are left behind where they may be painful during sexual arousal.
2 *Clitoral recession.* Clitoral recession is an appro-

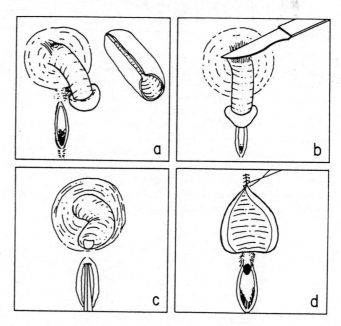

Fig. 44.1 Clitoral recession. (a) The skin of the clitoral shaft has been removed, leaving the glans intact. (b) The suspensory ligament is transected. (c) A tunnel extending from just above the urethral meatus to the clitoral incision is created, and the clitoris is pulled through with a clamp, burying the shaft. (d) The skin incision is closed, leaving only the glans visible. (Modified from Lattimer JK. *J Urol* 1961; 85: 113.)

priate cosmetic operation for individuals who have only moderate clitoral enlargement [6]. The procedure consists of burying the clitoral shaft and bringing the glans out just above the urethral orifice and is illustrated in Figure 44.1.

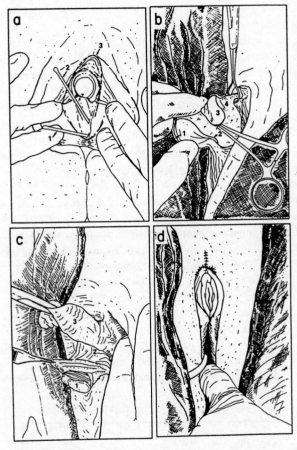

Fig. 44.2 Clitoroplasty. (a) Skin incision for clitoroplasty. 2 is cue tip in urethra, 1 is cue tip in blind vagina. (b) Dissection of clitoral shaft (4) leaving neuromuscular bundle (2) intact. Skin (3) will be removed along with clitoral shaft, leaving glans (1) attached to neuromuscular bundle. (c) Clitoral shaft (3) has been divided just above glans (1). Neurovascular bundle is preserved along with glans. The crurae will be dissected off the pubic ramus, leaving no remnants. (d) The glans clitoris has been attached to the periosteum of the symphysis pubis with four 00 polyglycol sutures and the skin incision has been closed, leaving normal appearing genitalia.

3 *Clitoroplasty*. Clitoroplasty is the most commonly utilized surgical procedure for management of clitoral enlargement [7]. This procedure is illustrated in Figure 44.2. The patient shown is a 14-year-old individual who was reared as female. Genitalia were ambiguous at birth, and the karyotype is 46,XY. Laboratory data are consistent with Reifenstein's syndrome. In Figure 44.2a an incision has been made in the ventral clitoral skin, which will be excised. In Figure 44.2b, the neurovascular bundle has been separated from the clitoral shaft, and the shaft has been transected just above the glans. Note in Figure 44.2c that the clitoral crura are dissected to their origins, and the clitoral shaft is excised. The glans is then sutured to the periosteum of the symphysis pubis, and the skin is closed, producing a near normal cosmetic result (Fig. 44.2d). The author has had considerable experience with the latter procedure and the results are consistently good. This procedure can be carried out on children at a quite young age, thus avoiding any psychologic discomfort because of the genital abnormalities.

In summary, the techniques presently available allow for satisfactory cosmetic and functional results for restoration of normal size to an abnormally enlarged phallus.

REFERENCES

1 Jirasek JE. *Development of the Genital System and Male Pseudohermaphroditism*. Johns Hopkins University Press, 1971: 3–23.
2 Wilson JD, Griffin JE, George FW, Leshin M. The role of gonadal steroids in sexual development. *Recent Prog Horm Res* 1981; 37: 1.
3 Grumbach MM, Conte FA. Disorders of sexual development. In: Wilson JD, Foster DW, eds. *Williams's Textbook of Endocrinology*. WB Saunders, 1985: 312–401.
4 Money J, Ehrhardt AA. *Man and Woman, Boy and Girl*. Johns Hopkins University Press, 1972: 176–194.
5 Gross RE, Randolph J, Crigler JF. Clitorectomy for sexual abnormalities. *Surgery* 1965; 59: 300.
6 Lattimer JK. Relocation and recession of the enlarged clitoris with preservation of the glans: an alternative to amputation. *J Urol* 1961; 85: 113.
7 Graves KL, Wilson EA, Greene JW. Surgical techniques for clitoral reduction. *Obstet Gynecol* 1982; 59: 758.

Adrenal insufficiency

WILLIAM J. BUTLER

The adrenal glands are paired structures located at the upper poles of the kidneys. The gland is divided into two distinct regions, the cortex and the medulla. Within the cortex there are three functional zones: the outer zona glomerulosa, the zona fasciculata, and the zona reticularis. Each of these zones is responsible for the synthesis of specific hormones. The glomerulosa is mainly involved in aldosterone biosynthesis and the inner fasciculata–reticularis zone is the site of cortisol and androgen biosynthesis. The medulla is involved in catecholamine metabolism and will not be further discussed in this chapter.

ADRENAL STEROID HORMONES

The primary glucocorticoid produced in the adrenal gland is cortisol (Fig. 45.1). It functions as a regulator of intermediary metabolism. This includes promotion of the conversion of proteins to carbohydrates (gluconeogenesis), storage of glycogen, and effects on lipid metabolism. Mineralocorticoids, of which aldosterone is the most potent, are responsible for fluid and electrolyte metabolism. Absence of both glucocorticoid and mineralocorticoid function is responsible for the symptomatology seen in adrenal insufficiency.

Glucocorticoid metabolism is under hypothalamic and pituitary regulation. Corticotropin-releasing hormone (CRH) is a 41 amino acid polypeptide synthesized in the median eminence of the hypothalamus and released into the portal vessels to the anterior pituitary. In the pituitary it is responsible for synthesis of a preprohormone, proopiomelanocortin (POMC). This precursor molecule is cleaved to a 39 amino acid peptide, adrenocorticotropic hormone (ACTH). Other cleavage products include β-lipotropin and the endorphins. ACTH is secreted in a pulsatile fashion with diurnal variation, peaking in the early morning hours and reaching a nadir in the evening. This variation accounts for the diurnal

pattern of cortisol production seen in the peripheral blood. Cortisol exerts negative feedback on ACTH production, probably by decreasing cellular responsiveness to CRH.

Aldosterone is under control of the renin–angiotensin system. Renin is released from the renal juxtaglomerular cells in response to alterations in blood volume, plasma sodium concentration, and sympathetic nervous system stimulation. It acts on a substrate, angiotensinogen, to produce angiotensin I which is then converted to angiotensin II in tissues such as the pulmonary vascular endothelium. Angiotensin II stimulates aldosterone synthesis.

ADRENOCORTICAL INSUFFICIENCY

Adrenal hypofunction may result either from intrinsic disease of the adrenal glands (primary adrenal insufficiency, Addison's disease) or secondarily from insufficient secretion of ACTH by the pituitary gland (secondary adrenal insufficiency). Adrenal insufficiency may be either acute (Addisonian crisis) or chronic. The pathophysiology of primary adrenal insufficiency results from deprivation of both glucocorticoid and mineralocorticoid effects. There is loss of salt and plasma volume, diminished cardiac output, and decreased renal perfusion. In secondary adrenal insufficiency aldosterone metabolism is not affected.

ETIOLOGY OF PRIMARY ADRENAL INSUFFICIENCY

Addison's disease results from the destruction of both adrenal cortices. The three major causes are autoimmune destruction, infiltration by infectious diseases, and metastatic neoplasia. Approximately two-thirds of cases are due to circulating antibodies directed against adrenal cortical tissue. This may occur as isolated adrenal insufficiency or in com-

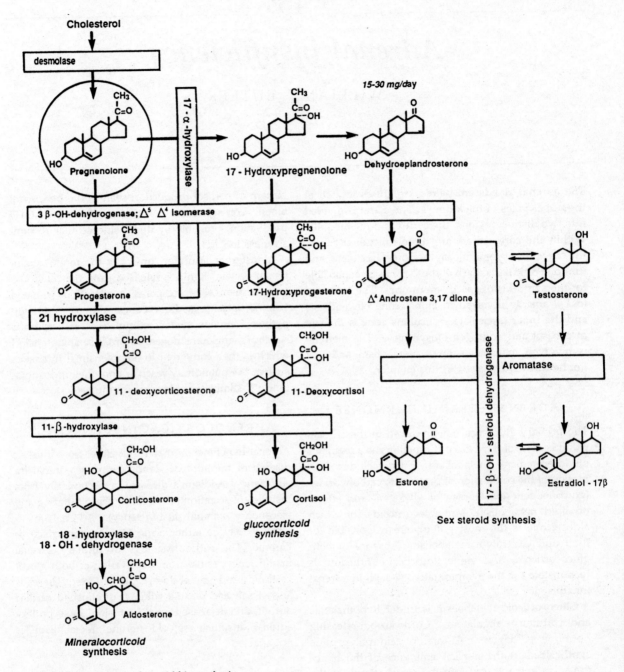

Fig. 45.1 Pathways of steroid biosynthesis.

bination with other autoimmune endocrinopathies such as premature ovarian failure or hypothyroidism. Autoimmune polyglandular syndrome type I is an autosomal recessive condition encompassing Addison's disease, hypoparathyroidism, and chronic mucocutaneous candidiasis. Autoimmune polyglandular syndrome type II (Schmidt's syndrome) is characterized by Addison's disease, autoimmune thyroid disease, and insulin-dependent diabetes mellitus and is inherited in an autosomal dominant fashion.

In past years, tuberculosis was the most common cause of adrenal insufficiency. Although it is still the predominant infectious cause, other infiltrative diseases such as histoplasmosis and coccidioido-mycosis are seen more frequently. Patients with acquired immunodeficiency syndrome (AIDS) are susceptible to adrenal failure secondary to cyto-megalovirus, cryptococcus, and *Mycobacterium avium/intracellulare* infections. Metastatic disease from primary neoplasms of the lung, breast, or lymphoma may not uncommonly involve the adrenals. Rarer causes of adrenal insufficiency may be intraadrenal hemorrhage secondary to septicemia (Waterhouse–Friderichsen syndrome) or anticoagulant therapy. Certain drugs such as ketoconazole or etomidate may block adrenal steroidogenesis by inhibiting cytochrome P450-dependent enzymes involved in steroidogenesis. Aminoglutethimide and O, p'-DDD can be used to induce a medical adrenalectomy.

ETIOLOGY OF SECONDARY ADRENAL INSUFFICIENCY

Pituitary ACTH deficiency may result from any injury to the pituitary gland. It may be isolated or part of a panhypopituitary picture. It also may occur following prolonged administration of exogenous glucocorticoid preparations. Such suppression may last several months.

CLINICAL SIGNS AND SYMPTOMS

The presentation of adrenal insufficiency is deter-mined by the rapidity of onset of the adrenal failure (Table 45.1). Adrenal crisis is characterized by severe volume depletion, hypotension, and azotemia. Pro-found shock may result. Chronic adrenal insufficiency may exhibit only subtle symptomatology and be difficult to diagnose. The patient's complaints are nonspecific but the hyperpigmentation of mucous membranes and in areas of skin flexion is a helpful diagnostic sign. This is absent in secondary adrenal insufficiency. The symptoms of volume depletion including the severe electrolyte imbalance and hypotension are more marked in primary adrenal insufficiency.

DIAGNOSIS

A decision tree for evaluation of adrenal insufficiency is shown in Figure 45. 2. Neither plasma cortisol nor urinary free cortisol determinations are adequate for diagnosis for adrenal insufficiency. Direct serum radioimmunoassay for ACTH will differentiate elevated levels as seen in primary adrenal insuf-ficiency but will not differentiate normal from low values and therefore is not useful in assessing ACTH reserve. The rapid ACTH stimulation test can be performed as an outpatient at any time of day, does not require fasting, and can be performed in con-junction with initiation of therapy. A basal plasma cortisol level is obtained and then 0.25 mg of cosyn-tropin (a synthetic derivative of ACTH containing its first 24 amino acids) is given by intravenous injection. Serum cortisol levels are drawn at 30 and 60 min. A normal result is a basal cortisol level greater than 10 μg/dl with a rise of at least 7 μg/dl or to a value of 18 μg/dl or greater 1 hour after cosyntropin injection. An abnormal response can be due to primary or secondary adrenal insufficiency. This is because in secondary adrenal insufficiency the adrenal may become relatively unresponsive to acute stimulation with ACTH. Serum ACTH determination by radio-immunoassay will allow differentiation with elevated ACTH values usually exceeding 80 pg/ml in primary adrenal insufficiency.

To overcome the relative refractoriness of the adrenal gland in secondary adrenal insufficiency, a prolonged ACTH stimulation test may be performed.

Table 45.1 Signs/symptoms of adrenal insufficiency

Acute	Chronic
Lethargy/confusion	Weakness/fatigue
Hypotension/shock	Hypotension
Nausea/vomiting	Weight Loss
Dehydration	Hyperpigmentation
Hyponatremia/hyperkalemia	Anorexia/nausea/vomiting
Abdominal pain	Irritability
Hypothermia	Electrolyte imbalance

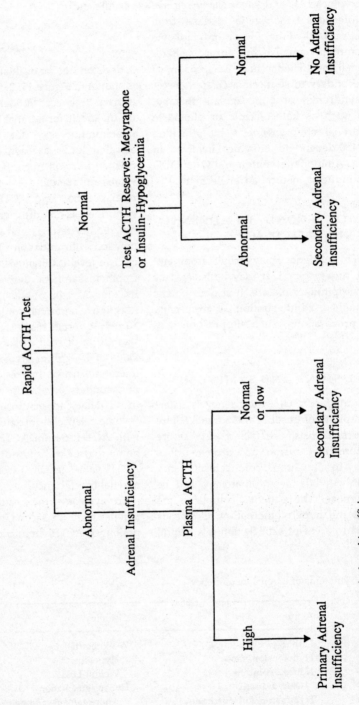

Fig. 45.2 Diagnosis of adrenal insufficiency.

Baseline 24-hour urine collection is assayed for 17-hydroxycorticosteroids and then 0.25 mg of cosyntropin is infused intravenously over an 8-hour period on each of the next 3 days. Plasma cortisol levels are measured at 8.00 a.m. and 4.00 p.m. and a final 24-hour urine collection for 17-hydroxycorticosteroids is obtained on the third day. A normal result should show increased plasma cortisol levels by 15–40 µg/dl over baseline. The 24-hour 17 hydroxycorticosteroids should increase 15–40 mg per 24 hours. The absolute values obtained are not as important as showing a significant rise in glucocorticoid synthesis.

An adequate response to the rapid ACTH stimulation test does not rule out inadequate pituitary reserve to respond to stress. To test pituitary responsiveness directly CRH 1–2 µg/kg can be given and plasma ACTH can be measured at 15 min intervals from baseline to 120 min. The clinical utility of CRH testing has not yet been established, but in general patients with pituitary disease exhibit a blunted response. Indirect stimulation of ACTH reserve can be accomplished using either insulin-induced hypoglycemia or metyrapone. Hypoglycemia is induced by injecting 0.05–0.15 units of regular insulin per kg body weight to induce blood glucose to fall 50%, to less than 40 mg/dl. A normal plasma cortisol will rise to 1.5 times the pretreatment level with a rise of at least 10 µg/dl and a maximum level greater than 20 µg/dl at 60 min. Metyrapone inhibits 11β-hydroxylase and therefore blocks cortisol synthesis, removing endogenous feedback inhibition of ACTH. An overnight metyrapone test is performed by administering a dose of 2–3 g at midnight and measuring 11-deoxycortisol and cortisol at 8.00 a.m. the following day. A normal result will have a plasma deoxycortisol greater than 7 µg/dl. A plasma cortisol level of less than 10 µg/dl indicates adequate enzyme inhibition by the drug and therefore a valid test. A more prolonged test involves measuring baseline 24-hour urine 17-hydroxycorticosteroids and then administering 750 mg of metyrapone by mouth every 4 hours for 24 hours. Subsequent 24-hour urinary 17-hydroxycorticosteroids (collected the next day) should show a threefold increment (increase 10–40 mg/24 hours). Serum 11-deoxycortisol concentration should rise to greater than 10 µg/dl with plasma cortisol falling to less than 6 µg/dl. By following the decision tree in Figure 45.2 a diagnosis of primary or secondary adrenocortical insufficiency or normal adrenal function is possible.

A risk of using these feedback tests to assess pituitary ACTH reserve is that the induced stress or block in cortisol synthesis may precipitate an acute adrenal crisis. Appropriate safeguards should be to have both 50% glucose for injection and intravenous hydrocortisone preparations available for the duration of each study.

Other diagnostic testing may be directed towards the determination of the etiology of the adrenal insufficiency. Computed tomography scans of the adrenals may demonstrate enlarged glands compatible with infectious infiltrates or metastatic diseases. A decrease in the size of the adrenals is consistent with autoimmune disease. More specific diagnosis may be obtained by needle biopsy of the glands. Other appropriate studies should be done to diagnose tuberculosis, other infectious diseases, and associated endocrine deficiencies.

TREATMENT

The treatment of acute adrenal insufficiency is a medical emergency. Volume repletion should begin with normal saline with 5% dextrose and may require several liters of fluid replacement. Glucocorticoid replacement with intravenous hydrocortisone 100 mg every 8 hours is essential. Should a rapid ACTH screening test be desired, initial therapy may begin with 10 mg of dexamethasone phosphate. This will not interfere with serum cortisol assays. Obviously, therapy should also address any etiologic or precipitating factors such as septicemia. Maintenance therapy should be initiated when the patient is stabilized. This is the same as the treatment for chronic adrenal insufficiency. Full replacement dosage of glucocorticoids is cortisone acetate 25 mg each morning and 12.5 mg each afternoon or equivalent glucocorticoid (prednisone 5 mg each morning and 2.5 mg each afternoon). Not all patients with primary adrenal insufficiency will require mineralocorticoid replacement because of significant mineralocorticoid activity in these synthetic steroids. Should hypotension or hyperkalemia develop, fluorocortisone in a dosage of 0.05–0.1 mg/day orally can be added.

During periods of illness or other stress the cortisone dosage should be increased two- to threefold. Coverage for acute stress episodes like surgery should be equivalent to the treatment of acute adrenal insufficiency, hydrocortisone 100 mg i.v. every 8 hours. Patients with chronic adrenal insufficiency should carry identification describing their medical condition, such as a medic alert bracelet. Patients on chronic treatment need to be monitored for blood pressure and electrolyte levels. The most common side-effect of oral steroid therapy is gastrointestinal upset. This may be minimized by taking a daily medication dosage with meals.

FURTHER READING

Bondy PK. Diseases of the adrenal cortex. In: Wilson JD, Foster DW (eds). *Williams Textbook of Endocrinology*, 7th edn. WB Saunders, 1985; 816–890.

Kannan CR. Diseases of the adrenal cortex. *Disease-a-Month*, 1988; 34: 601–674.

Schlaff WD. Dynamic testing in reproductive endocrinology. *Fertil Steril* 1986; 45: 589–606.

Part IVD
Endocrinologic abnormalities: The ovary

46

Polycystic ovarian syndrome

KAREN D. BRADSHAW & BRUCE R. CARR

INTRODUCTION

Women with polycystic ovarian syndrome (PCOS) may present with complaints of hirsutism, infertility, or disturbances of the menstrual cycle (abnormal bleeding or amenorrhea). Diagnosis can be made with some certainty and therapy can be directed toward alleviating the principal symptom or complaint.

Historically, hyperandrogenism and polycystic ovaries were described as early as the nineteenth century. It was not until 1935 that a syndrome was identified and subsequently named for Stein and Leventhal who first associated amenorrhea, obesity, and hirsutism with polycystic ovaries [1]. Subsequent morphologic, biochemical, and endocrinologic studies by numerous investigators in women with polycystic ovaries has led to the conclusion that PCOS is a complex, heterogeneous disorder with diverse clinical and biochemical features. Proposed pathogenetic mechanisms for PCOS include primary abnormalities of the hypothalamic–pituitary unit, the ovary, and the adrenal. Recent clinical observations also demonstrate a strong association between insulin resistance with resultant hyperinsulinemia and hyperandrogenism.

CLINICAL OVERVIEW

Although the diagnosis of PCOS is frequently made in hyperandrogenic women, it is somewhat difficult to establish a rigorous clinical definition due to the heterogeneity of the disorder. However, in an analysis of 100 women [2] with histologically documented polycystic ovaries the most common features of histories were:

1 Mean age at menarche (12.3 years) close to the mean of 12.9 years found in the normal population. Although rare, 10% of women with PCOS present with primary amenorrhea.

2 Menstrual irregularity consisting of anovulatory bleeding or secondary amenorrhea.

3 Onset of excessive hair growth either before or around the time of menarche.

4 Considered overweight among the patient's peers prior to menarche.

The frequency of various clinical manifestations of patients with PCOS is summarized in Table 46.1 [3].

On physical examination, hirsutism, acne, and oily skin (manifestations of androgen excess) are common. The ovaries may be bilaterally enlarged on pelvic examination. Frank virilization (clitoromegaly, deep voice, temporal baldness, male habitus) is uncommon and, if present, other causes of androgen excess such as ovarian or adrenal tumors must be ruled out.

The incidence of hyperandrogenism, insulin resistance, and acanthosis nigricans approaches 50% of all women with functional hyperandrogenism with serum testosterone >1 ng/ml. Acanthosis nigricans or localized areas of velvety gray-brown hyperpigmentation is seen in the subgroup of patients who exhibit insulin resistance, and is a dermatologic manifestation of the chronic hyperinsulinemia. It presents as a mossy, verrucous, hyperpigmented

Table 46.1 Frequency of clinical manifestations of proven cases of polycystic ovary syndrome ($n = 1079$). (Adapted from [3])

Symptoms	Frequency (%)
Infertility	74
Hirsutism	69
Amenorrhea	51
Obesity	41
Functional bleeding	29
Corpus luteum at surgery	22
Virilization	21

skin that usually develops over the nape of the neck, in the axillae, beneath the breasts, and other body folds. Skin tags are often found in or near areas of acanthosis.

Bilaterally enlarged ovaries with a smooth pearly-white thickened capsule are frequently found. On cut section, multiple follicular cysts surrounded by abundant ovarian stroma are found throughout the cortex of the ovary. Subcapsular cysts are lined with a reduced number of granulosa cells, with early stages of antrum formation. On higher power, hyperplasia of the theca interna with luteinization is seen. In electron microscopic studies of the polycystic ovary, the basal lamina that separates the theca interna from the granulosa is increased in thickness.

ETIOLOGY

A critical concept is that the majority of cases of functional ovarian hyperandrogenism have a multi-factorial etiology. Disturbances of at least six major systems may contribute to the development of PCOS syndrome: (1) the hypothalamic–pituitary unit; (2) the ovary; (3) the periphery, including the liver, skin, and adipose tissue; (4) the adrenal gland; (5) insulin resistance; and (6) genetic causes. The exact cause and initiating event are still unknown. In concert, the interactions of these major systems lead to a vicious cycle whereby the initiation of PCOS and functional hyperandrogenism leads to its perpetuation. Within the cycle there is inappropriate gonadotropin secretion with an elevated luteinizing hormone : follicle-stimulating hormone (LH:FSH) ratio secondary to chronically elevated and acyclic estrogen feedback on the hypothalamic–pituitary system. Increased gonadotropin-releasing hormone (GnRH) pulsatile secretion, in addition to elevated estrogen levels and ovarian inhibin levels, leads to preferential increases in plasma LH levels and inhibition of FSH. The LH-dependent hyperplasia of the theca cells leads to associated hypersecretion of ovarian androgens. High insulin levels in the insulin resistant PCOS patient may also stimulate ovarian androgen production. Androgen excess leads to inhibition of sex hormone binding globulin (SHBG) production with increased free androgen and estrogen levels. Excess androgens are aromatized to estrogens in peripheral extra-glandular sites such as adipose tissue, resulting in self-perpetuation of the cycle. Estrogens are not secreted directly by the ovary, but are formed from androgens in extraglandular sites. As a result, inadequate follicular maturation, anovulation, and increased follicular atresia occur.

DIAGNOSIS AND LABORATORY EVALUATION

The diagnosis is essentially a clinical one based on the following criteria: (1) varying degrees of menstrual irregularity (amenorrhea or anovulatory bleeding; (2) hirsutism; and (3) obesity.

All symptoms are first noted at the time of expected menarche. The laboratory findings include higher circulating levels of estrone, testosterone, androstenedione, dehydroepiandrosterone, dehydroepiandrosterone sulfate, and reduced levels of estradiol. In contrast to the characteristic picture of fluctuating hormone levels in the normal cycle, a steady state of gonadotropins and sex steroids is associated with persistent anovulation. The LH:FSH ratio, both biologic and immunologic, is elevated and usually greater than 3:1. However, 20% of women with PCOS will have a ratio close to 1:1.

TREATMENT

The treatment of PCOS is dependent on the desires of the patient and includes: (1) infertility — ovulation induction; (2) hirsutism — oral contraceptive pills, GnRH analogs, spironolactone; and (3) disturbances of the menstrual cycle (amenorrhea or abnormal uterine bleeding) — oral contraceptive pills or progestogen withdrawal.

Infertility — ovulation induction

The majority of women with PCOS and infertility can be successfully treated with some mode of therapy that improves the LH:FSH ratio, or decreases intra-ovarian androgen. The initial therapy for obese patients is to lose weight. If not successful and if the patient remains anovulatory with evidence of endogenous estrogen activity, the first treatment is clomiphene citrate. Clomiphene citrate is an orally active, nonsteroidal drug whose structure resembles diethylstilbestrol (DES). Clomiphene citrate is an antiestrogen and its mechanism of action is believed to result in release of pituitary FSH. It acts primarily by binding hypothalamic estrogen receptors, thereby displacing endogenous estrogen and stimulating FSH release. Both FSH and LH secretion increase following clomiphene citrate, allowing for recruitment and selection of a dominant follicle. Ovulation usually occurs within 7 days after the completion of treatment. A 50–70% ovulation rate is found in patients receiving clomiphene, but pregnancy figures are only about 40%. The multiple pregnancy rate averages about 7% and the miscarriage rate is slightly higher than that seen in the general population.

Patient selection is crucial for successful therapy. As the key feature of clomiphene is to lower the estrogenic signal to the hypothalamus and pituitary, there must be significant endogenous estrogen present. The presence of copious cervical mucus or a positive withdrawal to a progestin challenge confirms an estrogenic milieu. Evaluation of both partners is also important to screen for male factor infertility or the presence of tubal disease.

Therapy with clomiphene is begun with 50 mg given for 5 days beginning from the third to the fifth day of bleeding (Fig. 46.1). Cycles may be either spontaneous or induced by progestin withdrawal. Ovulation and pregnancy rates are similar in day 3

through day 5 start up with clomiphene. Ovulation prediction and documentation should be performed. The basal body temperature charting is an inexpensive marker and a biphasic elevation indicates that ovulation has occurred. Urinary LH monitoring by means of commercially available kits is a convenient means of predicting the timing of ovulation. Patients are instructed to begin testing on cycle day 12. Twice-daily monitoring is most accurate and ovulation occurs within 12–24 hours after LH peak. Timed intercourse or intrauterine insemination with washed husband's sperm is then performed. Confirmation of follicular development and ovulation is also accomplished by ultrasonography or midluteal progesterone levels of 10 ng/ml or greater.

If ovulation does not occur clomiphene dosage is increased by increments of 50 mg daily and ovulation and luteal phase documentation is performed. As long as an adequate response is noted and there are no unusual side-effects, clomiphene therapy is

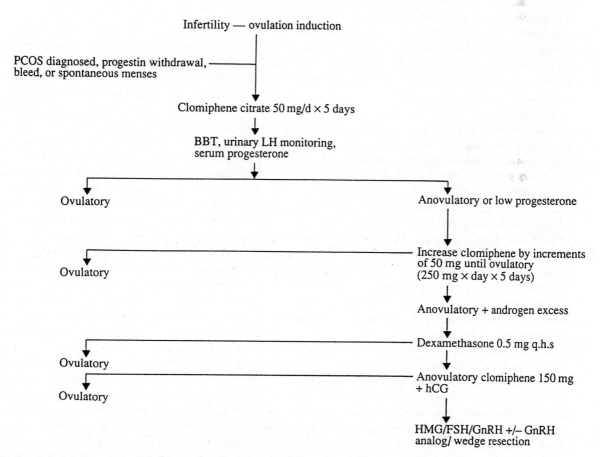

Fig. 46.1 Flow diagram for ovulation induction in women with PCOS.

continued usually for 3–6 months. If pregnancy has not occurred at that time other causes of infertility are reassessed.

Side-effects of clomiphene citrate are hot flashes, vaginal dryness, and headaches. About 50% of patients conceive at the 50 mg dose, another 20% at 100 mg, and another 15% at the 150–200 mg dose levels. If ovulation is not obtained with a dose of 150–250 mg, one option is to add dexamethasone 0.5 mg each evening. This treatment decreases adrenal androgen production and may increase the patient's sensitivity to clomiphene, particularly if the level of dehydroepiandrosterone sulfate is elevated. The dexamethasone is maintained daily until pregnancy is diagnosed.

In patients who do not conceive with clomiphene or clomiphene plus dexamethasone, pelvic sonography is indicated to document normal follicular development. If a normal-sized follicle is observed but ovulation fails to occur, human chorionic gonadotropin (hCG) (10 000 U i.m.) is given when the leading follicle reaches 18 mm diameter. Although extended clomiphene regimens have been proposed for the difficult patient, this approach requires estrogen monitoring, and is often unsuccessful in achieving pregnancy. More commonly, in modern practice these patients are treated instead with gonadotropins.

Bilateral ovarian wedge resection was an early effective treatment for anovulation. The purpose of wedge resection is to decrease the ovarian production of androgens, either by reducing the amount of steroid-producing tissue, or by temporarily interfering with the ovarian blood supply. The response to ovarian wedge resection is variable. Some patients resume ovulation permanently; however, most become anovulatory and some patients fail to respond at all. The risk of adhesion formation with wedge resection probably exceeds 10%. Recently, reports of laparoscopic surgical treatment of polycystic ovaries, either by electrocautery or laser, appear to be similar to results obtained with traditional wedge resection [4].

Human menopausal gonadotropin (hMG) treatment is indicated for the treatment of anovulation in patients refractory to clomiphene, or in whom clomiphene is unlikely to be effective. Some patients with PCOS are exquisitely sensitive to the effects of hMG, and are likely to develop hyperstimulation. Prior to beginning an hMG treatment cycle, a pelvic sonogram looks for adnexal cysts which might be mistaken for follicles later in the cycle.

Purified FSH is approved for use in clomiphene-resistant PCOS patients with elevated LH levels. The rationale for FSH use is to increase follicle development without the presumably deleterious effects of LH on ovarian androgen production. Ovulation, pregnancy, and complication rates are similar to results obtained with hMG, and no study has unequivocally shown an advantage of FSH over hMG. hMG and FSH therapy is initiated by daily increases in dose using 1–6 A over 7–14 days of therapy. The estrogen levels and follicle size are monitored until a ripe follicle is identified and ovulation is triggered with hCG (5000–10 000 units). The risks of hMG and FSH include multiple pregnancy (20%) and hyperstimulation (10–20%). If these methods fail to induce ovulation, then pretreatment with GnRH analogs may be effected. Recently the use of GnRH analogs, followed by GnRH given by a portable infusion pump, has resulted in ovulatory cycles in some women with PCOS.

Hirsutism

PCOS is often associated with increased androstenedione and testosterone secretion from the ovary and is the most common etiology for androgen excess. Patients with PCOS usually give a history of peripubertal onset of increased hair growth, and irregularity of menses. The hirsutism may or may not be progressive; occasionally, some evidence of virilization may be present. This history of peripubertal onset is vital in the diagnosis of PCOS, as a recent, rapid progression of hirsutism or virilization requires a more intensive search for other causes of androgen excess, such as tumor formation. The evaluation of women with hirsutism or virilization is presented in Figure 46.2.

Hirsutism is an excessive growth of hair in women which occurs in specific androgen-sensitive areas of the body such as the face, lower back, chest, buttock, areola, inner thigh, linea alba, and external genitalia and pubic hair areas. The therapeutic approach to androgen excess must be tailored to individual patients and etiologies.

Treatment of hirsutism falls into two main categories: medical and cosmetic. Medical therapy includes: (1) therapy directed toward suppression of the secretion of androgens by the ovary or adrenal, includes treatment with oral contraceptives, glucocorticoids, and GnRH analogs; and (2) therapy with antiandrogens that act at the level of the hair follicle or sebaceous gland. Cosmetic therapy such as plucking,

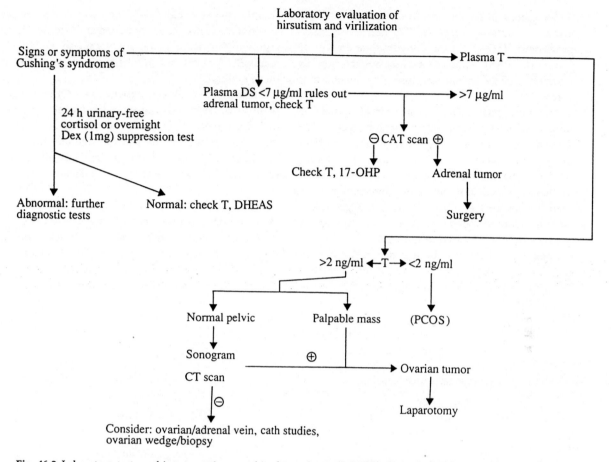

Fig. 46.2 Laboratory tests and interpretations used in the evaluation of hirsutism and virilization. DHEAS, dehydroepiandrosterone sulfate; T, testosterone; 17-OHP, 17-hydroxyprogesterone; PCOS, polycystic ovarian syndrome. (From Carr BR. Disorders of the ovary and female reproductive tract. In: Wilson JD, Forest DE, eds. *Williams Textbook of Endocrinology*. Philadelphia: Saunders, 1991: 780.)

waxing, shaving, depilatory creams, and electrolysis is frequently used in combination with medical therapy.

The ideal response is eradication of hirsutism, but alleviation of hirsutism is the more usual outcome. Treatment should be continued for 8–10 months before it is deemed ineffective. As the rate of hair growth increases in the summer, therapy may need to continue longer before judgment is made. Electrolysis or depilatory therapy should be added to treatment regimens for patients who are quite concerned about their cosmetic appearance.

Combination oral contraceptives (OCs) act to decrease androgen excess both by inhibiting ovarian production of androgens (by suppression of pituitary gonadotropin release) and by stimulating hepatic synthesis of SHBG, which in turn decreases the level of unbound testosterone. An OC formulation with substantial estrogen (50 µg) as well as progestin effects will maximize both hepatic SHBG production and pituitary suppression. Thus, the newer triphasic OCs are probably not as effective as higher-dose pills for treatment of the hirsute patient. OC use also provides for prophylaxis against the development of endometrial hyperplasia in the anovulatory hirsute woman. If OCs are contraindicated, medroxyprogesterone acetate (Provera 10–30 mg orally each day) usually suppresses LH and results in decreased androgen production.

Dexamethasone (0.25–1.0 mg each evening) is effective in decreasing the production of androgens from the adrenal. It seems logical to consider dexamethasone treatment for hirsute women who have adult-onset adrenal hyperplasia. In the majority of patients, lowering of elevated adrenal androgen level is associated with an improvement in androgen excess symptoms, especially acne. 17-hydroxy-progesterone (17-OHP) and dehydroepiandrosterone sulfate (DHEAS) levels can be assessed at monthly intervals until the therapeutic dose of dexamethasone is reached.

Antiandrogens interfere with target tissue androgen effects by competing for intracellular androgen receptors, and they may inhibit androgen biosynthesis as well. Spironolactone (50–100 mg b.i.d.) is the most effective antiandrogen available in this country, and clinical improvement may be seen within 2–3 months of therapy. Cyproterone acetate is another potent androgen antagonist, but it is currently not marketed in the USA.

Depilatory creams may be superior to shaving as a mechanical method of hair removal as the regrowing hair has a softer, subtle tip as opposed to the bristly stubble of shaven hairs. Waxing may allow a greater area of hair growth to be removed at one time and as regrowing hairs are in the anagen phase, no stubble results. Folliculitis and skin irritation may occur with these methods.

Electrolysis relies on destruction of the dermal papillae by electrical vibrations and effects permanent hair removal. This therapy should be delayed for 9–10 weeks following medical therapy to insure synchronization of terminal hairs. Side-effects include scarring, pigmentation, and infection.

Disturbances of the menstrual cycle

When uterine bleeding occurs in subjects with PCOS, it is unpredictable with respect to time of onset, duration, and amount, and on occasion the bleeding can be severe. The dysfunctional uterine bleeding in this disorder is usually due to estrogen-breakthrough.

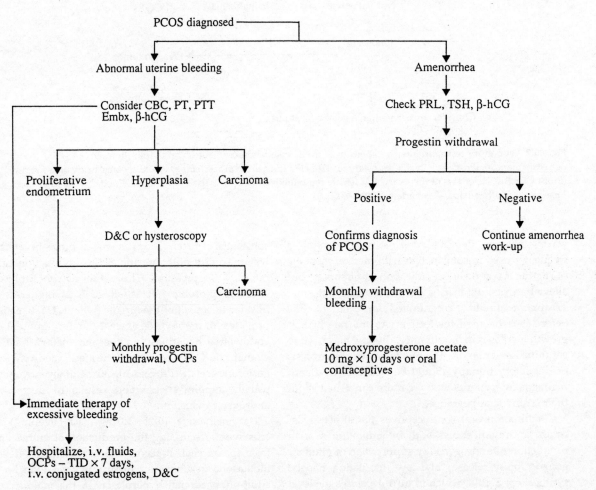

Fig. 46.3 Treatment of disturbance of the menstrual cycle in women with PCOS.

The anovulatory endometrium (with the absence of luteal progesterone) is in a chronic estrogen-stimulated proliferative state. This thickened tissue bleeds irregularly and sheds incompletely.

In treating dysfunctional uterine bleeding due to anovulation it is important first to stabilize the endometrium before allowing a controlled bleeding episode (Fig. 46.3). This can be accomplished by several methods. On an outpatient basis administration of high-dose combined estrogen–progestin OCs are usually successful in stopping bleeding. One pill is given three times daily for 7 days. Bleeding usually ceases and then either a withdrawal bleed is allowed or the patient continues on one OC pill for 21 days and is then allowed to withdraw. Progestin therapy for 10 days will result in a relatively complete sloughing of the endometrial lining and is useful in the estrogen-primed individual. For patients with severe bleeding, anemia, or other medical disorders, intravenous conjugated estrogens may be used to stabilize a denuded endometrium. Conjugated estrogens in a dose of 25 mg i.v. every 6 hours for up to 24 hours will cause estrogen-stimulated growth and repair of a raw denuded lining. It is then necessary to allow for a controlled bleeding episode, as with the use of OC pills. In patients who continue to bleed despite medical therapy, dilatation and curettage is necessary to control bleeding and for tissue diagnosis.

Amenorrhea is frequently a chronic problem and long-term therapy is essential. If contraception is not needed, cyclic medroxyprogesterone acetate 10 mg daily for the first 10 days of each month will allow for scheduled bleeding. Low-dose OCs provide both contraception and endometrial stabilization.

Endometrial hyperplasia and carcinoma may develop as a result of chronic unopposed estrogen exposure and is diagnosed by endometrial biopsy. A fractional curettage or hysteroscopically directed biopsy is necessary when hyperplasia is present to rule out coexisting carcinoma. Progesterone therapy — medroxyprogesterone acetate 20 mg daily for 6 months — and repeat sampling are recommended for endometrial hyperplasia. In all patients with PCOS who are obese, diet, weight loss, and exercise have been shown to be beneficial. Diets low in fat and high in fiber and carbohydrates are recommended. Reduction in weight loss reduces androgen levels and insulin resistance and may result in resumption of ovulatory cycles.

REFERENCES

1 Stein IF, Leventhal ML. Amenorrhea associated with polycystic ovaries. *Am J Obstet Gynecol* 1935; 29: 181–191.
2 Yen S. The polycystic ovary syndrome. *Clin Endocrinol* 1980; 12: 177.
3 Goldzieher JW, Axelrod LR. Clinical and biochemical features of polycystic ovarian disease. *Fertil Steril* 1963; 14: 631.
4 Greenblatt E, Casper RF. Endocrine changes after laparoscopic ovarian cautery in "polycystic" ovarian syndrome. *Am J Obstet Gynecol* 1987; 156: 279–285.

FURTHER READING

Barbieri RL, Smith S, Ryan KJ. The role of hyperinsulinemia in the pathogenesis of ovarian hyperandrogenism. *Fertil Steril* 1988; 50: 197–212.
Barnes R, Rosenfield RL. The polycystic ovary syndrome: pathogenesis and treatment. *Ann Intern Med* 1989; 110: 389–399.
Daniell JF, Miller W. Polycystic ovaries treated by laparoscopic laser vaporization. *Fertil Steril* 1989; 51: 232–236.
Franks S. Polycystic ovary syndrome: a changing perspective. *Clin Endocrinol* 1989; 31: 87–120.
McKenna TJ. Pathogenesis and treatment of polycystic ovary syndrome. *N Engl J Med* 1988; 318: 558–562.

47

Resistant ovary syndrome

MINNA R. SELUB & CHARLES B. HAMMOND

Resistant ovary syndrome was originally described by Jones and DeMoraes-Ruehsen, who named the entity Savage syndrome, after their first patient with this disorder [1]. It was later defined by the triad of endogenous hypergonadotropinism, hyporeceptivity of the ovaries to an excessive stimulation with exogenous human gonadotropins, and the presence of apparently normal ovarian follicles (follicular ovarian failure). It differs from classical ovarian failure, in which ovarian follicles are absent or severely reduced. In this chapter we will attempt to provide the reader with an understanding of the symptom of amenorrhea and of its work-up. In addition, we hope to define further the subgroup of patients who have resistant ovary syndrome and to discuss its possible etiologies and its appropriate therapies.

DIAGNOSIS

Amenorrhea is defined as primary (no menses by age 16) or secondary (absence of previously established menses for an interval of 1 year or longer). Initially, the evaluation of the amenorrhea should be thorough and include a complete history and physical examination (Table 47.1). In structurally normal women (who possess a uterus), in order to begin to establish a diagnosis the usual first tests done are serum follicle-stimulating hormone (FSH) and luteinizing hormone (LH). In those patients with normal gonadotropin values, causes for the menstrual disturbance other than ovarian failure are likely. Elevated values of gonadotropins (greater than 40 mIU/ml) suggest ovarian failure has occurred.

Patients with premature ovarian failure, usually defined as being younger than 40 years, usually present with amenorrhea and may complain of infertility or the symptoms of hypoestrogenism. Women with ovarian failure have been estimated to comprise between 1 and 3% of the general population. In fact, the disorder appears to be more com-

Table 47.1 Evaluation of young women with signs and symptoms of ovarian failure

Thorough history and physical examination

Obtain baseline bone density evaluation

LH, FSH, and E_2 assays on at least two occasions

Leukocytic karyotype

Antithyroglobulin and antimicrosomal antibodies, T_4, TSH

Complete blood count with differential, erythrocyte sedimentation rate, total serum protein and albumin : globulin ratio, rheumatoid factor, antinuclear antibody, fasting blood glucose, a.m. cortisol, serum calcium and phosphorus

LH, luteinizing hormone; FSH, follicle stimulating hormone; E_2, estradiol; T_4, thyroxine; TSH, thyroid stimulating hormone.

mon than appreciated previously, though it is likely that the wider availability of gonadotropin determinations has increased the frequency with which it is detected.

To prove a patient is hypergonadotropic, elevated levels of the gonadotropins FSH and LH should be documented on at least two occasions. Some investigators have suggested that the presence (or absence) of withdrawal bleeding in response to a progestin challenge obviates the need to measure basal FSH levels in amenorrheic women. This does not, however, appear to be a reliable method of determining ovarian failure, since almost half of affected individuals experienced withdrawal bleeding in response to exogenous progestin in a recent series by Rebar and Connolly [2]. Because the absence of menses from ovarian failure may be attributable to either decreased ovarian reserve, as in premature ovarian failure (also called premature menopause), or resistant ovary syndrome (follicular ovarian failure),

RESISTANT OVARY SYNDROME

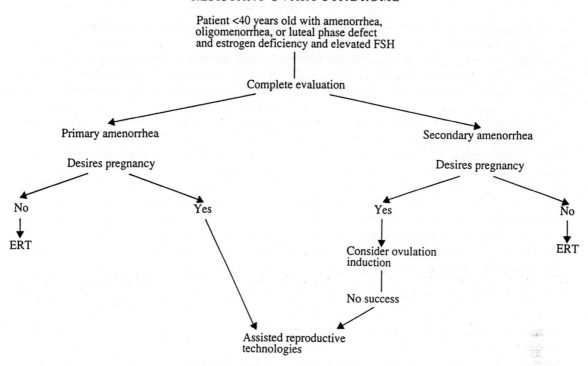

Fig. 47.1 Evaluation of young patients with evidence of ovarian failure, or luteal phase defect.

it has been suggested that these terms be condensed to the term hypergonadotropic amenorrhea, at least when initially encountering such patients. This group may include both primary and secondary amenorrhea patients.

Serum estradiol (E_2) should be obtained more than once during the course of the work-up, as well. Variability in the basal concentrations of estrogens among affected patients is great and the anticipated low circulating concentrations of estrogens characteristic of ovarian failure are not always present. This corresponds to the growing body of literature documenting evidence of follicular activity, ovulation, and even pregnancies occasionally occurring in women with confirmed hypergonadotropic amenorrhea. Thus, the measurement of serum LH, FSH, and E_2 concentrations on a number of occasions may be of prognostic value in determining if any ovarian follicles remain. At least some hope can be offered to infertile women with hypergonadotropinism if an increase in E_2 greater than 50 pg/ml or an LH:FSH ratio of greater than 1.0 is noted, suggesting some follicular activity remains. This is true since the vast majority of circulating E_2 is secreted by granulosa cells which are part of follicles containing oocytes. On the other hand, failure to

document elevations in E_2 may not preclude the existence of remaining oocytes.

Other laboratory studies which may be useful in helping to discern the etiology of ovarian failure includes a leukocytic karyotype, complete blood count with differential, sedimentation rate, total serum protein and albumin:globulin ratio, rheumatoid factor, antinuclear antibody, fasting blood sugar, morning cortisol, serum calcium and phosphorus, L-thyroxine (T_4), thyroid-stimulating hormone (TSH), antithyroglobulin, and antimicrosomal antibodies.

Ovarian failure associated with chromosomal abnormalities appears to be much more common in patients with primary amenorrhea, with or without pubertal development, but may be found in patients with secondary amenorrhea. It is especially important to obtain a karyotype in such women younger than age 30. This is supported by the series by Rebar and Connolly [2] in which more than half the patients with primary amenorrhea had abnormal karyotypes. Twenty percent of the genetically abnormal group had Y chromosomes and dysgerminomas when first seen.

Ovarian destruction by various chemotherapeutic agents used to treat malignancies of childhood and the early adult years has become increasingly common. Alkylating agents will produce ovarian failure in perhaps 50% of women so treated. Interestingly, the hypergonadotropic amenorrhea which ensues may be only transient. Radiation therapy may result in hypergonadotropic amenorrhea, as well. Also, epidemiologic studies have revealed an inverse dose–response relationship between the number of cigarettes smoked per day and the age of menopause. In some women this may represent an environmental cause for ovarian failure, though the responsible agent is unknown. Polycyclic aromatic hydrocarbons have been shown to be toxic to oocytes in several animal systems. However, since the number of female smokers is so great and premature ovarian failure so uncommon, it is difficult to establish a correlation between the two. The possibility, though, cannot be dismissed in the absence of more definitive data.

Temporal relationships between development of secondary amenorrhea and infections such as chicken pox, severe shigellosis, mumps, and malaria have been reported. There are also specific metabolic diseases associated with ovarian failure, such as deficiency of 17α-hydroxylase, the intraovarian enzyme involved in estrogen biosynthesis and galactosemia, an extraovarian cause of aberrant ovarian function, resulting from a deficiency of the enzyme galactose-1-phosphate uridyl transferase, which is involved in galactose metabolism even before birth. Familial premature ovarian failure has also been reported and affected women should be encouraged to inform their daughters of the possibility of early menopause. A thorough history should suggest such etiologies.

Often, a cause for ovarian failure is not established with certainty. In theory, an ovarian biopsy should easily enable the clinician to distinguish between follicular resistance and depletion, but in reality this has not proven to be the case. Until recently, the absence of ovarian function in individuals with hypergonadotropic amenorrhea was considered irreversible. This belief was based on findings of a group who performed ovarian biopsies on individuals with FSH levels greater than 40 mIU/ml. These individuals found that these patients, without exception, had no viable follicles on ovarian biopsy. Although ovarian biopsy has been advocated in evaluating young hypergonadotropic patients to determine if follicles are present, sampling error, especially prevalent with the use of laparoscopy, may prevent accurate diagnosis. Also, there have been a number of reports of pregnancies in women whose ovarian biopsies showed an absence of oocytes. Indeed, oocyte number may be markedly diminished in most patients and it is even possible that the remaining oocytes will be removed by biopsy. Thus, once the clinician has reached the point in a particular patient's work-up where he or she has eliminated most of the previously mentioned causes for ovarian failure, rather than considering an ovarian biopsy to establish a definite diagnosis, attention should be directly solely on therapy. The endpoints for ovarian failure, hypoestrogenism and infertility, are the same regardless of the etiology. At this point in time, existing therapies do not vary with the cause, though investigation into the latter from an academic viewpoint may reveal new options for patients in the future.

ETIOLOGY

In most reported series, immune abnormalities are present in 20–40% of women with premature ovarian failure and vary greatly in the type identified. In fact, autoimmune disturbances of the ovary are suspected of being the major cause of intermittent ovarian failure in the majority of women presenting with hypergonadotropic amenorrhea. Ovarian failure has often been noted in patients with polyglandular endocrinopathies including hypoparathyroidism, hypoadrenalism, and mucocutaneous candidiasis, but it seems reasonable to surmise that autoimmune ovarian failure may occur independently, as well. From a practical standpoint, it is most important to rule out thyroid antibodies and evidence of parathyroid and adrenal dysfunction. The most common endocrine disturbance occurring in association with hypergonadotropic amenorrhea is hypothyroidism resulting from thyroiditis. Although rare, hypoadrenalism and hypoparathyroidism can occur and are potentially life-threatening. Since poor pregnancy performance has been associated with anticardiolipid antibodies, the measurement of these antibodies may be reasonable.

In patients with premature ovarian failure in whom the presence of ovarian follicles has been documented, the possibility of the secretion of altered molecular forms of gonadotropins that are biologically inactive cannot be excluded. However, if the existence of altered forms of gonadotropins is to account for the apparent ovarian resistance in such patients, then treatment with exogenous human menopausal and chorionic gonadotropins (hMG and hCG) should be successful in such individuals. Such responses seem to be extremely rare. It is also possible that the patient may harbor antigonadotropin antibodies or have altered gonadotropin metabolism. It has been suggested that the resistant ovary syndrome might represent an FSH receptor protein defect, a concept supported by the familial tendency observed. However, it is difficult to explain ovulatory menses and even pregnancies in patients prior to the onset of symptoms of ovarian failure on the basis of a receptor site defect present since birth. An acquired receptor deficiency, however, could explain such a course of events. In patients with primary amenorrhea, the pathogenesis of the disorder could also be explained by failure of the gonadotropinreceptor complex to activate a critical postreceptor step, or a defect in the molecules necessary for these steps themselves. Such failures could lead to accelerated atresia and premature ovarian failure and could also be inherited defects. The molecular genetic etiology of such defects would make them undetectable by the usual banding techniques employed in karyotyping.

The finding of a number of patients with a familial tendency to ovarian failure is also consistent with the well-recognized familial nature of autoimmune disorders in general. In those patients with or without other detectable autoantibodies, there may be unrecognized circulating autoantibodies to the surfaces of some ovarian cells. In a proportion of cases the fluctuating nature of the ovarian failure may represent the undetected presence of specific blocking antibodies to the gonadotropin receptors on the ovaries, similar to those found in myasthenia gravis patients. Or there may be a combination of blocking and stimulating antibodies, as found in patients with Graves disease. A circulating inhibitor of FSH receptor binding that behaves as an immunoglobulin G has been found in some patients with hypergonadotropic amenorrhea and myasthenia gravis, but further work is needed to detect the presence of such antibodies in other patients. Thus far, there has been no specific cytogenetic marker or human leukocyte antigen type associated with early ovarian failure. Modern immunologic and molecular genetic tools may enable such etiologies to be determined more precisely in the future, and this may have implications for management. Some autoimmune problems may be more easily reversible in their early stages by treatment with corticosteroids or plasmapheresis, for example [3].

THERAPY

Consideration of estrogen replacement therapy is warranted in patients found to have even intermittent hypergonadotropic amenorrhea. The majority of such women have signs and symptoms of estrogen deficiency. Greater than 50% have significantly decreased bone density. Twice as much estrogen is usually necessary in these younger individuals than is required in postmenopausal women to alleviate symptoms. Therapy with estrogen and a progestin, cyclic or continuous, should be prescribed to prevent endometrial hyperplasia. If withdrawal bleeding fails to occur, a pregnancy test should be obtained, though the chance of conception is remote in those patients who do not wish to be pregnant but are sexually active.

FERTILITY

The patient interested in fertility should be advised that her condition is almost always end-stage and the prospects for spontaneous future conception bleak. Though there is evidence of ovulation in about a quarter of patients following establishment of the diagnosis, at present, it is not known how to induce ovulation in those who desire pregnancy. Clomiphene citrate and hMG are unlikely to be effective. Rarely, massive doses of gonadotropins can elicit an ovarian response. Suppression of gonadotropins with gonadotropin-releasing hormone agonist followed by concomitant hMG has failed to improve pregnancy rates.

There have been many instances of ovulation and pregnancy observed during or following exogenous estrogen treatment, but since no controlled studies have been undertaken it is impossible to discern whether these events occurred during intervals of rebound in affected patients or if a causal relationship truly exists. In rats, E_2 has been shown initially to promote the ability of FSH to increase and maintain FSH receptors by increasing the number of granulosa cells per ovary. Estrogens also have an antiatretic effect and promote differentiation of granulosa cells, as well as enhancing the appearance of LH receptors induced by FSH. Ovulation induction schemes have been proposed based on speculations that in humans suppression of excess endogenous gonadotropins might result in increased follicular sensitivity to gonadotropins and that follicular development can begin once FSH receptors are induced by exogenous estrogen. Though some cases of ovarian failure may be reversible with such regimens, the patient must be made aware that fewer than 10% of patients conceive with this type of therapy [4].

The poor prognosis for one type of fertility in women with ovarian failure has recently been challenged by the first successful pregnancy following *in vitro* fertilization and embryo transfer (IVF-ET) using donated oocytes into such a patient treated with steroid replacement by an Australian team at Monash University. This is especially encouraging for women with ovarian resistance or failure presenting with primary amenorrhea, a group in whom no pregnancies have previously been reported. At IVF centers around the world, success rates among this group of patients are higher than in any other group. For every attempt, the chances of taking home an infant appear to be about one in three. Thus, women desiring pregnancy should be advised to consider the possibility of utilizing donor oocytes, or donor embryos. Gamete intrafallopian transfer (GIFT) using donor oocytes and husband's sperm, tubal embryo transfer (TET) using donor oocytes, and transfer to a patient of an embryo retrieved by uterine lavage following fertilization with the patient's husband's sperm in the donor's reproductive tract have also been reported. These approaches, which use the intratubal rather than an *in vitro* environment to support embryo development and facilitate transfer to the uterus, appear to have even higher pregnancy rates per treatment cycle, ranging between 36 and 54%. Clearly, the ability to perform tubal transfers in a less invasive fashion from the vagina, instead of the currently prevalent laparoscopic approach, will foster a more widespread use of such techniques and promote their acceptability. At such a point, future randomized studies among GIFT, IVF-ET, and TET will be necessary to demonstrate whether there are any significant differences between these techniques in success rates for patients lacking gonadal function in whom gamete or embryo donation is indicated [5].

Synchronization in patients without gonadal function with the donor's cycle is established by beginning with estradiol tablets on the first day of the donor's menstrual cycle. Stepwise increases in the E doses are given until the day of the donor's LH peak or hCG injection. Progesterone (P) is added to the E regimen beginning the next day. For IVF-ET, oocyte retrieval is usually performed on the second day and ET on the fourth day following the donor's

LH peak or hCG injection. If establishment of a pregnancy is not detected chemically, steroid support is withdrawn from the recipient. If her hCG levels are found to be progressively rising, an ultrasound examination is performed at about 6 weeks' gestation to identify an intrauterine pregnancy with fetal cardiac activity. E and P support are completely withdrawn about 16–17 weeks, or when serum levels of E_2 and P are clearly documented to be increasing independently of the administered drug doses, though the luteoplacental shift has been shown to occur as early as 7 weeks in these patients and even earlier in patients with twin pregnancies.

CONCLUSIONS

Hypergonadotropic amenorrhea is an enigmatic disorder that every obstetrician-gynecologist might see during the course of practice. Whether it is the result of ovarian resistance to gonadotropin or decreased ovarian follicular reserve, its treatment consists primarily of hormonal replacement to prevent premature bone loss. In patients desiring pregnancy, attempts at ovulation induction with estrogen and hMG regimens may be considered in those presenting with secondary amenorrhea, but are unlikely to succeed. The advent of assisted reproductive technologies incorporating ovum and embryo donation has drastically altered, and increased, the potential for childbearing in all patients without gonadal function, though subject to the emotional, ethical, legal, and political considerations inherent in such procedures.

REFERENCES

1 Jones GS, DeMoraes-Ruehsen M. A new syndrome of amenorrhea in association with hypergonadotropinism and apparently normal ovarian follicular apparatus. *Am J Obstet Gynecol* 1969; 104: 597.
2 Rebar RW, Connolly HV. Clinical features of young women with hypergonadotropic amenorrhea. *Fertil Steril* 1990; 53: 804.
3 LaBarbera AR, Miller MM, Ober C, Rebar RW. Autoimmune etiology in premature ovarian failure. *Am J Reprod Immunol Microbiol* 1988; 16: 115.
4 Check JH, Nowroozi K, Chase JS, Nazari A, Shapse D, Vaze M. Ovulation induction and pregnancies in 100 consecutive women with hypergonadotropic amenorrhea. *Fertil Steril* 1990; 53: 811.
5 Rotsztejn DA, Rehomi J, Weckstein LN *et al*. Results of tubal embryo transfer in premature ovarian failure. *Fertil Steril* 1990; 54: 348.

48

Premature ovarian failure

MARIAN D. DAMEWOOD

Premature ovarian failure is defined as the cessation of menses before age 40 in association with increased levels of gonadotropins and a hypoestrogenic state. Early ovarian failure has been observed for many years but the nature of its etiology has remained obscure [1]. Premature ovarian failure in some instances has been regarded as an autoimmune disorder in association with circulating antibodies to ovarian tissue.

It is helpful to think of premature ovarian failure as being related to defects in the oocyte or follicular apparatus and to consider the temporal development of these defects. Prenatally, there may be a lack of oocytes, a lack of migration of oocytes, or an accelerated atresia of germ cells occurring as a result of a genetic defect or chromosomal abnormality. In addition, during the prenatal stage defective ovarian differentiation may occur. Postnatally accelerated atresia of oocytes may continue, most commonly resulting from chromosomal anomalies, as well as destruction of germ cells, a resistant follicular apparatus, abnormal gonadotropins, or circulating antiovarian antibodies with associated autoimmune states.

Investigations to determine the location or nature of the specific ovarian tissue antigen(s) have suggested various cell types [2] within the ovaries such as the granulosa or interstitial cells, or the follicle-stimulating hormone (FSH) and luteinizing hormone (LH) receptor apparatus. Definitive tissue confirmation of the antigen has not, however, been established. Premature ovarian failure has been associated with other autoimmune states, e.g. polyglandular syndrome, [3] and antiovarian antibodies have been demonstrated in 18–30% of patients with Addison's disease, myasthenia gravis, Hashimoto's thyroiditis, or Graves disease.

THE INDIFFERENT STAGE

It is important to note when considering early gonadal development that there is an inherent tendency to feminize. Thus an ovary will differentiate unless a gonad is directed by testicular organizing factors regulated by the Y chromosome. Therefore gonadal differentiation is regulated by the fetal testis. The indifferent stage in the human embryo begins at approximately 5 mm crown—rump length and lasts until about 15 mm, the time when testicular differentiation begins. During this stage of gonadal development germ cell migration is essential to the development of the normal gonad. The germ cells are generally located beneath the coelomic epithelium, and can be found in the endodermic wall of the primitive gut, at stages beginning with the differentiation of the genital ridge. From the endodermic wall germ cells migrate to the gonadal site. The gonadal ridges are thus invaded by germ cells by the fifth to sixth week of development. If this process fails to occur and the germ cells fail to reach the urogenital ridge, the gonad fails to develop.

GONADAL DIFFERENTIATION: OVARY

Ovarian differentiation occurs later than that of the testis, at approximately the 15–17 mm embryo or 11–13 weeks of gestational age. The primitive undifferentiated gonad is derived from mesodermal coelomic epithelium in the urogenital cell ridge. At 5 weeks, germ cells migrate through the dorsal mesentery to this ridge. If this gonad does not become a testis, an ovary will develop. The first step in ovarian differentiation occurs at approximately 12 weeks with the beginning of meiosis of the oogonia. At approximately 9 weeks of embryonic life the oogonia in the anterior part of the ovary contact the rete cords which secrete a substance which acts in the inductive capacity, termed meiosis-inducing factor. At 11–12 weeks the germ cells enter meiotic prophase, transforming the oogonia into oocytes, and at 25 weeks the primordial follicle is seen with granulosa cells surrounding it with a definitive ovarian structure.

MATURATION OF OOCYTES

In the female the first meiotic division occurs prior to birth and the transformation of oogonia into primary oocytes begins at approximately 11–12 weeks. Oogonia continue to develop by mitotic division however and at approximately 20 weeks of gestation 6–7 million oogonial cells are present. The formation of oogonia ceases at approximately 7 months of gestation with these cells, now primary oocytes, entering the prophase of the first meiotic division (diplotene stage). At birth approximately 2 million primary oocytes with a surrounding layer of granulosa cells, or primordial follicles, are estimated to be present. However, the process of oocyte atresia continues after birth so essentially 200 000 are present at menarche.

Completion of the first meiotic division is held until prior to ovulation when the first polar body is extruded, and the second meiotic division is not completed until fertilization has occurred. When considering the numbers presented, beginning with 6–7 million oogonia at 5 months, 2 million primary oocytes at term, 200 000 at menarche, and approximately 400 at the climacteric the process of atresia is indeed operative through the lifespan of ovarian function (Fig. 48.1) [3]. Ovulation thus never occurs from 99.1% of follicles. It is unclear to which mechanism of follicular development and progression the natural atretic process is directed.

ABNORMALITIES OF GONADAL DEVELOPMENT AND DIFFERENTIATION

Abnormalities of gonadal development and differentiation in the embryonic state may be associated with: (1) defects in germ cell migration; (2) defects in ovarian differentiation; (3) defects in testicular differentiation; and (4) accelerated atresia of germ cells

Defects in germ cell migration
Complete lack of migration of the germ cell to the urogenital ridge is an infrequent cause of primary gonadal failure. This entity, if present, may be associated with an inherited reduction in germ cell

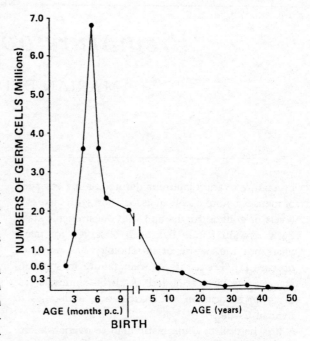

Fig. 48.1 Decline in the total number of germ cells in the human ovary from 6 months prenatal to the menopause. (Adapted from [3].)

endowment in cases of familial XX or XY gonadal dysgenesis. In this situation of a complete lack of germ cells, there is no induction of gonadal differentiation and a streak rather than a gonad is formed. In some cases germ cells do reach the urogenital ridge but in decreased numbers, which would lead to hypoplastic gonads and associated attrition of oogonia and premature ovarian failure in adult life. Some rare associations with increased germ cell number and migration to the urogenital ridge include the neurologic disorder myotonia dystrophica and the inherited enzyme disorder galactosemia. In galactosemia the level of galactose-1-phosphate uridyltransferase is reduced, with decreased oocyte numbers and possible interference in germ cell migration.

Defects in ovarian differentiation
Defects in ovarian differentiation are most often associated with the absence of two functioning X chromosomes. The malfunction of an X chromosome may occur as a consequence of a structural or genetic deletion. Most commonly referred to as gonadal dysgenesis, the most frequently recognized form is Turner's syndrome (Table 48.1). Turner's syndrome is associated with 45,XO chromosome complement

Table 48.1 Features of XO gonadal dysgenesis: Turner's syndrome

Phenotype	Short stature; sexual infantilism at puberty, somatic stigmata
External genitalia	Female
Internal genitatia	Female
Gonads	Streak
Inheritance	Sporadic; meiotic or mitotic nondisjunction
Karyotype	45,XO
Hormone profile	↑ Plasma LH and FSH concentrations
	↑ Plasma estradiol levels

LH, luteinizing hormone; FSH, follicle-stimulating hormone.

in patients with streak gonads present without oocytes. Pathologically, many tubal structures with degenerating ova and empty follicles are present. The mechanism by which the germ cells undergo a reduction in number is unknown. It has been postulated that the streak gonads may be due to a failure of follicular cells to surround the germ cell at the time when oogonial mitosis ceases and meiosis begins. This results in a failure of liberation of meiosis-inhibiting factor. Meiosis-inhibiting factor keeps the oocytes suspended in the prophase of meiosis I (which has been initiated by the rete signal meiosis-inducing substance). If the process of meiosis I is completed prematurely the oocytes degenerate. Oocyte atresia is accelerated in patients with Turner's syndrome, resulting in premature gonadal failure. Gonadal dysgenesis is a well-known entity with frequency estimated at one per 5000−7000 newborns. The karyotype 45,XO, however, is relatively rare with a frequency of occurrence of one in 10 000 live births. (Only 57% of patients with Turner's syndrome have the karyotype 45,XO.) The presence of more or fewer than two X chromosomes or of a structural abnormality in either X chromosome will result in premature gonadal failure and is often associated with other congenital anomalies. X chromosome mosaics, XO/XX, are well known and associated with primary or secondary amenorrhea. Patients with the 47,XXX karyotype also appear to have gonadal failure due to increased attrition of oocytes.

Gonadal dysgenesis in 46,XY individuals is significant in that these patients present with sexual infantilism and bilateral streak gonads. However, it is important to note that in 20−30% of these cases neoplastic transformation of the gonad may occur with resultant gonadoblastoma formation.

Accelerated germ cell atresia
There are other unusual circumstances where ac-

celerated germ cell atresia may occur in the female which include cases of abnormal forms of gonadotropins with immunologically active and biologically inactive LH or altered forms of immunoactive FSH and LH. Evidence also suggests that absence of the thymus gland may lead to accelerated follicular atresia in congenitally athymic girls who died before puberty [4]. It has been shown that thymic peptides can stimulate secretion of LH-releasing factor and thus LH, possibly accounting for the association of ovarian failure and thymic aplasia. Also galactosemia may result in increased oocyte atresia, with possibly alteration of the carbohydrate moieties of LH and FSH as the mechanism of ovarian follicular inactivity.

ABNORMALITIES IN OOCYTE MATURATION AND DEVELOPMENT: PREMATURE OVARIAN FAILURE

The processes of accelerated germ cell atresia or destruction of germ cells can occur postnatally and result in premature ovarian failure or premature menopause in the adult. Afollicular or primary ovarian failure has already been described and is most often associated with abnormal sex chromosome complement. The follicular type of ovarian failure which will be described in detail here is defined by the presence of numerous primordial follicles or follicles in various stages of maturation. This may be due to accelerated atresia and destruction of oocytes from extrinsic causes, resistance to circulating gonadotropins, or circulating antiovarian antibodies.

GONADOTROPIN-RESISTANT OVARY SYNDROME (RECEPTOR DEFECT)

In 1969 Jones and de Moraes-Rueshen described a syndrome of premature ovarian failure with hypogonadotropic amenorrhea and a normal follicular apparatus [5]. The ovaries were found to be resistant to gonadotropin stimulation. Diagnostic criteria for the gonadotropin-resistant ovary syndrome include the presence of primary or secondary amenorrhea in conjunction with secondary sexual development and Müllerian structures (Table 48.2). A 46,XX karyotype is noted with numerous primordial follicles on ovarian biopsy. Gonadotropins are elevated and the ovaries are usually resistant to exogenous gonadotropins. The most accurate criteria for detection of ovarian failure and ovarian resistance are elevated gonadotropin concentrations with no ovarian response as determined by clinical shift, estradiol, or ultrasound (during induction of ovulation with human menopausal gonadotropin). Current theories regarding the etiology of this syndrome of gonadotropin insensitivity include an abnormal FSH molecule, an FSH receptor defect, or abnormal responses of target cells. The gonadotropin-resistant ovary syndrome is one of the few situations of premature ovarian failure in which the appropriate high-dose gonadotropin therapy may in some cases result in pregnancy and thus it is important to maintain strict criteria of diagnosis.

17-HYDROXYLASE DEFICIENCY

The rare syndrome of 17-hydroxylase deficiency consists of those patients with sexual infantilism and primary amenorrhea associated with increased gonadotropin concentrations [6]. The 17-hydroxylase enzyme is essential not only for the synthesis of cortisol but also for the formation of gonadal hormones and adrenal steroids. Deficiency of this enzyme system is manifested in both adrenal and gonadal abnormalities. The affected individuals have increased levels of deoxycorticosterone and progesterone and they present with hypertension and hypokalemic alkalosis. Ovarian tissue from patients such as these

shows numerous primordial follicles and complete failure of normal follicular maturation.

ENVIRONMENTAL CAUSES OF OOCYTE LOSS (DESTRUCTIVE AGENTS)

Destruction of oocytes extrinsically is most frequently due to physical causes. Irradiation of the ovaries with 800 rad in 3 days is sufficient to induce ovarian failure. Patients irradiated for Hodgkin's disease receive 400—500 rad to the ovaries over 4—6 weeks [7]. In approximately 50% of patients, permanent amenorrhea occurs. Low-dose chronic irradiation of less than 25 rad will not cause sterility in human females (Table 48.3). Radiation therapy results in hypergonadotropin and hypoestrogenism within 4—8 weeks of therapy (Fig. 48.2). Several antitumor agents such as cyclophosphamide are associated with ovarian failure [8]. Viral illnesses such as mumps oophoritis have been postulated by some investigators to be responsible for premature ovarian failure.

AUTOIMMUNE ETIOLOGY OF PREMATURE OVARIAN FAILURE

Circulating antibodies to ovarian tissue have been demonstrated in the sera of patients with premature ovarian failure [2]. In several studies 18—30% of patients with premature ovarian failure had associated autoimmune disorders including Hashimoto's thyroiditis, Graves disease, Addison's disease, myasthenia gravis, hyperparathyroidism, pernicious anemia, and mucocutaneous candidiasis [1] (Table 48.4). These patients have been grouped by the term suggested by Coulam (polyglandular syndrome) [1]. All patients in the series had a 46,XX chromosome complement and several patients, on ovarian biopsy, had evidence of lymphocytic infiltration of the ovaries. Theories regarding etiology

Table 48.2 Diagnostic criteria for the gonadotropin resistant ovary syndrome

History	Primary or secondary amenorrhea
	Absence of autoimmune disease
Physical	Uterus and vagina present
Laboratory	Elevated FSH and LH
	46,XX karyotype
Pathology	Numerous primordial follicles on ovarian biopsy

FSH, follicle-stimulating hormone; LH, luteinizing hormone.

Table 48.3 Effects of ionizing radiation on ovarian function. (Adapted from [7])

Ovarian dose	Results
60	No deleterious effect
150	No deleterious effect in young women; some risk for sterilization in women older than 40
250–500	In women aged 15–40, 60% permanently sterilized; remainder may suffer temporary amenorrhea. In women older than 40, 100% permanently sterilized
500–800	In women aged 15–40, 60–70% permanently sterilized; remainder may experience temporary amenorrhea. No data available for women over 40
>800	100% permanently sterilized.

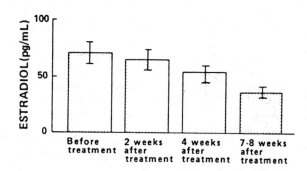

Table 48.4 Premature ovarian failure: commonly associated autoimmune conditions

Addison's disease
Chronic lymphocytic thyroiditis
Chronic mucocutaneous candidiasis
Graves disease
Hypoparathyroidism
Idiopathic thrombocytopenic purpura
Myasthenia gravis
Pernicious anemia
Vitiligo

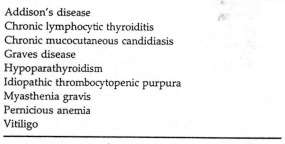

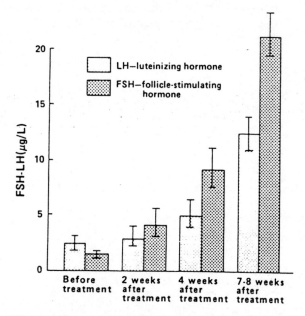

Fig. 48.2 Changes in gonadotropins and estradiol values after radiation therapy to the pelvis. (Adapted from [7].)

or mechanism for autoimmunity in ovarian failure include genetic factors, antireceptor antibodies, and/or specific tissue antigens in the ovary, including the theca interna or granulosa cells. Several techniques have been developed to determine the presence of circulating antibodies in premature ovarian failure, including immunofluorescence and ligand-binding methods. Since autoimmune ovarian failure will result in a lack of ovarian follicular development in a hypoestrogenic state it is important to diagnose this entity early and begin the appropriate hormone replacement therapy. Some patients may respond to high-dose glucocorticoid therapy and induction of ovulation can possibly be attempted.

EVALUATION AND THERAPY

Premature ovarian failure is suspected in a patient presenting with primary or secondary amenorrhea with an associated hypoestrogenic clinical picture.

CHAPTER 48

Table 48.5 Evaluation of premature ovarian failure patients. (Adapted from [4])

Complete history and physical examination

Maturation index
Karyotype

Complete blood count with differential, sedimentation rate, total serum protein and albumin:globulin ratio, rheumatoid factor, antinuclear antibody

Serum calcium and phosphorus, a.m. cortisol

T_4, TSH, antithyroglobulin, and antimicrosomal antibodies

Weekly serum LH, FSH, and estradiol ×4

Open ovarian biopsy (?)

T_4, thyroxine; TSH, thyroid-stimulating hormone; LH, luteinizing hormone; FSH, follicle-stimulating hormone.

A complete evaluation of the patient includes several steps [4] (Table 48.5).

Ovarian biopsy should be performed only in those situations where premature menopause, iatrogenic ovarian failure, gonadotropin resistance, or auto-immune oophoritis is suspected and should be reserved for the patient who desires to confirm the presence of oocytes prior to an attempt at induction of ovulation.

Hormone replacement therapy with cyclic estrogen and progesterone is indicated in those patients with no ovarian follicular function. Treatment schedules include conjugated or micronized estrogens 0.625–1.25 mg a day from days 1 to 25 of each month with addition of a progestogen on days 16 through 25. This cyclic regimen will alleviate the frequency of symptoms of estrogen deficiency in the young woman so affected [9].

REFERENCES

1 Coulam CB. Premature gonadal failure. *Fertil Steril* 1982; 38: 645–655.
2 Damewood MD, Zacur HA, Hoffman G, Rock JA. Circulating antiovarian antibodies in premature ovarian failure. *Obstet Gynecol* 1986; 68: 850–854.
3 Baker TG. Radiosensitivity of mammalian oocytes with particular reference to the human female. *Am J Obstet Gynecol* 1971; 110: 746.
4 Rebar RW. Hypergonadotropic amenorrhea and premature ovarian failure. *J Reprod Med* 1982; 27: 197–186.
5 Jones GS, de Moraes-Ruehsen M. A new syndrome of amenorrhea in association with hypergonadotropism and apparently normal ovarian follicular apparatus. *Am J Obstet Gynecol* 1969; 104: 597–600.
6 Biglieri EG, Herron MA, Brust N. 17-Hydroxylation deficiency in man. *J Clin Invest* 1966; 45: 1946–1954.
7 Ash P. The influence of radiation on fertility in man. *Br J Radiol* 1980; 53: 271.
8 Damewood MD, Grochow L. Prospects for fertility after chemotherapy or radiation for neoplastic disease. *Fertil Steril* 1986; 45: 443.
9 Damewood MD. What factors underlie premature ovarian failure? *Contemp Obstet/Gynecol* 1990; 35: 31.

Part V

The breast

Abnormal breast examination

MARIA D. ALLO

Breast cancer is a common disease affecting one of every 10 women in the USA within her lifetime. Consequently, fear of breast cancer is one of the most frequent reasons women seek medical advice. Symptoms of breast pain, mass, nipple discharge, and skin and nipple changes are the most common presenting complaints (Fig. 49.1).

BREAST PAIN

Breast pain which is cyclic in nature is most likely related to fibrocystic change. However, breast pain associated with a movable, well-circumscribed mass should be needle aspirated. Emanation of fluid defines it as a cyst which should be aspirated dry. If no fluid returns, the lesion is a solid mass in which case fine-needle aspiration can be done. Most well-circumscribed movable solid lesions are benign fibroadenomas. However, occasionally, particularly in perimenopausal and postmenopausal women, these lesions may represent breast cancers.

BREAST MASSES

All breast masses require evaluation and, if suspicious, require biopsy. Patients should be instructed to be alert to solitary lumps, particularly ones which are hard and have irregular borders. These lumps are usually nontender and patients can be reassured that breast pain is usually not a major symptom of breast cancer. Biopsy incisions should be made in the direction of skin lines and with consideration of the potential for segmental resection or mastectomy. Should the lesion be malignant, the area of the biopsy incision would need to be incorporated into the resected specimen. Fine-needle aspiration provides an excellent noninvasive method for evaluating breast lumps. A needle of small caliber is inserted into the lump and cells are aspirated and studied cytologically. Because there may be a sampling error,

it is sometimes necessary to take multiple samples within the same lump. An experienced pathologist is needed to interpret the cytology.

NIPPLE DISCHARGE

Nipple discharge is frightening to the patient but is usually associated with benign disease. Galactorrhea (milky nipple discharge in the absence of pregnancy or lactation) has multiple causes. The most significant problem associated with galactorrhea is pituitary micro- or macroadenoma. For this reason, patients presenting with galactorrhea should have blood drawn for serum prolactin levels. There are many other causes of galactorrhea, including other forms of benign hypothalamic—pituitary dysfunction (e.g., Forbes—Albright syndrome), chronic renal disease, hypothyroidism, and drugs such as pheno-thiazines, tricyclic antidepressants, dopamine antagonists and agonists, and oral contraceptives which may be responsible for abnormal prolactin levels and associated galactorrhea. Reflex stimulation of the breast is a frequent cause of benign galactorrhea. The so-called jogger's nipple syndrome is an example of one kind of mechanical stimulation resulting in nipple discharge. Sometimes a measure as simple as having a patient refit her bra may cure galactorrhea by removing mechanical stimulation from garments that compress or continually rub against the breast. Nonmilky brown discharge which tests positive for blood, or which is frankly bloody, usually indicates intraductal papilloma. About 30% of the time associated malignancy is present.

Bloody discharges require evaluation and consideration for duct excision. In examining a patient with bloody nipple discharge, it is important to ascertain whether the discharge is unilateral or bilateral, and which duct or ducts are involved. Green, yellow, or nonmilky white discharges are associated with low-grade chronic infection of the

CHAPTER 49

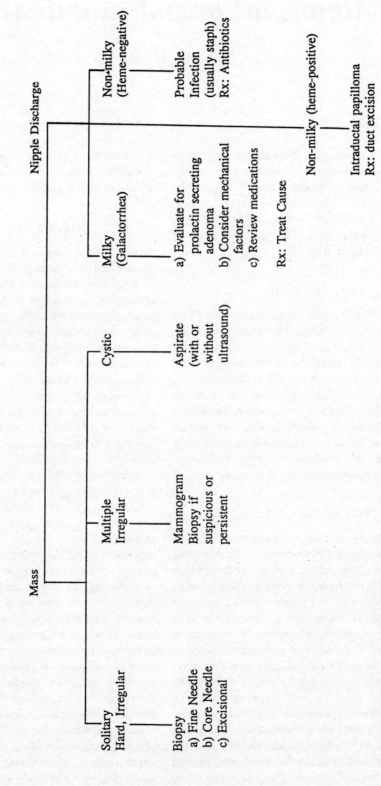

Fig. 49.1 Decision making tree for an abnormal breast examination.

304

ducts that is generally responsive to antibiotics. This is seen in older women with ductal ectasia and young women with fibrous mastopathy. Acute infection presenting as diffuse cellulitis or frank abscess may present with a sticky, yellow, purulent discharge from the nipple that most commonly cultures *Staphylococcus aureus*.

NIPPLE AND SKIN CHANGES

All patients who have change in appearance of the skin overlying the breast or nipple require evaluation. Significant findings include dimpling of the skin, retraction of skin, and nipple inversion in which the nipple had not been previously inverted. Any of these may signify fairly advanced breast cancer.

PHYSICAL EXAMINATION OF THE BREAST

The examination of the breasts should be carried out in both the sitting and supine positions. Patients should be stripped to the waist to allow thorough inspection prior to palpation. Inspection should include looking for asymmetry of the breasts, tension on the breast skin, and skin lesions with particular attention to the preareolar area. Scaly skin lesions about the nipple might indicate Paget's disease which is often associated with intraductal carcinoma.

Next, the breasts are palpated in an orderly manner. The specific method of palpation is not important as long as it is organized so as not to miss any major parts of the breast. By using variable finger pressure, deeper or more superficial lesions can be delineated and not missed. After initial palpation, a second examination is carried out with the patient's hands placed on her hips, and shoulders relaxed. Final palpation is then done with the arms raised above the head. At this time lymph nodes are palpated in the axillary and superclavicular regions. Next, the examination as described above is repeated in the supine position. In patients presenting with nipple discharge, the nipple should be squeezed to release the discharge.

MAMMOGRAPHY

Yearly mammography is recommended by the American Cancer Society for all women over age 50. At age 35–40 a baseline mammogram is recommended. Between age 40 and 50, examinations are recommended every 1–2 years. In a woman with a family history of premenopausal breast cancer consideration may be given to mammography beginning at an earlier age. However, because of the density of the younger breasts these mammograms are not always very revealing. Careful clinical examinations are probably as good a screening device as X-ray in younger women. A mass which is dense and has irregular margins is mammographically suspicious for carcinoma. Peripheral spiculations are frequently present. Mammographic signs of breast cancer include small masses, calcifications, and some subtle and indirect signs which will be discussed later. There are some rare forms of breast cancer which can present as well-circumscribed nodules. These look very much like benign cysts or fibroadenomas on mammogram and need to be carefully evaluated clinically. Specifically, papillary carcinomas can arise in cysts and dilated lactiferous ducts. Colloid carcinomas, found mostly in postmenopausal women, may appear as well-circumscribed lesions that are sharply separated from surrounding tissue. It cannot be emphasized enough that these lesions must be evaluated clinically by needle aspiration, excisional biopsy or, if deep, by sonography to delineate a cystic from a solid mass. A negative mammogram does not preclude cancer in a breast in which a suspicious lump has been palpated. Approximately 15% of malignant mass lesions do not appear mammographically as such, either because underlying thick breast parenchyma obscures them or because their radiodensity is comparable to that of the normal breast.

Mammography is important in the detection of cancer because of its ability to demonstrate clusters of microcalcifications which may indicate malignancies which are not palpable because of their small size. These calcifications are usually numerous and vary in size and shape. Generally the presence of six or more microcalcifications in a cluster would warrant a biopsy and often, because of the nonpalpable nature of these lesions, biopsies need to be done with radiographic needle localization. In contrast to small microcalcifications, a number of conditions can produce nonspecific calcifications which may actually be in skin, or benign calcifications related to trauma or epithelial hypoplasia. Nonclustered calcifications usually indicate a benign condition such as sclerosing adenosis. In situations where the significance of calcifications is equivocal, magnification views are helpful. Secondary mammographic features such as skin thickening, skin or nipple retraction, or enlarged axillary nodes are not very helpful since most of the time a clinical examination has already indicated these findings. Indirect mammographic signs of malignancy include single dilated ducts, architectural distortions in the breast, asymmetric densities or densities which appear to be changing from one study to the next. Architectural distortions are usually the result of previous breast surgery and often have spiculations emanating from the radial scar that are extremely difficult to differentiate from scirrhous carcinomas. These must be carefully evaluated by the surgeon and radiologist in order to rule out malignant disease. Asymmetric densities also need to be evaluated clinically. Sometimes cone compression views are helpful to distinguish true architectural distortion from projectional asymmetry related to positioning of the patient. It is important that asymmetric densities being considered for biopsy be identifiable on two different mammographic projections. In a woman who has had a previous mammogram, it is imperative that comparison be made to the original mammogram. Evolution of a previously noted density may indicate early breast cancer.

SURGICAL TREATMENT OPTIONS FOR BREAST DISEASE

The initial invasive procedure is done in order to make a definitive diagnosis. Three options are currently used: fine-needle aspiration cytology, core needle biopsy, and excisional biopsy. All can be performed with local anesthesia with or without intravenous sedation.

Fine-needle aspiration cytology
This was described earlier under breast masses.

Core needle biopsy
A piece of tissue from the lump is extracted using a Tru-cut or other available biopsy needle. Often several samples are taken. The patient undergoing biopsy by this method should be aware that excisional biopsy may be required if an adequate sample cannot be obtained by this method. Very soft tumors, those with necrotic centers, and some with a large mucinous component, may not be amenable to biopsy by this method.

Excisional Biopsy
Excisional biopsy refers to local excision of the tumor grossly without regard to microscopic margins of resection. For lesions which are found mammographically and are not palpable, localization of the area to be biopsied can be done radiographically immediately prior to the biopsy. A mammogram of the excised specimen can confirm successful excision of the lesion.

DEFINITIVE PROCEDURES FOR LOCAL MANAGEMENT OF MALIGNANT LUMPS

Once diagnosis has been made options for definitive local management are considered. Because several options exist, some of which involve nonsurgical specialists, most practitioners no longer do a one-stage (biopsy and, if positive, proceed to mastectomy) approach. Possibilities for local management include radical mastectomy, modified radical mastectomy, and limited resection plus radiotherapy.

Radical mastectomy
Radical mastectomy, once the gold standard, is currently limited to situations where the tumor extends through the pectoralis fascia. This procedure differs from modified radical mastectomy in that the pectoralis muscle is removed along with the breast and axillary contents. Removal of this muscle leaves a considerable cosmetic, if not also a functional, deformity. Studies looking at outcome in women with tumors not violating the pectoralis fascia show no survival advantage for women undergoing this more extensive procedure. For this reason it has been largely abandoned.

Modified radical mastectomy
This refers to removal of the entire breast down to and including the pectoralis fascia with level I and II dissection (dissection of the axillary contents from the tail of the breast inferiorly, beneath the pectoralis minor medially, the latissimus dorsi muscle laterally and the axillary vein superiorly). For any resectable lesion this procedure should be offered as an option. At the present time it represents the standard against which local procedures are compared.

Limited surgery with radiotherapy
For stage I and some higher-stage tumors, limited surgery with postoperative radiotherapy has been

shown to compare favorably with mastectomy with respect to outcome. It has the advantage of preserving the breast with good cosmetic results. The major selection issue is whether the primary tumor can be resected without significant cosmetic deformity. The lesions most amenable to conservative management are the lateral upper quadrant lesions. For subareolar and very medial lesions, especially on patients with small breasts, one must weigh the cosmetic results achievable against those obtainable with mastectomy and reconstruction. Likewise some women with very large or very pendulous breasts may opt for mastectomy of the affected breast with reconstruction and mastopexy or reduction mammoplasty of the contralateral breast. It is important that patients considering limited resection and radiation confer with the radiotherapist prior to making a final decision since technical and logistic considerations pertinent to the radiation therapy may significantly influence the therapeutic decision. It is also important that the surgeon and radiation therapist work closely together. For example, the decision to give a boost dose of radiation to the area of the lesion is partially predicated on the extent of resection, and the ability to boost requires accurate depiction of the tumor's location within the breast. In general the amount of radiation required for treatment is inversely proportional to the amount of surgery performed.

An axillary dissection is performed for purposes of staging, and if there are clinically suspicious nodes to remove the metastatic disease. Although some authors have advocated node sampling, most authors still recommend level I and II node dissection as the gold standard.

Chemotherapy

The preceding sections have dealt with management of local disease. In the presence of disease outside the breast, systemic therapy is indicated. Because many regimens and combinations are rapidly changing, details as to various protocols and dosages will not be included here. Suffice it to say that the decision about procedure to manage local disease is independent of the decision to use chemotherapy.

FURTHER READING

Fisher B, Bauer M, Margolese R et al. Ten year results of a randomized clinical trial comparing radical mastectomy and total mastectomy with or without radiation. N Engl J Med 1985; 312: 674–681.

Horgan PG, Waldon D, Mooney E et al. The role of aspiration cytologic examination in the diagnosis of carcinoma of the breast. Surg Gynecol Obstet 1991; 172: 290–297.

Kurtz JM, Jacquemier J, Amabric R et al. Breast conserving therapy for macroscopically multiple cancers. Ann Surg 1990; 212: 38–44.

Nicastri GR, Reed WP, Dziura BR. The accuracy of malignant diagnosis established by fine needle aspiration cytologic procedures of mammary masses. Surg Gynecol Obstet 1991; 172: 457–464.

Progress Symposium – Benign Breast Disorders. Fibrocystic disease? Nondisease? Or ANDI? World J Surg 1989; 13: 667–815.

Stolter A, Atkinson EN, Fairston BA et al. Survival following locoregional recurrence after breast conservation therapy for cancer. Ann Surg 1990; 212: 166–172.

Tabar L, Fagerberg CIG, Gad A et al. Reduction in mortality from breast cancer after mass screening with mammography: randomized trial from the breast cancer screening working group of the Swedish National Board of Health and Weltare. Lancet 1985; 1: 829–832.

50

Breast pain

RICHARD B. DAMEWOOD

INTRODUCTION

Breast pain is a common problem, often resulting in the presentation of women to their physicians. Frequently, the degree of pain is minimal and the patient may desire assurance that it is not a manifestation of breast cancer. Alternatively, the pain may be so severe that the patient is seeking symptomatic relief as well as diagnosis. For this reason, physicians assessing women with breast pain must have a plan for both diagnosis and therapy.

DIFFERENTIAL DIAGNOSIS

As discussed previously, breast cancer is an important consideration in the differential diagnosis of any breast symptom, and breast pain is no exception. However, it is relatively rare that breast cancer presents primarily as breast pain. On the other hand, simple gross breast cysts frequently present as acute onset of a localized pain, usually accompanied by an easily palpable mass found in the area of tenderness. Breast abscesses may also present as an area of localized pain, usually with other obvious signs of inflammation. Surprisingly, on occasion a patient referred for the evaluation of breast pain may be pregnant. It is exceedingly important to consider this possibility in all women of reproductive age, since a mammogram may be obtained during the evaluation of the patient's problem.

Other causes of breast pain include Tietze syndrome, Mondor's disease, and cervical spine disease. Tietze's syndrome is a form of costochondritis characterized by tenderness directly over the costochondral junction associated with swelling. Other forms of idiopathic costochondritis are recognized which do not involve swelling. The etiology of these entities is uncertain and they may be refractory to therapy, though nonsteroidal antiinflammatories are often prescribed. Mondor's disease is a form of superficial thrombophlebitis of the veins of the breast. An indurated cord in the breast, especially over the lateral surface, is observed. The cord can often extend beyond the breast on to the chest wall, which may assist in differentiating the problem from other causes of an indurated area in the breast. The etiology is most likely traumatic and the cord usually resolves spontaneously or may improve with nonsteroidal antiinflammatory agents. Cervical disk problems may lead to radicular pain referred to the breast area. These cases are usually associated with pain radiating to areas outside the breast as well. Appropriate radiologic and neurologic evaluation establishes the source of the pain.

Finally and commonly, the source of breast pain is determined to be in the diagnostic category of mastalgia. Presentations may range from cases of mild cyclic breast pain, which are essentially physiologic, to cases of severe debilitating pain. The correlation between the pathologic entities associated with the term fibrocystic disease and the clinical entity of mastalgia is tenuous and uncertain. Studies in general have failed to link the two in a consistent manner and for this reason it is best to consider mastalgia as a clinical entity.

Generally, two patterns of mastalgia are recognized [1]. The first consists of cyclic pain usually peaking in the luteal phase. The pain tends to be bilateral, poorly localized, and associated with diffuse nodularity in the upper outer quadrants. In Preece's study at the Cardiff Mastalgia Clinic [1], approximately 75% of the patients fit this category. Because this presentation resembles an exaggerated version of breast changes that are felt to be physiologic in relation to the menstrual cycle, it is natural that theories about the origin of this problem have concentrated on a hormonal basis. Imbalance between estrogen and progesterone production is one suggested mechanism. Estrogen in the form of estradiol is the hormone responsible for breast duct proliferation, increased ductal cell activity, and stimulation of the periductal connective tissue. Progesterone has both synergistic and antagonistic actions with respect to estrogen, acting synergistically with estrogen on the acinar stuctures to complete their differentiation but antagonistically on the ductal cells by promoting cellular differentiation and mitotic rest [2]. It is theorized that an imbalance in estrogen production relative to progesterone production leads to overstimulation of ductal cells and the surrounding stroma. This, in turn, results in breast pain with a cyclic component. Thus, a form of luteal-phase defect may be responsible for this form of mastalgia. Clinical studies of this possibility have produced mixed results. A second possible hormonal mechanism for breast tenderness has been suggested to be prolactin and at least one study has shown a small basal elevation of prolactin levels in patients with cystic disease [3].

The second group of patients with mastalgia have pain which is unrelated to the menstrual cycle [1]. The pain is continuous and tends to be unilateral and localized. Fewer patients present with this entity, it may be difficult to differentiate such pain from other causes of focal pain. The etiology is uncertain but focal unilateral mastalgia is less responsive to hormonal therapy.

DIAGNOSIS

The usual history and physical examination with emphasis on the preceding considerations should help place the patient's symptoms into a general category (Fig. 50.1). Discrete palpable masses will require aspiration. This will allow immediate diagnosis and treatment of a gross cyst or an aspiration cytology of a solid discrete nodule. A solid nodule will warrant an excisional biopsy, even in the event of a benign cytology, because of the possibility of sampling error.

Mammography is frequently indicated to rule out underlying nonpalpable lesions. In women of reproductive age it is important to be sure there is no chance of ongoing pregnancy prior to performing the study. Mammography will be more productive in older patients due to the replacement of dense glandular tissue by fat, allowing increasing resolution by the technique, and due to the naturally increasing incidence of significant lesions with age. Younger women will frequently show increased breast parenchyma and density on mammogram and this is of

questionable relevance with regard to the patient's breast pain other than the possibility that lesions might be obscured. As always, any discrete palpable abnormality should be surgically excised even in the presence of a normal mammogram, because of the approximately 10—15% incidence of breast cancers which may be missed on mammogram.

Ultrasound examination of the breast may be very useful when evaluating breast pain. The primary role of ultrasound is to differentiate solid from cystic areas of breast parenchyma. Ultrasound examination of a focal area of breast tenderness which is normal to palpation may reveal clear evidence of multiple or solitary cysts. Palpable lesions which are not aspirated because of patient refusal or technical difficulties may be evaluated by ultrasound. If the lesion is clearly cystic, ultrasound-guided aspiration or medical therapy may be attempted. Other modalities of diagnosis such as thermography or breast transillumination have not gained widespread acceptance and their current role is limited.

TREATMENT

As noted previously, breast pain of nonbreast etiology is treated according to the source of the pain. Infections of the breast are treated with the appropriate combination of antibiotics and surgical drainage. Solid lumps associated with pain are treated by excision, primarily to establish that they are benign. Any residual symptoms can then be addressed with medical therapy, as outlined in the following section.

Acute isolated cyst formation deserves separate comment. The pain associated with this condition is generally due to distention of the breast parenchyma by the swollen cyst. Aspiration will relieve these symptoms. Though these cysts are rarely associated with malignancy, characteristics which are felt to warrant surgical excision include bloody cyst fluid, solid residual mass after aspiration, and recurrence of the same cyst multiple times. Further medical therapy for an aspirated cyst which meets criteria for benignity is indicated for those patients who have a history of multiple recurrent cysts over a short period of time and who desire an alternative to multiple aspirations, or patients whose risk for breast cancer is high and in whom multiple cysts might mask an early cancer.

The remaining patients fall into the category of primary mastalgia. For the majority of these patients no therapy will be necessary once they are assured that

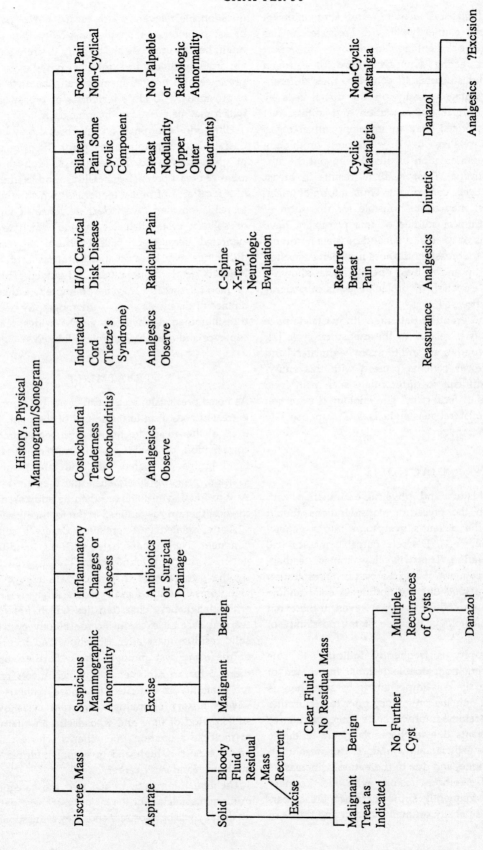

CHAPTER 50

Fig. 50.1 Decision making tree for breast pain.

there is no evidence of cancer. Other patients will be interested in therapeutic options to the degree that the therapy's side-effects do not outweigh benefits.

Therapy may be initiated with analgesics, usually in the form of nonsteroidal antiinflammatory agents. Occasionally, low doses of diuretics given premenstrually will have a dramatic effect on mastalgia. Dietary measures such as abstinence from caffeine or other methylxanthine-containing agents have been suggested as a possible therapy. Although some studies have shown a possible correlation between caffeine intake and fibrocystic disease, other studies have been inconclusive and no definitive proof is available that caffeine abstinence will improve mastalgia [4]. Nevertheless, caffeine abstinence is a relatively innocuous measure and in some patients does seem to improve symptoms. Various vitamins have also been suggested as a possible therapy for mastalgia. Of these, vitamin E has shown the most promise. In a manner similar to caffeine, early less poorly controlled studies seemed to indicate that vitamin E significantly improved fibrocystic disease. However, follow-up controlled studies failed to confirm this effect [5].

Hormonal therapy may be effective for severe mastalgia. As noted previously, this has been primarily effective in those patients with the cyclic form of mastalgia. The only Food and Drug Administration-approved therapy for mastalgia is danazol. Danazol is an androgenic heterocyclic steroid with marked antigonadotropic effects. Clinical trials in the use of danazol for mastalgia have demonstrated a significant decrease in breast symptomatology in 70–90% of patients with doses from 50 to 400 mg/day [6]. This effect may be seen after several weeks of therapy and some patients will experience a complete cessation of symptoms. Nodularity of the breasts may decrease as well, though less noticeably. Patients treated with danazol may develop the full spectrum of side-effects inherent in the use of this drug, which include weight gain, acne, increase in hirsutism, and oily skin. Though it is reported that these problems are low in incidence and tolerated well, many patients refuse therapy with danazol when apprised of these possible side-effects.

Other hormonal regimens suggested for therapy of mastalgia have included the prolactin-decreasing agents bromocriptine and progesterone. The use of these agents is obviously rooted in the previously mentioned theories concerning the origin of cyclic mastalgia. Clinical trials with both agents have been performed with some success, but neither regimen has been studied enough to be recommended as standard therapy.

Therapy for the second pattern of mastalgia is more problematic. Analgesics may provide some relief. Hormonal therapy has generally not been shown to be effective. If the pain is truly localized or associated with a trigger point, surgical resection of the area would seem to be a logical option. However, the success rate for this is estimated to be only about 50% [7]. A more effective therapy for this clinical entity awaits better understanding of the etiology of the problem.

CONCLUSIONS

Breast pain is significant for both the psychologic effect of its implication for the patient and for the degree to which the pain physically affects the patient. A careful history and physical examination, complemented by appropriate diagnostic procedures, should allow the physician both to reassure most patients and to offer effective therapeutic options.

REFERENCES

1 Preece PE, Hughes LE, Mansel RE et al. Clinical syndromes of mastalgia. Lancet 1976; 2: 670–673.
2 Mauvais-Jarvis P, Sitruk-Ware R, Kuttenn F et al. Luteal phase insufficiency: a common pathophysiologic factor in development of benign and malignant breast disease. In: Bulbrook RD, Taylor DJ, eds. Commentaries on Research in Breast Disease. New York: Alan R. Liss, 1979: 25–59.
3 Cole EM, Sellwood RA, England PC et al. Serum prolactin concentrations in benign breast disease throughout the menstrual cycle. Eur J Cancer 1977; 13: 597–603.
4 Ernster VL, Mason L, Goodson WH et al. Effects of caffeine-free diet on benign breast disease: a randomized trial Surgery 1982; 91: 263.
5 London R, Sundarum GS, Murphy L et al. The effect of vitamin E on mammary dysplasia. Obstet Gynecol 1985; 65: 104.
6 Brookshaw JD. Danazol treatment of benign breast disease: a survey of USA multicentre studies. Postgrad Med J 1979; 55 (suppl 5): 52–58.
7 Mansal RE. Diagnosis and treatment of mastalgia. In: Grundfest-Broniatowski S, Esselstyn CB, eds. Controversies in Breast Disease. New York: Marcel Dekker, 1988: 72.

51

Mammography: diagnosis and screening

BERNARD E. ZELIGMAN

Several decades of clinical experience with breast imaging, during which mammographic image quality has improved significantly while radiation doses have decreased greatly, have culminated in widespread acceptance of mammography while some other modalities proposed for breast imaging have failed to live up to their promise. Mammography is now the major modality for breast imaging and is the only imaging method suitable to screen for cancer.

This discussion is an orientation of the role of mammography in the diagnostic setting and of the management of various findings that may be discovered during screening. In both settings, a clinician who optimally uses this important imaging technique not only should appreciate the effectiveness of mammography but also should be aware of its limitations.

MAMMOGRAPHY WHEN A MASS IS PALPABLE

Although mammography is mainly a screening tool, a mammogram should be obtained if a woman with a palpable mass is of "cancer age" — certainly if she is at least 40 years old and probably if she is in her 30s (Fig. 51.1). The mammogram should precede open biopsy or needle aspiration because hematoma and edema from biopsy can alter the mammographic appearance of the breast and because postbiopsy tenderness may preclude the vigorous compression necessary for a good mammogram.

The major purpose of the mammogram is to detect any clinically occult finding in either breast, in addition to the palpable mass, that might be malignant. The mammogram is, therefore, used mainly for screening even when a mass is palpable. The mammogram also may provide some impression about whether the mass is malignant and, if malignant,

may help assess the extent of cancer in the breast.

A basic principle is that the mammogram should not be obtained to determine if aspiration or biopsy of the palpable mass can be avoided. Actually, a mammogram occasionally does prove that a palpable mass is benign but too seldom for this to be a purpose of the mammogram. If the mammogram shows that the mass contains fat, the mass is a lipoma, hamartoma, galactocele, oil cyst, or intramammary lymph node. One other mammographic mass appearance is reassuring enough to avoid further evaluation: a well-circumscribed mass containing macrocalcifications is almost always a fibroadenoma [1].

These definitely benign masses by mammography are the exception to the rule. Cancer often produces a mammographic abnormality indistinguishable from benign disease and sometimes shows nothing abnormal at all. The false-negative rate of mammography for a palpable cancer, at least with routine mammographic views, is about 20% [2]. While special views may decrease this false-negative rate, the rate remains significant. Unless one of these uncommon definitely benign masses by mammography corresponds to the palpable mass, the mammogram should be followed by evaluation with one or more modalities: aspiration for fluid, ultrasound to look for cystic characteristics, fine-needle aspiration cytology, core needle biopsy, or open biopsy. With these occasional exceptions, the basic rule is that when a mass is palpable, a mammogram negative for a mass or for malignancy should be ignored.

The role of mammography is different when a woman with a palpable mass is in her teens or 20s because a mammogram provides less benefit with more risk than when a woman is older. At this age, the possibility is less that the palpable mass is malignant or that an incidental clinically occult cancer exists; mammography is less capable of demonstrating masses because the breasts tend to be more radiodense; and the breasts are more susceptible to

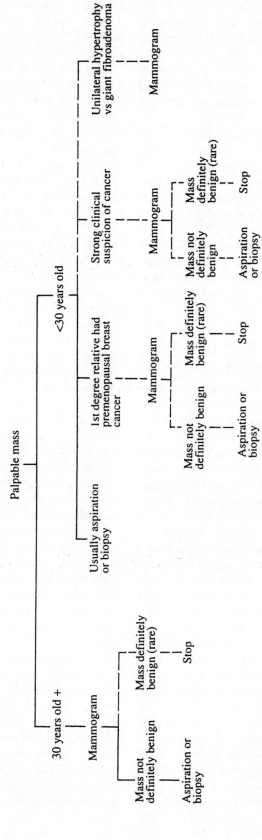

Fig. 51.1 Mammography when a mass is palpable. Dashed lines indicate common pathways.

radiogenic cancer. For most women under 30, the mass should be evaluated without a mammogram unless biopsy reveals malignancy. This approach is recommended not because the palpable mass couldn't be cancer — it could be and needs further evaluation — but because the small possibility that the mammogram will alter management does not justify the radiation exposure and expense [3].

Mammography should be the first step to evaluate a palpable mass when a woman is under 30 only: (1) if clinical suspicion that the mass is cancer is very high; (2) if first-degree relatives of the patient have had breast cancer before menopause — a family history that indicates the patient is at high risk of developing cancer at a young age; or (3) if, when one breast of an adolescent is much larger than the other, physical examination fails to distinguish between unilateral increased volume of normal breast tissue (unilateral adolescent hypertrophy) and a neoplasm (usually a giant fibroadenoma).

CLINICALLY OCCULT MAMMOGRAPHIC FINDINGS

Mammography has somewhat limited value for diagnosis but is effective for screening. Breast cancer usually is detectable mammographically before it is detectable clinically, and this earlier detection permits breast conservation therapy more often than when cancer is more advanced and probably results in modestly decreased mortality [4]. Although mammography usually detects cancer first, physical examination detects cancer first about 10% of the time and should be part of a screening regimen.

The basic principle of mammographic screening results from this high sensitivity of mammography for detecting cancer and from the fact that most women who develop breast cancer have no special risk factors. Recommendations for biopsy for mammographic findings stand on their own. When biopsy is recommended because of a mammographic finding, the absence of any finding suggestive of cancer on physical examination and the absence of any special risk factors for breast cancer are irrelevant; biopsy always should be done.

Management of a nonpalpable mammographic finding which raises suspicion of malignancy is based on the probability that the finding is malignant, that is, the predictive value of that finding for malignancy. Biopsy is indicated when the probability of malignancy is significant enough to warrant the physical morbidity, psychological stress, and financial cost of biopsy. Mammographic follow-up is chosen, instead, for findings that are only occasionally malignant [5].

Even with mammographic follow-up of minimally suspicious findings, most mammographic findings that lead to biopsy turn out to be benign because many cancers, especially early ones, are mammographically indistinguishable from benign disease. The malignant rate for biopsies performed because of mammographic findings has varied in published series from about 10% to about 40% and at the University of Colorado (unpublished data) has been 20%, a rate similar to the reported rate of malignancy when biopsies are performed because of palpable masses. Just as an 80% false-negative cancer rate is accepted for biopsies of palpable masses, a similar false-negative rate for mammographic findings should not cause recommendations for biopsies to be ignored.

Comparison to previous mammograms a woman may have had is the first step when a mammographic finding raises concern about cancer. When a somewhat suspicious but probably benign finding is unchanged for several years, the finding is almost always benign. Also, recognizing one sign of cancer — a new density — obviously requires old films. Interpretation of a mammogram should be deferred until comparison films are available, even if waiting for films from another facility is required.

When a finding on routine mammographic views raises concern about malignancy, the next step after comparison to any previous mammograms is often more mammography. Additional views — often with magnification — may clarify the probability of, or extent of, malignancy. With a high-volume, rapid throughput approach to screening, in which mammograms are not reviewed until after screenees have left the mammography facility, such mammographic problem-solving is accomplished on a return visit.

A new technique could alter current management of mammographic findings. Mammographically guided needle biopsy, performed either as aspiration cytology or as core needle biopsy [6], is less expensive and less invasive than open biopsy and has been introduced in some centers with the hope that negative needle biopsies can obviate some open biopsies. In addition, positive needle biopsies might allow the initial surgery for a mammographic finding to be more suitable for cancer than routine biopsy sometimes is. The accuracy of this technique is still unclear, and the discussion that follows will not include its possible future role.

Clinically occult cancer usually presents as a mass or as a group of microcalcifications, each accounting for about 40% of cases. Less common mammographic presentations are an asymmetric density, distorted architecture, an asymmetrically prominent duct, skin thickening, and a new density [7].

Masses (Fig. 51.2)

Any single or dominant mass raises suspicion of malignancy. The less sharply circumscribed the mass, the more likely the mass is malignant. The classic appearance of cancer is a spiculated mass; spiculated masses are almost always cancer and require biopsy (Fig. 51.3). Any nonspiculated mass with irregular margins also requires biopsy.

A mass with fairly sharp margins could be a cyst, and ultrasound examination is performed next, as long as the mass is large enough — about 1 cm or larger — that ultrasound is likely to be productive. About 25% of masses that might be cysts by mammography are proved cystic by ultrasound [8] and require further evaluation only under unusual circumstances. Some disagreement exists about these circumstances, but the author recommends cyst aspiration or excision: (1) if the ultrasound appearance of the cyst raises the possibility of cystic carcinoma; (2) if the clinical setting is unusual for a benign cyst, such as a single cyst in otherwise fatty breasts of a postmenopausal woman not on hormone replacement; or (3) if the patient is at very high risk for cancer, such as if she has a personal history of breast cancer.

If a mass, rather than cystic by ultrasound, is either solid or inapparent, or if the mass is too small to be evaluated by ultrasound, the margins and size of the mass by mammography determine the next procedure. A mass that is not sharply circumscribed should be excised. With sharply circumscribed masses, some disagreement exists about the probability of cancer and optimal management. Because the probability of malignancy with well-circumscribed masses may be as high as 5% and because the prognosis is worse for large cancers than for small cancers, the author recommends biopsy of any well-circumscribed mass that is solid or inapparent by ultrasound and that is over 1 cm in diameter [9]. Those masses under 1 cm are followed mammographically.

The probability of cancer decreases as masses become more numerous. With multiple, relatively well-circumscribed masses, mammographic follow-up is recommended. However, a mass that looks considerably different from the others, especially if much less well circumscribed, should be evaluated as if it is solitary.

Microcalcifications (Fig. 51.4)

The management of microcalcifications is determined by their number, morphology, and distribution within the breasts. The general principle is that the more irregular and pleomorphic the calcifications are and the more focal their distribution, the greater is the probability of cancer.

The most common appearance of microcalcifications that raises concern about malignancy is a single cluster. Because about 20% of clusters of microcalcifications are malignant (Fig. 51.5), biopsy is warranted for all single clusters of microcalcifications unless their characteristics strongly suggest benignity. Cancer is very unlikely if the calcifications: (1) are ring-shaped; (2) form horizontal lines or "cups" when viewed with a horizontal X-ray beam — an indication that the calcium is in small cysts; (3) are round or oval with little pleomorphism; or (4) are in the skin — an absolute sign of benignity.

Management decisions about microcalcifications in other distributions can be more problematic and are more difficult to outline, but here are some examples. Microcalcifications limited to one region of one breast are managed like a cluster. Bilateral diffuse or symmetrically distributed microcalcifications are generally regarded as benign, but in the rare situation in which their morphology is "wild," that is, very pleomorphic or pleomorphic and distributed in a way to suggest an intraductal location (a linear and branching pattern), biopsy is indicated.

Asymmetric density

Mammographically, normal breasts tend to be mirror images: fibroglandular tissue is symmetrically distributed within the fat of each breast. Asymmetrically prominent density in one part of one breast is uncommonly malignant, and mammographic follow-up is usually indicated. However, if a palpable mass or thickening or mammographically abnormal architecture is located in the region of asymmetry, while the finding is still often benign, the probability of cancer is high enough to warrant biopsy.

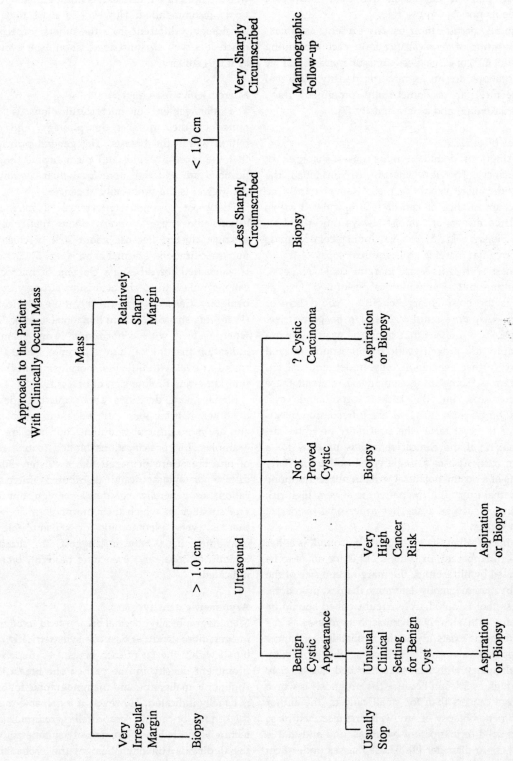

Fig. 51.2 Management of mammographic masses. Clinically occult mass.

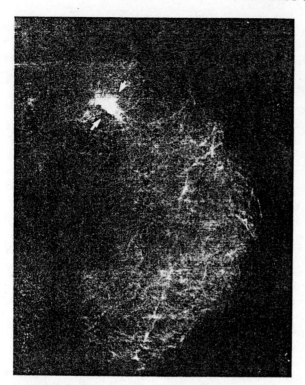

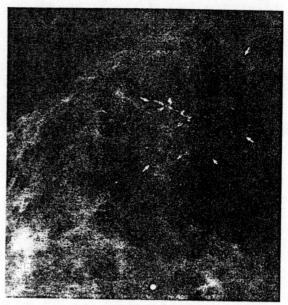

Fig. 51.4 These microcalcifications are highly predictive of cancer. Irregular, pleomorphic rods, their arrangement in a linear and branching pattern indicates an intraductal location. Intraductal carcinoma.

Fig. 51.3 This nonpalpable spiculated mass was, as expected, malignant. Infiltrating duct carcinoma.

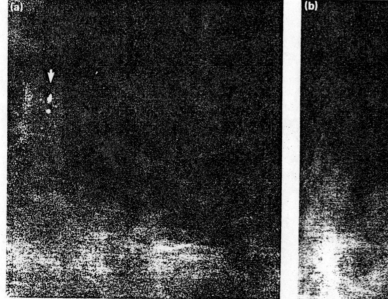

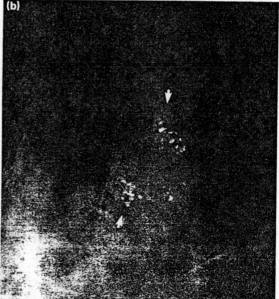

Fig. 51.5 Most clusters of microcalcifications that come to biopsy are less specific than that in Figure 51.4. (a) and (b) have about a 20% probability of cancer: (a) is infiltrating duct carcinoma; (b) is benign.

Distorted architecture

This finding refers to architecture that is spiculated or that exhibits lines oriented in a direction not explained by normal septa. While distorted architecture is usually benign, cancer is the cause often enough that biopsy is indicated (Fig. 51.6) unless a benign cause, such as surgical scar, is apparent from clinical correlation.

Single prominent duct

This finding is much more often benign than malignant, and mammographic follow-up is usually appropriate. If the prominent duct produces a discharge suggestive of cancer, the probability of malignancy is great enough that the duct should be excised.

Skin thickening

Skin thickening may accompany other signs of cancer, but this discussion is about skin thickening without other signs. Numerous benign processes can thicken the skin of the breast, but if clinical correlation does not provide a benign explanation, cancer must be considered. If breast cancer is the cause, cancer cells are often located in the dermal lymphatics and may be there even if inspection of the breast does not show inflammatory carcinoma.

If mastitis is suspected clinically — an uncommon situation in the screening setting — antibiotic therapy can be tried. If mastitis is not suspected clinically; if the skin thickening does not resolve with antibiotic therapy; or if the patient wants diagnosis without delay, biopsy of the skin should be done.

New density

The breasts of women in the age group undergoing mammography usually do not develop densities that are new since previous mammograms. Although often benign, any single new density raises suspicion of malignancy. Because in the author's experience new densities frequently decrease in size or disappear during brief (6 weeks to 3 months) mammographic follow-up, he recommends this short follow-up unless the characteristics of the new density are very suspicious of cancer. If the new density does not resolve at least partially during brief follow-up, biopsy is generally indicated.

REFERENCES

1 Homer MJ. Imaging features and management of characteristically benign and possibly benign lesions. *Radiol Clin North Am* 1987; 25: 939–951.
2 Edeiken S. Mammography and palpable cancer of the breast. *Cancer* 1988; 61: 263–265.
3 Williams SM, Kaplan PA, Petersen JC, Lieberman RP.

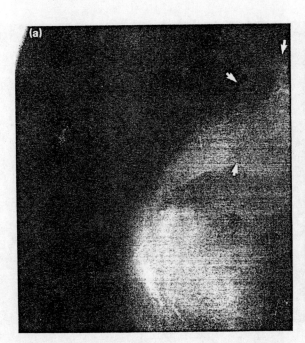 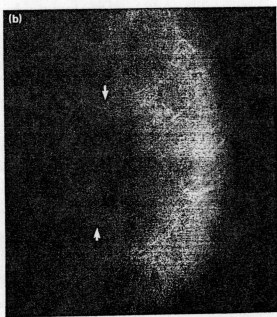

Fig. 51.6 This patient had a nonpalpable region of spiculated architecture in each breast: (a) in the right breast, was malignant; (b) in the left breast, was benign.

Mammography in women under age 30: is there clinical benefit? *Radiology* 1986; 161: 49–51.

4 Morrison AS. Review of evidence on the early detection and treatment of breast cancer. *Cancer* 1989; 64: 2651–2656.

5 Brenner RJ, Sickles EA. Acceptability of periodic follow-up as an alternative to biopsy for mammographically detected lesions interpreted as probably benign. *Radiology* 1989; 171: 645–646.

6 Parker SH, Lovin JD, Jobe WE *et al*. Stereotactic breast biopsy with a biopsy gun. *Radiology* 1990; 176: 741–747.

7 Sickles EA. Mammographic features of 300 consecutive nonpalpable breast cancers. *Am J Roentgen* 1986; 146: 661–663.

8 Hilton SW, Leopold GR, Olson LK, Willson SA. Real-time breast sonography: application in 300 consecutive patients. *Am J Roentgen* 1986; 147: 479–486.

9 Marsteller LP, Shaw de Paredes E. Well defined masses in the breast. *Radiographics* 1989; 9: 13–37.

Evaluation and management of galactorrhea and nipple discharge

KAYLEN M. SILVERBERG

INTRODUCTION

Galactorrhea and nongalactorrheal nipple discharge are very common symptoms in women presenting with breast abnormalities. Nipple discharge is second in frequency only to a palpable lump, with a reported incidence of 7.4% in those patients eventually taken to surgery. However, in the general population it appears to occur much more commonly than this figure would indicate. In Japan, where mass screening for breast cancer has been performed since 1977, over 13% of the female population has been found to have nipple discharge. The incidence of galactorrhea unrelated to breast feeding is probably even higher.

The most serious concern surrounding nipple discharge is its assumed association with breast cancer. In a 1966 review, Barnes reported a 4–52% incidence of cancer in women with a discharge. More recent and more extensive data suggest that this association is much more rare. In Japan, only 0.2% of more than 20 000 women with nipple discharge were subsequently found to have breast cancer. In North America and Europe, where the incidence of breast cancer is significantly higher, still only 4–12% of women with secretions have an underlying carcinoma. Regardless, any discharge not associated with pregnancy or lactation should be considered abnormal and warrants evaluation.

ETIOLOGY

Galactorrhea is characterized by a white, milky discharge and is usually, though not always, bilateral. Galactorrhea can be diagnosed on physical examination by expression of the breast tissue in a radial manner from the outside of the breast toward the nipple, and is most easily elicited with the breast in a dependent position. If a discharge is produced, it can be placed on a slide and observed on medium to high power under the microscope. Identification of round lipid droplets of varying sizes is diagnostic of galactorrhea. The most common cause of galactorrhea is related to hyperprolactinemia, discussed in Chapter 24. Other possible causes include hypothyroidism with associated increased prolactin, chest wall trauma or infection such as shingles, or breast stimulation from sexual relations or other causes. Additionally, as many as 20% of parous women may have expressible galactorrhea, particularly if they have breast-fed in the past. The incidence of this complaint decreases in proportion to the interval from last breast-feeding. If the galactorrhea is a result of hyperprolactinemia, treatment should be directed as discussed in Chapter 24. If it is a result of irritation to the breast or the chest wall, the source of the problem should be identified and eliminated if possible. If no etiology can be found and the prolactin level is normal, the patient can simply be reassured. If the symptoms are unacceptable to her, low doses of bromocriptine can be considered and will likely ameliorate or eliminate the symptoms.

The nongalactorrheal causes of nipple discharge are far more numerous and the diagnosis and management is less straightforward. The bulk of this chapter will focus on such discharge which can result from something as simple as a poorly fitting bra causing continuous nerve stimulation of the breast, to more complex entities such as duct ectasia, infection, or neoplasia. The most common causes of nipple discharge are listed below:

1 Fibrocystic breast disease.
2 Mastitis.
3 Duct ectasia.
4 Papilloma.
5 Carcinoma.

Fibrocystic disease

Fibrocystic disease may be a unilateral or bilateral condition. More commonly, the discharge is unilateral and serous. Although some patients present because of pain, most are asymptomatic. Demographic data suggest that 75–80% of patients are Caucasian and their mean age is 43–45 years.

Mastitis

This condition occurs almost exclusively in women of child-bearing age. These patients usually present complaining of pain, fever, and tenderness. Culture of the discharge usually grows *Staphylococcus aureus*.

Duct ectasia

Duct ectasia is perhaps the most common cause of nongalactorrheal nipple discharge. It results from dilatation of the terminal lactiferous ducts. A lipid fluid builds up within the duct, causing local inflammation and discharge. This condition is frequently bilateral, and multiple ducts within each breast may be involved. Nipple hygiene is often poor in these patients; however, culture of the discharge is sterile. The median age of these patients is 35–40 years.

Duct papilloma

Papillomas are usually found in middle-aged women, with a median age of 55–60 years. They are almost always unilateral and produce discharge from a single duct. Approximately 60% of the discharges will be bloody, and 30–35% will be serous. Twenty percent of affected patients will also present with a palpable mass.

Carcinoma of the breast

Breast cancer typically presents in the sixth to seventh decade of life. It is almost exclusively a unilateral disease at the time of presentation, and only rarely will patients present because of a nipple discharge. When they do, however, the discharge may be bloody, watery, serosanguineous, or serous.

DISCHARGE CLASSIFICATION

The first step in the evaluation of nipple discharge is to determine whether the secretions are spontaneous or whether they are elicited only with manual expression. The latter, nonspontaneous discharges are frequently the result of medications such as oral contraceptives, tranquilizers, and some antihypertensives, and may be associated with hyperprolactinemia. If the serum prolactin level is normal, then these patients can be reassured, as recent literature suggests that nonspontaneous discharge is only rarely associated with underlying pathology.

The next step in the patient with a spontaneous discharge is to ensure that the secretion is indeed coming from a mammary duct and not from the areola or surrounding tissue. Several clinical entities, such as herpes simplex infection, eczema, Montgomery gland abscesses, or mammary duct fistulas, can result in secretions resembling true nipple discharge. In addition, nipple inversion or repetitive trauma (i.e., resulting from aerobics or jogging) can mimic a true discharge.

Once the source of the secretion has been established, the discharge must be characterized. Until recently, most texts have referred to three types of discharge: clear, serous, or bloody. However, in an excellent review of this subject, Leis *et al.* [1] described six types of nongalactorrheal nipple discharge. Accurate classification of the secretions will frequently aid in determining the patient's diagnosis. Purulent discharge most frequently results from infection, such as mastitis. The discharge is unilateral in 80% of cases, and approximately 20% have either noticeable induration or a mass present in the affected breast.

Patients will frequently present with a colored, sticky discharge, most commonly indicative of duct ectasia or comedomastitis. This discharge is usually greenish, but it may alternatively be yellow, brown, or gray. It is frequently associated with pruritis, pain, and/or thickening of the nipple and the areola. Occasionally, an odor may be associated with the discharge. Clear, watery discharge occurs infrequently. However, in at least one large study, it was the type of discharge most commonly associated with the coexistence of a malignancy. A yellow-tinged serous secretion is the most common type of nongalactorrheal nipple discharge. It is usually associated with fibrocystic breast disease, but has also been noted in association with intraductal papillomas, mastitis, and, rarely, cancer. A pink-tinged serosanguineous discharge is a nonspecific finding. It has been associated with everything from fibrocystic breast disease to papillomas to cancer. Historically, the most worrisome type of discharge has been the bloody discharge. It is more commonly associated with papillomas, however, than with malignancy. In one large series, only 24% of patients with bloody discharge had breast cancer, compared to 40% or more who were found to have a papilloma.

CYTOLOGY

Once a discharge has been characterized, if it is multicolored and emanates from multiple ducts, then the patient can be reassured that she has duct ectasia. There is no need to proceed with cytologic or mammographic evaluation in these patients due to the risk of a false-positive result. Treatment, consisting of daily nipple hygiene using antiseptic solutions and avoidance of nipple stimulation, should be promptly instituted.

Cytologic evaluation should be performed on all other types of discharge. Although more than 90% of these examinations will yield negative or nonspecific findings, the presence of either numerous white blood cells or malignant cells can be diagnostic. If white blood cells are encountered, then the fluid should be sent for culture and sensitivity.

A review of the literature demonstrates that cytology for breast cancer has a sensitivity of 40–60%. In other words, if breast cancer is present, it will be detected on cytologic examination about half of the time. If malignant cells are identified, then the likelihood that the patient truly has a malignancy is approximately 90–95%, i.e., there is a false-positive rate of 5–10%. Cytologic sensitivity increases markedly if suspicious results, or cases in which atypical cells are present, are included in the positive category. There are also data that suggest that the evaluation of multiple smears increases the sensitivity. In addition, a preliminary report has suggested that carcinoembryonic antigen estimation from the discharge fluid may be a useful adjunct to the detection of breast cancer. Unfortunately, with regard to malignancy detection, the overall results from nipple discharge cytology are not as good as those obtained from fine-needle aspiration.

MAMMOGRAPHY

If cytology reveals the presence of either malignant cells or a nonspecific combination of foam cells and benign duct cells against a proteinaceous background, then the next step should be mammography. This is important in the patient with suspected malignancy in order to rule out the presence of a concurrent lesion in the contralateral breast. Likewise, in the patient with negative cytology, mammography may prove effective in identifying a nonpalpable lesion.

The Breast Cancer Detection Demonstration Project identified 3557 cancers in 280 000 women over a 5 year period. Of these, 41.6% were detected by mammography alone in patients without a palpable mass. The most common criticism of mammography is the significant false-positive rate, which can be as high as 40%. This can be markedly reduced, however, through the use of second opinions. Although mammography alone can be reasonably expected to miss 10–15% of underlying malignancies, when both cytology and mammography are negative the risk of missing a breast cancer falls to 5% or less. All patients with either malignant duct cells noted on cytology or a suspicious mass on mammography should be taken to the operating room for appropriate surgical management.

GALACTOGRAPHY

Galactography is a radiologic procedure that enables visualization of individual lactiferous ducts. It has been recommended for all patients who present with nipple discharge and have negative cytology and mammography. It should most certainly be performed on those patients with bloody nipple discharge, unless cytology or mammography is positive, as it is especially effective at diagnosing intraductal papillomas.

TREATMENT

As described above, nonspontaneous nipple discharge should be evaluated with a serum prolactin level. If this is abnormal, patients should be evaluated for hyperprolactinemia as described previously. If the prolactin level is normal and there is no palpable mass, then patients can be managed expectantly. Approximately 50% of these patients will continue to have a discharge for several years. In the event that the discharge is persistent or particularly bothersome, then patients may be tried on an empiric course of bromocriptine. Euprolactinemic galactorrhea is a well-known entity, and may well represent a subset of hyperprolactinemia. The standard prolactin assay measures only one of the four bioactive forms of prolactin. Therefore, a normal serum prolactin level does not truly exclude hyperprolactinemia.

Patients diagnosed with duct ectasia should be treated with nipple hygiene, consisting of an antiseptic solution such as Phisohex or Betadine applied to the nipple for 5 min daily. In addition, all nipple stimulation and manipulation should be avoided.

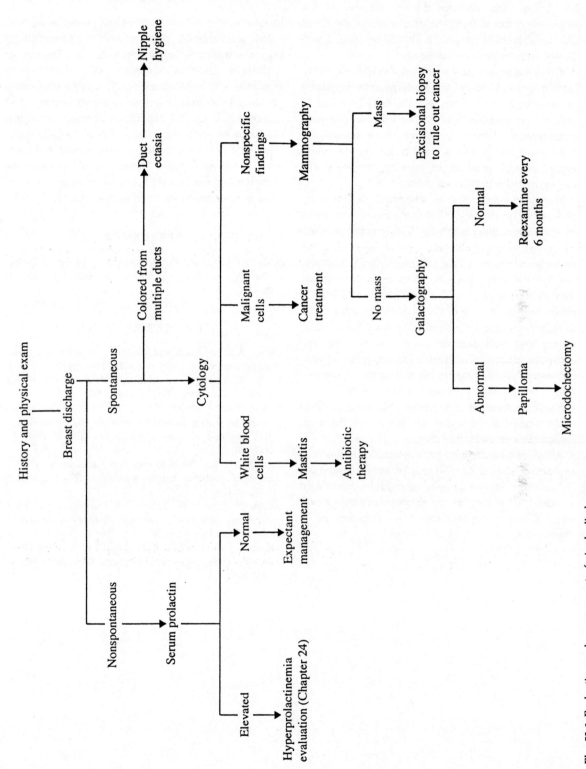

Fig. 52.1 Evaluation and management of nipple discharge.

Those patients diagnosed with mastitis should be treated with antibiotic therapy directed at the organism cultured from the discharge. In the event that an abscess is present, it should be treated surgically with incision and drainage.

When malignant cells are noted on cytologic examination, patients should still undergo mammography as described above. They should then be taken to surgery for excisional biopsy or other appropriate management. Likewise, patients with nonspecific cytologic findings and a mass noted on mammography should proceed to surgery for excisional biopsy in order to rule out cancer.

When galactography is abnormal, a microdochectomy, or removal of the abnormal lactiferous duct, is routinely performed. This treatment effectively removes papillomata. In the event that the entire work-up, including galactography, is negative, yet the discharge persists, then microdochectomy may also be indicated. This procedure can be facilitated through the use of either one of two methods. First, patients can be instructed to paint the affected nipple with collodion for several days. This will allow the duct producing the discharge to become distended, facilitating microdochectomy. Alternatively, if the abnormal duct is easily identified, one can instill a solution of methylene blue into the duct at the time of surgery. This solution will fill the duct, facilitating complete dissection.

All other patients who have a completely negative evaluation should be reexamined every 6 months. In addition, mammography should be performed annually for as long as the abnormal discharge persists. These recommendations are summarized in Figure 52.1.

CONCLUSIONS

In summary, both galactorrhea and nongalactorrheal nipple discharge are very common symptoms affecting women of child-bearing age and older. The former is likely to reflect an abnormality of prolactin secretion or simply to be a temporary, though sometimes prolonged, sequela of previous breast-feeding. The potential etiology and implication of nongalactorrheal discharge are more complex. Although usually indicative of a benign disorder, it may herald the presence of breast cancer. Therefore, all spontaneous nongalactorrheal breast discharge warrants a complete evaluation, as outlined in this chapter.

REFERENCE

1 Leis HP Jr, Greene FL, Cammarata A, Hilfer SE. Nipple discharge: surgical significance. *South Med J* 1988; 81: 20–26.

FURTHER READING

Barnes AB. Diagnosis and treatment of abnormal breast secretions. *N Engl J Med* 1966; 275: 1184–1187.

Devitt JE. Management of nipple discharge by clinical findings. *Am J Surg* 1985; 149: 789–791.

Inaji H, Yayoi E, Maeura Y et al. Carcinoembryonic antigen estimation in nipple discharge as an adjunctive tool in the diagnosis of early breast cancer. *Cancer* 1987; 12: 3008–3013.

Johnson TL, Kini SR. Cytologic and clinicopathologic features of abnormal nipple secretions. *Diagn Cytopathol* 1991; 7: 17–22.

Knight DC, Lowell DM, Heimann A, Dunn E. Aspiration of the breast and nipple discharge cytology. *Surg Gynecol Obstet* 1986; 163: 415–420.

Takeda T, Matsui A, Sato Y et al. Nipple discharge cytology in mass screening for breast cancer. *Acta Cytol* 1990; 34: 161–164.

53

Suppression of lactation

KAYLEN M. SILVERBERG

INTRODUCTION

Breast-feeding has become increasingly popular in the USA since reaching a nadir in 1970. At that time, only 25% of women were breast-feeding 7 days postpartum. By 1985, that figure had risen to approximately 60%, with over 25% of women continuing to breast-feed their infants through 5 months of age. For the 40% who do not initiate breast-feeding and for the others who discontinue at various intervals, the optimal method to suppress lactation is an issue of some concern.

PHYSIOLOGY

Many hormones interact during pregnancy to prepare the human breast for lactation. In addition to the primary hormones (estrogen and prolactin) insulin, growth hormone, and thyroxine play supportive roles. The breast is actually capable of milk secretion as early as the second trimester. By that time, the necessary enzymes and specialized cellular organelles have developed within the mammary epithelium, probably in response to human placental lactogen (hPL). As parturition approaches, lactose, casein, and α-lactalbumin are synthesized at a more rapid rate.

At parturition, there is a marked change in the maternal hormonal milieu. This period is characterized by a significant fall in progesterone and hPL levels, with a concomitant rise in prolactin, oxytocin, glucocorticoids, and estrogen. Current evidence suggests that removal of the placental steroids, especially progesterone, serves to initiate lactogenesis. Estrogen levels, too, must fall postpartum to enable lactation to occur.

Soon after delivery, colostrum is secreted in response to suckling. By the fourth postpartum day, however, milk production and secretion predominate. Despite an optimal hormonal milieu, nipple stimu-lation is essential for continued milk production. The frequency and intensity of this stimulation are the major determinants for the maintenance of lactation. Once stimulated, impulses travel from the nipple, through the afferent mammary nerve fibers, to the hypothalamic intraventricular and supraoptic nuclei. In response to this stimulus, the hypothalamus coordinates the release of prolactin and oxytocin from the anterior and posterior pituitary gland, respectively. With continued regular breast-feeding, the basal prolactin level remains significantly elevated for the first 2 weeks postpartum. The level then gradually declines to normal by the fourth postpartum month. Each feeding episode, however, continues to cause a transient increase in prolactin secretion, though this too becomes attenuated by the sixth postpartum month.

SUPPRESSION OF LACTATION

Nonpharmacologic mechanisms

Avoidance of nipple stimulation is the simplest and most cost-effective method of lactation suppression (Fig. 53.1). Several mechanisms are responsible for this effect. First, without this stimulation, the milk ejection reflex and, hence, prolactin secretion are reduced. This leads to a fall in milk production. Second, inhibition of the milk ejection reflex leads to incomplete emptying of the breast, alveolar distention, and disruption of the secretory ability of the alveolar epithelium.

Breast-binders (or tight bras) have been used to cause mechanical compression of the breast, inhibit nipple stimultion, and hasten alveolar distention. Although effective, their use is commonly associated with breast engorgement and pain. These symptoms can frequently be ameliorated through the simultaneous use of ice packs and mild analgesics.

CHAPTER 53

Suppression of Lactation

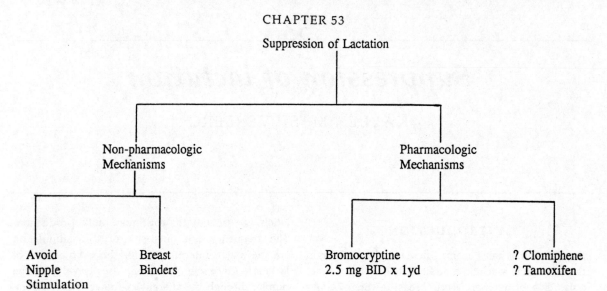

Fig. 53.1 Steps to avoid the suppression of lactation.

Pharmacologic mechanisms

Bromocriptine

Bromocriptine is a lysergic acid derivative developed in 1967 specifically as an inhibitor of prolactin secretion. It was introduced in the USA in 1978, and in 1980 the Food and Drug Administration (FDA) approved it for use in the prevention of physiologic lactation. Once absorbed from the gastrointestinal tract, this dopamine agonist binds to central dopamine receptors, causing inhibition of pituitary prolactin secretion.

When administered very early in the postpartum period, bromocriptine lowers prolactin levels to normal within 24–48 hours. In addition, it will prevent the initiation of lactation and prevent breast engorgement and mastodynia. Bromocriptine is also effective at suppressing lactation when therapy is initiated following a course of breast-feeding. In this situation, however, up to 25% of women experience rebound breast engorgement when treated for only 8 days.

The most effective oral dosage regimen for lactation suppression is 2.5 mg twice daily for 14 days postpartum. Some investigators have advocated an additional 2.5 mg given once daily for a third week of treatment. An injectable form of long-acting bromocriptine microspheres has been shown to be both safe and effective in several European studies. It is administered as a single injection of 20–50 mg soon after delivery. The 50 mg dose is associated with the lowest incidence of breast engorgement and rebound

lactation. This formulation has not been approved for use in the USA.

The most common side-effects of bromocriptine are nausea and orthostatic hypotension, which usually occur shortly after the initiation of treatment. Tolerance to these symptoms develops rapidly, and these adverse reactions can be minimized by beginning therapy with food shortly before bedtime. Other less common side-effects include headache, constipation, fatigue, and abdominal cramping. Controlled trials have demonstrated bromocriptine's efficacy when compared to placebo, breast-binders, estrogens, and estrogen–androgen combinations.

Over the past several years, occasional reports in the literature have implicated bromocriptine usage in the development of postpartum seizures, hypertension, and strokes. Its safety and efficacy in the treatment of hyperprolactinemia and galactorrhea have not been seriously questioned, however. In June 1988, an FDA advisory committee reviewed these reports and stated that although bromocriptine was effective at suppressing and preventing postpartum lactation, no drug should be routinely used for this indication. In August 1988, a large retrospective epidemiologic study demonstrated no causal relationship between the use of bromocriptine and the occurrence of postpartum seizures. The data were insufficient to determine whether or not there was an association with postpartum strokes. A more recent report evaluated the association between bromocriptine usage and the development of postpartum hypertension. In this study of over 1800 consecutively delivered patients, bromocriptine was found to increase the risk of postpartum hypertension in only those patients who had developed antepartum pregnancy-induced hypertension.

In June 1989, the FDA Advisory Committee on Fertility and Maternal Health Drugs recommended that all manufacturers of medications used routinely to prevent postpartum lactation should voluntarily remove this indication from product labeling. The Committee did not, however, withdraw FDA approval from these medications. This decision has created considerable controversy, and bromocriptine remains available for use in the suppression of postpartum lactation.

Estrogens

Estrogens were first used in the late 1930s to suppress lactation. The exact mechanism of this effect is unknown, but it appears that the site of action must be the breast itself, as estrogen stimulates rather than suppresses prolactin secretion. Animal studies support this theory, as direct intramammary injection of estrogen suppresses lactation, whereas intrapituitary injection stimulates milk production.

Over the years, numerous preparations and dosing regimens of estrogens have been employed with inconsistent results. TACE (chlorotrianisene) capsules were approved for this indication in the USA until 1989. At that time, following the FDA's recommendation, its manufacturer withdrew lactation suppression from product labeling. When used, estrogen treatment should be initiated prior to or just following delivery, as estrogens cannot effectively suppress milk secretion once lactation has been initiated. In addition, a high incidence of rebound breast engorgement, excessive lochia, and thromboembolic phenomena demonstrated in several large epidemiologic studies further complicate its routine use.

Antiestrogens

Both clomiphene citrate and tamoxifen have been used for the suppression of postpartum lactation, though neither has been extensively studied. The mechanism of action of these drugs is inhibition of prolactin secretion. Although two clomiphene studies have demonstrated effective suppression of prolactin, only one reported significant inhibition of lactation.

Tamoxifen has been evaluated in two European studies, one a large placebo-controlled, double-blind trial. Both reports suggest that, when given shortly after delivery, tamoxifen is both safe and effective. No serious side-effects were observed in either study, and lactation was suppressed in up to 92% of women studied.

Estrogen—androgen combinations

Despite the pitfalls of estrogen cited above, estrogen—androgen combinations have been commonly used to suppress lactation. Androgens appear to inhibit prolactin secretion, and various preparations have been reported to be effective for this indication. Deladumone was the formulation approved for use in the USA until the FDA's 1989 recommendation. Although neither serious side effects nor virilization from the large dosages of androgens used have been reported, rebound lactation has been documented in 40% of patients treated. In addition, as with pure estrogen preparations, therapy must be initiated either before or immediately following delivery.

Other medications

Numerous other formulations have been employed for lactation suppression. Prostaglandin E_2 reduces serum prolactin levels when given in the early puerperium, and it has been reported to suppress lactation effectively with less rebound breast engorgement than does bromocriptine. It is not effective when given once breast-feeding has been initiated. Pharmacologic doses of pyridoxine (vitamin B6) have been reported to suppress serum prolactin levels; however, nutritionally relevant doses (0.5—4 mg/day) are ineffective at suppressing either serum prolactin levels or lactation. Other medications, such as diuretics, need further evaluation, as do recent reports concerning the use of terguride (a dopamine agonist available in Europe) and selenium disulfide.

CONCLUSIONS

For the majority of patients who do not desire to breast-feed their newborns, tight bras, combined with avoidance of nipple stimulation, afford relief from breast engorgement until prolactin levels fall. For those women who do experience mastodynia and/or significant engorgement, ice packs can be used in conjunction with the binders. If this regimen is ineffective, bromocriptine can be used; the therapy should be continued for at least 14 days. Further FDA action may be taken in the near future, but until that time, bromocriptine retains its governmental approval. Although it should not be used either routinely or in women with antenatal pregnancy-induced hypertension, in select cases it can be relied upon to be both safe and effective for the suppression or prevention of postpartum lactation.

FURTHER READING

Kaplan CR, Schenken RS. Endocrinology of the breast. In: Mitchell GW Jr, Bassett LW, eds. *The Female Breast and Its Disorders*. Baltimore: Williams & Wilkins, 1990.

Katz M, Kroll D, Pak I, Osimoni A, Hirsch M. Puerperal hypertension, stroke, and seizures after suppression of lactation with bromocriptine. *Obstet Gynecol* 1985; 66: 822–824.

Kochenour NK. Lactation suppression. *Clin Obstet Gynecol* 1980; 23: 1045.

Vance ML, Evans WS, Thorner MO. Diagnosis and treatment. Drugs five years later. Bromocriptine. *Ann Intern Med* 1984; 100: 78–91.

Watson DL, Bhatia RK, Norman GS, Brindley BA, Sokol RJ. Bromocriptine mesylate for lactation suppression: a risk for postpartum hypertension? *Obstet Gynecol* 1989; 74: 573–576.

Part VI
Pregnancy and pregnancy prevention

54

Threatened abortion

DAVID L. KEENAN

Threatened abortion continues to be a frequently encountered diagnostic problem for the practicing physician. This term is used to describe vaginal bleeding during the first half of gestation. Approximately 20−25% of women will encounter this type of bleeding during a pregnancy. The true incidence is difficult to know since it often goes unreported to the physician. On the other hand, very early sensitive tests for β-human chorionic gonadotropin (β-hCG) affect the data in the opposite direction.

Threatened abortion is most commonly the first stage of a spontaneous abortion, although only approximately one-half of patients will proceed from threatened abortion to spontaneous abortion. Moreover, threatened abortion can be very frustrating to both the patient and physician since very little can be done to intervene in a therapeutic manner. This is true unless, of course, the patient has a previously documented luteal-phase defect by endometrial biopsy; this should be treated with progesterone supplementation.

Bleeding is more often encountered in the first trimester than later in pregnancy (Fig. 54.1). While the scope of this chapter is limited to the discussion of threatened abortion, the topics of inevitable, incomplete, missed, and habitual abortion are also mentioned to add another perspective in discussing the main topic. Inevitable abortion refers to the condition of dilatation of the cervix in the presence of ruptured membranes. A missed abortion is a term describing the retention of a dead fetus, which died during the first 20 weeks of pregnancy, for a period of 4 weeks or more. Habitual abortion is defined by three or greater consecutive spontaneous abortions. An incomplete abortion describes the retention of a portion of the placenta within the uterus during a spontaneous abortion. Vaginal bleeding is commonly seen with all of these conditions [1].

Vaginal bleeding at the time of the expected menstrual period might be physiologic, as was suggested by Hartman in 1929 in his studies of rhesus monkeys [2]. Vaginal bleeding at that time was referred to as the placental sign and resulted from leakage of blood from the uterine glands to the uterine cavity and then passed through the cervix to the vagina. Hartman observed bleeding starting from 13 to 20 days after the date of mating and lasting approximately 3 weeks.

The exact mechanism or pathophysiology of spontaneous abortion is not clear. Pathologic studies show bleeding into the decidua basalis. The embryo is partially or completely detached. It is postulated that expulsion of the embryo is caused by uterine contractions stimulated by the embryo as a foreign body within the uterus. Chromosomal abnormalities such as autosomal trisomies and monosomy X (45,X) are the most commonly identified anomalies seen in approximately 50% of all spontaneous abortions. Moreover, blighted ova are seen in approximately 50% of abortuses. Blighted ova are characterized by the absence of any fetus inside the gestational sac. Euploid abortions, where chromosomal complement is normal, occur more often around 13 weeks of gestation while aneuploid abortions occur earlier — around 8 weeks of gestation. The possible causes are extensive and include infection, hyperthyroidism, diabetes mellitus, environmental toxins such as tobacco, alcohol, and radiation, immunologic, laparotomy, leiomyomas, intrauterine adhesions, and *in utero* exposure to diethylstilbestrol.

Threatened abortion is often accompanied by a cramping pain which mimics menstrual cramps or even a lower backache. Commonly the bleeding is the first sign of threatened abortion and it is followed by the crampy abdominal pain. The pain may be perceived in various locations such as in the lower back, deep in the pelvis, or anteriorly, and is of various types. These include repetitive contractions suggestive of labor, a dull ache, or perception of pressure or discomfort. Unless the pain resolves, the

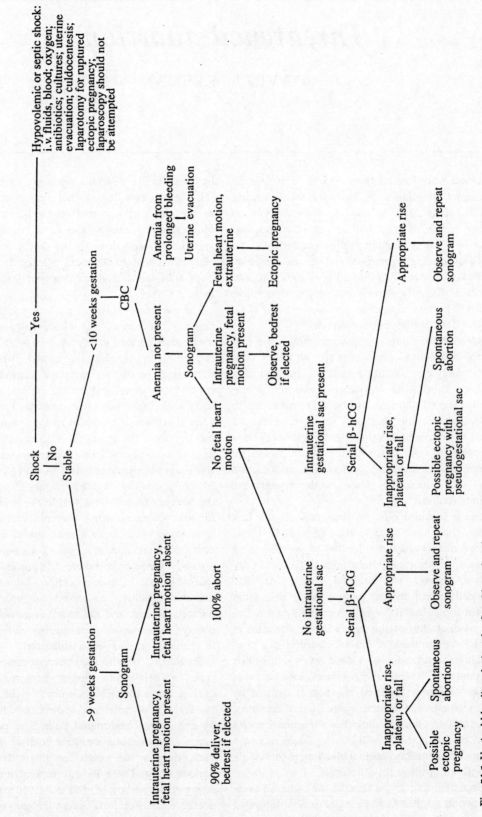

Fig. 54.1 Vaginal bleeding during the first 20 weeks of pregnancy.

chances of maintaining the pregnancy are diminished.

Clinical decisions in caring for a patient with threatened abortion are best made after informing the patient of her particular situation and getting a good idea of how she feels. It is not necessary to intervene if the patient is stable and wants to continue the pregnancy. The patient should be informed that bleeding may continue for several weeks. There is no increased incidence of congenital anomalies or growth retardation, and she should be so informed. However, the patient should know that she is at increased risk of preterm birth and concomitant lower birthweight and increased perinatal mortality. A relative risk of 2 was shown by Batzofin and colleagues that patients with threatened abortion were more likely to deliver prior to 37 weeks of gestation [3]. Moreover, the perinatal mortality rate was three times higher in patients with threatened abortion.

All patients who have vaginal bleeding during the first half of pregnancy do not have a threatened abortion. Vaginal bleeding may arise from many other sources. Hopefully, however, pregnant patients will report any notice of vaginal bleeding so that

they can be evaluated. Unless the patient is in shock with hypovolemia secondary to brisk bleeding, it is important to take a thorough history, especially if you are seeing the patient for the first time. Important subjective data needed are included in Table 54.1. The most important piece of information is to know that the patient actually is pregnant, how and when it was diagnosed, and the gestational age of the pregnancy.

Just as in any clinical situation, a thorough physical examination is equally important and will be necessary to differentiate disorders presenting with vaginal bleeding such as vaginitis, cervicitis with postcoital bleeding, cervical cancer, inevitable abortion, incomplete abortion, septic abortion, or ectopic pregnancy. Table 54.2 gives a list of pertinent objective findings to note on physical examination.

Although tests such as vaginal smears, cultures, and Pap smears are beneficial, three laboratory tests are usually used as the cornerstone in making the correct diagnosis. These include a complete blood count (CBC), quantitative level of β-hCG in the blood, and a pelvic sonogram. In addition, it might be necessary to obtain repeat tests over time.

With all of the data in hand, the physician can begin to focus on the correct diagnosis. Missed abortion can be accurately diagnosed by ultrasound. Incomplete abortions are usually seen in conjunction with profuse vaginal bleeding and are readily diagnosed when the cervix is examined and noted to be

Table 54.1 Important historical data

Age, last menstrual period, previous menstrual period
Date and method by which pregnancy was diagnosed
Onset, color, quantity of bleeding
Postcoital bleeding
Leakage or gush of fluid
Passage of tissue or fetus
Onset, nature, consistency, location of pain
Previous obstetric history, previous abortion, ectopic
   pregnancies
Use of oral contraceptive pills, minipill, presence of
   intrauterine device
Incompetent cervix, Müllerian anomalies
Luteal-phase defect
Vaginal discharge, sexually transmitted diseases, pelvic
   or vaginal infections
Abnormal Pap smears
Tubal surgery, tubal ligation, recent laparotomy
   to disturb corpus luteum
Diethylstilbestrol exposure *in utero* (family history
   of spontaneous abortions)
Hyperthyroidism, diabetes mellitus
Medications
Environmental or workplace exposure
Radiation, tobacco, alcohol
History of uterine leiomyomas, especially submucous
Asherman's syndrome
History of attempted abortion or self-instrumentation

Table 54.2 Salient features of the physical examination

Vital signs, orthostatic changes
Abdominal examination to exclude acute abdomen
Complete pelvic examination
   Quantity of blood loss
   Vaginitis
   Cervicitis
   Cervical polyp
   Gross cervical lesion of cervical cancer
   Presence of intrauterine device string
   Cervical dilatation
   Cervical effacement
   Ruptured membranes
   Products of conception in the cervical canal
   Uterine size and change in size over time from previous
      examination (compatibility with last menstrual period)
   Uterine tenderness
   Adnexal mass or tenderness
   Cul-de-sac mass or tenderness
   Presence of fetal heart tones

---

dilated with fragments of placental tissue in the canal. They can often be easily pulled free using forceps, causing prompt diminution of blood loss. Otherwise urgent evacuation of the uterus is necessary.

Patients presenting with vaginal bleeding and hypovolemic shock are, if not experiencing an incomplete abortion, likely to have an ectopic pregnancy with hematoperitoneum. After initial fluid resuscitation with intravenous fluids and blood products, culdocentesis can be performed promptly to secure the diagnosis of hematoperitoneum with probable ruptured ectopic pregnancy. Laparotomy should be performed to isolate the source of blood loss. Laparoscopy should not be attempted in the face of hypovolemic shock. Febrile patients with septic abortions also need immediate attention with intravenous fluid resuscitation, cultures, and administration of antibiotics followed by uterine evacuation.

Patients of a less emergent nature with vaginal bleeding can be divided into two groups, according to Jouppila and colleagues, who have written extensively on the diagnosis and outcome of threatened abortion [4]. In their studies patients seen after 9 weeks of gestation should have a sonogram performed. The demonstration of fetal heart motion predicted a 90% chance of continuation to delivery. The absence of fetal heart motion after 9 weeks of gestation is indicative of a 100% chance of abortion. Approximately one-half of these patients will spontaneously abort. This group is comprised of patients with blighted ova, incomplete abortion, molar pregnancy, missed abortion, inevitable abortion, and ectopic pregnancy.

Patients earlier in pregnancy — usually between 5 and 9 weeks of gestation — are more difficult to diagnose. In addition to a sonogram, quantitative β-hCG levels in the blood are the most helpful in the differential diagnosis. Frequently it is useful to get a repeat β-hCG value 48 hours after the initial sample. Most patients with a normal pregnancy should have a minimum increase of 66% over 48 hours' time. With β-hCG values of 6000 mIU/ml or greater, abdominal sonography should demonstrate an intrauterine gestational sac if present. Transvaginal sonography can often demonstrate this at even lower levels of β-hCG. According to Jouppila et al. [4], pathologic levels of β-hCG on the first determination portend abortion in 93% of cases. On the other hand normal values of β-hCG are not totally predictive since only 74% proceed to delivery. It is important to

note that a blighted ovum is often seen with normally rising β-hCG values through 11 weeks of pregnancy, but that the diagnosis is made by the repeated sonogram which continues to show an empty gestational sac. Threatened abortion is a diagnosis of exclusion and should only be made after life-threatening conditions such as ectopic pregnancy are resonably excluded. No hard and fast rules can be made that apply to every clinical situation; however, with the use of serial sonograms, β-hCG values, and physical examinations, the patient can be correctly counseled and forewarned about the possible outcome of her pregnancy. A summary of diagnoses that must be excluded are: (1) ectopic pregnancy; (2) hydatidiform mole; (3) adnexal torsion; (4) cervical cancer.

Little can be done in the way of therapeutic options for threatened abortion. Evacuation of the uterus is suggested if bleeding continues with resulting anemia. Remember that approximately 50% of these patients will advance to spontaneous abortion and that the onset of pain increases the likelihood of this. Some patients will desire evacuation of the uterus after being informed of increased risks of preterm delivery and perinatal mortality.

Progesterone as a treatment for threatened abortion should be reserved for those patients who have a luteal-phase defect previously documented by endometrial biopsy. Progesterone supplementation is given most commonly by vaginal suppository or intramuscularly by injection. It is important to know that synthetic progestational agents such as Provera should not be given during pregnancy since they may cause virilization of a female fetus and, moreover, have not been shown to be effective in treatment.

In addition to pelvic rest, bedrest has been advised for women with threatened abortion as far back as the time of Hippocrates [5]. Even though the effectiveness of bedrest on the outcome of threatened abortion has never been firmly settled, most current obstetric textbooks recommend it. This is reflected in the practice of obstetrics where the majority of obstetricians suggest bedrest for patients with the diagnosis of threatened abortion. Even though many physicians do not think that it is an effective treatment, they are concerned that they might be blamed for a possible ensuing spontaneous abortion if they do not prescribe bedrest.

Diddle et al. studied the question of the effectiveness of bedrest for threatened abortion in 1953. This study examined 1452 women with threatened abortion. Although the patients were placed into three groups based on complete hospital bedrest, partial bedrest, and continuing normal daily activities, there was no standardized treatment for the medications which they received, such as barbituates, vitamin E, progesterone, stilbesterol, and thyroid. Nevertheless, it is interesting to note that while 59% of the complete bedrest group and 81% of the partial bedrest group proceeded to spontaneous abortion, only 54% of the women who continued their normal daily routine advanced to miscarriage. While the medications given to these patients complicates drawing definite conclusions from this study, the results lend no proof to the recommendation of bedrest for threatened abortion.

While it is unlikely that the continued recommendation of bedrest for threatened abortion will change in the near future, the physician should realize that there is room for individualized decision on the part of the patient since bedrest has a considerable impact on medical disability, family dynamics, and economic hardships. Moreover, this emphasizes the need for prompt diagnosis in the case of nonviable pregnancies so that treatment may be instituted and morbidity reduced.

REFERENCES

1 Cunningham FG, MacDonald PC, Gant NF. *Williams Obstetrics*, 18th ed. Norwalk: Appleton and Lange, 1989; 489–532.
2 Hartman CG. Uterine bleeding as an early sign of pregnancy in the monkey (*Macacus rhesus*), together with observations on the fertile period of the menstrual cycle. *Bull Johns Hopkins Hosp* 1929; 44: 155.
3 Batzofin JH, Fielding WL, Friedman EA. Effect of vaginal bleeding in early pregnancy on outcome. *Obstet Gynecol* 1984; 63: 515.
4 Jouppila P, Huhtaniemi I, Tapanainen J. Early pregnancy failure: study by ultrasonic and hormonal methods. *Obstet Gynecol* 1980; 55: 42.
5 Crowther C, Chalmers I. Bed rest and hospitalization during pregnancy. In: Chalmers I, Enkin M, Keirse MJNC, eds. *Effective Care in Pregnancy and Childbirth*. New York: Oxford University Press, 1989: 624–625.
6 Diddle AW, O'Connor KA, Jack R, Pearse RL. Evaluation of bedrest in threatened absortion. *Obstet Gynecol* 1953; 2: 63–67.

55

Ectopic pregnancy

STEVEN J. ORY

Ectopic pregnancy is an increasingly prevalent complication of reproductive endocrinology and infertility therapy. Since 1970, the year in which the Centers for Disease Control began to record the number of ectopic pregnancies diagnosed in US hospitals, there has been a fivefold increase in the rate of ectopic pregnancies per 1000 live births. During the same interval there has been a steady decline in mortality. In 1987 only 30 women died in the USA from ruptured ectopic pregnancies, producing a 0.03% mortality rate. Although the number of deaths from ectopic pregnancies has steadily declined, it is still considered the second leading cause of maternal mortality. Several factors have contributed to the epidemic of ectopic pregnancy, including the epidemic of sexually transmitted diseases which began in the 1960s, wider application of tubal reparative procedures, and enhanced diagnostic capabilities. The availability of sensitive assays for human chorionic gonadotropin (hCG), high-resolution ultrasonography, and the aggressive use of laparoscopy have led to more frequent and earlier diagnosis. It is probable that a significant number of early ectopic pregnancies escaped clinical detection in the past and spontaneously resolved as tubal abortions at an early stage. Twenty years ago fewer than 10% of ectopic pregnancies were diagnosed prior to tubal rupture. Presently, many centers are intervening before rupture in over 90% of cases.

Patients with suspected ectopic pregnancies typically present in one of two ways. An increasing number of patients being prospectively followed are at high risk for ectopic pregnancy because of a previous history of pelvic inflammatory disease, prior ectopic pregnancy, or tubal surgery. A variety of new diagnostic modalities are available for early diagnosis and surveillance. The second group of patients typically present with more advanced ectopic gestations and have more obvious evidence of tubal

pregnancy. Pelvic pain is the most common presenting symptom and these patients usually require rapid evaluation and treatment.

EARLY DIAGNOSIS GROUP

Patients who are known to be at high risk and who are having regular menses are advised to have confirmation of pregnancy with a quantitative serum hCG determination within 2–3 days of missed menses. Serum hCG determinations are positive in greater than 99% of intrauterine and ectopic pregnancies. Once pregnancy is confirmed, additional diagnostic modalities, including serum progesterone determination and sonograms, are helpful (Fig. 55.1).

A single serum progesterone determination is helpful in distinguishing normal intrauterine pregnancies from ectopic pregnancies and nonviable intrauterine pregnancies. Values greater than 15 ng/ml are predictive of viable intrauterine pregnancy, although successful pregnancies with values as low as 5 ng/ml have been described. Pregnancies associated with progesterone levels less than 15 ng/ml are usually ectopic pregnancies or inevitable abortions. Progesterone determinations are not helpful in distinguishing ectopic pregnancies from inevitable abortions.

Pelvic sonograms are helpful in detecting intrauterine pregnancies and effectively help establish a diagnosis of ectopic pregnancy by exclusion. The discriminatory zone was originally defined in 1981 as a range of serum hCG concentration between 6000 and 6500 mIU/ml (International Reference Preparation; IRP) above which a gestational sac could be consistently noted with transabdominal ultrasonography [1]. Patients lacking gestational sacs presumptively had ectopic pregnancies. Patients with hCG levels below 6000 mIU/ml (IRP) do not have gestational sacs which could be consistently visualized with transabdominal ultrasonography.

Use of transabdominal ultrasonography significantly enhanced diagnostic capabilities, but the diagnosis was usually established at 6 weeks' gestation or later, when the hCG levels exceeded 6500 mIU/ml (IRP). The advent of transvaginal ultrasonography has permitted the detection of intrauterine gestational sacs 1 week earlier when the hCG levels are approximately 1400 mIU/ml (IRP) or 900 miu/ml (Second International Standard; 2nd IS).

Further refinement of the discriminatory zone has been complicated by variations in the sensitivity of various assays and significant differences in the two available reference standards. The IRP is currently the most commonly used reference standard and utilizes a highly purified source of hCG. The 2nd IS, which paradoxically is the older reference standard, contains substantial amounts of α- and β-subunits in addition to intact hCG and is less suitable as a standard for radioimmunoassays. Several radioimmunoassays still use the 2nd IS as a reference preparation and comparable concentrations of hCG will be reported as lower with the 2nd IS.

In the absence of a detectable gestational sac, other ultrasound findings may be suggestive of ectopic pregnancy. The presence of a complex adnexal mass is associated with ectopic pregnancy in 85% of cases and the predictive value of this finding increases to over 90% in patients who also have free peritoneal fluid. The sensitivity of transvaginal ultrasonography is considerably greater than transabdominal studies in the delineation of adnexal masses and early gestational sacs.

Asymptomatic pregnant patients who have not had their site of implantation determined may be prospectively followed with serial hCG determinations. Retrospective studies have established a normal hCG doubling time of 1.98 days and abnormal pregnancies are associated with less than a 66% increase in hCG levels within a 2-day interval. These pregnancies usually represent ectopic pregnancies or inevitable abortions, but approximately 15% of normal intrauterine pregnancies are associated with abnormal hCG increases. A recent prospective study found a much lower specificity and sensitivity.

THERAPEUTIC OPTIONS

A variety of therapeutic options exist for patients with early asymptomatic ectopic pregnancies. Each option confers unique benefits and risks to the patient and should be presented to the patient in comprehensive discussion as soon as the diagnosis of ectopic pregnancy is seriously entertained. Patients not interested in subsequent fertility should not be treated conservatively and exposed to the risk of future ectopic pregnancies. Those electing conservative approaches should be advised that they will incur a 15–30% risk of future ectopic pregnancies and a 5% risk of persistent trophoblastic disease.

Generally, the diagnosis of ectopic pregnancy can be established within 1 week of confirmation of pregnancy. Many patients with early ectopic pregnancy undergo spontaneous tubal abortion and their course may be evident by declining hCG levels. The risk of tubal rupture and significant intraabdominal bleeding is low when the hCG level is less than 1000 mIU/ml (IRP). Patients with declining hCG values below 1000 mIU/ml (IRP) can be prospectively followed without intervention. Generally, laparoscopy is required for confirmation of the diagnosis and this should be undertaken when the diagnosis is suggested by ultrasound, persistent suboptimal serial hCG increases, or alteration in clinical status. Although patients experiencing spontaneous tubal abortion typically have mild lower pelvic discomfort of 1–2 days' duration, significant pelvic pain necessitates proceeding to laparoscopy or laparotomy.

Patients desirous of subsequent fertility should be treated conservatively. Linear salpingostomy is the treatment of choice for unruptured ampullary ectopic pregnancy and segmental resection for unruptured isthmic ectopic pregnancies. Fimbrial expression should be reserved for those patients who are already undergoing spontaneous tubal abortion. Vigorous fimbrial expression of intact ampullary ectopic pregnancies has been associated with a higher rate of persistent and recurrent ectopic pregnancy. Patients who have completed child-bearing, who have incurred tubal rupture or uncontrolled bleeding from the implantation site, or who have substantial anatomic distortion of the tube, making subsequent function unlikely, should be treated with salpingectomy. Although previous studies suggested that the rate of recurrent ectopic pregnancies was comparable in patients treated with salpingectomy and conservative procedures, more thorough recent studies have confirmed that patients treated with conservative techniques have a twofold higher risk of recurrent ectopic pregnancy. If the patient is hemodynamically unstable, it is most expeditious to proceed directly to laparotomy rather than try to attempt surgery through the laparoscope. In addition, patients with primary contraindications to laparoscopy and those with dense adhesions obscuring the pelvis or between the affected tube and the pelvic sidewall should be treated via laparotomy. Previously, some clinicians used size criteria for resection of ectopic pregnancies, but with the availability of morcellators and other techniques for removal of large amounts of tissue, size alone need not be a contraindication to a laparoscopic approach provided that hemostasis can be assured.

Other therapeutic options for early ectopic pregnancy include systemic methotrexate therapy and salpingocentesis. Presently, there appears to be little advantage in treating with methotrexate if laparoscopy is necessary for the confirmation of the diagnosis and the capability for laparoscopic treatment exists. Some centers have the capability of reliably making the diagnosis of early ectopic pregnancy by ultrasound and have documented the efficacy of systemic methotrexate. Methotrexate 1 mg/kg intramuscularly on alternating days and leucovorin

0.1 mg/kg administered intramuscularly on intervening days is approximately 95% effective for treating unselected ectopic pregnancies and is near 100% effective when limited to patients with early ectopic pregnancies. Alternatively, a single outpatient intramuscular dose of 50 mg/m² without leucovorin has also been recently documented to be effective.

Several authors have described a technique of injection of the tubal gestational sac with a variety of agents including methotrexate, potassium chloride, and prostaglandin $F_{2\alpha}$ and have applied the term salpingocentesis to this procedure. A needle is typically passed via a transvaginal ultrasound needle guide or at the time of laparoscopy into the gestational sac. This treatment appears to be effective, but concerns regarding local tissue effects of inflammatory agents such as methotrexate and potassium chloride have not been resolved. Its use is not recommended in patients seeking additional fertility.

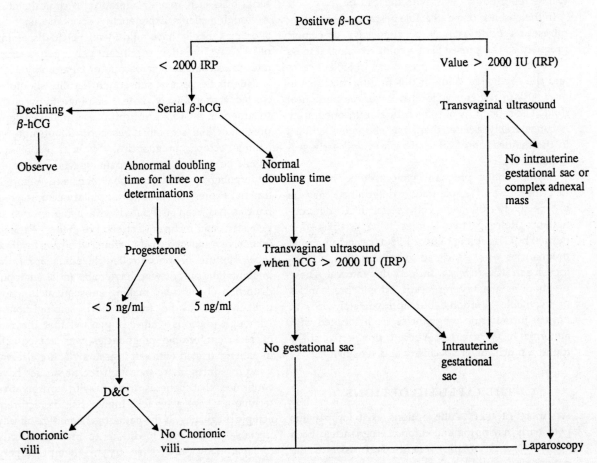

Fig. 55.1 Prospectively followed patients. Development of significant pain moves the patient to stage 2 (Fig. 55.2).

ECTOPIC PREGNANCY

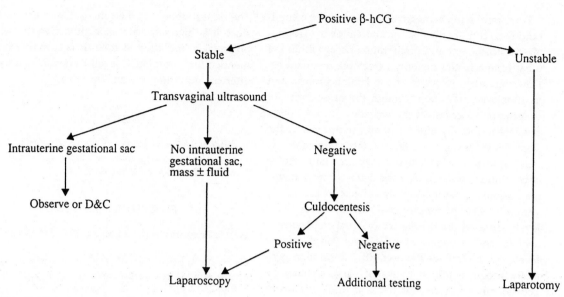

Fig. 55.2 Emergency room presentation with pain.

SYMPTOMATIC PATIENTS

Historically, the most typical clinical presentation of patients with ectopic pregnancy include the classic triad of pelvic pain, menstrual irregularity, and a palpable adnexal mass. Patients who are not being prospectively followed and those with limited health care access still commonly present with these clinical features at a more advanced stage. The likelihood of early spontaneous tubal abortion is less in this group and they usually require early clinical intervention.

Patients presenting in the emergency room with pelvic pain or menstrual irregularity should have a quantitative hCG determination performed (Fig. 55.2). In urgent circumstances a qualitative assay will suffice if the results of the quantitative study will be delayed. If positive, a pelvic sonogram is useful in excluding complicated intrauterine pregnancies and other pelvic pathology. A pregnant patient with significant pelvic pain without evidence of an intrauterine pregnancy should be evaluated with laparoscopy. Culdocentesis may be helpful in determining whether or not a patient needs to go to surgery immediately in a select few cases when the ultrasound findings are equivocal. Positive culdocentesis is highly predictive of ectopic pregnancy. Serial hCG testing is rarely appropriate in this circumstance. Dilatation and curettage may be helpful to identify chorionic villi in nonviable pregnancies prior to laparoscopy.

Most of these patients require surgical therapy.

Although some authors have successfully used systemic methotrexate therapy in advanced ectopic pregnancies, the failure rate with methotrexate is higher and these patients typically have a more complicated and protracted course. Often it is not possible to have the result of the quantitative hCG value back before surgery is performed, making this parameter unavailable for patient selection. The intraoperative choice of surgical procedures is made in the same manner as for those patients diagnosed with earlier ectopic pregnancies. However, more symptomatic patients will present with tubal rupture and advanced ectopic pregnancies, necessitating salpingectomy more often.

SPECIAL CIRCUMSTANCES

The more prevalent use of fertility agents has dramatically increased the incidence of multiple gestations and heterotopic (combined intrauterine and ectopic) pregnancies. The incidence of heterotopic pregnancy was previously determined to be one in 30 000, calculated as the product of the incidence of multiple pregnancies and ectopic pregnancies. As noted previously, both entities are now more common and particularly so in high-risk groups receiving fertility therapy. This possibility should be considered and patients with atypical clinical courses should be carefully followed with serial hCG levels and sonograms after treatment.

CHAPTER 55

Persistent ectopic pregnancy is a unique complication of conservative surgical treatment. Trophoblastic attachment and proliferation occur within the tubal lumen in the majority of ectopic pregnancies. However, early invasion of the lamina propria and trophoblastic dissection through the muscularis not uncommonly occurs. In this instance, it may not be possible to identify effectively and remove all of the trophoblastic tissue at the time of linear salpingotomy. Persistent trophoblastic tissue may gradually resolve or continue to proliferate. If the latter occurs, patients may re-present with symptoms of ectopic pregnancy within 2 weeks of conservative surgery. Serum hCG levels are a reliable marker of residual trophoblastic activity and patients with declining or plateauing levels can be followed expectantly. Resolution generally occurs within 6 weeks of surgery, but may occasionally be more protracted. If hCG levels continue to rise, additional therapy should be undertaken. Options include a second attempt at conservative surgery — which is not recommended because the same limitations are likely to continue to exist — salpingectomy, or systemic methotrexate therapy.

The latter option is becoming the most popular since it is highy effective and preserves the fertility potential of the affected tube. It is currently recommended that serum hCG levels be obtained at weekly intervals until they are undetectable.

REFERENCES

1 Kadar N, DeVoe G, Romero R. Discriminatory hCG zone: its use in the sonographic evaluation for ectopic pregnancy. *Obstet Gynecol* 1981; 58: 156.

FURTHER READING

Ectopic Pregnancy — United States, 1987. *MMWR* 1990; 39: 401.
Garcia A, Aubert J, Sama J, *et al*. Expectant management of presumed ectopic pregnancies. *Fertil Steril* 1987; 48: 395–400.
Leach RE, Ory SJ. Modern management of ectopic pregnancy. *J Reprod Med* 1989; 34: 324–338.
Stovall TG, Ling FW, Carson SA, Busler JE. Nonsurgical diagnosis and treatment of tubal pregnancy. *Fertil Steril* 1990; 54: 537–540.

56

Recurrent abortion

JOHN F. RANDOLPH JR

INTRODUCTION

A common definition for the diagnosis of recurrent abortion is three or more pregnancy losses occurring prior to 20 weeks' gestation. The terms primary recurrent abortion and secondary recurrent abortion can be utilized but do not change the diagnostic evaluation or therapeutic program. Primary recurrent abortion applies when no viable offspring have been delivered, whereas secondary recurrent abortion describes losses following at least one successful pregnancy. Approximately 3% of all women who conceive will suffer at least three spontaneous abortions.

An important part of the clinical management of couples with recurrent pregnancy loss is patient education and counseling, especially regarding the risk of subsequent losses. Older estimates of the risk of future losses based on the number of previous losses were calculated on incorrect assumptions and greatly exaggerated the risks. Clinical studies have demonstrated a 20−26% risk of a third abortion after two spontaneous losses, a 32% risk of a fourth abortion after three losses, and 50% risk of another abortion after four or more losses. In general, a diagnostic evaluation will identify a problem associated with recurrent abortion in about two-thirds of couples completely studied. In couples with no identifiable problem associated with recurrent abortion approximately two-thirds will have a live birth within 3 years [1].

CAUSES OF RECURRENT ABORTION

At least five major categories of disorders have been associated with recurrent abortion. These include genetic, anatomic, endocrinologic, infectious, and immunologic abnormalities. This section will briefly discuss the pathophysiology of each.

Genetic

Abnormal gestational karyotypes have been identified in about two-thirds of spontaneous abortions studied, with trisomies accounting for the majority followed by polyploidies and monosomies. Genetic studies of couples with two or more spontaneous abortions have noted a 7.2% frequency of parental karyotype [2]. The majority of karyotypic abnormalities were balanced translocations in one of the parents, resulting in the risk of passage of unbalanced genetic material to a conceptus with the resulting loss. Appropriate genetic counseling can provide some estimate to the couple of the likelihood of further losses.

Anatomic

Congenital or acquired Müllerian structural abnormalities are found in 15−30% of women with recurrent abortions. The congenital anomaly most associated with recurrent abortion is a uterine septum, a Müllerian resorption defect. Excision of the septum, or metroplasty, restores a normal viable pregnancy rate.

Müllerian fusion defects such as a bicornuate uterus or uterine didelphys are typically associated with problems later in pregnancy such as preterm labor and premature delivery. Similarly, *in utero* diethylstilbestrol (DES) exposure has been associated with problems in the mid and late trimesters due to cervical incompetence and premature delivery.

Acquired anatomic defects include intrauterine scarring, or synechiae, and uterine leiomyomas. Synechiae are usually iatrogenic and typically occur after a pregnancy-related instrumentation of the uterus, particularly in the presence of infection. Submucous myomas have been theorized to exert hemodynamic, hormonal, or mechanical influences on a pregnancy and result in early losses.

CHAPTER 56

Endocrinologic

Endocrine causes of recurrent abortion, whether overt endocrinopathies or ovulatory abnormalities, have been reported in 5–25% of women with recurrent losses. Most overt endocrinopathies, such as diabetes mellitus or thyroid disease, must be clinically apparent before an effect on reproductive function is seen. Currently, unless diabetes mellitus is obvious and uncontrolled, it is unlikely to be a significant factor and does not require formal screening. Significant thyroid disease is usually symptomatic and authorities debate the utility of routine screening. There is no place for empiric thyroid replacement therapy in the treatment of recurrent abortion. Hyperprolactinemia associated with normal menstrual function in the absence of galactorrhea plays an uncertain role in recurrent pregnancy loss. It is generally treated if noted due to the uncertainty.

Ovulatory abnormalities without another obvious endocrinopathy comprise the majority of women with endocrinologic causes for recurrent abortion. The long-standing concept of a luteal-phase defect due to inadequate progesterone secretion in the luteal phase of the cycle and subsequent failure to support an early pregnancy has become a fixture in the evaluation of couples with recurrent abortions [3]. A broader view of ovulatory dysfunction resulting from abnormal folliculogenesis, an inadequate corpus luteum, or a poor endometrial response may be a more useful approach to the evaluation and treatment of couples with recurrent pregnancy losses.

Infections

There is some evidence that *Ureaplasma urealyticum* is associated with recurrent abortions in humans based on a greater frequency of positive cultures in women with recurrent losses and an improvement in the viable pregnancy rate after treatment of the infection [4]. There is little or no evidence to support an association between any other organism and recurrent abortion.

Immunologic

Immunologic associations with recurrent pregnancy loss can be grouped into autoimmune and alloimmune causes. Autoimmunity as a source of recurrent abortions has been associated with the presence of antiphospholipid antibodies in the mother, specifically lupus anticoagulant or anticardiolipin antibody, resulting in a tendency to thrombosis with infarction of trophoblast and eventual pregnancy loss. Alloimmunity in recurrent pregnancy loss has been theorized to result from parental genetic similarity with failure of the mother to recognize the fetus as foreign. Blocking antibodies do not develop to protect the pregnancy and it is subsequently lost due to the resultant cytotoxic maternal response. The exact relationship of alloimmunity to recurrent pregnancy loss has not been firmly established and therapy has been generally provided at a few major centers.

EVALUATION

The traditional approach to the evaluation of couples with recurrent abortion required three spontaneous losses before a work-up due to the statistical likelihood of success after one or two losses. In view of the modern tendency to delay pregnancy for social reasons and the overall decrease in family size, it may be judicious to undertake an abbreviated or complete evaluation after only two losses dependent upon the clinical situation (Fig. 56.1).

History and physical

A detailed reproductive history is vital to the complete evaluation of couples with habitual abortion and should include a full menstrual history, complete obstetric history, the gestational ages of losses, any studies performed on the abortus, any operative intervention associated with pregnancy, and any complications of successful pregnancies. A history or symptoms of connective tissue diseases or endocrinopathies should be obtained. Attention should also be paid to any family history of pregnancy losses or congenital anomalies.

The physical examination should pay particular attention to the thyroid gland for evidence of thyroid disease, the breasts for the presence of galactorrhea, the skin and muscoskeletal system for evidence of connective tissue diseases, and the pelvis for signs of Müllerian anomalies.

Initial laboratory studies

At the time of the initial evaluation a number of studies should be obtained to expedite the evaluation. Karyotypes should be obtained from both partners. Thyroid-stimulating hormone (TSH) and prolactin should be obtained from the woman to rule out subclinical endocrinopathies. Lupus anticoagulant (or partial thromboplastin time) and anticardiolipin antibody should be obtained to screen for autoimmune-

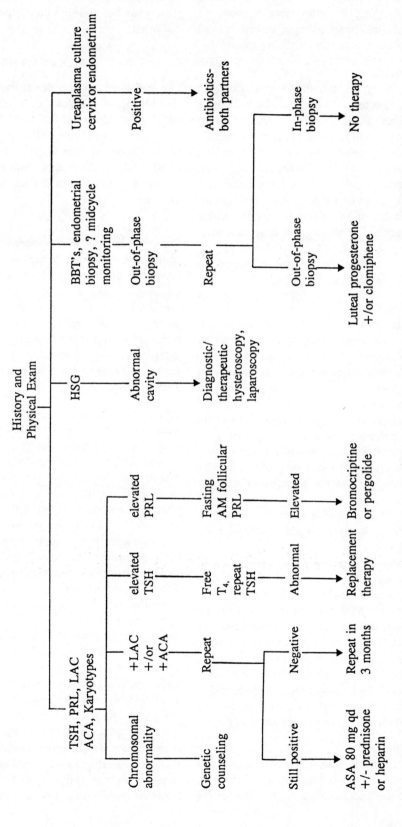

Fig. 56.1 Decision making tree for the evaluation and treatment of couples with recurrent abortion. TSH, thyroid stimulating hormone; PRL, prolactin; LAC, lupus anticoagulant; ACA, anticardiolipin antibody; HSG, hysterosalpingogram; BBT, basal body temperature.

CHAPTER 56

associated recurrent pregnancy loss. Some authors recommend obtaining an antinuclear antibody in addition but this relatively nonspecific test has an uncertain association with recurrent abortion.

Anatomic evaluation

A hysterosalpingogram should be performed in the follicular phase to avoid the risk of irradiating a recent conceptus. Slow insufflation during fluoroscopic viewing provides the most sensitive method of detecting filling defects suggestive of myomas, polyps or synechiae. A classic Y-shaped cavity indicates a Müllerian defect but does not determine whether it is a fusion or a resorption defect. Laparoscopic evaluation of the external uterine fundus is currently required to distinguish a septate from a bicornuate uterus. Ultrasonography has proved promising in the evaluation of anatomic defects and may ultimately replace laparoscopy.

Ovulatory evaluation

The current standard for evaluation of normal ovulation includes basal body temperature monitoring and late luteal endometrial sampling. Late luteal decidualized endometrium serves as a bioassay of adequate estrogen priming and cumulative progesterone exposure and is felt to be a reflection of ovulatory adequacy. If the endometrium lags behind the expected histologic development by 2 or more days, the biopsy is felt to be out of phase and suggestive of a luteal-phase defect. Out of phase biopsies in two consecutive cycles are required to establish the diagnosis. The biopsy should be performed approximately 12 days after ovulation, as timed by urinary luteinizing hormone testing or basal body temperatures.

Due to criticisms of endometrial biopsies as subjective and insensitive indicators of ovulatory adequacy, other methods have been utilized to determine normal ovulation. Midluteal serum progesterone levels have been utilized but criticized as being too variable and without an accepted standard. Midluteal urinary progesterone levels may prove to be a more useful measure. Midcycle follicular monitoring with ultrasonogrpahy and associated endocrinologic measurements is being evaluated as a potentially more sensitive measure of ovulatory adequacy.

Infectious evaluation

Cultures for *Ureaplasma urealyticum* can be obtained from the cervix at the time of the initial evaluation or directly from the endometrium at the time of the endometrial biopsy. Routine screening for other pathogens has no scientific support unless clinically indicated.

TREATMENT

The treatment for couples with recurrent abortion should logically follow complete evaluation and address all abnormalities discovered. It must be emphasized to the couple that the goal of treatment is to restore the normal successful pregnancy rate of 80–85% per conception. Subsequent losses must be evaluated in the context of the normal spontaneous loss rate.

Genetic treatment

Genetic treatment at the current time is limited to counseling the couple regarding the potential for a successful pregnancy and alternative approaches to building a family. If the genetic defect is paternal in origin then donor insemination should be mentioned as an alternative source of sperm. If the defect is maternal in origin, oocyte donation can now be considered since it is becoming increasingly available. Embryonic genetic diagnosis and therapy will not be available for some time.

Anatomic treatment

Congenital or acquired Müllerian structural anomalies require surgical therapy for correction. Most procedures can be performed endoscopically and it is practical to plan for definitive surgery at the time of surgical diagnosis. Since laparoscopy remains the standard approach to evaluate further Müllerian anomalies identified by hysterosalpingography and simultaneous laparoscopic monitoring is recommended during operative hysteroscopy, it is prudent to plan for hysteroscopic surgery at the time of diagnostic laparoscopy.

Septate uteri have been associated with a 90–95% abortion rate in couples with recurrent losses. Hysteroscopic metroplasty has been reported to reduce the loss rate to 10–13%, comparable to abdominal approaches [5]. A number of instruments can be used, including flexible scissors, electrocautery, and laser, all with comparable results. As with most endoscopic procedures, patients undergo outpatient surgery with minimal recovery time. The hysteroscopic approach avoids the complications of a laparotomy as well as postoperative adhesion formation interfering with conception and transfundal scarring, necessitating a cesarean section for delivery. Complications can occur and include uterine perforation, incomplete resection, and pulmonary edema from fluid overload due to extravasation of distending media.

Nonseptate Müllerian anomalies rarely are an indication for surgical therapy with uterine unification, usually only if no other abnormalities can be identified. Synechiae are best handled with the hysteroscopic approach, utilizing any of the methods available for metroplasty. Success depends in large part on the degree of intrauterine adhesions and the ability both to restore a normal uterine cavity and to regenerate a normal endometrium. Abdominal myomectomy is an acceptable technique for significant fibroids, especially if the cavity is distorted. The relationship of myomas not distorting the cavity to recurrent abortion has not been clarified. Hysteroscopic resection of myomas is appropriate for pedunculated intracavitary tumors but an uncertain approach for submucous or transmural myomas.

Endocrinologic treatment

All obvious endocrinopathies should be corrected with optimization of therapy for diabetes or thyroid disease. Biopsy-proven luteal-phase defects can be treated by several methods. Progesterone can be administered in the luteal phase of the cycle, beginning 3 days after the urinary luteinizing hormone surge, on the second day of temperature elevation, or on day 16 of the cycle, and continued for 12 days. Progesterone can be given as an intramuscular injection, as vaginal suppositories, or as micronized capsules in doses of 25–400 mg b.i.d. A traditional approach is 25 mg suppositories b.i.d. Clomiphene citrate can also be used instead of or in addition to luteal progesterone and typically is given as 25–100 mg daily for 5 days in the follicular phase of the cycle. If these therapies are unsuccessful, then human menopausal gonadotropins can be used.

Hyperprolactinemia should be treated with a dopamine agonist, either bromocriptine or pergolide. The dose should be slowly titrated to the minimum that will control the serum prolactin level.

Infections

Should the couple demonstrate culture-positive *Ureaplasma* then antibiotic therapy for both partners should be instituted, utilizing tetracycline, erythromycin, or another antibiotic with good coverage for the organism. Some authors recommend prophylactic treatment of all partners with recurrent abortion rather than routine cultures.

Immunologic treatment

Positive maternal antiphospholipid antibodies have been treated with a variety of therapies with a significant improvement in pregnancy success. Glucocorticoids were initially used in immunosuppressive doses. Prednisone 40–60 mg/day was commonly required to depress serum antibody levels. Low-dose daily aspirin has become relatively standard to help counteract the thrombotic tendency in patients with antiphospholipid antibodies. The dose is 80 mg/day or one children's aspirin. Heparin 7500 U b.i.d. is also being utilized in some centers with some success, oftentimes combined with aspirin therapy. Other therapies are being tested. It is advisable to initiate therapy before conception is attempted.

Therapy for alloimmune problems has generally involved attempts to establish blocking antibodies in the mother by immunization with paternal or third-party cells or tissue. The safety, efficacy, and clinical indications for such therapy are currently being investigated in a number of centers.

CONCLUSIONS

Recurrent abortion is a devastating form of infertility punctuated by periods of joy, hope, and anxiety followed by great frustration, anger, and depression. A clinical reason for recurrent abortion can be found most of the time and information and/or treatment provided. The practitioner is encouraged to evaluate couples completely, treat all identified problems, and to caution couples that the goal of therapy is to restore the normal chance for a healthy baby.

REFERENCES

1 Parazzini F, Acaia B, Ricciardiello O, Fedele L, Liati P, Candiani GB. Short-term reproductive prognosis when no cause can be found for recurrent miscarriage. *Br J Obstet Gynaecol* 1988; 95: 654.

2 Boue A. Spontaneous abortions and cytogenetic abnormalities. In: Behrman SJ, Kistner RW, Patton GW, eds. *Progress in Infertility*, 3rd edn. Boston: Little Brown & Co., 1988: 783.

3 McNeely MJ, Soules MR. The diagnosis of luteal phase deficiency: a critical review. *Fertil Steril* 1988; 50: 1.

4 Stray-Pedersen B, Eng J, Reikvam TM. Uterine mycoplasma colonization in reproductive failure. *Am J Obstet Gynecol* 1978; 130: 307.

5 March CM, Israel R. Hysteroscopic management of recurrent abortion caused by septate uterus. *Am J Obstet Gynecol* 1987; 156: 834.

57

Antiphospholipid antibodies and pregnancy loss

MICHELLE PETRI

BACKGROUND

A family of autoantibodies — antiphospholipid antibodies — have been identified that are associated with a clinical syndrome of: (1) venous thrombosis; (2) arterial thrombosis; (3) pregnancy losses; and (4) thrombocytopenia [1]. The clinical syndrome can occur in parts, so that women may present with pregnancy losses alone [2]. The clinical syndrome is not limited to patients with systemic lupus erythematosus; many women will have no autoimmune symptoms or signs [2].

The two antiphospholipid antibodies of clinical importance are the lupus anticoagulant (LA) and anticardiolipin antibody (ACL). The LA, the first antibody described, obtained its confusing name because it interferes with *in vitro* clotting tests, producing a prolongation of tests such as the activated partial thromboplastin time (aPTT). *In vivo*, however, it is associated with a hypercoagulable state. Bleeding from the LA is very rare, and usually is due to a second defect, such as thrombocytopenia, factor deficiency, or vascular abnormality.

ACL, more recently described, has an equally unfortunate name. It is highly unlikely that the antibody is primarily directed against cardiolipin, which is found inside of mitochondria. Instead, the antibody may be directed against negatively charged phospholipids, such as those found on endothelial cells or against a phospholipid—cofactor complex. ACL is measured by enzyme-linked immunosorbent assay (ELISA), not by coagulation tests. Results will be given in standard deviations above the mean or in international units.

Although patients may make both antibodies and the two antibodies are associated with the same clinical syndrome, they are not the same. Thus, it is necessary to measure both LA and ACL in patients suspected of having the antiphospholipid antibody syndrome.

PATHOGENESIS

Although associated with a hypercoagulable state, it is not at all clear that antiphospholipid antibodies are causally related to the antiphospholipid antibody syndrome. They may be epiphenomena, with the causative factor or factors yet to be identified.

Several mechanisms have been proposed by which antiphospholipid antibodies might lead to a hypercoagulable state. First they may lead to an imbalance in the prostacyclin/thromboxane pathway. Second, they may bind to or activate platelets. Third, they may interact with control proteins in the coagulation cascade, including protein C, protein S, and possibly apolipoprotein H. Fourth, they may inhibit fibrinolysis. Lack of understanding of the mechanism of action has hampered identification of the most appropriate treatment. Both antiplatelet agents and anticoagulation with heparin and warfarin have been used for patients with venous and/or arterial thrombotic events.

In women with the antiphospholipid antibody syndrome who present with pregnancy losses alone, it is unclear whether a hypercoagulable state is necessarily the mechanism of pregnancy loss. Although some placentas are small with thrombi, many do not show pathologic abnormality [3].

PREVALENCE OF ANTIPHOSPHOLIPID ANTIBODIES AND RISK OF FETAL LOSS

In patients with systemic lupus erythematosus, antiphospholipid antibodies are commonly found. In one cross-sectional study, 7% of lupus patients had the lupus anticoagulant and 25% had the ACL [4]. Because patients with lupus can transiently have antiphospholipid antibodies, longitudinal studies have shown much larger percentages of patients having one or more antiphospholipid antibodies at some point in time. Women with systemic lupus erythematosus have, on average, a 25% chance of pregnancy loss. In lupus, pregnancy loss is multifactorial, with contributions from active lupus, renal disease, and antiphospholipid antibodies. The presence of antiphospholipid antibodies is a major predictor of pregnancy loss in both prospective and retrospective studies [1,5]. However, patients with lupus may have normal pregnancies, even in the presence of and without treatment of antiphospholipid antibodies.

Studies of normal young women have shown that approximately 2% have anticardiolipin antibody [6]. The prevalence of antiphospholipid antibodies is increased in women who have idiopathic habitual abortion, with frequencies of 10% or higher [5–7]. Antiphospholipid antibodies may be transient, appearing only during pregnancy, making it difficult to measure accurately prevalence figures. Women with idiopathic habitual abortion and antiphospholipid antibodies have had pregnancy loss in all three trimesters [6,7], although there may be an association with late pregnancy loss in particular. As in patients with lupus, normal pregnancies, without treatment, have occurred in some women with antiphospholipid antibodies and past pregnancy losses.

INDICATIONS OF SCREENING FOR ANTIPHOSPHOLIPID ANTIBODIES

Screening for antiphospholipid antibodies is recommended for women contemplating pregnancy with; (1) systemic lupus erythematosus, other connective tissue diseases, or autoimmune symptoms or signs such as a biologic false-positive test for syphilis; (2) a history of venous or arterial thrombosis; (3) a poor obstetric history, including two or more spontaneous abortions, or any second-trimester loss or late intrauterine death; and (4) thrombocytopenia.

Antiphospholipid antibodies may appear transiently during pregnancy and, therefore, be missed if screening is performed between pregnancies. Repeat testing is recommended as soon as pregnancy is confirmed and at monthly intervals thereafter.

CHOICE OF LABORATORY TESTS

The LA is measured with coagulation assays. The aPTT has the advantage of being widely available, but is neither specific nor sensitive for the LA [6]. Better tests for the LA are phospholipid poor and require careful preparation of the plasma sample.

Excellent tests for the LA include: (1) recalcified clotting time; (2) modified Russell viper venom time; (3) kaolin clotting time; and (4) platelet neutralization procedure. Because the lupus anticoagulant is heterogeneous, no one assay is capable of identifying all patients with the antibody. If possible, two different tests should be employed. The Russell viper venom test is not affected by rising levels of factor VIII during pregnancy.

ACL is measured using an ELISA assay. A polyclonal assay or an immunoglobulin G ACL (the most important isotype) are both adequate. The assay can be performed on either serum or plasma.

In a patient in whom antiphospholipid antibodies are found, a search for subclinical or occult connective tissue disease should be undertaken. The antinuclear antibody test is usually positive in women with systemic lupus erythematosus, but is also positive (in titers up to 1:640) in 20% of normal women [6]. Other autoantibody tests include anti-Ro (associated with congenital heart bock), anti-La, anti-Sm, anti-RNP, and anti-DNA.

TREATMENT DILEMMAS

It is not surprising, given the lack of knowledge of the mechanism of action of antiphospholipid antibodies or even if the antibodies are causally related to pregnancy loss, that treatment regimens are controversial and constantly changing. The major source of controversy is whether the aim of treatment during pregnancy should be immunosuppression (i.e., prednisone) or anticoagulation (the antiplatelet agent aspirin or heparin). In nonpregnant patients with venous or arterial thrombosis alone, anticoagulation alone is usually used. In nonpregnant patients with thrombosis and lupus, anticoagulation is recommended with sufficient prednisone to control other manifestations of lupus.

Treatment of women without prior pregnancy losses
In a woman with no prior pregnancy losses, the finding of antiphospholipid antibodies does not require treatment. Multiple reports of normal pregnancies exist despite the presence of the lupus anticoagulant or antiphospholipid antibodies.

Treatment of women with prior pregnancy losses
The first issue to be faced is treatment or no treatment. Unfortunately, there is no current test to predict which women with antiphospholipid antibodies will

benefit from treatment and no way to decide whether prednisone, aspirin, anticoagulation, or all three, are preferable. In a recent randomized, controlled trial, prednisone and aspirin were as effective as subcutaneous heparin and aspirin, but rates of pre-eclampsia and maternal morbidity were higher in the prednisone arm [8].

The second issue is whether to commence treatment before conception. Certainly, a daily baby aspirin can be started when pregnancy is contemplated. However, beginning prednisone prior to conception exposes the woman to the hazards of prednisone (including infection, hypertension, diabetes, osteopenia, and avascular necrosis of bone) for an unacceptably long period of time.

The third issue is to pick a regimen to follow and to decide how to "fine-tune" that regimen during the pregnancy. Most physicians have followed some variation of the regimen of Lubbe et al. [9], using a daily baby aspirin and prednisone in doses from 20 to 40 mg a day. However, it is perfectly acceptable to use a daily baby aspirin alone as the first treatment attempt. There is no correct dose of prednisone. However, high doses of prednisone, in the 60 mg range, are not associated with better outcomes. Because therapy with subcutaneous heparin and aspirin appears to have less maternal morbidity, it may become the preferred treatment.

Adjustment of the regimen during pregnancy cannot be done on a logical basis. Because there is no direct evidence that the antiphospholipid antibodies are causally related to pregnancy loss, it is not necessary to completely abolish their presence with immunosuppressive therapy. In general, the LA appears to be more sensitive to suppression by prednisone than ACL. However, rising titers of antibodies are of concern and are often used as the basis for an increase in the prednisone dose or addition of another agent.

If the woman has had both a prior pregnancy loss or losses and a thrombotic event, subcutaneous heparin is used with or without prednisone and, often, a daily baby aspirin. Warfarin is not used because of its teratogenic potential. In women without thrombotic events, a pregnancy loss on aspirin and prednisone therapy might lead to the use of subcutaneous heparin on the "next try." No correct dose of subcutaneous heparin exists. Doses employed are usually larger than prophylactic subcutaneous

heparin, but less than that needed to achieve full anticoagulation. In many women with the lupus anticoagulant, the aPTT is prolonged prior to treatment and, therefore, cannot be used to monitor therapy.

Experimental regimens include the use of plasmapheresis or intravenous immunoglobulin. In the choice of any regimen, the pregnant woman and her physicians must weigh the potential side-effects to the woman of the treatment versus the emotional cost of pregnancy loss. Figures available on the success rate of any treatment regimen range from 60% to 75%, but published case series are overly optimistic. Multiple failures have occurred on prednisone, baby aspirin, and even subcutaneous heparin.

REFERENCES

1 Harris EN, Chan JKH, Asherson RA et al. Thrombosis, recurrent fetal loss, and thrombocytopenia: predictive value of the anticardiolipin antibody test. Arch Intern Med 1986; 146: 2153–2156.
2 Branch W, Scott JR, Kochenour NK et al. Obstetric complications associated with the lupus anticoagulant. N Engl J Med 1985; 313: 1322–1326.
3 Lockshin MD, Druzin ML, Goei S et al. Antibody to cardiolipin as a predictor of fetal distress or death in pregnant patients with systemic lupus erythematosus. N Engl J Med 1985; 313: 152–156.
4 Petri M, Rheinschmidt M, Whiting-O'Keefe Q, Hellmann D, Corash L. The frequency of lupus anticoagulant in systemic lupus erythematosus: a study of 60 consecutive patients by activated partial thromboplastin time, Russell viper venom time, and anticardiolipin antibody. Ann Intern Med 1987; 106: 524–531.
5 Cowchock S, Smith JB, Gocial B. Antibodies to phospholipids and nuclear antigens in patients with repeated abortions. Am J Obstet Gynecol 1986; 155: 1002–1010.
6 Petri M, Golbus M, Anderson R, Whiting-O'Keefe Q, Corash L, Hellmann D. Antinuclear antibodies, lupus anticoagulant, and anticardiolipin antibody in idiopathic habitual abortion: a controlled prospective study of 44 women. Arthritis Rheum 1987; 30: 601–606.
7 Maier DB, Parke A. Subclinical autoimmunity in recurrent aborters. Fertil Steril 1989; 51: 280–285.
8 Cowchock FS, Reece EA, Balaban D, Branch DW, Plouffe L. Repeated fetal losses associated with antiphospholipid antibodies: a collaborative randomized trial comparing prednisone with low-dose heparin treatment. Am J Obstet Gynecol 1992; 166: 1318–1323.
9 Lubbe WF, Butler WS, Palmer SJ, Liggins GC. Fetal survival after prednisone suppression of maternal lupus anticoagulant. Lancet 1983; I: 1361–1363.

58

Recurrent abortion: immunotherapy

JOSEPH A. HILL

Human reproduction is biologically inefficient as 70% of conceptions fail to achieve viability. Approximately 50% of these are lost prior to the first missed menses. Clinically detectable spontaneous abortion occurs in 10–20% of all human pregnancies. The risks of recurrence have been tabulated to be 24% after one miscarriage, 26–30% after two, 32–34% after three consecutive losses, and 36–40% after four spontaneous abortions.

Recurrent abortion, defined by the occurrence of three or more spontaneous abortions prior to the 20th week of gestation, occurs in one in 300 pregnancies. Recurrent abortion is therefore a clinically important medical problem. Many etiologies have been proposed (Table 58.1). All except chromosomal abnormalities in the couple experiencing recurrent abortion are controversial. The cause in the majority of couples is unexplaind [1]. Many immunologic theories have been proposed to explain recurrent abortion (Table 58.2), for viviparous reproduction is an immunologic enigma since the conceptus contains paternal and unique differentiation antigens that are genetically foreign to the maternal host. An assumption has been that initial contact of the conceptus with the maternal immune system occurs at implantation. However, even prior to implantation the developing conceptus is supported and bathed in the immunologically dynamic milieu of uterine and tuboperitoneal fluid [2]. Despite the many theories that have been proposed for immunologic recurrent abortion there remain few direct substantive data [3]. Nevertheless, immunotherapy for recurrent abortion has promulgated, often more by outcome of therapy than by elucidation of basic pathophysiologic mechanisms.

Both immunostimulating and immunosuppressive therapies (Table 58.3) have been implemented, depending upon whether the maternal immune system is believed to be either hyporesponsive or hyperresponsive to paternal–fetal antigens. Immunostimu-

Table 58.2 Immunologic theories of recurrent spontaneous abortion

Suppressor cell and suppressor factor deficiency
Induction of major histocompatibility antigen expression
Blocking antibody deficiency
Antiphospholipid syndrome
Immunodystrophism (cytokine-mediated immunologic attack)

Table 58.1 Potential etiologies of recurrent spontaneous abortion

Cause	Percentage
Endocrinologic	17
Anatomic	10
Chromosomal	5
Infectious	5
Humoral immune	3
Unknown	60

Table 58.3 Immunotherapy for recurrent spontaneous abortion

Immunostimulating
    Leukocyte transfusions
    Immunoglobulin transfusions
    Seminal plasma suppositories

Immunosuppression
    Corticosteroids
    Aspirin
    Heparin
    Progesterone
    Pentoxifylline
    Cyclosporine

lating therapy is based on three suppositions: (1) there is an antifetal maternal cellular immune response that develops in all pregnancies that must be blocked; (2) blocking antibodies develop in all successful pregnancies that prevent antifetal immunity; and (3) in the absence of blocking antibodies abortion occurs. Unfortunately, there is no direct evidence to support these suppositions. Cause-and-effect relationships are difficult to ascribe, yet pathologic evidence is inconclusive whether immunologic abortion occurs. Blocking antibodies are also not demonstrable in all successful pregnancies. In fact only 40–60% of multigravid women make such immunoglobulin effectors (reviewed in [3]).

The rationale for immunostimulating therapy involving leukocytes, immunoglobulin or seminal plasma has been based on reports of increased human leukocyte antigen (HLA) sharing, trophoblast–lymphocyte cross-reactive (TLX) antigen similarities, and hyporesponsive mixed-lymphocyte culture (MLC) reactivities between partners experiencing recurrent abortion. The underlying hypothesis is that antigenic similarities between mating partners abrogate maternal recognition of paternal–fetal antigens, thus preventing blocking antibody formation. Theoretically, then, by overriding the maternal immune system with leukocytes, exogenous immunoglobulin, or third-party seminal plasma, the presumed antifetal maternal cellular immune attack would be blocked, thus allowing successful gestation. Basic and clinical research has been unable to provide direct evidence to substantiate this theory. Reports regarding HLA sharing are generally retrospective and without population-based controls. However, one prospective, population-based study in Hutterites has conclusively demonstrated that HLA sharing is not associated with recurrent abortion [4]. Animal studies also do not support this concept since inbred strains have achieved successful pregnancies for generations.

Theories involving the concept of TLX are also controversial because of the finding that the polyclonal antisera that originally defined TLX are identical to CD46, a marker for membrane cofactor protein (MCP), a complement receptor [5]. Therefore, rather than TLX functioning as an essential maternal recognition structure involving idiotype and antiidiotype hypotheses, the characterization of TLX as CD46 implies that its function is to bind complement, thus preventing complement-mediated attack of the developing trophoblast. CD46, not surprisingly, is

also present on a wide range of other cells including leukocytes and sperm, thus explaining the cross-reactive nature of the antisera that defined TLX. The concept that MLC hyporesponsiveness is a marker for immunologic recurrent abortion is also questionable since MLC hyporesponsiveness is an inconsistent finding in women with recurrent abortion but, more importantly, MLC hyporesponsiveness is present in many couples with successful pregnancies. The presence or absence of antipaternal cytotoxic antibody is also not a good marker for determining the success or failure of pregnancy. HLA typing, antipaternal cytotoxic antibody testing, and MLC determinations are therefore unnecessary as they have neither diagnostic nor therapeutic value.

As the scientific rationale for immunostimulating therapy becomes more dubious, patient expectations and belief in the efficacy of this therapy have become the new rationale for its use. Therapeutic efficacy can only be proven in double-blinded, appropriately controlled trials. One double-blinded placebo-controlled trial has been published supporting leukocyte immunization [6]. However, two other double-blinded placebo-controlled trials have been unable to demonstrate a therapeutic benefit of leukocyte immunization over placebo [7,8]. The double-blinded nature of the study indicating efficacy has been questioned due to the inappropriately low success rate with placebo (37%) as compared to epidemiologic data indicating a 60% chance of successful pregnancy even after four prior spontaneous abortions [9].

Intravenous α-globulin has been used for replacement therapy in women with humoral immune deficiency and to treat both autoimmune diseases (chronic immune thrombocytopenic purpura (ITP) and alloimmune disorders (Rh sensitization) in pregnancy. The mechanisms are unclear, although feedback inhibition of fetal antibody synthesis, Fc-receptor target cell blockade in both mother and fetus, and blockade of Fc-mediated transplacental antibody transport have been proposed (discussed in [10]). Its use in pregnancy is anecdotal. The rationale for its use in women with recurrent spontaneous abortion other than due to Rh disease and ITP has not been elucidated. Appropriate dosage, frequency of administration, and potential efficacy in randomized placebo-controlled trials have yet to be determined.

Third-party seminal plasma suppositories have also been recommended as therapy for recurrent abortion. The rationale for its use is unclear but involves the belief that TLX antibodies are present in semen. The finding that TLX is equivalent to CD46, a complement receptor found on sperm and not in seminal plasma, makes the rationale for its use even less clear.

Immunostimulation therapy may not necessarily be innocuous (Table 58.4), although not all investigators have reported adverse sequelae. Potential adverse reactions include anaphylaxis, serum sickness, and sensitization produced by administration of foreign cells or antigens. Graft-versus-host reactions in immunized women and fetal growth retardation in their progeny are other concerns. The transmission of infectious organisms such as hepatitis, human immunodeficiency virus, cytomegalovirus, and toxoplasmosis are other possibilities.

Immunosuppressive therapy (Table 58.3) has also been proposed for recurrent spontaneous abortion based on the concept that an adverse maternal immune response, whether humoral (antibody-mediated) as occurs in the antiphospholipid syndrome or cellular (cytokine-mediated) as occurs with immunodystrophism, can cause recurrent abortion. Women who develop antiphospholipid antibodies are at increased risk for pregnancy loss. Antiphospholipid antibodies are autoantibodies directed against negatively charged phospholipids and comprise the lupus anticoagulant, anticardiolipin antibody, and the biologically false-positive test for syphilis. The lupus anticoagulant and anticardiolipin antibody are the most clinically relevant regarding thrombosis and recurrent abortion. The lupus anticoagulant is most often detected by activated partial thromboplastin time elevation or an elevated Russell viper venom time. The highest prevalence of antiphospholipid antibodies is in women with autoimmune disease, especially systemic lupus erythematosus. The basic hypothesis is that these autoantibodies prevent the formation of prostacyclin by inhibiting the release of arachidonic acid

Table 58.4 Potential risks of immunostimulating immunotherapy

Anaphylaxis
Serum sickness
Sensitization
Graft-versus-host disease
Inability to receive donor organs
Infection
Intrauterine growth retardation

from endothelial phospholipids. The inhibition of prostacyclin, a potent vasodilator and antithrombolic compound, could be responsible for the thrombotic events observed in some women with antiphospholipid antibodies. Decidual vasculopathy and placental infarction could result, culminating in fetal growth retardation, stillbirth or recurrent abortion. Placental pathologic evidence has not substantiated this hypothesis in all cases of fetal loss where elevated antiphospholipid antibodies have been detected. There are many false-positive reactions with antinuclear antibody assessment and they are not necessarily associated with elevated antiphospholipid antibodies. Therefore, antinuclear antibody testing is not necessary in women with recurrent abortion.

Therapy with low-dose aspirin (80 mg/day) and prednisone in doses of 20–80 mg/day has been implemented in women with high-titer antibodies in an effort to inhibit the formation of thromboxanes while not lowering prostacyclin levels and to lower autoantibody titers. Studies have not been able to confirm that lowering autoantibody titers has a beneficial effect on pregnancy outcome [11]. Potential side-effects of corticosteroid treatment include adrenal insufficiency, severe acne, glucose intolerance, impaired wound healing, cushingoid facies, platelet abnormalities and aseptic necrosis of the hip. Therefore low-dose aspirin may be a better therapeutic choice than corticosteroid therapy for women with antiphospholipid antibodies. Heparin has also been recommended due to its effects on cellular immunity and in decreasing thrombosis. Its use, however, remains controversial as optimal dosage and timing of administration have not been determined.

The hypothesis that soluble products of activated immune cells (cytokines) can induce immunodystrophism is as yet relatively untested, but offers a potential new mechanism for immunologic recurrent abortion. This hypothesis is based on aberrant cell-mediated immunity to reproductive antigen (sperm or trophoblast) stimulation of immune cells residing in female reproductive tissues. A byproduct of this activation is the secretion by stimulated immune cells of soluble factors (cytokines), some of which may be toxic to the developing conceptus. An association has been made between the occurrence of these embryotoxic and trophoblast-toxic factors in nonpregnant women with a history of recurrent abortion [12]. Further studies are needed to determine the clinical relevance of this association and to determine whether immunosuppressive therapy can ameliorate pregnancy loss by decreasing the ability of maternal immune cells to become activated by offending reproductive antigens.

Progesterone is essential for the maintenance of pregnancy. Since the 1950s progesterone has been used for its endocrinologic effects of supplementing the corpus luteum in cases of luteal-phase insufficiency. In concentrations attained at the maternal—fetal interface progesterone is also immunosuppressive [13]. Due to its essentially anecdotal use for the past 30 years, progesterone has never been tested in a double-blind placebo-controlled manner for recurrent abortion. Newer agents with immunosuppressive capabilities, such as pentoxifylline and cyclosporine, offer therapeutic possibilities. However, at this time, neither adequate nor well-controlled studies in pregnant women have been published documenting safety and efficacy. Therefore, their use cannot be currently advocated.

CONCLUSIONS

An intact maternal immune system is not required for successful gestation, yet immunologic mechanisms may be involved in reproductive failure. Before considering an immunologic diagnosis for recurrent abortion, potential chromosomal, anatomic, and endocrinologic etiologies must be eliminated (Table 58.5). Current evidence supports the rationale for obtaining antiphospholipid antibodies (anticardiolipin antibody and lupus anticoagulant) and for prescribing low-dose aspirin and possibly heparin for women found to have sustained high titers. Current evidence does not support a rationale for

Table 58.5 Evaluation of recurrent spontaneous abortion

Karyotype of both partners

Hysterosalpingogram (followed by hysteroscopy/laparoscopy if indicated)

Luteal-phase endometrial biopsy with concomitant serum progesterone

Thyroid function studies (TSH, T_4)

Anticardiolipin antibody

Lupus anticoagulant (aPTT or Russell viper venom time).

TSH, thyroid-stimulating hormone; T_4, thyroxine; aPTT, activated partial thromboplastin time.

obtaining antinuclear antibodies, antipaternal cytotoxic antibodies, MLC reactivities or HLA profiles. Further work is needed before embryotoxic and trophoblast-toxic factor assessment is clinically justified or available.

Safe and effective treatment modalities are needed for couples experiencing recurrent abortion. The rationale for therapy, however, must be scientifically well founded. Practicing physicians should refrain from utilizing or recommending immunotherapy for recurrent abortion until the rationale of such therapy has been proven and the safety and efficacy of potential regimens have been scientifically tested in double-blind, randomized, appropriately controlled trials.

REFERENCES

1 Hill JA, Raviniker VA, Recurrent abortion. In: Ryan KJ, Barbieri RL, Berkowitz RS, eds. *Kistner's Gynecology: Principles and Practice*. New York: Year Book; 1989: 406–430.
2 Hill JA, Anderson DJ. Evidence for the existence and significance of immune cells in male and female reproductive tissues. *Immunol Allerg Clin North Am* 1990; 10: 1–12.
3 Hill JA. Immunological mechanisms of pregnancy maintenance and failure: a critique of theories and therapy. *Am J Reprod Immunol* 1990; 22: 33–42.
4 Ober C, Martin AO, Simpson JL. Shared HLA antigens and reproductive performance among Hutterites. *Am J Genet* 1983; 35: 994–1004.
5 Purcell DFJ, McKenzie IFC, Johnson PM. CD46 (Huly-m5) antigen of humans includes the trophoblast leukocyte antigen (TLX) and the membrane cofactor protein (MCP) of complement. *Immunology* 1990; 70: 155–161.
6 Mowbray JF, Gibbings C, Liddell H, Reginald PW, Underwood JL, Beard RW. Controlled trial of treatment of recurrent spontaneous abortion by immunization with paternal cells. *Lancet* 1985; i: 941–944.
7 Cauchi MN, Lim D, Young DE, Kloss M, Papparell RJ. Treatment of recurrent aborters by immunization with paternal cells — controlled trial. *Am J Reprod Immunol* 1991; 25: 16–17.
8 Ho HN, Gill TJ, Hsieh HJ, Jiang JJ, Lee TY, Hsieh CY. Immunotherapy for recurrent spontaneous abortions in a Chinese population. *Am J Reprod Immunol* 1991; 25: 10–15.
9 Alberman E. The epidemiology of repeated abortion. In: Beard RW, Ship F, eds. *Early Pregnancy Loss: Mechanisms and Treatment*. New York: Springer Verlag, 1988: 9–17.
10 Sacher RA, King JC. Intravenous gamma-globulin in pregnancy: a review. *Obstet Gynecol Surv* 1988; 44: 25–34.
11 Branch DW, Scott JR, Kochenour WK, Hershgold E. Obstetric complications associated with the lupus

anticoagulant. *N Engl J Med* 1985; 313: 1322.

12 Hill JA, Anderson DJ, Polgár K, Harlow BL. Evidence of embryo- and trophoblast-toxic cellular immune response(s) in women with recurrent spontaneous abortion. *Am J Obstet Gynecol* 1992; 166: 1044–1052.

13 Clemens LE, Siiteri PK, Stites DP. Mechanisms of immunosuppression of progesterone on maternal lymphocyte activation during pregnancy. *J Immunol* 1979; 122: 1978–1985.

Intrauterine contraceptive devices and their complications

RONALD T. BURKMAN

Although a number of intrauterine devices (IUDs) have been described historically, it was not until 1960 with the introduction of the Lippes loop that the modern-day era began. The 1960s and 1970s saw the evolution of a variety of inert and medicated devices. Unfortunately, as the knowledge base relative to risks expanded, coupled with the occurrence of the Dalkon shield controversy, the 1980s saw a marked decline in their use in the USA. This chapter will briefly review the types, mode of action, indications, event rates, and minor sequelae for the two devices currently available in the USA and also discuss in greater detail the potential serious sequelae.

TYPES OF IUD

Both devices used in the USA are T-shaped, being around 36 mm in length and 32 mm in diameter. The Progestasert-T is made from a special polymer that contains a reservoir of 38 mg of progesterone. The progesterone is released at a rate of about 65 μg daily; contraceptive efficacy is maintained for 1 year. The Paragard or T-Cu-380A is wound with 300 mm^2 of fine copper wire on its vertical arm and 40 mm^2 on each horizontal arm. The device slowly releases copper ions; contraceptive efficacy is maintained for 6 or more years.

MODE OF ACTION

There are a number of suggested, though unproven, theories regarding the mode of action of IUDs. The most common theory is that IUDs inhibit endometrial implantation of the blastocyst through mechanical interference, local inflammatory responses, interference with endometrial maturation, or through release of prostaglandin. Other studies suggest that some IUDs are spermicidal, can interfere with maturation of ova, reverse the direction of tubal cilia, or disrupt the capacitance qualities of cervical mucus.

INDICATIONS

The major indication for IUDs is pregnancy prevention, although occasionally they have been used to prevent reaccumulation of endometrial synechiae following surgical treatment of Ashermann's syndrome. The most appropriate candidates for IUD use are parous, monogamous women who are at low risk for sexually transmitted diseases or salpingitis. Women who highly desire future child-bearing; who have small or abnormally configured uterine cavities, e.g., leimyomas or congenital abnormalities; who have heavy menses, undiagnosed gynecologic problems, or who have experienced difficulties with IUDs in the past are not ideal candidates. The manufacturer's guidelines and consent forms should be closely followed relative to screening, counseling, insertion techniques, and follow-up in order both to reduce the potential for adverse sequelae and also to reduce the likelihood of medicolegal action should a serious problem develop.

EVENT RATES

The Progestasert-T has a failure or pregnancy rate of about 1.8–2.5 pregnancies per 100 woman-years while the Paragard has a pregnancy rate of 0.5–1.0 over 4 years of use. Significantly, about 25% of the Progestasert-T pregnancies are ectopic; very few of the Paragard pregnancies are extrauterine. About 20% of IUD users request removal during the first 3 months due to dysmenorrhea or bleeding. The continuation rate after 1 year's use of the Paragard is about 70%; the requirement for removal and reinsertion of the Progestasert-T and the accompanying cost limit its continued use after 1 year. IUD expulsions occur at rates ranging between 5 and 25%, with most occurring in the first 3 months of use.

MINOR SEQUELAE

Menometrorrhagia is the most frequent complaint of IUD users; most users experience an increase in menstrual blood loss of between 20 and 100% from preinsertion levels while Progestasert-T wearers have their average flow reduced by about 40%. Use of nonsteroidal antiinflammatory agents appears to reduce the amount of menstrual blood loss. Persistent complaints need evaluation and/or occasionally IUD removal. Although the etiology of increased bleeding is unknown, investigators have suggested that the bleeding is due to surface irritation or to increased concentrations of plasminogen inactivators in the endometrium leading to interference with the fibrinolytic system [1,2]. Abdominal cramping or dysmenorrhea is highest just after insertion, although there are reports that suggest that this is less of a problem with the Progestasert-T. The use of a paracervical block or nonsteroidal antiinflammatory drugs will reduce discomfort during insertion; persistent or severe pain should suggest the possibility of perforation or inappropriate positioning of the device in the uterine cavity. The possible occurrence of acute salpingitis or pelvic inflammatory disease (PID) must always be considered when evaluating a patient with this complaint, particularly during the first few days or weeks after insertion.

POTENTIAL SERIOUS SEQUELAE

The major potential sequelae associated with IUD use of particular interest to a reproductive endocrinology–infertility specialist include pelvic infection, tubal infertility, spontaneous abortion, and ectopic pregnancy.

Pelvic infection and tubal infertility

Acute salpingitis (PID) is the most common of the serious sequelae associated with IUD use. In major epidemiologic studies, the overall relative risk of acute salpingitis among IUD users compared to nonusers of IUDs ranges between 1.2 and 4.5 [3,4]. It is important to recognize in comparing various studies that the presence of other risk factors, e.g., young age, past PID, multiple sexual partners, influences risk of this complication; when data are adjusted, the overall relative risk often falls to between 1.0 and 2.0. In particular, for monogamous, married women, the risk of salpingitis associated with IUD use appears to be only slightly higher than the risk experienced by women who use no contraception.

Further, use of contraception protective against salpingitis, e.g., barrier methods, oral contraceptives, by large numbers of women in study comparison groups will also bias the relative risk estimate such that it will reflect both the risk associated with IUD use as well as the protective effect of the contraceptive method. Data from the largest multicenter study conducted in the USA suggest that the greatest risk of salpingitis occurs around the time of insertion (about fourfold), with the relative risk declining dramatically after the first month of use to between 1.0 and 2.0 [5]. The limited data published to date regarding use of prophylactic antibiotics at the time of insertion suggest that some benefit might occur with their use. Figure 59.1 provides a brief algorithm for managing patients with suspected salpingitis.

Hospitalization should be liberally utilized, particularly if the diagnosis is uncertain and/or if a surgical emergency such as appendicitis cannot be excluded; if there is a suspected abscess; with pregnancy; with severe illness; with failure to follow, respond to, or tolerate outpatient treatment regimens; and with inability to arrange follow-up within 72 hours of initiating treatment. In addition, most authors also recommend IUD removal soon after start of antibiotic therapy.

The role of *Actinomyces israeli* in infections associated with IUD use has been investigated in several studies. It appears that these uncommon infections are seen with long use of IUDs, particularly inert devices, With the current practice of using medicated or copper-bearing devices for shorter periods of time, the significance of these infections in the future is unclear.

Two US studies have associated past IUD use with risk of subsequent tubal infertility [6,7]. Relative risks for past IUD users compared to nonusers ranged between 2.0 and 2.5. Users of the Dalkon shield had risks substantially higher (three- to sixfold); past copper IUD users had relative risks of 1.5–2.0. Mongamous, parous women who were older than age 25 years and who had used a copper IUD did not appear to have an increased risk of tubal infertility. Data from one of the studies also support the notion that women can experience significant tubal damage yet be unaware of a preceding episode of salpingitis. For example, the relative risks of tubal infertility for women experiencing an episode of salpingitis while wearing an IUD versus women recalling no episodes of salpingitis during or after IUD use were 3.0 and 2.6, respectively.

CHAPTER 59

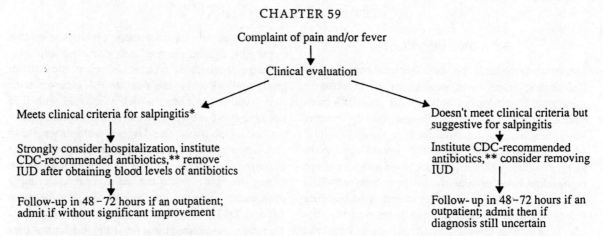

Fig. 59.1 Pelvic infection algorithm for IUD users. * Clinical criteria for diagnosis of salpingitis. All of items below are necessary: direct abdominal tenderness with or without rebound; cervical/uterine motion tenderness; and adnexal tenderness. Plus one or more of the following: cervical gram stain suggests gonorrhea; temperature greater than 38°C; leucocytosis greater than 10 000; purulent material (contains numerous WBCs) in peritoneal cavity noted by culdocentesis or at diagnostic laparoscopy; pelvic abscess/inflammatory complex noted on examination or by ultrasonography. (Modified from [6].) ** Centers for disease control guidelines for antibiotic treatment of salpingitis. *Inpatient therapy*: Cefoxitan 2 g i.v. q 8 hours or Cefotetan 2 g i.v. q 12 hours (or cephalosporin equivalent) *plus* Doxycycline 100 mg p.o. or i.v. q 12 hours. An alternate is Clindamycin 900 mg i.v. q 8 hours *plus* Gentamycin 2 mg/kg loading dose i.m. or i.v followed by 1.5 mg/kg q 8 hours. The above regimens continued for a minimum of 48 hours after clinical improvement. After discharge continue Doxycycline 100 mg p.o. q 12 hours for 10−14 days. *Outpatient therapy*: Cefoxitan 2 g i.m. *plus* Probenicid 1 g p.o. or Ceftriaxone 250 mg i.m. (or equivalent cephalosporin) *plus* Doxycycline 100 mg p.o. q 12 hours for 10−14 days or Tetracycline 500 mg p.o. q 6 hours for 10−14 days. (Modified from [7].)

Spontaneous abortion and ectopic pregnancy

As already noted, contraceptive failure or pregnancy is an uncommon occurrence with today's IUDs. However, when pregnancy does occur there are two potential considerations: spontaneous abortion and ectopic pregnancy. There are data from several sources to support the finding that when a pregnancy occurs with an *in situ* IUD, the risk of spontaneous and even septic abortion is increased [8]. Most studies estimate the spontaneous abortion rate to be about 50%, with the risk of infection increased about 20-fold if the IUD is left in place. IUD removal in the first trimester reduces the risk of spontaneous abortion by about one-half and virtually eliminates the risk of septic abortion. Therefore, pregnant women should be counseled to have IUDs removed, when the strings are visualized, if a pregnancy occurs. For women desiring a pregnancy termination, removal can be accomplished concomitantly with the procedure. If the strings are not visualized, pelvic ultrasonography often can localize the device. It has been suggested by some that the use of "tail-less" IUDs may reduce the risk of spontaneous abortion and even infection. Available data are unable fully to clarify these issues. Further, any benefit would have to be weighed

against the problems associated with difficulty in following an IUD user.

It has been noted by some investigators [9] that approximately 5% of the pregnancies that occur in association with IUD use are ectopic — a rate about five times that found in the general population. However, it is important to recognize that, with the exception of the Progestasert-T, IUD use as opposed to nonuse of contraception protects against ectopic pregnancy. For example, in a sample of 1000 unprotected couples followed over 1 year, about 800 pregnancies would occur, of which 8 would be ectopic. If that same group utilized a Paragard IUD for 1 year, 20 pregnancies, including one ectopic gestation would be expected. In other words, because IUDs are highly effective in preventing pregnancy overall, the risk of ectopic pregnancy is also small.

REFERENCES

1 Burkman RT. *Handbook of Contraception and Abortion*. Boston: Little, Brown, 1989.
2 Treiman K, Liskin L. IUDs — a new look. In: *Population Reports, Population Information Program*. Baltimore: The Johns Hopkins University, 1988.

3 Grimes DA. Intrauterine devices and pelvic inflammatory disease: recent developments. *Contraception* 1987; 36: 97–109.

4 Lee NC, Rubin GL, Boruckki R. The intrauterine device and pelvic inflammatory disease revisited: new results from the Women's Health Study. *Obstet Gynecol* 1988; 72: 1–6.

5 Burkman RT and the Women's Health Study. Association between intrauterine device and pelvic inflammatory disease. *Obstet Gynecol* 1981; 57: 269–276.

6 Hagar D, Eschenbach DA, Spence MR, Sweet RL. Criteria for diagnosis and grading of salpingitis. *Obstet Gynecol* 1983; 61: 113.

7 Sexually transmitted disease guidelines. September 1989. *MMWR* 1989; 38: 58.

8 Cramer DW, Schiff I, Schoenbaum SC *et al*. Tubal infertility and the intrauterine device. *N Engl J Med* 1985; 312: 941–947.

9 Daling JR, Weiss, Metch BJ *et al*. Primary tubal infertility in relationship to use of an intrauterine device. *N Engl J Med* 1985; 312: 937–941.

10 Foreman H, Stadel BV, Schlesselmann S *et al*. Intrauterine device usage and fetal loss. *Obstet Gynecol* 1981; 58: 669–677.

11 Ory HW and the Women's Health Study. Ectopic pregnancy and intrauterine contraceptive devices: new perspectives. *Obstet Gynecol* 1981; 57: 137–147.

60

Oral contraceptives: initial selection and management of menstrual side-effects

RICHARD P. DICKEY

Figure 60.1 is a decision-making tree for the selection and management of menstrual side-effects. An initial physical examination should reveal no abnormality of blood pressure, thyroid, breasts, heart, liver, uterus, cervix, including Pap test, or extremities. A cardiac risk profile, consisting of total cholesterol, high-density lipoprotein (HDL), low-density lipoprotein (LDL), cholesterol, and triglyceride, should be performed if the patient has a personal or family history of cardiovascular disease or diabetes, or is ≥35 years of age. A mammogram should be performed if the patient is ≥35 years of age.

The patient being considered for oral contraceptive (OC) use should have none of the absolute contraindications to OC use shown in Table 60.1. If relative contraindications exist (Table 60.2). OCs may be used with caution, providing patients are followed with appropriate laboratory and physical testing. Ideally, patients with relative contraindications should use nonhormonal methods of contraception. Note that age ≥40 is no longer a contraindication for use in women who do not smoke cigarettes.

OC use bestows many benefits besides contraception (Table 60.3). Therapeutic uses of OCs include treatment of irregular menses, heavy menstrual bleeding, painful menses, premenstrual syndrome, and prevention of recurrent ovarian cysts. Also, OCs are useful in the treatment of hirsutism, due to ovarian androgens. OCs are especially useful in polycystic ovarian syndrome, where they provide a three-fold benefit of regulating menses, suppressing

Table 60.1 Absolute contraindications to oral contraceptive use

Known or suspected pregnancy

Present or past history of deep vein thrombophlebitis or thrombolic disorders

Undiagnosed genital bleeding

Present or past history of:

  Cerebral, vascular, or coronary artery disease or myocardial infarction

  Known or suspected carcinoma of the breast

  Known or suspected estrogen-dependent neoplasia

  Benign or malignant liver tumor which developed during the use of oral contraceptives or other estrogen-containing products

Table 60.2 Relative contraindications to oral contraceptive use

Insulin-dependent diabetes

Past history of chemical, gestational diabetes

Any cardiac or renal dysfunction

Type II hyerlipidemia (hypercholesterolemia)

Migraines or vascular headaches

Impaired liver function, recent hepatitis, or mononucleosis (within 1 year)

Psychotic depression

Hypertension

Varicose veins

Cholestatic jaundice during pregnancy

Sickle cell disease or sickle C disease

Breast-feeding

Ulcerative colitis

Nonrheumatic cardiovascular disease of a first-order relative before age 50

Immobilization of an extremity

Cigarette smoking if age ≥35

Any chronic disease which worsened during previous pregnancy

ORAL CONTRACEPTION

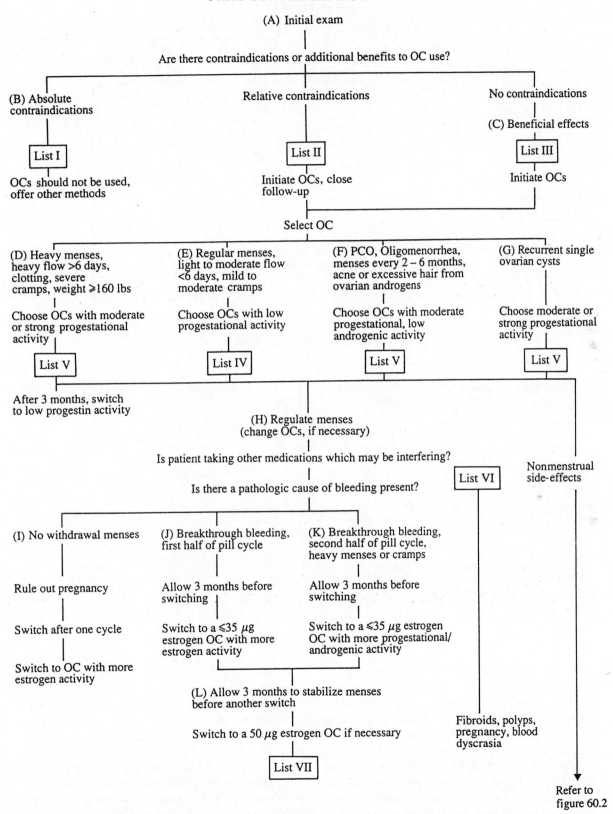

(A) Initial exam

Are there contraindications or additional benefits to OC use?

(B) Absolute contraindications

Relative contraindications

No contraindications

(C) Beneficial effects

| List I | List II | List III |

OCs should not be used, offer other methods

Initiate OCs, close follow-up

Initiate OCs

Select OC

(D) Heavy menses, heavy flow >6 days, clotting, severe cramps, weight ≥160 lbs

Choose OCs with moderate or strong progestational activity

(E) Regular menses, light to moderate flow <6 days, mild to moderate cramps

Choose OCs with low progestational activity

(F) PCO, Oligomenorrhea, menses every 2 – 6 months, acne or excessive hair from ovarian androgens

Choose OCs with moderate progestational, low androgenic activity

(G) Recurrent single ovarian cysts

Choose moderate or strong progestational activity

| List V | List IV | List V | List V |

After 3 months, switch to low progestin activity

(H) Regulate menses (change OCs, if necessary)

Is patient taking other medications which may be interfering?

Is there a pathologic cause of bleeding present?

List VI

Nonmenstrual side-effects

(I) No withdrawal menses

Rule out pregnancy

Switch after one cycle

Switch to OC with more estrogen activity

(J) Breakthrough bleeding, first half of pill cycle

Allow 3 months before switching

Switch to a ≤35 μg estrogen OC with more estrogen activity

(K) Breakthrough bleeding, second half of pill cycle, heavy menses or cramps

Allow 3 months before switching

Switch to a ≤35 μg estrogen OC with more progestational/ androgenic activity

(L) Allow 3 months to stabilize menses before another switch

Switch to a 50 μg estrogen OC if necessary

Fibroids, polyps, pregnancy, blood dyscrasia

List VII

Refer to figure 60.2

Fig. 60.1 Oral contraceptives: initial selection and management of menstrual side-effects. (*Continued next page.*)

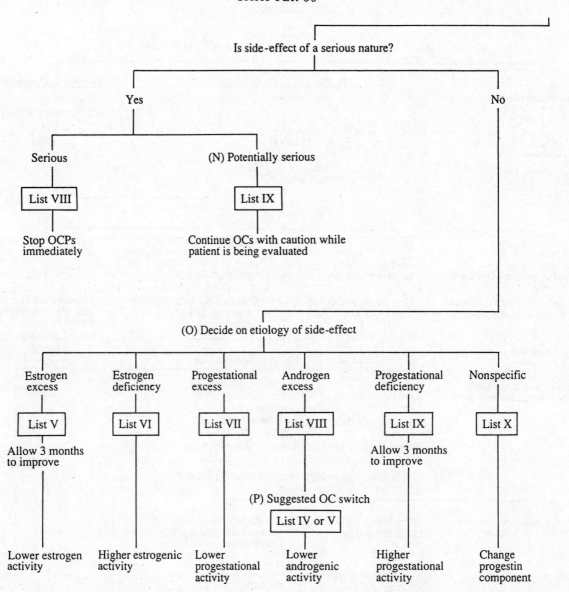

Is side-effect of a serious nature?

Yes — No

Serious — (N) Potentially serious

List VIII

Stop OCPs
immediately

List IX

Continue OCs with caution while
patient is being evaluated

(O) Decide on etiology of side-effect

Estrogen excess — Estrogen deficiency — Progestational excess — Androgen excess — Progestational deficiency — Nonspecific

List V — List VI — List VII — List VIII — List IX — List X

Allow 3 months to improve — Allow 3 months to improve

(P) Suggested OC switch

List IV or V

Lower estrogen activity — Higher estrogenic activity — Lower progestational activity — Lower androgenic activity — Higher progestational activity — Change progestin component

Fig. 60.1 (*Continued*)

symptoms of androgen excess, and reducing the incidence of endometrial cancer due to unopposed estrogen effect. OCs conserve future reproductive capability by reducing the incidence of endometriosis, pelvic inflammatory disease (PID), and uterine fibroids.

Ideally, all patients should use OCs which contain ≤35 μg estrogen and a progestin with progestational and androgen activity ≤0.5 mg norethindrone/day. These doses have been repeatedly demonstrated to have no adverse effects on serum lipids and thus may

be considered to be least likely to cause immediate or long-term adverse cardiovascular effects.

The progestational, androgenic, estrogenic, and endometrial activity of ≤35 μg estrogen OCs is shown in Table 60.4 and of 50 μg estrogen OCs in Table 60.5. Note that individual progestins differ in both their progestational activity and their ratio of androgenic to progestational activity. Progestins also either add to or antagonize estrogenic activity. OCs with similar amounts but different types of progestins and the same amount of estrogen may

ORAL CONTRACEPTION

Table 60.3 Beneficial side-effects of oral contraceptive use

Decreased incidence of:
  Pregnancy, all types
  Irregular menses
  Premenstrual syndrome
  Menstrual cramps
  Breast cysts
  Uterine fibroids*
  Benign ovarian cysts
  Ovarian cancer
  Endometrial cancer
  Pelvic inflammatory disease*
  Endometriosis*
  Rheumatoid arthritis
  Iron-deficiency anemia
  Acne and hirsutism due to ovarian androgen

* These conditions have an adverse effect on future reproductive capability.

differ in progestational, androgenic, or estrogenic activity. Endometrial activity is the result of the composite effect of all progestational, androgenic,

and estrogenic effects. Endometrial activity is represented in Tables 60.4 and 60.5 as the percentage of patients who have spotting during the third cycle of OC use.

Patients with excessively heavy menses, clotting and marked menstrual pain, and patients weighing ≥160 lb (72 kg) initially require moderate to strong activity to control menses (Table 60.2). After 3 months, patients on stronger progestins should be switched to pills with the equivalent of ≤0.5 mg norethindrone.

Patients with polycystic ovarian syndrome (PCOS) or androgens of ovarian origin require both moderate progesterone activity and low androgen activity. After one cycle, a switch to an OC with lower progestational activity may be attempted.

Patients with recurrent ovarian cysts due to anovulation require moderate to strong progesterone activity to prevent cyst recurrence. Use of moderate to strong progestational OCs must continue as long as OCs are used.

Low-dose OCs result in unsatisfactory menstrual cycles initially in as many as 40% of patients. Men-

Table 60.4 Properties of oral contraceptives containing ≤35 μg estrogen

	Progestin	Estrogen activity	Progestational activity	Androgen activity	Spotting and bleeding: 3rd cycle
Low progestational /low androgen activity					
Brevicon	NE	42	0.5	0.15	14.6
Modicon	NE	42	0.5	0.15	14.6
Nelova 5/35	NE	42	0.5	0.15	14.6
Ovcon 35	NE	40	0.4	0.17	11.0
Triphasic					
Ortho Novum 7/7/7	NE	48	0.8	0.25	12.2
Tri-Norinyl	NE	40	0.7	0.23	14.7
Tri-Levlen	LN	28	0.5	0.29	15.1
Tri-Phasil	LN	28	0.5	0.29	15.1
Moderate progestational/moderate androgen activity					
Genora 1/35	NE	38	1.0	0.34	14.7
Levlen	LN	25	0.8	0.46	14.0
Loestrin 1/20	NA	13	1.2	0.53	29.7
Lo-Ovral	NG	25	0.8	0.46	9.6
Nelova 1/35	NE	38	1.0	0.34	14.7
Nordette	LN	25	0.8	0.46	14.0
Norethin 1/35	NE	38	1.0	0.34	14.7
Norinyl 1/35	NE	38	1.0	0.34	14.7
Ortho Novum 1/35	NE	38	1.0	0.34	14.7
Moderate progestational/low androgen activity					
Demulen 1/35	ED	19	1.4	0.23	37.4

NE, norethindrone; LN, levonorgestrel; NA, norethindrone acetate; NG, nogestrel; ED, ethynodiol diacetate.

361

Table 60.5 Properties of oral contraceptives containing 50 µg estrogen

	Progestin	Estrogen activity	Progestational activity	Androgen activity	Spotting and bleeding: 3rd cycle
Moderate progestational/low androgen activity					
Demulen 1/50	ED	26	1.4	0.21	13.9
Moderate progestational/moderate androgen activity					
Genora 1/50	NE	32	1.0	0.34	10.6
Norethin 1/50	NE	32	1.0	0.34	10.6
Norinyl 1/50	NE	32	1.0	0.34	10.6
Norlestrin 1/50	NA	39	1.2	0.53	13.6
Ortho Novum 1/50	NE	32	1.0	0.34	10.6
Ovcon 1/50	NE	50	1.0	0.34	11.9
High progestational/high androgen activity					
Loestrin 1.5/30	NA	14	1.7	0.80	25.2
Norlestin	NA	16	2.7	1.30	5.1
Ovral	NG	42	1.3	0.80	4.5

ED, ethynodiol diacetate; NE, norethindrone; NA, norethindrone acetate; NG, norgestrel.

strual irregularities are the most common reason patients give for discontinuing OCs. Bleeding events (spotting, or breakthrough bleeding equal to menses) ordinarily decrease in subsequent cycles until a plateau is reached in the third cycle of use. All patients should be told to expect some intermenstrual bleeding during the first two cycles as they become adjusted to the lower amounts of estrogen and progestin in OCs. After the third cycle, if still bleeding, a switch can be made to an OC with greater endometrial activity, usually without having to increase the estrogen dose above 35 µg, Before switching OCs, first determine that there are no drugs present which interfere with OC activity (Table 60.6). Also, check that there are no pathologic reasons for bleeding, such as abnormal pregnancy, submucosal leiomyoma, endometriosis, polyps, or blood dyscrasia.

Patients who fail to have withdrawal bleeding between OC cycles will not improve in subsequent cycles and should be switched to another OC after one cycle.

After three cycles, patients with bleeding in the first half of the OC cycle require a switch to an OC with more estrogen activity.

Patients with bleeding in the second half of the OC cycle and those with persistent heavy menses or severe menstrual pain require a switch to OCs with more progestational or androgenic activity after three cycles.

Table 60.6 Drugs which reduce the efficacy of oral contraceptives

Anticonvulsant and sedative Drugs
Antimigraine preparations
Barbiturates
 Carbamazepine
 Ethosuximide
 Phenobarbital
 Primidone
Benzodiazepines
Chloral hydrate
Ethotoin
Mephenytoin
Phenytoin

Antiinfection
Ampicillin
Chloramphenicol
Co-trimoxazole
Griseofulvin
Metronidazole
Neomycin
Nitrofurantoin
Penicillin
Rifampin
Sulfonamide
Tetracycline

Other
Clofibrate

After the swith to an OC with higher progestational or androgenic activity, allow three cycles for improvement before a further change. When switching to an OC with higher estrogen activity, the improvement should be apparent in the first cycle. A second or even third switch is sometimes necessary before the OC best suited for a particular patient is discovered. Rarely, patients may require a switch to an OC with 50 µg estrogen to regulate menses. Unless OCs are being used therapeutically for management of heavy menses, PCO syndrome, or recurrent ovarian cysts, consideration should be given to using other forms of contraception, rather than to using an OC with 50 µg of estrogen.

The first step in the management of any non-menstrual side-effect is to decide if it indicates the presence or potential development of a serious illness. When symptoms of serious side-effects occur, OCs should be discontinued immediately (Table 60.7). Upon discontinuing OCs, it is important to recommend other methods of contraception, such as condom and/or foam.

Other symptoms, shown in Table 60.8, indicate the possibility of a less serious illness, and OCs can be continued for a brief time while the diagnosis is confirmed.

For other nonlife-threatening side-effects, it is first necessary to determine their probable cause. Most

Table 60.7 Serious side-effects related to oral contraceptive use*

Symptom	Possible cause
Loss of vision, proptosis, diplopia, papilledema	Retinal artery thrombosis
Unilateral numbness or weakness or tingling	Hemorrhagic or thrombotic stroke
Severe chest pains, left arm or neck pain	Myocardial infarction
Hemoptysis	Pulmonary embolism
Severe leg pains, tenderness or swelling, warmth or palpable cord	Thrombophlebitis
Slurring of speech	Hemorrhagic or thrombotic stroke
Hepatic mass or tenderness	Liver neoplasm

* Pills should be stopped immediately.

Table 60.8 Potentially serious side-effects related to oral contraceptive use*

Symptom	Possible cause
Absence of menses	Pregnancy
Spotting or breakthrough bleeding	Cervical, endometrial, or vaginal cancer
Breast mass, pain, or swelling	Breast cancer
Right upper quadrant pain	Cholecystitis, cholelithiasis, or liver neoplasm
Midepigastric pain	Thrombosis of abdominal artery or vein, myocardial infarction, or pulmonary embolism
Migraine (vascular or throbbing) headache	Vascular spasm which may precede thrombosis
Severe nonvascular headache	Hypertension, vascular spasm
Galactorrhea	Pituitary adenoma
Jaundice, pruritus	Cholestatic jaundice
Depression	Vitamin B_6 deficiency
Uterine size increase	Leiomyomas, adenomyosis, pregnancy

* Pills may be continued with caution while the patient is being evaluated.

OC side-effects are related to excess or deficiency of either the estrogen (Table 60.9) or the progestational component of the pill. Some side-effects such as allergic reactions and gastritis may be related to the "inert" ingredients, such as milk byproducts, present in OCs. Estrogen- and progestin-related side-effects are similar to those symptoms which occur naturally, although sometimes due to pathologic conditions during periods of hormonal excess or deficiency. Symptoms due to excess of the progesterone component may be either progestational, as occurs during later pregnancy, or androgenic, as occurs in PCOS patients. Symptoms of natural estrogen excess occur during these first 10 weeks of pregnancy.

After determining the probable cause, the next step is to decide if a switch to a different OC is needed. It will be possible to treat some side-effects without changing medication, for instance, by reducing salt or calorie intake for edema or weight gain. Side-effects due to estrogen excess will often improve

CHAPTER 60

Table 60.9 Symptoms of estrogen excess

General symptoms	Reproductive system
Chloasma	Breast cystic changes
Chronic nasal pharyngitis	Cervical extrophy
Gastric influenza and varicella	Dysmenorrhea, menstrual cramps
Hayfever and allergic rhinitis	Hypermenorrhea, menorrhagia, heavy flow, and clots
Urinary tract infections	Increase in breast size
Premenstrual syndrome	Mucorrhea
Bloating	Uterine enlargement
Dizziness—syncope	Uterine fibroid growth
Edema	
Headaches (cyclic)	*Cardiovascular system*
Irritability	Capillary fragility
Leg cramps	Cerebrovascular accident
Nausea and vomiting	Deep vein thrombosis hemiparesis (unilateral weakness and numbness)
Visual changes (cyclic)	Telangiectasias
Weight gain (cyclic)	Thromboembolic disease
	Vascular headaches (migraine)

spontaneously within three OC cycles. Those related to progestin or androgen excess and those due to estrogen deficiency become more severe with continued cycles of OC use. Most side-effects which do not improve spontaneously or after symptomatic treatment may be reduced or eliminated by switching to another OC with less or more estrogen, progesterone, or androgen activity. A switch to an OC with less activity should be made at the start of the next cycle. A switch to an OC with more activity can be made at any time.

Approximately 15% of patients will be unable to tolerate any OC or will not be able to take one of the "safe" low-dose OCs.

FURTHER READING

Dickey RP. *Managing Contraceptive Pill Patients*, 6th ed. Durant: CIP, 1990.

Dickey RP, Dorr CH III. Oral contraceptives: selection of the proper pill. *Am J Obstet Gynecol* 1969; 33: 273.

Dickey RP, Stone SC. Progesterone potency of oral contraceptives. *Am J Obstet Gynecol* 1975; 18: 2.

Dickey RP, Chihal HJW, Peppler R. Estrogen potency of oral contraceptive pills. *Am J Obstet Gynecol* 1975; 121: 75.

Godsland IF, Crook D, Wynn V. Low-dose oral contraceptives and carbohydrate metabolism. *Am J Obstet Gynecol* 1990; 163: 348.

Swyer GIM, Little V. Potency of progestogens and oral contraceptives: further delay-of-menses data. *Contraception* 1982; 26: 23.

61

Diabetes in pregnancy

OLIVER W. JONES III

Pregnancy is a condition of glucose intolerance. This has been attributed to the hormonal mechanisms that provide for nutrients to promote fetal growth. The hormones primarily responsible for this state are human placental lactogen (hPL), prolactin (PRL), and cortisol. Therefore, women who are diabetic or are predisposed to diabetes will exhibit exacerbation of their disease or show evidence of new-onset glucose intolerance.

Two classification systems for diabetes in pregnancy are currently in use. The more recent system is that of the National Diabetes Data Group [1] which divides pregnant diabetic women into three categories: insulin-dependent (type I), noninsulin-dependent (type II), and gestational diabetes (GDM). The older system is White's classification [2] based on duration of disease and organ involvement. The National Diabetes Data Group nomenclature will be used here.

Type I diabetics are those women who are essentially insulin-deficient. Following a glucose challenge they fail to release insulin. This can be shown by a lack of increase in C-peptide immunoreactivity following a 400 kcal meal. These women tend to be younger, of normal body habitus, and prone to ketoacidosis. In contrast the type II diabetic still retains endogenous insulin production but fails to produce adequate amounts in response to a glucose challenge. In addition, these women tend to be obese but are not prone to diabetic ketoacidosis. When not pregnant, weight reduction will often decrease their insulin requirements. The woman with gestational diabetes has a condition of reversible glucose intolerance brought on by the change in hormonal milieu produced by pregnancy. This condition is very unlikely to occur prior to 20 weeks' gestation and usually resolves in the postpartum period. Approximately 1–3% of all pregnant women will develop gestational diabetes.

SCREENING FOR DIABETES

All pregnant women should be evaluated for diabetes at their initial prenatal visit (Fig. 61.1). Those with significant risk factor such as previous gestational diabetes, macrosomic (>4100 g) babies, unexplained fetal demise, infant with a congenital anomaly, polyhydramnios, family history of diabetes, obesity, overt symptoms of diabetes or abnormal laboratory values (glycosuria, fasting plasma glucose ≥105 mg/dl or 2-hour post-prandial glucose ≥120 mg/dl) should receive a 3-hour 100 g glucose tolerance test.

The current recommendation is that prenatal screening in women without previous history or risk factors for gestational diabetes be conducted at 24–28 weeks. The preferred method is the 50 g oral glucose load given at random (i.e., nonfasting) with a plasma glucose measured after 1 hour. A value greater than 150 mg/dl is abnormal. However, this is not diagnostic of glucose intolerance. Those women with a positive screening test proceed to the 3-hour 100 g glucose tolerance test following a fast. Exceeding two or more of the following venous plasma values constitutes an abnormal test: a fasting of 105, a 1-hour of 190, a 2-hour of 165 and a 3-hour of 145 mg/dl. Those women who had a positive screening test but a negative 3-hour test should have a repeat 3-hour glucose tolerance test at 32 weeks to detect delayed development of glucose intolerance. Similarly, those patients with a significant prior history but a negative 1-hour 50 g test should have a repeat screen at 32 weeks and if positive then proceed with the 3-hour glucose tolerance test.

MANAGEMENT

Ideal management of the pregnant diabetic patient should begin with preconceptual counseling, education, and control of her diabetes. More commonly, the diabetic patient discovers her pregnancy because

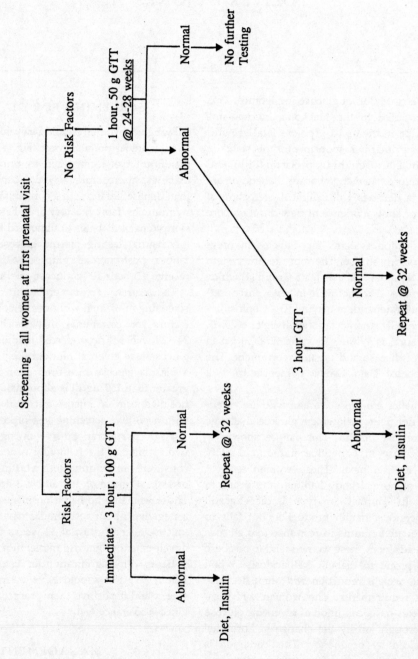

Fig. 61.1 Management of diabetes in pregnancy.

of sudden difficulty controlling her serum glucose with the onset of gestation. The type I diabetic may even present in diabetic ketoacidosis. Therefore, it is important to rule out pregnancy in the diabetic woman of reproductive age who develops this complication.

A team approach is very useful in maximally utilizing the resources available for the care of diabetic pregnant women. This would include the obstetrician, an internist (diabetologist), nurse, social worker, and access to particular subspecialists such as an ophthalmologist and nephrologist. Because the care of the pregnant diabetic is labor-intensive, a clinic nurse whose only responsibility is the diabetic patients is very useful. This person can provide a contact point in the clinic for questions and education when the physician is unavailable.

Frequent office visits (weekly at least) are essential to maintain continued good control once it has been established. During the visit the weekly home glucose tests are reviewed and appropriate adjustments in insulin dosage are made. In addition, this allows early attention and treatment of complications (urinary tract infections, poor glycemic control, renal disease, retinal complications, hypertension, etc.).

Standard screening measures also apply to the diabetic patient. This particularly includes the maternal serum α-fetoprotein test and subsequent ultrasound examination if indicated for detection of neural tube defects. Ultrasound is also useful in diagnosis of fetal cardiovascular, skeletal, genitourinary, and gastrointestinal defects associated with diabetes. In addition, ultrasound measurements of the fetus every 3 weeks can be used to monitor growth and aid in detection of macrosomia.

DIET

Appropriate diet for the diabetic patient has always been a major part of their management. Consultation with a nutritionist will greatly facilitate dietary recommendations and instructions for the patient. The current recommendation is restriction of glucose and alcohol with 50–60% of the daily diet made up of complex carbohydrates, 12–20% made up of protein, less than 10% in the form of saturated fatty acids and the remainder of fat from monounsaturated sources. Suggested caloric intake is 2000–2400 kcal/day with some adjustment downward (1500–1700 kcal/day) for the obese gestational diabetic. For the obese woman pregnancy should not be a time of weight

reduction and sufficient calories should be provided to allow fetal growth. Using these guidelines the frequency and number of meals and snacks can be adjusted on an individual basis to meet lifestyle and activity demands. In particular, ethnic variations in diet should be considered to aid in compliance and to prevent exceeding the caloric guidelines.

INSULIN

With the discovery of insulin diabetic management was revolutionized. Along with diet control this provides the mainstay of treatment for the diabetic patient. With the availability of recombinant DNA-derived human insulin, beef and pork preparations should no longer be used. The primary advantage of the human insulin is reduced maternal antibody formation and thus decreased likelihood of developing resistance to insulin therapy.

The most common insulin regimens utilize a combination of short-acting (regular insulin) and intermediate-acting (NPH or Lente). Regular insulin given subcutaneously usually has a peak response within 30–60 min with a duration of action up to 6 hours. NPH should produce a maximal decrease in blood glucose at about 8 hours from the time of injection, with activity lasting up to 24 hours. However, responses to insulin may vary in that activity may be delayed or prolonged. Therefore, individual responses need to be monitored to insure adequate dosing.

For the type I diabetic a suggested insulin regimen is two-thirds of the 24-hour requirement administered in the morning as a combination of 60% NPH and 40% regular. The remaining one-third is injected prior to dinner as a combination of 50% NPH and 50% regular insulin. Typically, two injections of insulin per day provides adequate control of blood glucose. However, some patients may require more frequent injections with additional regular insulin to maintain good control. As in the dietary management, it is important to tailor the insulin requirements of each patient on an individual basis.

The suggested insulin regimen for the type II diabetic or the gestational diabetic in whom diet alone is inadequate to control blood glucose depends on maternal weight (Fig. 61.2). The obese patient should receive regular insulin prior to each meal, whereas the normal-weight patient should receive a similar split dose as the type I diabetic with two-thirds the daily requirement in the morning (60% NPH and

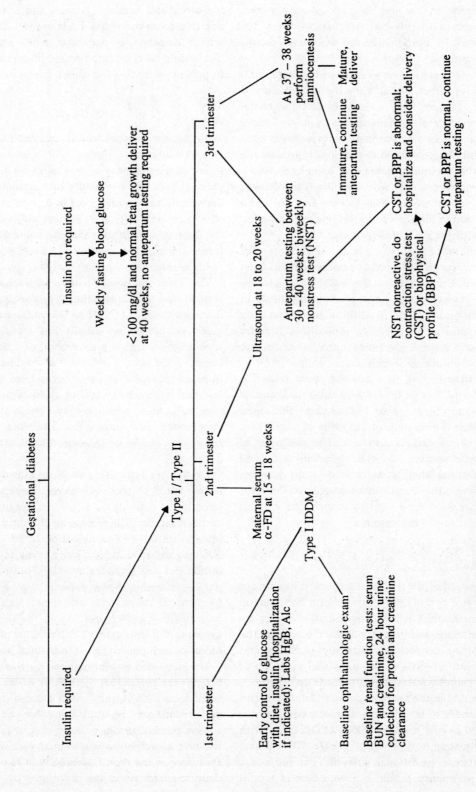

Fig. 61.2 Algorithm for care of patient with gestational diabetes.

40% regular). The remaining one-third is injected prior to dinner and divided between regular and NPH, based on individual needs.

Glucose monitoring for the gestational diabetic who does not require insulin should be a 2-hour postprandial blood glucose obtained at the weekly clinic visit. Those patients on insulin therapy are best managed with home glucose monitoring. There are several types of electronic glucose meters available for patient use and the patient should be instructed appropriately. Blood glucose values should be measured at a minimum fasting, before lunch, before dinner, and prior to bedtime on a daily basis. If the patient suspects hyperglycemia or hypoglycemia then additional tests can be done. The daily record is then reviewed at the weekly clinic visit for trends in blood glucose and the need for adjustment in insulin dose.

The goal of insulin therapy during pregnancy is very good control of blood glucose. Ideally, fasting values less than 100 mg/dl and 2-hour postprandial values less than 120 mg/dl are desired. However, this cannot be achieved in all patients. Overzealous use of insulin also carries with it the risk of significant hypoglycemia, particularly in those patients with long-standing diabetes and weak counterregulatory mechanisms (glucagon and epinephrine release) in response to decreased blood glucose.

ANTEPARTUM TESTING AND DELIVERY

The patient with gestational diabetes who does not require insulin can be allowed to continue her pregnancy to 40 weeks' gestation without necessitating antepartum testing. At 40 weeks' gestation delivery is recommended.

Recommendations when to begin antepartum testing for women receiving insulin vary between 30 and 34 weeks' gestation depending on the severity of the diabetes. Patients should undergo a nonstress test twice weekly. If the nonstress test is nonreactive than either a contraction stress test or biophysical profile is performed. Based on the results of the latter tests the patient is either hospitalized for further observation and/or delivery or continues with antepartum testing.

If there is no evidence of fetal compromise or deteriorating maternal health then type I and type II diabetics undergo amniocentesis at 37–38 weeks' gestation to assess fetal lung maturity. A lecithin : sphingomyelin ratio greater than 2.5 with a phos-

Table 61.1 Recommended insulin infusion rates depending on blood glucose values

Blood glucose (mg/dl)	Insulin Infusion rate (U/h)
<100	0.5
100–140	1.0
141–180	1.5
181–220	2.0
>220	2.5

phatidylglycerol value greater than 3% is considered mature. If the fetal lungs are mature, then the patient is delivered electively at 37–38 weeks.

The various methods (clinical and sonographic) of estimating fetal weight are notoriously inaccurate late in gestation. However, the incidence of shoulder dystocia has been reported to be 3% in fetuses with estimated fetal weight of 4100–4500 g and 8% in fetuses greater than 4500 g. It is recommended that if the estimated fetal weight is greater than 4500 g and the abdominal circumference measures greater than the 95th percentile, a primary cesarean section be considered.

Intrapartum euglycemia may reduce the incidence of neonatal hypoglycemia. This may be achieved in a variety of ways. Perhaps the easiest method utilizes intravenous infusion of insulin via a pump. For an elective induction, the patient withholds her morning insulin injection. Intravenous access is obtained and an infusion of D5W or D5 normal saline is started at 100–125 ml/h to provide glucose for the fetus. Insulin is then infused from a pump at a rate of 0.25–2.0 U/h with blood glucose values checked every hour. Recommended infusion rates depending on blood glucose values are shown in Table 61.1. The intravenous infusion of insulin allows quick adjustments in insulin with rapid maternal response.

DIABETIC KETOACIDOSIS

Diabetic ketoacidosis is a problem most frequently associated with the type I diabetic pregnant woman and is potentially life-threatening for the mother and the fetus (fetal mortality 50–90%). The instigating event is usually decreased insulin precipitated by infection. Initially, plasma glucose and ketoacids (acetoacetic and β-hydroxybutyric) increase due to impaired tissue uptake of ketones, hepatic ketone production, and lipolysis from increased production of catecholamines and other stress hormones. This results in an osmotic diuresis followed by dehydration, impaired ability to excrete ketones, and increased hyperosmolality. As the disease progresses there is worsening metabolic disturbances, hypotension, coma, and subsequent death.

Clinically these patients may present with hyperventilation, fruity odor on their breath, normal or altered mental status, abdominal pain, nausea, and vomiting. Laboratory tests reveal a plasma glucose greater than 300 mg/dl and positive serum ketones. Arterial blood gas measurements are consistent with a metabolic acidosis: pH less than 7.30 and HCO_3 less than 15 mmol/l.

If detected early and in a mild state, ketoacidosis may be readily reversed with judicious rehydration and insulin replacement. However, in the advanced situation more aggressive therapy may be indicated. In these situations a perinatologist and/or internist/diabetologist should be consulted for assistance in the management of the patient.

FETAL AND NEONATAL COMPLICATIONS

With the use of insulin, development of sensitive antepartum testing, application of a team approach to prenatal care and the ability to assess pulmonary maturity, perinatal mortality in the diabetic population has been reduced from 30% in the 1940s to a current 2–5%. Congenital malformations account for 30–40% of the perinatal deaths. Abnormalities in glucose metabolism during the first 8 weeks of embryo development may account for these significant defects. Poor preconceptual and early conception glucose control, as indicated by a hemoglobin A1c (glycosylated hemoglobin) greater than 8.5%, has an associated 22% fetal morbidity/mortality rate.

With proper management the incidence of macrosomia and associated birth trauma can be reduced. However, insulin and diet control has to be achieved prior to 32 weeks' gestation for potential prevention of macrosomia. Other associated neonatal complications are respiratory distress syndrome, polycythemia with hyperviscosity, hypoglycemia, hypocalcemia, hypomagnesemia and hyperbilirubinemia. Therefore, pediatric involvement at the time of delivery is important.

CONCLUSIONS

Diabetes in pregnancy is not a rare disease. With current techniques the maternal and fetal morbidity and mortality have been significantly reduced from previous years. Once the diagnosis is made, strict glucose control with diet and insulin is essential. In addition, timely attention to any sign or symptom of complicating disease is important in keeping these patients healthy and out of the hospital. At the time of labor and delivery appropriate insulin management will reduce maternal and neonatal complications. The time and effort spent with these patients prior to conception, and during the course of the pregnancy and delivery, are more than paid back by the gratification of a healthy mother and baby.

REFERENCES

1 National Diabetes Data Group. Classification and diagnosis of diabetes mellitus and other categories of glucose intolerance. *Diabetes* 1979; 28: 1039–1057.
2 White P. Diabetes mellitus in pregnancy. *Clin Perinat* 1974; 331–347.

FURTHER READING

Barss VA. Diabetes and pregnancy. *Med Clin North Am* 1989; 73: 685–700.
Creasy RK, Resnik R (eds). *Maternal–Fetal Medicine: Principles and Practice*, 2nd edn. Philadelphia: WB Saunders, 1989: 925–988.
Gabbe SG, Niebyl JR, Simpson JL (eds). *Obstetrics: Normal and Problem Pregnancies*, 2nd edn. New York: Churchill Livingstone, 1986: 1097–1116.
Hollingsworth DR. *Pregnancy, Diabetes and Birth: A Management Guide*. Baltimore: Williams & Wilkins, 1984.
Rathi M. *Current Perinatology*. New York: Springer-Verlag, 1988: 99–141.

Thyroid disease and pregnancy

GEORGE R. SAADE

Thyroid disease occurs more commonly in women of reproductive age. It may interfere with the reproductive process, complicate an ongoing gestation, or develop in the postpartum period.

THYROID DISEASE AND REPRODUCTION

Reproductive function can be affected by changes in thyroid homeostasis. The spectrum includes menstrual irregularities, corpus luteum dysfunction, anovulation, and recurrent abortions. The most common thyroid disorders, Graves disease and chronic lymphocytic thyroiditis or Hashimoto's disease, are secondary to an autoimmune disorder which may also be the cause of the reproductive dysfunction, either solely or in combination with the hormonal abnormalities. The thyroid disorder may be subclinical or overt.

Hypothyroidism and reproductive dysfunction

Primary hypothyroidism has been associated with ovulatory dysfunction through its effect on the hypothalamic dopaminergic feedback system. Both dopamine and thyrotropin-releasing hormone (TRH) are increased in these cases, leading to stimulation of the lactotrophs and hyperprolactinemia. In addition, hypothyroid patients have been noted to have reduced levels of sex hormone-binding globulin (SHBG), resulting in elevated free testosterone levels, and contributing to the menstrual irregularities and ovulatory dysfunction seen in these patients. Thyroid hormone replacement reverses all these changes. Measurement of thyroid-stimulating hormone (TSH) should be part of the initial evaluation of all patients with hyperprolactinemia, whether associated with ovulatory dysfunction or not (Fig. 62.1).

Hypothyroidism has been implicated in recurrent miscarriages. Some studies have shown a twofold increase in spontaneous abortion with hypothyroidism, and improved outcome following thyroxine (T_4) replacement. It is important to note, however, that lower total T_4 and higher TSH levels in these cases could have been secondary to decreasing estrogen and human chorionic gonadotropin (hCG) levels in a failing pregnancy, with resultant decrease in T_4-binding globulin (TBG) and in the thyrotropic effect of hCG. A recent prospective study showed that total T_4 and TBG were lower, but free T_4 the same in patients who had spontaneous abortion as compared to those who continued their pregnancy [1]. Another study showed that women with thyroid autoantibodies have a higher rate of miscarriage regardless of their thyroid function status [2].

Hypothyroidism should be treated before conception. Thyroid hormone however is not recommended for therapy of patients with recurrent abortions unless it is associated with hyperprolactinemia or luteal-phase defect secondary to occult or overt hypothyroidism, as described above. As part of the attempt to uncover an autoimmune cause for repeated miscarriages, checking the patient for thyroid autoantibodies, along with lupus anticoagulant and anticardiolipin antibody, should be considered.

Hyperthyroidism and reproductive dysfunction

Figure 62.2 outlines the recommended steps in the diagnosis and management of hyperthyroidism.

Thyrotoxicosis increases SHBG and total circulating estrogens and androgens. Because of the increase in SHBG, however, free estradiol is probably decreased. These hormonal changes are proportional to the degree of thyrotoxicosis which, when severe, can lead to tonically elevated luteinizing hormone (LH) and follicle-stimulating hormone (FSH) and to loss of the feedback modulation necessary for normal ovulatory function. The weight loss and debilitation found in severe thyrotoxicosis also contribute to

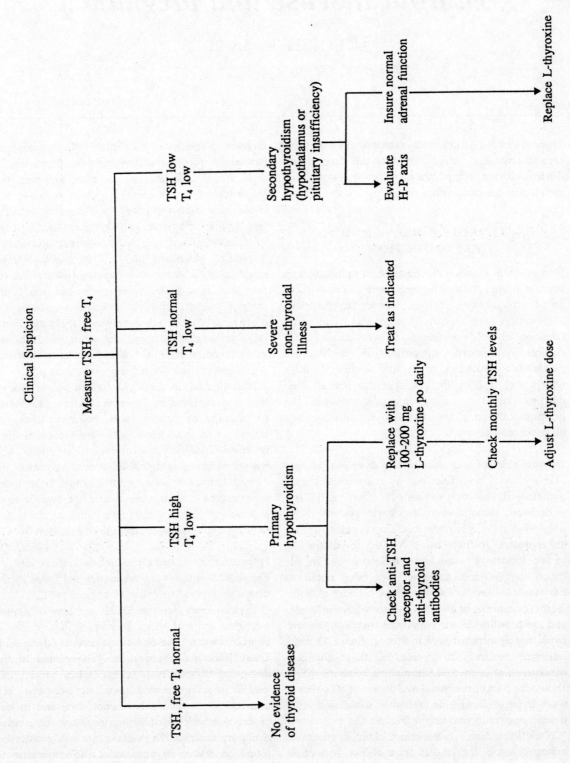

Fig. 62.1 Hypothyroidism in pregnancy.

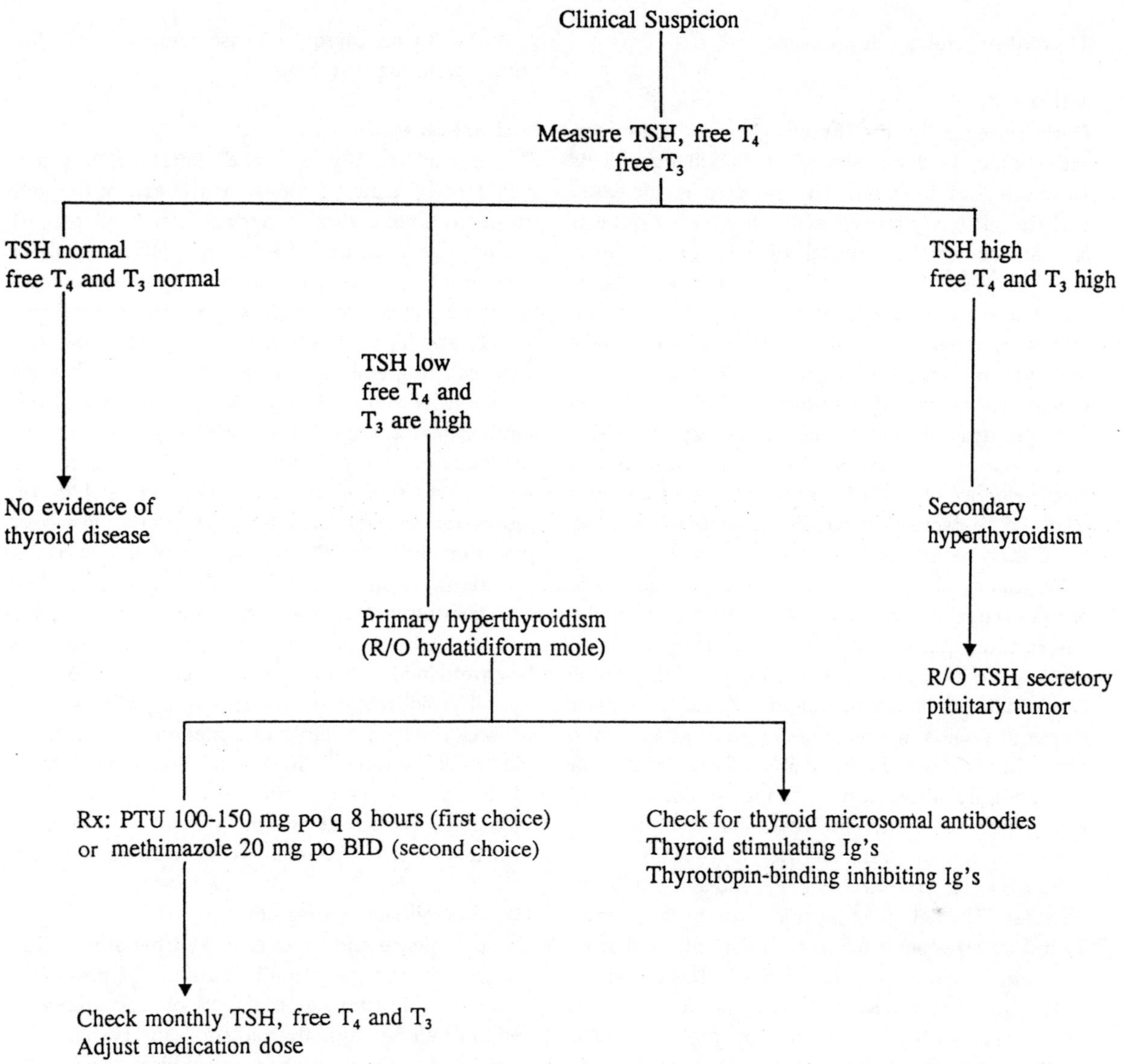

THYROID DISEASE

Clinical Suspicion

Measure TSH, free T$_4$
free T$_3$

TSH normal
free T$_4$ and T$_3$ normal

No evidence of
thyroid disease

TSH low
free T$_4$ and
T$_3$ are high

Primary hyperthyroidism
(R/O hydatidiform mole)

Rx: PTU 100-150 mg po q 8 hours (first choice)
or methimazole 20 mg po BID (second choice)

Check for thyroid microsomal antibodies
Thyroid stimulating Ig's
Thyrotropin-binding inhibiting Ig's

Check monthly TSH, free T$_4$ and T$_3$
Adjust medication dose

TSH high
free T$_4$ and T$_3$ high

Secondary
hyperthyroidism

R/O TSH secretory
pituitary tumor

Fig. 62.2 Hyperthyroidism in pregnancy.

the ovulatory dysfunction. Most cases do not reach this level before detection and, consequently, most hyperthyroid patients are ovulatory.

Increased rates of spontaneous abortion have been reported in patients with hyperthyroidism, most commonly in the severe cases. Some of these reports showed no difference in miscarriage rates between treated and untreated cases, raising the possibility that an underlying autoimmune disorder may be responsible for both the thyrotoxicosis, most commonly from Graves disease, and the miscarriages.

THYROID DISEASE IN PREGNANCY

Thyroid disease has been estimated to complicate about 0.5% of all pregnancies. Hypothyroidism is more common than hyperthyroidism, and autoimmune disorders are the major causes of thyroid disease in pregnancy and the puerperium. The appropriate management of thyroid diseases in pregnancy depends on the understanding of maternal—placental—fetal thyroid physiology during gestation.

CHAPTER 62

Thyroid physiology in pregnancy

Maternal

During pregnancy, the thyroid gland is in a hyperactive state, as demonstrated by the changes in its structure and function. Thyroid size is increased and the histology reflects active hormone synthesis and secretion. This physiologic response to pregnancy depends on multiple factors and is aimed at maintaining a euthyroid state. Starting in the first trimester, renal tubular reabsorption of iodide falls and urinary excretion increases. In areas where dietary iodine is not abundant, the thyroid gland compensates by increasing iodine uptake. This increased uptake persists until 1 week postpartum. The incidence of goiter in pregnancy varies between 5 and 70% depending on the geographic area and the dietary iodine status.

Pregnancy also affects the thyroid function tests, with the changes starting in the first trimester and the values returning to nonpregnant levels by the sixth week postpartum. In the serum, triiodothyronine (T_3) and T_4 are bound mainly to TBG and to a lesser extent to T_4-binding prealbumin (TBPA) and albumin with only 0.03% of T_4 and 0.3% of T_3 in the free, or metabolically active form. Owing to the effect of estrogens on the liver, TBG levels increase progressively throughout pregnancy up to twofold in the third trimester. In contrast, TBPA and albumin levels decrease. The net effect is an increase in total serum T_3 and T_4. To estimate the more important free thyroid hormone levels, the free T_4 index (FTI) has been used in the past. This test however is significantly affected by changes in the thyroid-binding proteins and is partly responsible for the contradictory findings in earlier reports concerning the changes in free thyroid hormone during gestation. Whenever available, the analog, or preferably the newer nonanalog free T_4 assays, should be used in pregnancy. Using these tests, the free T_4 and free T_3 levels show an initial rise in the first trimester and a progressive decline throughout the remainder of pregnancy. The changes in TSH levels show a reversed trend, with an early drop and a late progressive rise. The initial rise in free hormone and the drop in TSH are secondary to the thyrotropic effect of hCG, which has a TSH bioactivity of 0.7 μU TSH/U hCG and a peak level around 10 weeks' gestation. It should be noted that, despite the hormonal changes described above, serum TSH, free T_3, and free T_4 levels in a pregnant patient with no thyroid disease remain within the normal nonpregnant range.

Fetal and placental

The human fetal thyroid gland starts to concentrate iodide and secrete hormones at the end of the first trimester. Until that time, normal fetal development, notably the fetal nervous system development, is dependent on the minute amount of maternal thyroid hormone that crosses the placental barrier. Total and free T_4 and T_3 fetal serum levels start out low and increase progressively during the second half of gestation, with a reciprocal change seen in rT_3. The synthesis and secretion of fetal thyroid hormone are dependent on the maternal iodine supply. In addition to iodine deficiency causing fetal goiter, iodine excess may cause fetal goiter after 36 weeks' gestation when the thyroid autoregulation to iodine (Wolff–Chaikoff effect) matures in the fetus. TSH can be detected in the fetal pituitary and serum starting at 8 weeks' gestation. Serum level remains low until midgestation when it rises into the adult hypothyroid range of 10–15 μU/ml, with a small drop close to term. Early in gestation, TSH is under placental TRH regulation since fetal hypothalamic TRH secretion matures after 20 weeks. Thyroid hormones, TSH and TRH have been found in the amniotic fluid and the levels generally reflect fetal serum levels.

Hypothyroidism in pregnancy

The prevalence and main causes of hypothyroidism depend on the geographic location. In developed countries, it is estimated that 0.3% of pregnancies are complicated by hypothyroidism with Hashimoto's thyroiditis, idiopathic hypothyroidism, and post-ablative hypothyroidism accounting for more than 90% of the cases. On a global basis and in developing countries, hypothyroidism may be more prevalent, with iodine deficiency being the leading cause.

The clinical diagnosis of hypothyroidism during pregnancy may be difficult since many of the symptoms and signs, such as cold intolerance, weight gain, paresthesias, fluid retention, integument changes, delayed relaxation of deep tendon reflexes, slow pulse rate, and goiter may also be seen in normal pregnancies. If hypothyroidism is suspected, maternal serum TSH and free T_4 levels should be checked. Due to the physiologic changes described above, total serum T_4 is not useful for the diagnosis or management of thyroid diseases during pregnancy.

An elevated TSH is the most sensitive indicator of hypothyroidism in pregnancy. If TSH and free T_4 are normal, then the patient is not hypothyroid. A normal TSH and a low free T_4 can be seen in severe nonthyroidal illness. If both are low, secondary hypothyroidism should be ruled out and the pituitary–hypothalamic axis should be evaluated to rule out other hormonal deficiencies. If primary hypothyroidism is confirmed, then the patient should be checked for anti-TSH receptor and antimicrosomal thyroid antibodies in search for an autoimmune etiology. Of these, the anti-TSH receptor-blocking antibody is probably the most important, since its presence is associated with fetal and neonatal hypothyroidism. The prenatal diagnosis of fetal hypothyroidism using funipuncture has been reported in these patients [3], in addition to patients on anti-thyroid medications and patients who inadvertently received ablative radioisotope therapy.

The effect of pregnancy on the disease depends on the cause. Autoimmune thyroid diseases may improve during gestation with a decrease in thyroid antibody titer and postpartum relapse. Hypothyroidism from other causes tends to worsen during pregnancy because of the increased demand on the thyroid gland and the increased renal clearance of iodine.

The maternal and fetal effects of hypothyroidism depend on its cause, severity, and time of onset. In cases of iodine deficiency, the fetal wastage rate may be as high as 30%, with cretinism noted in the surviving offspring of untreated mothers. Lower fetal wastage rates are seen with other etiologic causes. In autoimmune causes, transient neonatal hypothyroidism secondary to transplacental passage of thyroid-blocking antibodies has been noted in about 1% of cases. As described above, the maternal thyroid hormone status during embryogenesis is critical, with increased incidence of neurologic sequelae noted in neonates whose mothers were hypothyroid during that period. As to the severity, the incidence of maternal complications in overt hypothyroidism is 40%, with low birth weights and fetal death from abruption occurring in 30 and 12%, respectively, while patients with subclinical hypothyroidism have only one-third as many complications.

The diagnosis and optimal treatment of hypothyroidism should be achieved as early as possible. In patients with no evidence of cardiovascular dis-ease, replacement therapy should be started with 100–200 µg L-thyroxine orally once daily (approximately 1 µg per lb maternal body weight). The dose should be adjusted to keep the TSH, which should be checked monthly, in the midnormal range. In patients with severe hypothyroidism and underlying heart disease, treatment should be started with a lower dose, 25–50 µg daily, and increased every 2–4 weeks until TSH levels are back within normal. In rare cases of *de novo* secondary hypothyroidism, the adrenocortical function should be evaluated before initiating thyroid hormone replacement, which could provoke an acute adrenal crisis in patients with unrecognized adrenal insufficiency. Patients already on T_4 therapy should be continued on it, with adjustments made according to TSH. If the original indication is unclear, it is advisable to wait until the postpartum period before stopping treatment, then reevaluating 6 weeks later. There have been no untoward fetal effects from *in utero* exposure to L-thyroxine. Reported breast milk levels vary, depending on the determination method used, from none found, to clinically insignificant low levels. Consequently, breast-feeding is not contraindicated in mothers on thyroid hormone replacement.

Hyperthyroidism in pregnancy

A total of 0.2% of pregnant women have hyperthyroidism, with Graves disease being the most common cause. Toxic multinodular goiter and toxic solitary nodule are much less common causes but, together with Graves disease, account for more than 90% of the cases. Another rare cause of hyperthyroidism in pregnancy is thyroiditis which, early in its course, can be associated with transient thyrotoxicosis before the onset of hypothyroidism.

The symptoms and signs of hyperthyroidism, such as heat intolerance, sweating, palpitation, fatigue, and goiter, are also found in normal pregnancies. The diagnosis may be suggested by an inadequate weight gain or by the presence of ophthalmopathy, but it essentially relies on laboratory evaluation. Free T_4, free T_3, and TSH should be measured. Measurement of free T_3 is important since in some cases of hyperthyroidism free T_4 is only slightly elevated or normal. Typically, however, both free T_4 and T_3 are elevated and TSH is suppressed. If TSH levels are elevated, then the rare situation of secondary hyperthyroidism with a TSH-secreting tumor should be considered. In cases where primary hyperthyroidism is confirmed, the maternal serum should be checked for thyroid microsomal antibodies, thyroid-stimulating immunoglobulins, and thyrotropin-binding inhibiting immunoglobulins which may be predictive of the development of maternal post-partum thyroid dysfunction and of fetal or neonatal thyrotoxicosis. This also applies to patients with previously diagnosed and treated primary hyper-thyroidism regardless of their thyroid function status during gestation. Finally, it should be mentioned that radioisotope thyroid scanning should not be performed during pregnancy and, if used postpartum, breast-feeding should be interrupted for at least 46 days when radioactive iodine is used and for 24 hours when pertechnetate is used.

Graves disease tends to improve in late pregnancy and to relapse postpartum. This is probably secondary to the decrease in helper T lymphocytes and in thyroid antibodies seen during gestation.

As to the effect of hyperthyroidism on pregnancy, an increased incidence of fetal anomalies, preterm deliveries, perinatal mortality, maternal heart failure, and peripartum thyroid storm was found in patients with uncontrolled disease. In addition, thyrotoxicosis increases insulin requirements during pregnancy and may interfere with the control of gestational diabetics. Recent reports seem to refute the previously held belief that thyrotoxicosis is a cause of hyperemesis gravidarum. The increased free T_4 levels seen in these cases only represent a physiologic response and correlate with higher levels of hCG, which in turn correlate with the severity of the nausea and vomiting. Finally, about 1% of neonates born to mothers with Graves disease will have transient thyrotoxicosis secondary to transplacental passage of TSH receptor-stimulating antibodies. These antibodies may be present irrespective of the mother's clinical status or previous therapy.

The first line of therapy for primary hyperthyroidism in pregnancy is medical. The thiourea derivatives propylthiouracil (PTU), methimazole, and carbimazole, which is metabolized to methimazole, have been used. All cross the placenta and are excreted in breast milk. PTU is less lipid-soluble and more highly protein-bound, therefore, its placental transfer may be lower. Because of this and the additional benefit of blocking the peripheral T_4 to T_3 conversion, PTU is the drug of choice in pregnancy. The initial dose is 100–150 mg orally every 8 hours to control the maternal thyrotoxicosis. Once this is achieved, the

dose is adjusted to the lowest possible that maintains the mother's T_4 level in the upper normal range. The patient should be followed with monthly free thyroid hormone and TSH determinations.

Methimazole is the drug of second choice and is used in patients who develop a reaction to PTU. Because of its longer half-life, it can be given once or twice daily for a total of up to 40 mg. Maternal side-effects of thiourea derivatives include skin rashes, pruritis, nausea, fever, lymphadenopathy, and agranulocytosis. All of these are reversible and, except for agranulocytosis, cross-sensitivity between PTU and methimazole does not usually occur. Agranulocytosis occurs in about 5% of patients, usually suddenly after 1–2 months of therapy. All patients receiving thiourea derivatives should be warned to report any fever, sore throat, or other symptoms of infection. As to the fetal effects, about 1% will develop transient neonatal hypothyroidism and goiter.

Surgical treatment of primary thyrotoxicosis in pregnancy should be reserved for patients with poor drug compliance, intolerable side-effects or goiters causing pressure symptoms, and is most safely performed in the second trimester. Thyroid function tests should continue to be checked in these patients postoperatively since some may develop hypothyroidism. Their fetuses and neonates would continue to be at risk for thyroid dysfunction from transplacental transfer of thyroid antibodies regardless of the maternal status.

As for β-adrenergic blocking drugs and cold iodides, their use in pregnancy should be limited to short periods, along with thionamides in preparation for subtotal thyroidectomy or in the acute management of thyroid storm. Radioiodine treatment is contraindicated in pregnancy since it crosses the placenta and, after 10 weeks' gestation, is concentrated by the fetal thyroid. The fetus may develop hypothyroidism in addition to the effects of whole-body radiation.

Finally, the immediate treatment of thyroid storm, a rare but life-threatening emergency characterized by hyperpyrexia, tachycardia, hypotension, and delirium, must be mentioned. Therapy should be aggressive and should be initiated as soon as the patient starts to decompensate, without waiting for definite diagnostic criteria. In cases with no heart failure, propranolol is given to block the peripheral effects of thyroid hormone. The initial dose is 1 mg/min i.v. for 2–10 min followed by 20–80 mg orally every 4 hours. The aim is to reduce the maternal heart rate to 100 beats/min. At the same time, thyroid hormone production should be reduced using PTU and iodide. PTU is given in doses of up to 400 mg orally every 8 hours. If oral medication cannot be given, methimazole 30–40 mg rectally every 8 hours may be substituted for PTU. Iodide 36–180 mg is given orally or intravenously every 8 hours as sodium or potassium iodide. Dexamethasone 1 mg orally or intramuscularly every 6 hours may be added to prevent adrenocortical insufficiency and to inhibit peripheral T_4 to T_3 conversion. In addition, oxygen, sedatives, antipyretics, and fluid hydration should be given according to the clinical situation. Because aspirin displaces the protein-bound thyroid hormone, acetaminophen is the preferred antipyretic in patients with a thyroid storm. Any precipitating cause, such as infection, must be treated vigorously.

Nodular thyroid disease in pregnancy

Diffuse thyroid enlargement is commonly seen in pregnancy and represents a physiologic response. Thyroid nodules on the other hand require investigation to rule out malignancy which is found in 15–20% of single thyroid nodules. Thyroid function tests should be ordered to rule out a toxic solitary nodule. Since radioisotope scanning is contraindicated in pregnancy, and ultrasound cannot give a firm pathologic diagnosis, the next step in the workup is a fine-needle aspiration of the nodule. Adequate material can be obtained in 93% of aspirates. False positives are extremely rare and false-negative results occur in 5–10% of cases. If the diagnosis remains unclear then excisional or open biopsy of the nodule is required. A benign euthyroid nodule can be followed up or suppressed with L-thyroxine. It should be noted that even malignant nodules may decrease in size with suppression and therefore this may not be used to differentiate between malignant and benign nodules.

The treatment of choice for primary thyroid carcinoma is surgery which can be performed in the second or third trimester. Radioactive iodine therapy should be withheld until after delivery. Surgery may be delayed until the postpartum period in cases where the diagnosis was made close to term. The common belief is that thyroid carcinoma is unaffected by pregnancy and that a previous history of thyroid carcinoma is not a contraindication to pregnancy. Recent reports however have questioned this notion.

THYROID DISEASE IN THE PUERPERIUM

Previously diagnosed autoimmune thyroid diseases tend to improve during pregnancy and relapse after delivery. Postpartum thyroiditis syndrome, however, represents a spectrum of thyroid dysfunction occurring in the puerperium. The prevalence varies between 2 and 16%, depending on the criteria and screening tests used for diagnosis. Risk factors include cigarette smoking, increased iodine intake, and previous personal or family history of thyroid disease. It is an immunologic disorder characterized by a chronic lymphocytic thyroiditis and associated with human leukocyte antigen types DR3, DR4, and DR5. About 50% of patients with thyroid microsomal antibodies in early pregnancy ultimately develop postpartum thyroiditis, and testing for this antibody is a cost-effective screening method.

These patients usually present 3–6 months after delivery with a painless goiter, and signs and symptoms of mild to moderate thyroid dysfunction. The dysfunction may be either hyper- or hypothyroidism, or one followed by the other. In addition to the abnormal thyroid hormone profile, the laboratory findings include a positive thyroid microsomal antibody and, in contrast to Graves disease, a low thyroidal radioiodine uptake.

Except in rare cases or patients with repeated episodes, the disease is transient and a return to euthyroid state occurs within a year. Most cases require no or only symptomatic treatment. If prescribed, therapy should be discontinued and the thyroid function reassessed 6–12 months later. Up to 50% of patients with postpartum thyroiditis may have a recurrence following a subsequent pregnancy.

The puerperium should be a time for careful scrutiny with respect to the development of new-onset thyroid dysfunction.

REFERENCES

1 Ross HA, Exalto N, Kloppenberg PWC, Benraad TJ. *Thyroid hormone binding in early pregnancy and the risk of spontaneous abortion. Eur J Obstet Gynecol Repr Biol* 1989; 32: 129–136.

2 Stagnaro-Green A, Roman SH, Cobin RH *et al*. Detection of at-risk pregnancy by means of highly sensitive assays for thyroid autoantibodies. *JAMA* 1990; 264: 1422–1425.

3 Davidson KM, Richards DS, Schatz DA, Fisher DA. Successful *in utero* treatment of fetal goiter and hypothyroidism. *N Engl J Med* 1991; 324: 543–546.

FURTHER READING

Becks GP, Burrow GN. Thyroid disease and pregnancy. *Med Clin North Am* 1991; 75: 121–150.

Mori M, Amino N, Tamaki H *et al*. Morning sickness and thyroid function in normal pregnancy. *Obstet Gynecol* 1988; 72: 355–359.

Nikolai TF, Turney SL, Roberts RC. Postpartum lymphocytic thyroiditis: prevalence, clinical course, and long-term follow-up. *Arch Intern Med* 1987; 147: 221–224.

Thorpe-Beeston JG, Nicolaides KH, Felton CV *et al*. Maturation of the secretion of thyroid hormone and thyroid-stimulating hormone in the fetus. *N Engl J Med* 1991; 324: 532–536.

Wenstrom KD, Weiner CP, Williamson RA, Grant SS. Prenatal diagnosis of fetal hyperthyroidism using funipuncture. *Obstet Gynecol* 1990; 76: 513–517.

Zakarija M, McKenzie M, Eidson MS. Transient neonatal hypothyroidism: characterization of maternal antibodies to the thyrotropin receptor. *J Clin Endocrinol Metab* 1990; 70: 1239–1246.

Part VII

Evaluation of the infertile couple

Assessing and monitoring ovulation

EMMETT F. BRANIGAN & MICHAEL R. SOULES

INTRODUCTION

All infertile women should receive an evaluation of their ovulatory status regardless of whether they have regular cycles or menstrual dysfunction. The characteristics of her menstrual cycle are a good reflection of the ovulatory status of a given woman. A patient has regular menses (eumenorrhea) if uterine withdrawal bleeding occurs at 21–36-day intervals. Oligomenorrheic cycles are ones where the intervals are greater than 36 days and amenorrhea is the absence of menses for 6–12 months. Between 10 and 25% of female infertility is due to ovulation disorders. These include both anovulation and oligoovulation. The patients generally present with symptoms of either amenorrhea or oligomenorrhea.

Abnormal menstrual function can be a symptom reflecting both an ovulation problem and an underlying medical condition. Therefore when menstrual dysfunction (amenorrhea or oligomenorrhea) is present, a thorough evaluation should follow. The evaluation of these conditions will be discussed briefly. If an infertile woman is eumenorrheic, the clinician can proceed directly to assess her ovulatory status.

Evaluation of menstrual dysfunction

Since amenorrhea or oligomenorrhea is frequently a symptom of a more serious underlying disease, they require a thorough evaluation before treatment of the anovulatory status. In the work-up many chronic diseases that can cause amenorrhea can be excluded simply by history and physical examination.

In women with secondary amenorrhea, the most common cause is pregnancy. If the serum concentration of β-human chorionic gonadotropin (β-hCG) is negative one should obtain thyroid function tests, serum prolactin and follicle-stimulating hormone (FSH) levels and administer a progestin challenge to complete the initial work-up.

In the patient with oligomenorrhea, prolactin and FSH levels as well as thyroid function tests should be determined. If abnormalities are detected then specific therapy can be instituted; if these are normal then ovulation induction can be initiated. However, most infertile women are eumenorrheic and have regular menses. In these women the clinican can proceed directly to the assessment of ovulation.

OVULATION ASSESSMENT

Ovulation is a key event in the ovarian cycle. Mastery of the methods for its identification is critical to the physician caring for the infertile couple. There are three important aspects of ovulation to evaluate: the occurrence, timing, and quality. No single test or measurement can simultaneously address all three of these issues. Therefore a variety of diagnostic tools are utilized to detect, predict, and confirm ovulation. Since clinicians are unable directly to observe ovulation, they rely on the various morphologic events and endocrine changes that occur in association with follicular rupture and extrusion of the oocyte to indirectly assess ovulation.

Detection of ovulation

Menstrual history
Most women who have regular menstrual periods every 21–36 days are ovulatory. A history of eumenorrhea correlates well with ovulation in approximately 90% of cases. When regular cycles are accompanied by midcycle mucorrhea and/or mittelschmerz, premenstrual symptoms, and dysmenorrhea, they are almost always ovulatory. However, while regular menses quite accurately predict ovulation, irregular menses cannot be relied upon to indicate anovulation. (Irregular cycles are those that occur every 21–40 days but each cycle length varies in relation to the others.) Approximately 75% of irregular

menstrual cycles are ovulatory. Therefore while a regular menstrual history is very helpful in assessing ovulatory status, an irregular menstrual history is an unreliable guide to ovulation.

Basal body temperature charting

The basal body temperature (BBT) chart is one of the least invasive and expensive methods to detect ovulation. The BBT is determined and charted by the woman recording her oral temperature each morning before getting out of bed. The most reliable BBTs are recorded after 6–8 hours of uninterrupted sleep.

The BBT chart is a graph that indicates the body's thermal response to progesterone in an ovulatory cycle. During the follicular phase of the cycle, the basal temperature averages 97.5°F and in the luteal phase it averages 98.1°F. This sustained rise in temperature during the luteal phase provides indirect evidence of ovulation. The BBT generally starts to rise simultaneously with the luteinizing hormone (LH) surge but a significant elevation above the follicular-phase temperature level does not occur until 2 days following the LH peak. It remains elevated until serum progesterone drops to less than 4 ng/ml.

Consistent biphasic BBT charts are a good indicator of ovulation. While monophasic charts usually indicate anovulation, exceptional women may not experience a temperature shift despite normal ovulation. The primary and best use of the BBT chart is for the retrospective documentation of ovulation. Other uses of the BBT chart include the following: (1) the duration of the luteal-phase temperature rise can give clues to the adequacy of the luteal phase; and (2) the BBT is useful as a guideline for scheduling tests and treatments during subsequent cycles. However, since the luteal-phase temperature rise occurs during ovulation it cannot be used to predict ovulation in the current cycle.

In summary, the BBT is a convenient method for detecting ovulation. When it is biphasic, it is a good indicator that ovulation occurred. It can give clues to the adequacy of the luteal phase and is useful in scheduling tests and other treatments in subsequent cycles. However, it is not useful in predicting ovulation during a particular cycle.

Serum progesterone

The most direct and accurate confirmation of follicular luteinization is the measurement of serum progesterone during the luteal phase. An increase in serum progesterone concentration above follicular-phase levels is generally accepted as evidence that ovulation has probably occurred. (*Note*: luteinization of a follicle can occur without prior extrusion of the oocyte-ovulation.) The lowest random serum progesterone value that is reliably associated with secretory endometrium on biopsy is 3 ng/ml. However, random midluteal progesterone levels of greater than 5 ng/ml are more certain evidence of luteinization of a follicle. Progesterone levels fluctuate in response to LH pulses during the luteal phase of the cycle. These fluctuations are quite pronounced and account for the fact that progesterone levels seem to have a wide variation. Even considering this variation, a serum progesterone above the indicated minimum is a very reliable indicator of ovulation.

For best results, the clinician should attempt to obtain a serum progesterone level in the midluteal phase (4–7 days prior to the predicted next menstrual period). The drawbacks to the serum progesterone as an indicator of ovulation are: (1) it requires a blood draw; (2) it is reliable only on a limited number of cycle days; (3) it is relatively expensive compared to a BBT chart; and (4) it indicates ovulation only in a single cycle.

Serial transvaginal ultrasounds

Transvaginal ultrasound is an excellent tool for detection of ovulation. Transvaginal ultrasound offers high-resolution images that do not require a full bladder, minimizing patient discomfort, and it is effective even in obese patients. Its use provides information on the progressive growth and development of the follicle and can pinpoint the day of ovulation. The disappearance of the dominant ovarian follicle as seen on daily ultrasound scans of the pelvis is now widely accepted as the best available indicator of the day of ovulation. The major drawback to ultrasound scanning for the routine detection of ovulation is the expense to the patient. Since the scans need to be repeated daily during the periovulatory period, this method is both time-consuming for the patient as well as expensive.

In summary, it is recommended that the clinician use a good menstrual history in combination with a BBT chart, a serum progesterone level, or a serial transvaginal ultrasound examination to detect ovulation in an infertile woman with regular menstrual cycles. The BBT chart is simple and provides information about several menstrual cycles but is dependent on patient compliance. While a series of BBT charts is quite reliable for the detection of ovulation, a critical serum progesterone level in the luteal phase is even more reliable. Its drawbacks are expense, timing, and information on only one cycle. A series of serial ultrasound scans of follicle development and rupture can clearly detect ovulation but the drawbacks attributable to a serum progesterone level are even more pronounced with this method.

Prediction of ovulation

Once the presence of ovulation has been detected, it is often important to be able to predict ovulation. Knowing the day of ovulation is clinically important for: (1) timing artificial insemination, sexual intercourse, and/or postcoital testing; (2) luteal phase testing; (3) embryo transfer timing in donor oocyte programs or embryo cryopreservation cycles; and (4) preventing conception in natural family planning. Several clinical parameters such as cervical mucus changes and the BBT nadir in the previous BBT chart recorded by regularly cycling women can be helpful in predicting the approximate day of ovulation. However, the LH surge, detected in plasma or urine, is generally accepted as being more accurate in predicting ovulation in a particular cycle.

The BBT charts of women with regular menstrual cycles that are consistent over time can be used retrospectively to predict reasonably the expected ovulation day in a future cycle. However, as cycle variability increases, the precision of this method markedly decreases. When the BBT nadir is not consistent, the temperature chart cannot reliably predict the day of ovulation. Similarly, cervical mucus changes around the time of ovulation can be used in conjunction with the BBT nadir further to improve the predictability. These methods, however, often cannot predict ovulation with enough precision to be clinically useful.

Detection of the LH surge in urine using a home testing kit is currently the most widely used method of predicting ovulation. There is a high degree of correlation between serum and urine LH measurements. It would be useful to review the timing and physiology of ovulation so the clinician can better understand the pertinence of detecting an LH surge. The peak plasma etradiol level occurs about 24–36 hours before ovulation. A sustained and relatively high estradiol leads to an acute increase in LH se-

cretion (the surge) via positive feedback on the hypothalamus and the anterior pituitary. The estradiol levels must reach a critical concentration (e.g., 200 pg/ml) and sustain it for 24–48 hours for positive feedback to occur. A smaller FSH surge also occurs simultaneously with the increase in LH. A small but acute increase in progesterone may actually trigger the LH surge. The LH surge leads to resumption of meiosis by the oocyte, luteinization of the granulosa cells, and follicle rupture. It is important to remember that LH is secreted in pulses by the anterior pituitary. If an attempt is made to detect the LH peak, pulsatile secretion must be taken into account. Since frequent multiple sampling would be necessary to detect the peak, the onset of the LH surge is used to predict ovulation rather than the LH peak itself. Various studies have defined the onset of the surge differently. An increase in daily serum LH values to 35 or 40 mIU/ml as well as an increase of 1.5 times previous daily values has been successfully used to define the onset of the surge. Regardless of how one defines the onset, the duration of the surge is about 36 hours. Ovulation is thought to occur 32–38 hours after the onset of the plasma LH surge. LH has a half-life of 20 min in the blood and is cleared into the urine.

Detection of the onset of the LH surge in serum using daily blood samples is not practical in the clinical setting. The use of urine samples allows a patient to perform these tests in a convenient manner. Home urine LH detection kit (also called ovulation predictor kits) all use an enzyme-linked immunosorbent assay (ELISA) system to identify LH in the urine. In the kits, one antibody is directed against the α-subunit of LH and a second monoclonal antibody is directed against the β-subunit of LH. One of the antibodies is attached to a bead or the test pad and the other is linked to an enzyme (usually alkaline phosphatase) that will convert a substrate from noncolored to colored. The concentration of LH is proportional to the amount of color produced. Most kits commercially available detect urine LH concentrations in the 20–40 mIU/ml range.

Urine LH kits have become the most widely used method of predicting ovulation because they are quick, reliable, and easy to use. They are relatively inexpensive compared to serum LH assays but expensive when compared to LH surge prediction using retrospective methods such as the BBT nadir. In consideration of the high correlation between serum and urine LH concentrations, most kits correctly predict ovulation in the 90–100% range when compared to serial serum LH values, and agree with ultrasound-detected ovulation (disappearance of the dominant follicle) 53–88% of the time.

These are some practical guidelines for the use of urine LH kits:

1 Since the LH surge tends to be initiated in the early a.m. hours (1200–0600 hours) it is recommended that the patient routinely check her urine in the evening beginning several days prior to the expected surge onset. Waiting until evening allows LH to accumulate in the urine during the day and thereby the evening assay becomes the first possible positive indication of impending ovulation.

2 Ovulation theoretically should occur approximately 24 hours after the LH surge is detected in urine (allowing a variable amount of time for LH to concentrate in the urine after the actual surge initiation in serum).

3 Once the day of ovulation has been predicted, then appropriate clinical measures can be taken (e.g., insemination).

4 Women should perform these tests at the same room temperature each day and they should limit their fluid intake.

5 The clinician and patient should remain aware of the approximate nature of these physiologic events as predicted by a daily urine LH test.

Assessment of the luteal phase

Finally, the assessment of the ovulatory process must include monitoring the function of the corpus luteum. Normal ovulation is a prerequisite for normal corpus luteum function. Proper functioning of the corpus luteum is necessary for implantation and maintenance of early pregnancy. Luteal-phase deficiency can cause infertility and can also lead to recurrent abortion. Patients with recurrent luteal-phase defects are deficient in either the amount or duration of progesterone secretion.

In the section on detection of ovulation, it was explained that certain random levels of progesterone indicated that ovulation had occurred. In that context, progesterone levels are used to confirm or deny ovulation — a yes or no situation. In this section on luteal-phase assessment, the focus is on a more subtle proposition — whether adequate amounts of progesterone are present.

While a BBT chart can sometimes imply the presence of luteal-phase deficiency, endometrial bi-

opsies and/or serial serum progesterone levels are necessary for an accurate diagnosis. Normal maturation of the endometrium during the secretory phase is a result of adequate progesterone secretion. Total progesterone secretion correlates well with endometrial dating.

Examination of the endometrium in the late luteal phase has become the standard clinical test for diagnosing luteal-phase deficiency. A difference of more than 2 days between the histologic endometrial dating and the chronologic dating based on the day of the onset of the next menstrual period in two or more cycles is the definition of a luteal-phase defect using this method. However, a major problem with endometrial biopsies is the fact that they are painful and expensive for the patient.

Single random serum progesterone levels alone cannot be used to establish a diagnosis of luteal-phase deficiency. The rather acute onset and decline of progesterone secretion by the corpus luteum indicates that daily samples would be needed to estimate accurately total progesterone production. Attempts to address this problem have tried repeated sampling during the midluteal phase of the cycle.

Using single midluteal progesterone levels, a serum level <10 ng/ml is an indication of a probable luteal-phase-deficient cycle. Three blood samples in the midluteal phase, with the sum of serum levels totaling <25 ng/ml gives a similar indication. However, serum progesterone levels are relatively expensive and are often difficult to time. Therefore, they are only recommended as a secondary method for the detection of luteal-phase deficiency.

Although the detection of luteal-phase deficiency is problematic, it remains an important aspect of ovulation assessment. Normal corpus luteum function is a good indication of normal ovulation.

FURTHER READING

Barratt CLR, Cooke S, Chauhan M, Cooke ID. A prospective randomized controlled trial comparing urinary luteinizing hormone dipsticks and basal body temperature charts with timed donor insemination. *Fertil Steril* 1989; 52: 394.

Blackwell RE. Detection of ovulation. *Fertil Steril* 1984; 41: 680.

Collins JA. Diagnostic assessment of the ovulatory process. *Semin Reprod Endocrinol* 1990; 8: 145.

Corsan GH, Ghazi D, Kemmann E. Home urinary luteinizing hormone immunoassays: clinical applications. *Fertil Steril* 1990; 53: 591.

Davis OK, Berkeley AS, Naus GJ, Gholst IN, Freedman

KS. The incidence of luteal phase defect in normal, fertile women determined by serial endometrial biopsies. *Fertil Steril* 1989; 51: 582.

Filicori M, Butler JP, Crowley WF. Neuroendocrine regulation of the corpus luteum in the human: evidence for pulsatile progesterone secretion. *J Clin Invest* 1984; 73: 1638.

Garcia JC, Jones GS, Wright GL. Prediction of the time of ovulation. *Fertil Steril* 1981; 36: 308.

Grimsted J, Jacobsen JD, Grinsted L, Schantz A, Steufoss HH, Nielsen SP. Prediction of ovulation. *Fertil Steril* 1989; 52: 388.

McIntosh JEA, Matthews CD, Crocker JM, Broom T, Cox L. Predicting the luteinizing hormone surge: relationship between the duration of the follicular and luteal phases and the length of the human menstrual cycle. *Fertil Steril* 1980; 34: 125.

Moghissi KS. Prediction and detection of ovulation. *Fertil Steril* 1980; 34: 89.

Rosenfeld DL, Garcia C-R. A comparison of endometrial histology with simultaneous plasma progesterone determinations in infertile women. *Fertil Steril* 1976; 27: 1256.

Shoupe D, Mishell DR Jr, Lacarra M *et al*. Correlation of endometrial maturation with four methods of estimating day of ovulation. *Obstet Gynecol* 1989; 73: 88.

Vermesh M, Kletzky OA, Davajan V, Israel R. Monitoring techniques to predict and detect ovulation. *Fertil Steril* 1987; 47: 259.

Wentz AC. Endometrial biopsy in the evaluation of infertility. *Fertil Steril* 1979; 33: 121.

Ultrasound in
reproductive endocrinology

GREGORY F. ROSEN

Transvaginal ultrasonography is revolutionizing office gynecology in a similar manner to the way that laparoscopic surgery is revolutionizing operative gynecology. In 1984, with the introduction of transvaginal ultrasound, ultrasound technologically was at the point that transabdominal visualization of ovaries was possible in the majority but not in all patients. Visualization of the ovaries in obese patients and patients with posteriorly placed ovaries was at times impossible. A full-bladder technique was employed because it was necessary to create an acoustic window to aid in visualization of the pelvic structure. Using the transvaginal approach, however, the transducer is placed within 3–5 cm of the ovaries in most patients. This allowed for markedly superior resolution of the anatomy and has greatly facilitated the interpretation of normal ovarian physiology and pathophysiology. Another advantage of transvaginal over transabdominal ultrasonography is that a full bladder is not a prerequisite. Not requiring a full bladder facilitates scanning of the patient from both a time perspective, i.e., there is no waiting for the bladder to fill, and from the patient's standpoint — not requiring a full bladder is much more comfortable.

Since transvaginal ultrasonography was introduced in 1984, when it was marketed primarily as a tool for monitoring controlled ovarian hyperstimulation for *in vitro* fertilization, its applications and merits have continued to expand in reproductive endocrinology and infertility. These uses now include: (1) documentation of ovulation in normal ovulatory cycles to simplify timing of postcoital tests and endometrial biopsies; (2) to confirm and localize early pregnancies; (3) to follow uterine pathology, i.e., uterine leiomyomas; (4) to evaluate pelvic masses; and (5) to follow physiologic and pathologic structures within the ovaries. The use of ultrasound in ovulation induction, *in vitro* fertilization, and ectopic pregnancies will be covered in other chapters throughout

this textbook. The remainder of this chapter will concentrate on the other topics as listed above.

WORK-UP OF THE INFERTILE COUPLE

The evaluation of the infertile couple involves the following sequence of tests: semen analysis, documentation of ovulation, postcoital testing, hysterosalpingogram, and laparoscopy. Transvaginal ultrasound can be used to document follicular growth and disappearance. Numerous studies have been performed that have shown that the dominant follicle grows at an average rate of 2–3 mm/day, reaching a mean diameter of approximately 20–24 mm or a longest single diameter of 22–26 mm prior to ovulation [1]. Ultrasound is considered the "gold-standard" of tools used to document ovulation. Ovulation can be documented by noting the disappearance of the dominant follicle, a significant decrease in follicle size (>2 mm), a marked increase in follicle size, or a change in the sonographic appearance of the follicular cyst. A follicular cyst is sonolucent (Fig. 64.1). A corpus luteum is sometimes filled with clot and therefore not sonolucent but irregularly echoed, giving it a "cobweb" appearance (Fig. 64.2). Serial ultrasound examinations can also be used to demonstrate normal follicle growth parameters, as mentioned above.

The ability to approximate when ovulation will occur is extremely useful for timing postcoital tests since the most common reason for a poor postcoital test is improper timing. The cervical mucus, i.e., the cervical score, is best the day before ovulation. Cervical mucus is commonly visible on ultrasound examination at this time (Fig. 64.3). Physiologically, this is because the onset of the luteinizing hormone (LH) surge, about 36 hours before ovulation, also marks a shift in steroid hormone production from estradiol to progesterone. Progesterone, through its

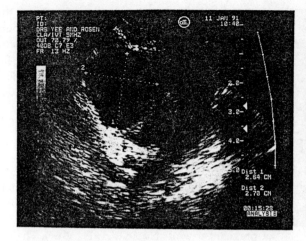

Fig. 64.1 Follicle cyst in the right ovary. Ovarian cortex is splayed to the right of the follicle.

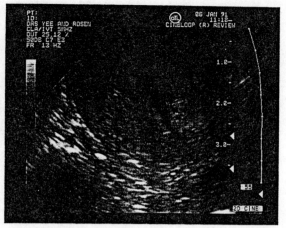

Fig. 64.3 A parasagittal scan of the cervix with the vagina at the point of the transducer. Note the cervical mucus (the black stripe).

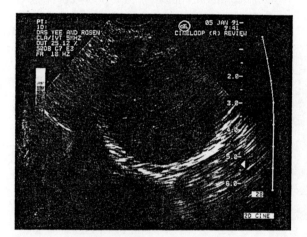

Fig. 64.2 Hemorrhagic corpus luteum in the right ovary. Note the "honey-comb" appearance.

antiestrogen effect, markedly decreases the production of favorable cervical mucus.

The presence of luteinized unruptured follicle syndrome is also a rare but potential finding in the work-up of the infertile couple. This finding in a single cycle is of no significant value. If it recurs, treatment with human chorionic gonadotropin (hCG) or clomiphene may be useful.

An example of optimizing use of the ultrasound in the work-up of the infertile couple would be under the following scenario: a woman presents to you with a history of infertility and regular 30-day cycles. She is asked to return to your office on day 13 for an ultrasound which shows a solitary follicle measuring 18 mm in the maximum diameter on her right ovary.

With the knowledge that follicles grow on the average of 2–3 mm/day and that follicle rupture occurs the day after reaching a maximal size of approximately 24 mm, she is asked to return 2 days later for a postcoital test and is instructed to have intercourse the evening prior to this visit. The postcoital test is then performed and, afterwards, the ultrasound is repeated to see whether or not the follicle has disappeared. If ovulation has occurred, a serum progesterone can be ordered 5–9 days later and/or endometrial biopsy can be performed on the 11th or 12th day postovulation. If she has not ovulated, she can be rescanned 1–2 days later to document follicle disappearance.

The endometrium can also be monitored throughout the menstrual cycle. Prior to ovulation, the consistency of the endometrium, per ultrasound, is very similar to the myometrium. There is, however, a line of demarcation between the endometrium and the myometrium which is readily visible (Fig. 64.4). Normal endometrium grows approximately 1–2 mm/day and usually is between 10 and 14 mm in thickness by the time of ovulation. The effect of progesterone is to luteinize the endometrium. A luteinized endometrium is ultrasonographically denser than the surrounding myometrium, i.e., in standard gray scale, the luteinized endometrium becomes whiter than the darker myometrium (Fig. 64.5).

Ultrasound can be used for timing of intrauterine insemination. Previous studies have compared basal body temperature (BBT) charts to urinary LH and to ultrasound in normal ovulatory women [2]. The

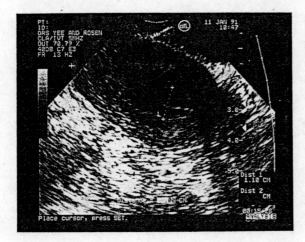

Fig. 64.4 A parasagittal scan of the uterus with the fundus pointing towards 3 o'clock. The proliferative endometrium is 1.1 cm thick and is approximately the same density as the surrounding myometrium.

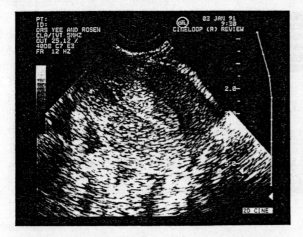

Fig. 64.5 A parasagittal scan of the uterus with the fundus pointing towards 4 o'clock. Secretory endometrium is usually denser (whiter) than the surrounding myometrium.

BBT nadir can occur up to 3 days before ovulation. Likewise, urinary LH may also be measurable up to 3 days before ovulation. This is important information since sperm that bypass the cervical mucus, i.e., with intrauterine insemination, have a life span of less than 24 hours. It is also important to note that there are no studies in the literature that look at urinary LH associated with the use of clomiphene citrate. It has been our experience that many patients on clomiphene citrate have blunted LH surges 2–8 days before ovulation. These blunted surges are of a significant height to trigger an LH color change but

are not significant enough to induce ovulation. If the human egg can be fertilized for at least 24 hours after ovulation, and our experience with *in vitro* fertilization indicates that eggs can be fertilized for up to 36 hours postovum retrieval, than performing intrauterine insemination on the day of follicle disappearance should be the most accurate method of timing this procedure.

EARLY PREGNANCY DETECTION

Numerous studies have shown that approximately 3 weeks postovulation an intrauterine gestational sac can be easily visualized in the great majority of pregnant patients (Table 64.1; Fig. 64.6). The differential diagnosis for not visualizing a sac at this time runs the gamut from poor dates (which is the most common etiology), to a poor-prognosis pregnancy, to an extrauterine gestation, or to physician error. We published a paper in 1990 that looked at the ability to predict pregnancy viability in previously infertile women by observing the time of appearance of a gestational sac and fetal cardiac activity

Table 64.1 Ultrasonographic findings in early pregnancy

Weeks postconception	Ultrasound findings
3	Gestational sac
3+	Yolk sac
4	Fetal pole ± cardiac motion
5	Must have cardiac motion
6	Crown–rump length 1.4–2.1 cm
8	Crown–rump length 2.6–3.4 cm

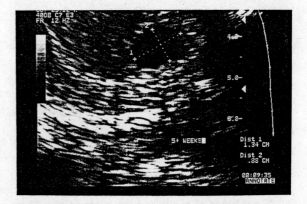

Fig. 64.6 A gestational sac at 3 weeks and 2 days postovulation.

Table 64.2 The probability of a previously infertile woman delivering a viable infant after observing the following ultrasonographic findings. (From [3])

Finding and weeks postovulation	Percentage
Gestational sac noted at 3 weeks	80
Cardiac activity noted at 4 weeks	94
No cardiac activity at 4 weeks but noted at 5 weeks	70
Cardiac activity noted again at 6 weeks with an appropriately sized fetus	97

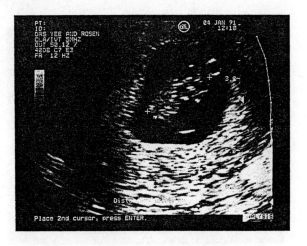

Fig. 64.8 A pregnancy at 6 weeks 2 days postovulation. Crown-rump length is 21 mm. Note that the yolk sac is superior and to the right on the fetus' head.

with weekly transvaginal ultrasound (Table 64.2) [3]. In a previously infertile woman, the predictive value of delivering a viable infant after observing a gestational sac at 3 weeks postconception was only 80%. Fetal cardiac motion was first observed 1 week later in over 75% of these pregnancies and in all of the remaining viable pregnancies by the fifth week postconception. When cardiac activity was first observed at 4 weeks postconception, 94% of these pregnancies delivered viable infants (Fig. 64.7). If cardiac activity was not observed at the 4-week examination but was *first* observed at the 5-week postconception scan, the chance of delivering a viable infant was only 70%. This makes good sense from an embryologic standpoint because the fetal

heart tubes coalesce and begin to pulsate at approximately $3\frac{1}{2}$ weeks postconception. If cardiac motion has not begun by the 4-week postconception scan, than it should be inferred that whatever caused this delay, whether it be genetic or environmental, should lead to a poorer prognosis regarding fetal viability. If an appropriate-sized fetus with cardiac motion is seen at 6 weeks postconception (approximately 15–19 mm crown–rump length) than the chance that this woman will deliver a viable infant rises to 97% and will remain so until delivery occurs (Fig. 64.8). By 6 weeks postconception, the fetus has an easily recognized head and body on transvaginal ultrasound. Movement of fetus can first be seen at this time. The four extremities are first easily seen by 7–8 weeks postconception. The normal herniation of the bowel into the umbilical cord occurs between 6 and 10 weeks postconception. This finding is expected and should cause no alarm (Fig. 64.9). Gross fetal anomalies are extremely difficult to detect in the first trimester and patients should be informed of this fact during these early examinations.

OVARIAN PHYSIOLOGY AND PATHOPHYSIOLOGY

Routine scanning of the ovaries results in finding many normal and pathologic entities that can be better observed and followed with transvaginal ultrasound than a physical examination alone. The sensitivity of ultrasound is far greater than one's hands with regard to detecting small ovarian neoplasms.

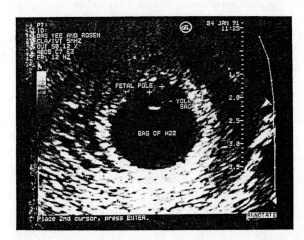

Fig. 64.7 A pregnancy at 4 weeks postovulation. Note the gestational sac measuring 17 mm in greatest diameter, a yolk sac and fetal pole.

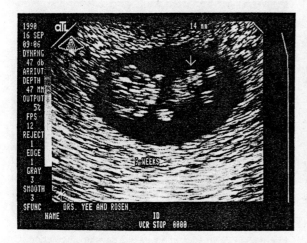

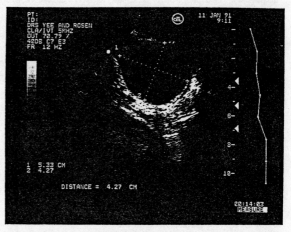

Fig. 64.9 A pregnancy at 7 weeks 2 days postovulation. The arrow is pointing at the normal herniation in the umbilical cord.

Fig. 64.11 A 5.33 × 4.27 serous cyst of the right ovary. Note that except for its size it is indistinguishable from a follicle cyst.

Endometriomas have a very classic appearance which the author describes as being like granite (Fig. 64.10). These are compared to other fluid-filled cysts such as serous cysts, corpora lutei, and follicular cysts whose centers are completely sonolucent (Fig. 64.11). Mucinous cysts have a honeycomb appearance which is very similar to a hemorrrhagic corpus luteum. Dermoids have many different ultrasonographic appearances depending on their contents.

Serial ultrasound examinations are an easy way to differentiate between the functional and non-functional ovarian cysts in a woman of reproductive age. The best time to repeat these examinations is in the very early follicular phase. If the patient is placed

on oral contraceptives, beware that the triphasic preparations are of insufficient strength to inhibit ovulation in 10–15% of women. This means that these oral contraceptives are of an inadequate dose to suppress gonadotropin secretion and therefore are not as likely to suppress a "functional" cyst. A moderate dose, monophasic preparation such as Ovral (50 μg ethinylestradiol and 0.5 mg norgestrel) should inhibit gonadotropin secretion and ovulation in almost all women.

UTERINE LEIOMYOMAS

Somewhere between 30 and 50% of all women in their later reproductive years have uterine leiomyomas. Classic indications for myomectomy versus hysterectomy will not be discussed in this chapter. Ultrasonographic visualization of these tumors is not a necessary prerequisite for any surgical procedure but a "picture" greatly facilitates the patient's understanding of the size and nature of the problem (Fig. 64.12). Serial scans can be extremely helpful in either demonstrating their growth or, if a gonadotropin-releasing hormone agonist is being utilized as a preoperative adjunct, their decrease in size. The larger the fibroids, the more significant the decrease in their size. As a rule of thumb, fibroids smaller than 2 cm usually respond poorly to these medications while fibroids larger than 4–5 cm respond dramatically. Since maximal reduction usually occurs by 8–12 weeks after starting these medications, our protocol is to get a baseline scan and then follow

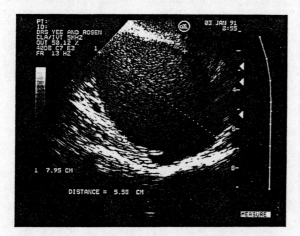

Fig. 64.10 A 7.95 × 5.58 cm endometrioma of the right ovary. Note the "granite-like" appearance of its contents.

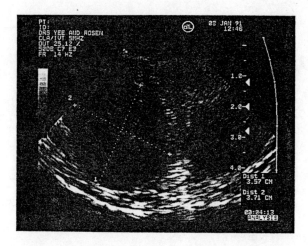

Fig. 64.12 Two fibroids: the largest is 3.71 × 3.57 cm.

these patients at monthly intervals until reduction of the fibroids has ceased. Surgery is then scheduled for the next 1–2 weeks while the patient is continued on the gonadotropin-releasing hormone agonist.

CONCLUSIONS

In conclusion, the ultrasound transducer is mightier than the hand and the routine use of ultrasound at annual gynecologic examinations will very soon become the norm! The best time for such an examination would be the very early follicular phase when follicular cysts are less than 1 cm in diameter. The use of routine annual ultrasound examinations will result in findings of subclinical pathology of both uterine and ovarian origin and more appropriate follow-up treatment. Cost-effectiveness does not necessarily need to be an issue once obstetrician-gynecologists own/lease their machines and view them not as potential money-makers but very practical and worthwhile adjuncts to routine healthcare in women.

REFERENCES

1 Yee B, Rosen GF. Monitoring stimulated cycles. In: Yee B, ed. *Infertility and Reproductive Medicine Clinics of North America*. Philadelphia: WB Saunders, 1990: 15–36.
2 Vermesh M, Kletzky OA, Davajan V, Isreal R. Monitoring techniques to predict and detect ovulation. *Fertil Steril* 1987; 47: 259.
3 Rosen GF, Silva PD, Patrizio P, Asch RH, Yee B. Predicting pregnancy outcome by the observation of early fetal cardiac motion with transvaginal ultrasonography. *Fertil Steril* 1990; 54: 260.

65

Luteal-phase defect

MARK GIBSON

INTRODUCTION

The diagnosis of luteal-phase defect acknowledges that endocrine function in an ovulatory cycle is not all or none in character, but can exhibit gradations which, at lower levels, may be insufficient to support normal fertility. Ordinarily employed clinical means for documentation of ovulation depend on confirmation of elevations in levels of progesterone or documentation of progesterone-dependent effects (basal body temperature (BBT) elevation, secretory transformation of the endometrium). The diagnosis of luteal-phase defect depends on the application of these means in a quantitative manner. Thus, three principal means for describing luteal function have been employed to identify luteal-phase defect, and it is as yet unclear which, if any, are of greatest clinical utility, and what their precise relationships are. The diagnosis of luteal-phase defect also depends upon the postulate that abnormalities of ovulatory endocrinology may occur repetitively in the same individual and be the cause of their infertility or the

cause of recurrent pregnancy loss. An outline of the approach to luteal-phase defect is shown in Figure 65.1.

PATHOPHYSIOLOGY AND CLINICAL FEATURES

Studies of the pathophysiology of luteal-phase defect often indicate that it originates in abnormal events during the antecedent follicular phase [1]. Observations of decreased follicle-stimulating hormone: luteinizing hormone (FSH:LH) ratios during folliculogenesis in spontaneously occurring luteal-phase defect cycles and the experimental creation of luteal-phase defect by perturbations in gonadotropin secretion during the early follicular phase lend support to this view. It may be most appropriate to view luteal-phase defect as a final common expression of disturbances at any of several sites in the reproductive endocrine axis and occurring during any of several possible phases of the cycle. While dyssynchrony between zygotic and endometrial events

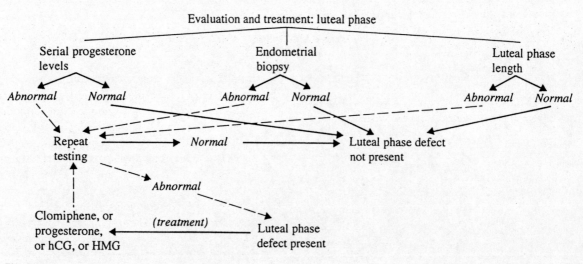

Fig. 65.1 Approach to luteal-phase defect.

is presumed important, the actual mechanisms by which infertility or pregnancy loss eventuate are not known and may differ in different forms of the disorder.

The incidence of luteal-phase defect in studies published about infertility clinic populations ranges from 5 to 10% [2]. Luteal-phase defect has been reported in association with modest elevations in prolactin, insufficient to interrupt ovulation completely. The athlete is at increased risk; studies have shown that a subset of high-performance athletes exhibit abnormal luteal function, and that the extent of abnormality is related to the contemporaneous level of training. Although luteal-phase defect is not a consistent feature of the cycles of the perimenopause, it has been associated with impending hypergonadotropic amenorrhea. Most importantly, however, there are no reliable clinical clues to the occurrence of the abnormality; it is usually an idiopathic disorder. There have been no menstrual or gynecologic features consistently associated with luteal-phase defect. The likelihood of diagnosis is not affected by cycle length, premenstrual symptoms, or bleeding pattern. Because the majority of diagnoses will be made in women without identifying clinical features, evaluation of luteal function should be part of the baseline work-up in any infertility investigation.

DIAGNOSIS (Table 65.1)

Endometrial Biopsy

The endometrial biopsy is the original technique described for evaluation of the luteal phase. It depends on careful histologic evaluation and assignment of a "date" to a late luteal-phase endometrial

biopsy, and careful correlation of the histologic date with the date expected from the occurrence of the next menses. It is critical in this convention to designate the day of onset of next menses as day 28, regardless of the cycle length, and to count back to the day of biopsy to derive the date expected for histology. There is substantial variance in values derived from dating the endometrial biopsy, and ideally the clinician will personally review the histology or insure that biopsies are read by a pathologist with experience and an interest in providing precise and accurate readings. While this method is a survivor of long clinical tradition, it does have unresolved weaknesses that are the subject of ongoing controversy.

1 The degree of lag in histologic date from chronologic date that can account for infertility or spontaneous abortion has not been clearly demonstrated.
2 The extent of the contribution of the error of the method of assigning histologic dates, and the choice of next menses, as opposed to day of LH surge as a reference to the likelihood of diagnosis, is not known.
3 The number of abnormal or normal cycles studied sufficient to justify or obviate therapy, respectively, remains to be resolved.

Despite these important issues, current clinical conventions are well established. An abnormal luteal phase is described when histology lags behind the expected value by more than 2 days. When it is documented that this is a recurrent abnormality (on two successive biopsies) the diagnosis of luteal-phase defect is made. An increasing number of studies are highlighting the sporadic nature of abnormal luteal phases in presumably normal women; therefore, diagnosis based on a single observation is unacceptable.

Progesterone levels

One of the most distressing inconsistencies in the topic of luteal-phase defect is the lack of clear correlation between progesterone measurements in the blood and the result of dating the endometrial biopsy. Explanations for this discrepancy include the facts that: (1) progesterone levels normally exhibit significant short-term variability; (2) progesterone is highly bound (to cortisol-binding globulin and albumin), leaving the free and biologically available fraction undetermined; and (3) some endometria may be less responsive than others to the effects of progesterone. Certainly single "spot" levels of progesterone during the luteal phase are insufficiently sensitive or specific

Table 65.1 Techniques for detection of luteal-phase defect

Technique	Description
Endometrial biopsy [2]	Histologic date more than 2 days behind date predicted by the onset of next menses
Serum progesterone [3]	Sum of all daily values from ovulation to menses less than 100 ng/ml per day
Luteal-phase length [4]	Number of days from LH surge to menses less than 12

LH, luteinizing hormone.

for the diagnosis of this disorder. Daily levels from ovulation until menses should usually sum to a value of 100 ng or greater in women with normal cycles and are frequently less than 100 in women with luteal-phase defect [3]. The necessary frequent sampling practices required to produce these observations are cumbersome clinically, and at the present cost of most assay systems, prohibitively expensive. This is all the more true in light of the fact that diagnosis of luteal-phase defect ideally depends on demonstration of a repetitive abnormality.

Luteal duration

In many instances, cycles with luteal defect by biopsy exhibit a shortended interval from ovulation to menses. This type of luteal defect (short luteal phase) may be a distinct entity, and can be identified using various markers for ovulation and measurement of the interval until subsequent menses. It has been best described from studies using daily hormonal measurements, but the use of urinary LH surge indicators to define the LH menstrual duration is more convenient and could be applied clinically. Basal temperature records are imprecise; their primary utility in diagnosis of luteal-phase defect is as a screening tool. An interval of 12 or more days from LH surge to menses (= [cycle day of menses] − [cycle day of LH surge]) is an appropriate threshold for diagnosis [4]. It is important to emphasize that not all instances of abnormal luteal function are associated with definitively shortened luteal phases, so that exclusion of the short luteal phase does not exclude the diagnosis of luteal-phase defect.

MANAGEMENT (Table 65.2)

At best, effective treatment of luteal-phase defect will restore the chance of pregnancy per cycle of effort to

Table 65.2 Therapeutic options in the treatment of luteal-phase defect

Progesterone vaginal suppositories	25–50 mg b.i.d.–t.i.d. commencing with ovulation
Clomiphene citrate	50 mg on days 5–9 of cycle
Human chorionic gonadotropin	10 000 IU to trigger or accompany ovulation and 5000 IU midluteal phase
Human menopausal gonadotropin	Per standard protocols

that of a normal couple, the mean time to conception under such conditions being on the order of four to five cycles. Thus, a trial of therapy can hardly be considered unsuccessful unless unproductive after at least a half a year, if not more. If other infertility factors remain unaddressed during this interval, considerable valuable time has been lost for the couple. Accordingly, treatment should be instituted in the context of a completed evaluation and a program of management that simultaneously addresses all abnormalities found in the work-up.

Once the diagnosis is made, a search for a specific cause of luteal-phase defect should be undertaken. Athleticism should be reevaluated, as one treatment option for such women is to reduce their training schedule. Prolactin levels should be determined, and hyperprolactinemia evaluated and treated specifically, if found. Luteal-phase defect may be a feature of evolving or impending frank ovarian failure in some instances, and would be detected by elevations of early follicular-phase FSH levels.

Treatment regimens comprise measures directed at enhancement of folliculogenesis, with clomiphene citrate or human menopausal gonadotropin (hMG), and measures directly treating the luteal phase with human chorionic gonadotropin (hCG) or progesterone vaginal suppositories. All of these therapies have been reported to be of benefit, although there are virtually no controlled trials demonstrating the superiority of any treatment over expectancy. Moreover, there are no comparative clinical trials which would direct the clinician toward a preferred initial treatment strategy in idiopathic luteal-phase defect. Because of these important short-comings in the clinical literature on this disorder the central and abiding principle of treatment is that effectiveness should be monitored, most often by endometrial histology, and the modality changed as necessary to achieve correction [5]. It has been clearly shown that the degree of correction of the underlying defect is a useful predictor of successful treatment.

Progesterone supplementation is usually given in the form of suppositories formulated in 25 or 50 mg doses and used two to three times daily. Treatment is begun once ovulation has occurred. The BBT and changes in cervical mucus can be observed to determine this point in time. Complementing these observations with LH detection might better assure timely institution of supplementation in those instances of luteal-phase defect where a delayed progesterone rise after ovulation is a feature of the pathophysiology.

Treatment is continued until menses occur. In a minority of patients, treatment will delay menses, in which case it is necessary to test for pregnancy before discontinuing suppository use. Progesterone supplementation is supported by a long clinical tradition and biopsies on treatment are corrected in as many as half of treated patients. However, progesterone vaginal suppositories are not marketed with approval from the Food and Drug Administration for this purpose, and must be prescribed outside of the customary rubric of using approved drugs for approved indications. Other drawbacks to therapy include annoyance with suppository use for many patients, and the cumbersomeness of excluding pregnancy each month for others.

Clomiphene citrate has nearly as long a track record of apparent utility in treating luteal-phase defect as does progesterone supplementation. Initial studies of endocrine profiles in induced ovulatory cycles with clomiphene citrate suggested that this agent could cause defective luteal function. Contemporary observations show that, when applied as a brief course, usually 50 mg daily on days 5–9 in already ovulatory women, clomiphene citrate is associated with higher preovulatory estradiol levels and higher postovulatory levels of progesterone than seen in spontaneous cycles. These steroid evaluations can be attributed to the increased numbers of preovulatory follicles and resulting corpora lutea seen with clomiphene citrate. The rationale for clomiphene citrate therapy is based on these observations, and on the considerable evidence that the roots of luteal dysfunction frequently can be traced to abnormalities of the endocrine physiology of early follicular phase. Success with clomiphene is more apparent in patients with evidence of marked ovulatory dysfunction (greater degrees of histologic lag). As with progesterone supplementation, repeat luteal-phase studies should be performed early in therapy, as correction of the disorder is not assured with clomiphene. Moreover, clomiphene interferes with cervical mucus production in many patients, and carefully timed postcoital evaluation of the cervical mucus is important early in therapy. While the prognostic significance of unfavorable cervical mucus rheology is difficult to pinpoint, the finding of poor cervical mucus on clomiphene citrate therapy should prompt consideration of alternative treatments. There are no published data to support increasing clomiphene doses if treatment at standard dosages does not correct the histologic defect.

Treatment with hCG has been described, but there is very little information on the clinical utility of this measure. Relative elevations in spot progesterone levels caused by hCG therapy may represent increased steroid synthesis and secretion by the corpus luteum. Alternatively, these elevations may be at least in part due to the continuous influence of the slowly cleared hCG overriding the intermittent gonadotropin signal afforded by the episodic secretion of LH. hCG is given intramuscularly in doses of 5000–10000 IU, once at the time of LH surge, or in concert with ovulation, and once again in the middle of the luteal phase. When used to provide the ovulatory signal, as is usually the case when it is used with clomiphene or hMG, it is given when lead follicular diameters reach 18 mm. It can be used to enhance clomiphene therapy, and is an obligatory element of hMG protocols. hCG alone cannot cause hyperstimulation syndrome: antecedent excess follicle recruitment is required for this to occur. Provided that excess follicle recruitment can be ruled out, hCG administration poses no specific risks of its own. Care should be taken in testing for pregnancy, as declining levels of hCG are detectable in the circulation for several days after injection.

Treatment with hMG involves greater risk and is more expensive, complex, and intrusive than other treatments for luteal-phase defect, and should be reserved for instances where other therapies have been shown to be inadequate. The "more is better" view of treatment is quickly tempered by the experience of supporting a couple through decisions regarding embryo reduction or the travails of pathologic multiple birth. There are couples for whom this is clearly the optimal treatment however. As with all treatments for luteal phase-defect, monitoring of the effectiveness of therapy, preferably by endometrial biopsy, is called for.

THE FUTURE

The practitioner should watch for emerging clarity in the definition of the techniques and thresholds for diagnosis of luteal-phase defect. The endometrial biopsy will be challenged by increasingly simple and inexpensive means for direct endocrine measurements. The true prognostic significance of any particular deviation from the expected will remain extremely difficult to determine. Future study may well also unveil distinct categories within this undoubtedly broad diagnostic grouping and beyond that, an understanding of which therapies to apply in each circumstance.

REFERENCES

1 DiZerega GS, Hodgen GD. Luteal phase dysfunction infertility: a sequel to aberrant folliculogenesis. *Fertil Steril* 1981; 35: 489–499.

2 McNeely MJ, Soules MR. The diagnosis of luteal phase deficiency: a critical review. *Fertil Steril* 1988; 50: 1–15.

3 Soules MR, McLachlan RI, Marit E, Dahl KD, Cohen NL, Bremner WJ. Luteal phase deficiency: characterization of reproductive hormones over the menstrual cycle. *J Clin Endocrinol Metab* 1989; 69: 804.

4 Lenton EA, Landgren B, Sexton L. Normal variation in the length of the luteal phase of the menstrual cycle: identification of the short luteal phase. *Br J Obstet Gynaecol* 1984; 91: 685–689.

5 Daly DC, Walters CA, Soto-Albors CE, Riddick DH. Endometrial biopsy during treatment of luteal phase defects is predictive of therapeutic outcome. *Fertil Steril* 1983; 40: 305–309.

66

Postcoital testing

BRUCE L. TJADEN

An important step in the investigation of the infertile couple is an evaluation of cervical function [1]. An integral part of this evaluation is the postcoital test (PCT). Also known as the Sims–Huhner test, the PCT is considered one of the five or six basic tests of the infertile couple [2,3]. Although most physicians who evaluate infertile patients recommend and perform the PCT on their patients, it is a poorly standardized, nonspecific, and insensitive test. The following discussion will outline the basic principles behind the PCT (Fig. 66.1) and define the controversy surrounding the test and its interpretation.

Approximately 200–500 million spermatoza are deposited in the vagina during a single coital episode. The sperm mix with the cervical mucus and under favorable conditions, prompt penetration of the cervical mucus occurs.

Cervical mucus is continually secreted by the epithelium of the endocervix [1]. Though frequently referred to as endocervical glands, technically the endocervix is lined not by glands but rather with an intricate system of clefts and grooves, giving the impression of glands. These crypts are filled with the secretory mucus of the epithelial lining. The quantity and quality of the mucus are intimately dependent upon the hormonal environment as determined by the ovarian cycle. There is a direct relationship between quantity of cervical mucus, its penetrability by sperm, and serum estradiol levels. Estradiol levels peak during the preovulatory period and it is at this time that the cervical mucus is most abundant and the most favorable for sperm penetration. It would seem logical that estradiol is responsible for the changes in cervical mucus; however, some observations do not support this contention, suggesting that other hormonal and nonhormonal factors may be important. Prolactin, produced in the anterior pituitary and also in the decidualized endometrium, is known to have water-regulatory effects in the

fetal membranes and may be an important factor in regulating the water content of cervical mucus.

Cervical mucus is a heterogeneous secretion, of which the most important consitituent is a hydrogel, rich in carbohydrates and consisting of mucin-type glycoproteins [1]. The physical properties of cervical mucus are a result of these mucins. Cervical mucus also contains amino acids, alkaline phosphatase, lactate dehydrogenase, estradiol, progesterone, prolactin, sodium chloride, lipids, mucin, organic salts, albumin, immunoglobulin A and G, glucose, and some trace elements [4].

Sperm penetrability begins on approximately cycle day 9 and increases over the next 4–5 days, peaking at ovulation and decreasing rather abruptly post-ovulation. The endocervical crypts act as a sperm reservoir, storing sperm then continually releasing them to the upper genital tract. The sperm are guided by the line of strain of the cervical mucus. Two to 3 days after ovulation sperm penetration is completely blocked.

The vagina and vaginal secretions are acidic (pH 3–4) – a property not favorable to sperm survival. In fact, sperm probably can survive no longer than 3–4 hours in the acidic environment of the vagina. In contradistinction, cervical mucus is considerably more alkaline (pH 6–8). Cervical mucus is believed to coat the upper vagina, increasing the pH and providing a much more hospitable environment, and favoring sperm survival.

Estrogenization increases not only the volume of cervical mucus but also the water content. By midcycle the cervical mucus is 95–98% water [4]. This change in water content of only 5% alters the ability of mucus to promote or inhibit sperm migration. The change in water content, along with the change in other biochemical parameters, increases the stretch-ability of cervical mucus (spinnbarkeit). Midcycle mucus will have a spinnbarkeit of 10–12 cm

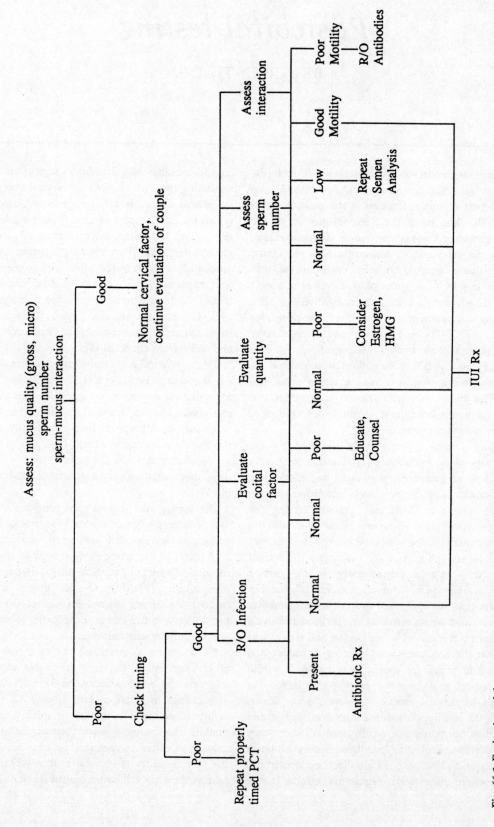

Fig. 66.1 Evaluation of the postcoital test. IUI, intrauterine insemination.

as compared to only 1—4 cm for mucus distant from ovulation or estrogenization. The relative water and salt concentrations of cervical mucus are, as previously described, cycle-dependent. When allowed to dry, midcycle mucus crystallizes, forming an aborization pattern. Mucus distant from ovulation or estrogenization will not fern upon drying.

The cellular content of cervical mucus is also cycle-dependent. Examination many days prior to ovulation and 2—3 days postovulation will reveal a rather opaque-appearing mucus, clouded because of high cellularity, mostly leukocytes. Again, as midcycle approaches the cellular content changes dramatically and preovulatory mucus is almost crytal clear and devoid of leukocytes, nearly acellular.

Given the above biochemical and physical properties of cervical mucus one can approach its evaluation in a systematic fashion. Clinical evaluation of cervical mucus includes determination of amount, viscosity, cellularity, pH, ferning, and spinnbarkeit.

TIMING

Because nearly all of the properties of cervical mucus are menstrual cycle dependent, timing of the examination is of utmost importance. Ideally, the examination should occur 1—2 days prior to ovulation. This can present problems for women with oligo-ovulation or anovulation. Repeating evaluations every other day may be beneficial. Urinary ovulation predictors are very useful. More sophisticated monitoring with estradiols and ultrasound tracking of follicular development can be performed but is rarely necessary for the evaluation of cervical function alone though it may be utilized if the patient is undergoing such monitoring for other indications. There is controversy surrounding the best time for evaluation postcoitus. Since one of the functions of the cervix appears to be as a reservoir for releasing sperm to the upper genital tract, most authors suggest 8—12 hours postcoitus as a reasonable time to perform the test, though a satisfactory test may be obtained 18—24 hours after the coital exposure. Some authors recommend only a 2—3 hour time lapse after coitus if a second evaluation is necessary.

TECHNIQUE

A multitude of methods have been described for performing the PCT, though none have been proven to be more beneficial or efficacious than the others.

The patient is placed in the dorsal lithotomy position as per usual for a gynecologic examination. A nonlubricated speculum is inserted into the vagina. Visual inspection of the vaginal vault and the cervix is done, noting the presence or absence of a vaginal pool and the amount and clarity of cervical mucus. A sample of the vaginal pool is aspirated into a small syringe, such as a tuberculin syringe. Using a separate syringe, samples of cervical mucus are taken from the ectocervix and the endocervix. All three samples are placed individually on to separate slides. Alternatively, other authors prefer to use a metal forceps placed into the endocervical canal; the forceps closed tightly to grasp, and then withdrawn to remove the cervical mucus, which is then placed on the glass slide. Still others prefer to use recently designed polyethylene catheters to take mucus samples from three levels of the endocervix. However these so-called fractional tests do not apper to be more reliable than the traditional Sims—Huhner test. In any event the aspirated or withdrawn cervical mucus is placed upon the glass slides and glass cover slips are then placed over the specimens. By slowly withdrawing one of the glass cover slips overlying the cervical mucus one can determine the stretchability or the spinnbarkeit, noting the number of centimeters the mucus will stretch prior to breaking. If cellular debris is found overlying the ectocervix, as occasionally happens, the cervix can be cleansed with saline and a cotton swab. Using metal forceps instead of a glass coverslip and glass slide can result in falsely low spinnbarkeit determinations [2].

The slides are then evaluated microscopically, initially under low power then under high power. Representative areas are identified. The number of sperm per high-powered field (hpf), their movement, and the type of movement are noted. Also noted is the amount of cellularity and acellular debris. Once completed, the slide is allowed to dry to determine the extent of aborization (ferning) which is determined with the microscope.

INTERPRETATION

The American Fertility Society has designed a scoring system to evaluate midcycle cervical mucus in conjunction with the PCT. The method assigns a score of 0—3 for each of five parameters: amount of cervical mucus, viscosity of cervical mucus, spinnbarkeit, ferning, and cellularity. Thus a total of 15 points is possible. A score of 10—15 is considered good,

5–10 unfavorable, and less than 5 hostile cervical secretions. pH should also be noted but is not part of the scoring system.

The amount or number of sperm necessary to qualify for a normal or adequate test has not been definitively established. Seibel [5] states that only two numbers are important: 0 sperm/hpf and >20 sperm/hpf. The American Fertility Society states [1]:

> In normal women, following coitus with a fertile man, more than 25 motile sperm (with 2–3+ motility) per high power field (400×) are commonly observed in the exocervical specimen; 10 or more sperm per high power field with a score of 3+ motility is considered satisfactory. Less than 5 sperm per high power field, particularly when associated with sluggish or circular motion, is an indication of oligoasthenospermia or abnormality of cervical mucus.

Under the American Fertility Society guidelines sperm motility is graded from 0 to 3, with immotile sperm given a 0, *in situ* motility a 1, sluggish motility a 2, and vigorous motility a 3.

Regarding the endocervical specimen, the American Fertility Society guidelines state [1]: "At 6–10 hours after intercourse, more than 10 sperm with adequate motility (3+) should normally be found per high powered field. A similar number of sperm is usually detected on a delayed test (13–24 hours after coitus)."

A recent review of publications on PCT studied six reports with sufficient information for evaluation [3]. As noted by these authors, the PCT is poorly standardized; each of the six reports evaluated used different systems for assessing sperm penetration and different definitions of normal. Sensivity, specificity, and the predictive value of abnormal and normal results were calculated. Sensitivity ranged from 0.09 to 0.71, specificity ranged from 0.62 to 1.00, predictive value of abnormal test ranged from 0.56 to 1.00, while the predictive value of a normal test ranged from 0.25 to 0.75. Sensitivity of the PCT is the ability of the test to detect infertile couples; 9–72% of the infertile couples were identified. Specificity of the PCT is the ability of the normal test to identify fertile couples: 62–100% of fertile couples were identified. The predictive value of an abnormal test is the ability to diagnose correctly infertile couples: two small studies had perfect predictive values for abnormal tests while the four larger studies ranged from 8 to 44%. The predictive value of a normal test is the ability of the PCT to identify correctly fertile couples: this ranged from 0.25 to 0.75: in other words, 75–25% of the diagnoses of fertility were incorrect. Likewise, the likelihood of pregnancy was not clearly related to the sperm concentration in aspirated cervical mucus; there was not a linear relationship between sperm density and pregnancy rates. Closer evaluation of the two largest studies reveals the predictive accuracy to be no better than flipping a coin. The authors of the review were unequivocal about their assessment that the PCT lacks validity as a test for infertility, the test should be used with greater selectivity and interpreted with greater caution [3].

Other tests for evaluation of sperm–mucus interaction have been described and include *in vitro* studies such as the capillary tube test, in which cervical mucus is aspirated into a flat capillary tube, one end of which is sealed. The open end is placed into a pool of freshly collected, liquified semen. The capillary tube can then be examined at different time intervals depending upon the type of study. Linear penetration and sperm density are recorded.

Similarly, a slide technique has been described utilizing fresh sperm and cervical mucus placed together on a glass slide and covered with a cover slip. At the junction of sperm and mucus, finger-like projections develop into the cervical mucus within a few minutes; subsequently, the sperm penetrate into the mucus. Sperm densities are recorded at various intervals; only those sperm clearly within the substance of the mucus are counted as having penetrated.

The results obtained by these techniques compare favorably with sperm concentration and motility as noted on traditional semen analyses.

Finally, sperm–mucus cross-match using the patient's mucus, her partner's semen, donor mucus, and donor semen can be performed. This determines which compartment — mucus or semen — is responsible for the abnormal PCT.

THERAPY

The PCT is not a substitute for a semen analysis. If religious preferences preclude masturbation as a means of collecting semen for analysis, a normal PCT can be considered as presumptive evidence of a normal male spermatogenesis and normal sperm function and may presumptively rule out male factors as a cause of infertility. However, a semen analysis is complementary to a PCT and therefore should be obtained on all couples.

Treatment of the abnormal PCT is contingent upon the findings of the test itself (see Fig. 66.1). Other such flow charts have been published. Probably the number one cause of an abnormal PCT is poor timing; thus, one must be sure to correlate the PCT with a menstrual calendar, basal body temperature chart, and possibly an ovulation predictor.

For an abnormal PCT — assuming that a semen analysis has been obtained and is normal — initially one should check timing. If the time in the cycle is deemed appropriate then one would repeat the PCT at a time closer to coitus, for instance 3—4 hours postcoitus rather than 10—12 hours postcoitus.

Persistently abnormal PCTs require further investigation. A poor quantity of and/or quality cervical mucus can be treated with exogenous estrogen, using Premarin 0.625 mg, ethinylestradiol 0.2 mg, or diethylstilbestrol. The estrogen is usually prescribed for 7—9 days, ceasing therapy 1 or 2 days prior to ovulation.

Highly cellular cervical mucus should be evaluated with cervical cultures and appropriate treatment should be rendered for positive cultures, followed by cultures to document test of cure.

When sperm are identified without purposeful movement, antibody testing (immune testing) should be performed and appropriate treatment rendered.

When a complete lack of sperm is persistently noted on PCT the couple should be evaluated for coital technique and/or sexual dysfunction.

REFERENCES

1 American Fertility Society. *Investigation of the Infertile Couple*. American Fertility Society, 1986, Birmingham, AL.
2 Zavos PM, Cohen MR. The pH of cervical mucus and the post coital test. *Fertil Steril* 1980; 34: 234.
3 Griffith CS, Grimes DA. The validity of the postcoital test. *Am J Obstet Gynecol* 1990; 162: 615—620.
4 McCoshen J. The role of cervical mucus in reproduction. Contemporary Obstet/Gynecol 1987; MAY: 94—117.
5 Seibel M. Work up of the infertile couple. In: Seibel M, ed. *Infertility, A Comprehensive Text*. East Norwalk: Appleton and Lange, 1990: 10—12.

FURTHER READING

Moghissi KS. Post coital test: physiologic basis, technique and interpretation. *Fertil Steril* 1976; 27: 117—129.

Hysterosalpingography

ALVIN M. SIEGLER

This chapter reviews the fundamentals for performing a proper hysterosalpingogram (HSG) and describes abnormalities encountered. Careful interpretation is essential so that the findings can be compared with endoscopic studies. Indeed, when the hysterogram is normal, it is unusual to find any significant intrauterine lesions at hysteroscopy. With normal fill and spill from both fallopian tubes, it is uncommon to find significant tubal disease. Salpingography has limitations, however, principally in its inability to detect periadnexal adhesions or significant endometriosis. Abnormal shadows must be interpreted in association with the history and physical examination.

An HSG is one of the basic procedures to perform before undertaking surgical correction of pelvic causes of infertility. Although this examination does not define the extent of certain conditions such as endometriosis and periadnexal adhesions, it does reveal the shape of the uterine cavity and characteristics of the tubal lumens as well as their patency. With the advent of modern diagnostic gynecologic techniques, including laparoscopy, endoscopy, ultrasonography, and magnetic resonance imaging, why contine to use the HSG? The HSG remains a nonoperative, simple, relatively painless screening procedure. Three recent books devoted primarily to HSG have been published and they represent comprehensive discussions of the subject [1-3].

INSTRUMENTS

Various cannulas have been used but the simplest and preferred one is the Jarcho type with an adjustable steel collar and rubber acorn. The acorn is fixed securely by means of a set screw in the metal collar located about 0.5 cm from the perforated end of the cannula.

HSG requires image intensification with spot films taken during television fluoroscopy for proper monitoring at propitious intervals. Indeed, four exposures can be recorded on one 10×12 film. By promptly developing the preliminary or scout film, the physician is able to decide on the proper exposure for subsequent films; pelvic calcifications or residual contrast material from a previous HSG become visible.

Media

All media used for HSGs contain iodine, some being soluble in water and others in oil. Both types have certain advantages and disadvantages and it is important for the physican to be aware of these characteristics because they influence the technique of the examination and the interpretation of the films. Water-soluble media pass through the uterus and tubes more quickly than oily media and greater amounts of it are needed. Only with water-soluble media can the healthy rugal folds evidenced by longitudinal dark lines be detected. In distally obstructed tubes, a dark line is often clearly visible when the endosalpinx is not severely damaged. An oily medium will not mix with the fluid in a hydrosalpinx, so that pearly cluster formations form in it.

TECHNIQUE

Although the technique, media, and instruments for HSG have improved, too many studies still cannot be interpreted, principally because of failure to attend to the relatively simple details of proper performance.

One can elicit the best pictures with fewest complications by gaining the confidence and cooperation of the patient, and gentle pelvic manipulation of the instruments. A tranquilizer may be used for a very apprehensive patient. Tubal occlusion caused by uterotubal spasm can result from stress or from irritation caused by the contrast material. Certain medications are reported to cause relaxation of the uterine musculature that envelops the interstitial tubal segment.

The time chosen for the HSG varies according to the patient's clinical condition, although most precedures are done in the first week after menses. The search for an incompetent isthmus probably should be done premenstrually, however, when physiologic contraction of the lower uterine segment is greatest. The cannula is filled with contrast material to flush out the air. After a tenaculum is fixed on the anterior cervical lip the cannula is inserted into the external cervical os and the two instruments are held together by the properly gowned physician. Some pressure should be maintained on the fluid-filled syringe but the study should be terminated in a patient who complains of increasing abdominal pain during the injection. Excessive contrast material exposes the patient needlessly to risk of mucosal or peritoneal irritation and prevents proper interpretation of the films. Insufficient fluid results in an incomplete study. A follow-up or drainage film is essential to observe the dispersions of the liquid medium. It should be taken about 30 min after removal of the instruments from the cervix if a water-soluble material is used. With oil-based substances, it is advisable to delay the drainage film until the following day because this medium does not disperse as rapidly in the peritoneal cavity.

The drainage or follow-up film
Peritioneal spill from a normal HSG is identified easily. The dispersion of the agent in the pelvis depends upon: (1) the type and amount of fluid used; (2) the degree of tubal patency; and (3) the presence or extent of significant periadnexal adhesions. Such adhesions can be discerned as a collection of medium in the lateral pelves and should not be mistaken for centrally placed fluid retained within the uterine canal or vagina. The interpretation of small, localized pelvic collections of contrast material caused by significant peritubal adhesions, fimbrial phimosis, or even hydrosalpinges can be difficult. Contrast material coming from one patent tube may obscure the configuration of the contralateral oviduct. When an oily material is used, it may be difficult to be certain whether the pearly clusters are in the cul-de-sac fluid or if they are enclosed in a hydrosalpinx. Some tubal configurations look normal initially, but the follow-up or drainage film may disclose localization of the contrast material. Sharply defined borders suggest that the contrast medium is confined

within the tube, while a "halo" configuration indicates periadnexal adhesions that allow some of the fluid to surround and outline the tubal wall.

Some adverse effects from HSG have been caused by faulty selection of patients and poor technique, but morbidity and sequelae occasionally result despite careful use.

INTERPRETATION OF RESULTS

The uterine cavity
Always begin the evaluation of the HSG by viewing the endocervical canal. Its serrated borders are caused by normal anatomic plicae palmatae. Abnormalities of the endocervical canal detectable by the HSG include polyps and adhesions which cause filling defects. The normal lower uterine segment has parallel borders that are usually regular. This segment may be unusually wide — >1 cm in an incompetent os. Diverticula may be congenital outpouchings or iatrogenic from a previous cesarean operation.

The normal uterine cavity has a triangular appearance with smooth borders. Physiologic alterations may cause various indentations along the lateral borders of the uterine shadow, but their persistence on sequential flims suggests an organic defect rather than a contraction. The upper border, the fundus, may be convex or saddle-shaped, and the cornua are generally pointed.

Congenital malformations
Uterine anomalies have been classified into several groups, each having particular characteristics and clinical sequelae. They represent a heterogeneous group of malformations that result from arrested development, abnormal formations, or incomplete fusion of the Müllerian ducts. Some malformations cause complications at menarche, during pregnancy, and in labor. Although malformed uteri do not prevent implantation or nidation, and most pregnancies proceed to term without difficulty, anomalies do increase the frequency of obstetric complications. A classification proposed by the American Fertility Society seems flexible enough to fit most possibilities [4]. The HSG is a screening procedure that gives one the initial clue to the possibility of a uterine anomaly. Ultrasonography and magnetic resonance imaging also have been used to evaluate several types of uterine anomalies.

On the HSG a true unicornuate uterus usually is displaced laterally. Since 80% of these women do not

CHAPTER 67

have a kidney on the contralateral side, an intravenous pyelogram or possibly an ultrasound is essential in such patients. The condition should be suspected whenever the uterus is displaced, pointing either to the left or right, with a poorly developed lateral fornix. This type of uterus must be differentiated from an incompletely filled cavity, an intense spasm of one horn, or a blockage by severe synechiae that prevent access to the opposite horn. A lateral film and uterine manipulation help to rule out the possibility of uterine spasm or an artifact caused by uterine torsion. Hysteroscopy and laparoscopy can substantiate the diagnosis and detect the presence of a rudimentary horn.

The so-called double uterus can be bicornuate or didelphic, the latter having two cervices, with or without a vaginal partition. HSGs of the didelphic uterus show two entirely separate uteri; the horns appear flexed toward each other or in opposite directions. Duplications of the uterus and vagina are caused by complete failure of the Müllerian ducts to fuse. Independent study of each horn will show the characteristic shadow of the unicornuate uterus. In such cases the Foley uterine catheter technique has advantage because the vaginal canal sometimes cannot accommodate two sets of instruments — cannulas and tenaculums.

The bicornuate uterus cannot be differentiated from the septate uterus by the HSG or hysteroscopy because the crucial diagnostic point lies in the configuration of the serosal surface. The division may be complete to the cervix, or partial, and the external surface reflects the character of this division. Imperfect absorption of the median partition results in paired uterine horns.

The septate uterus is either completely or partially divided by a longitudinal central septum. The length and width of the septum will cause different shadows on the HSG and, if complete, two separate, usually symmetric cavities are formed. A cannula inserted beyond the internal os can prevent adequate observation of one of the horns. Data suggest that women with a septate uterus are about twice as likely to abort as those with a bicornuate uterus. Both conditions must be differentiated from a fundal submucous myoma.

The arcuate uterus is a minor malformation in which the fundus appears concave, although the depth of the depression is <1.5 cm. The uterine cavity has smooth contours and symmetric horns. The hysterographic appearance can be verified hysteroscopically.

Another type of congenital uterine malformation has been described in some women who were exposed to diethylstilbestrol *in utero*. The uterus appears hypoplastic and T-shaped with indentations on its lateral borders. On hysteroscopic examination these radiologic changes can be explained by structural alterations within the myometrium that resemble submucous myomas. Bulbous cornual extensions often arise from the upper end of the uterine cavity.

Intrauterine adhesions
The HSG is the initial diagnostic test used to detect intrauterine synechiae. The defects can be single or multiple, variable in size and shape, central or marginal, and tend to persist on sequential films. Too much contrast material tends to obliterate these abnormal shadows. Intravasation, associated with multiple filling defects and a disorted but not enlarged uterine shadow, in a patient with a history of repeated early abortion and postabortal curettage followed by hypomenorrhea, is diagnostic of intrauterine adhesions. Amenorrhea is associated with a distorted uterine shadow revealing numerous intracavitary defects. Intrauterine adhesions cause filling defects that are usually sharply defined. Extensive or severe adhesions produce a distorted shadow associated with tubal occlusion or vascular intravasation. The defects must be differentiated from those caused by polyps, myomas, septa, and artifacts caused by air bubbles. With hysteroscopy the surgeon can ascertain the size and location of the adhesions and evaluate the surrounding endometrium. The HSG tends to overdiagnose rather than miss the presence of intrauterine adhesions.

Uterine tumors
When polyps are suspected, the medium should be instilled in fractional, small amounts so as not to overfill the cavity. Endometrial polyps may be large or small, single or multiple, pedunculated or sessile. A single polyp does not distort the triangular shape of the cavity, but multiple polyps producing larger defects cause some loss of the normal uterine outline. Disclosure of a polyp radiographically indicates the need for confirmation, and then a polypectomy under hysteroscopic control.

Submucosal and intramural myomas often enlarge and distort the shape of the uterine cavity and cause filling defects not easily obliterated by increments of the medium. Myomas may occlude the tubal ostia, cause abnormal uterine bleeding, and spontaneous

404

abortion. The HSG can detect these tumors and test tubal patency but the X-ray picture cannot show the size of the growth or its precise location. Hysteroscopy is advisable so that the gross characteristics of the myoma can be ascertained and a decision made concerning its possible resection hysteroscopically.

Submucous tumors, as well as endometrial tuberculosis, and intrauterine adhesions are among the predisposing causes of vascular intravasation. The patient's menstrual history and previous fertility furnish clues and aid in the differential diagnosis.

The fallopian tube
In the search for tubal patency, the endpoint of the HSG is either tubal filling and spill or increasing abdominal pain. If the tubes are not opacified on the HSG it is important to know: (1) if the cervix was occluded adequately; (2) the amount of contrast agent used; and (3) the reason for discontinuation of the procedure before tubal filling.

To differentiate spasm from organic disease the intramural segment should appear filled, that is, pointed rather than rounded, since it is uncommon to see proximal tubal obstruction caused by organic disease in the intramural segment. It may be difficult to differentiate isthmic from intramural obstruction on HSG because the myometrial width cannot be discerned radiographically. It may be helpful to remember the so-called thumb sign; if the thumb is placed at the cornu, its width will approximate that of the myometrium, the tubal shadow underneath the thumb representing the intramural segment.

Proximal tubal obstruction
Luminal fibrosis and salpingitis isthmica nodosa are the most common causes of proximal tubal obstruction. A prior tubal ligation, chronic salpingitis, tubal tuberculosis, or intraluminal debris can result in proximal tubal obstruction. The differential diagnosis can be made by observing the intramural and isthmic segments carefully to search for diverticula, filling defects, and luminal continuity. Salpingitis isthmica nodosa has a characteristic honeycombed appearance. Tuberculous salpingitis also affects the distal part of the tube, causing it to have a rigid pipestem appearance with terminal strictures.

Ostial salpingography is a technique used in patients who have proximal tubal obstruction diagnosed from a properly performed and adequately interpreted HSG and a confirmatory laparoscopy during which multiple attempts to overcome the obstruction by chromopertubation are made. This interventional radiographic procedure is advisable prior to an attempt at tubocornual anastomosis. Under fluoroscopic control, a 5.5 Fr catheter is wedged into the cornu with a J guidewire. After withdrawing the guidewire, 2–5 ml of a water-soluble contrast material is inserted through the catheter and into the uterotubal ostium. The indications for stopping the procedure are increasing abdominal pain, intravasation, or tubal filling and spilling. If the obstruction persists, an attempt is made at recanalization with a guidewire passed through a 3 Fr nylon catheter. Once the wire is thought to pass into the isthmic segment, the wire is removed and the catheter over it is passed into the area. About 2–3 ml of contrast medium is injected to test for tubal patency.

Tubal polyps create oval shadows in the intramural segment as the contrast fluid flows in a thin line above or below them. The remainder of the tube is normally patent in most patients and it is doubtful whether these tumors cause infertility. Sometimes they are seen at hysteroscopy; some have been excised at laparotomy through a small tubal incision. In most instances the diagnosis is made on the HSG in the course of an infertility study.

Distal tubal obstruction
Ampullary opacification indicates that the proximal tube is patent, although not necessarily normal. Although distally obstructed tubes sometimes have small club-shaped ends, they can reach as much as 4–5 cm in diameter, accommodating large amounts of fluid. Linear dark shadows seen within the lumen obtained with water-soluble media are formed by the rugae and their presence portends a better prognosis following neosalpingostomy than if they are not evident. Distal tubal obstructions have been classified into four groups based on the HSG findings, varying from degree I fimbrial phimosis to degree IV occlusion with ampullary diameter >25 mm. One of the prognostic factors following neosalpingostomy besides thickness of the tubal wall, the percentage of ciliated cells, and the morphologic condition of the tube is the degree of ampullary dilatation ascertained with HSG.

CONCLUSIONS

Despite the continued use of HSG, there remains a need for its review with amplification and clarification of abnormal findings. Many HSGs are technically unsatisfactory or poorly interpreted, so that it appears justified to offer suggestions to improve skills in performance and interpretation.

REFERENCES

1 Hunt RB, Siegler AM. *Hysterosalpingography: Techniques and Interpretation*. Chicago: Year Book, 1990.

2 Winfield AC, Wentz AC, eds. *Diagnostic Imaging of Infertility*. Baltimore: Williams & Wilkins, 1987.

3 Yoder IC. *Hysterosalpingography and Pelvic Ultrasound in Infertility and Gynecology*. Boston: Little, Brown, 1988.

4 The American Fertility Society. The American Fertility Society classifications of adnexal adhesions, distal tubal occlusion, tubal occlusion secondary to tubal ligation, tubal pregnancies, Müllerian anomalies, and intrauterine adhesions. *Fertil Steril* 1988; 49: 944.

68

Diagnostic and operative laparoscopy

ARLENE J. MORALES & ANA A. MURPHY

Laparoscopy is an essential tool for the gynecologist today. The technique of laparoscopy can be used for both diagnostic and operative purposes. This chapter will review the indications, contraindications, techniques, instruments, and complications of laparoscopy.

INDICATIONS

There is a wide variety of indications for laparoscopy as well as many yet-to-be-defined indications. The underlying theme is the need to evaluate the pelvis and/or abdomen. For diagnostic purposes, there are many signs, symptoms and clinical scenarios in which laparoscopy is an essential diagnostic component — pelvic pain (both acute and chronic), infertility, pelvic and/or adnexal mass (with some exceptions), second-look surgery (to assess results of prior surgeries), suspected ectopic pregnancy, and clarification of congenital Müllerian or Wolffian duct anomalies. Findings could include pelvic adhesions, endometriosis, adnexal torsion, adnexal tumors (both benign and malignant), uterine myomas, inflammatory exudate, fallopian tube disease, ectopic pregnancy, uterine anomalies, appendicitis, peritoneal surface disease, and other intraabdominal disease processes. There is a limited role of laparoscopy in the diagnosis, treatment, and follow-up of patients with gynecologic malignancy.

Indications for operative laparoscopy include therapy for many of the indications listed above, such as lysis of adhesions, myomectomy, resection of endometriomas, ablation of endometriosis, neosalpingostomy, removal of tubal, ovarian, or abdominal pregnancy, ovarian cystectomy, oophorectomy, as well as the most common indication of tubal sterilization.

CONTRAINDICATIONS

Absolute

There are absolute and relative contraindications to diagnostic and operative laparoscopy. The absolute contraindications include bowel obstruction, severe ileus, large abdominal mass, abdominal hernia, diaphragmatic hernia, severe cardiorespiratory disease and intraperitoneal hemorrhage causing cardiovascular instability and shock. The first two contraindications take into account the unacceptably high risk of bowel perforation. There is also an unacceptably high risk of perforation of a large abdominal mass and poor visualization. Patients with diaphragmatic hernias and severe cardiorespiratory disease may not tolerate the Trendelenburg position, creation of a pneumoperitoneum, or gaseous compression of large vessels. Time is of the essence in a patient with cardiovascular instability secondary to intraperitoneal hemorrhage; the safest, most efficient means of controlling hemorrhage must be pursued, and this is usually laparotomy. If a patient presents with septic shock obviously medical management and stabilization of the patient are of utmost concern. If a patient is septic and laparoscopy is needed for diagnosis, then preoperative antibiotics are required after stabilization.

Relative

Relative contraindications include extremes of body weight, intrauterine pregnancy, and ascites. Diagnostic laparoscopy is almost always possible, with some variation in techniques. Operative laparoscopy is usually not feasible in the morbidly obese because the ability to manipulate instruments through ancillary puncture sites is extremely limited by the large abdominal panniculus. Very thin patients also require modifications of techniques to avoid perforation of the abdominal aorta and other organs. The size of the uterus in a pregnant patient may present the same problems as an abdominal mass, described above. Patients with inflammatory bowel disease may have bowel adhesions and fistula formation which places them at higher risk for bowel perforation. Diagnostic laparoscopy in these patients should be approached with caution.

The role of laparoscopy, especially second-look surgeries for the evaluation of malignancies, has not been well defined. If hepatic adhesions or a surface lesion was suspected, laparoscopy may have a limited role. The etiology of the ascites would dictate whether laparoscopy is an appropriate tool of evaluation. A preoperative paracentesis may be beneficial to allow less compromise with creation of a pneumoperitoneum. Patients with suspected severe pelvic adhesive disease or a history of multiple abdominal surgeries are at increased risk for bowel and other organ perforation and injury. Open diagnostic laparoscopy should be considered.

TECHNIQUES OF LAPAROSCOPY

Preoperative visit
As in any surgical procedure, a thorough history and physical examination are the basis for patient care. Any particular medicines the patient is on should be reviewed as well as the particular needs of the patient, such as subacute bacterial endocarditis prophylaxis or stress coverage of steroids. Risk factors for surgical/anesthetic complications in general, such as cardiovascular–respiratory disease, bleeding diathesis or illicit drug use, must be obtained. Indications for the procedure must be reviewed with the patients in the process of informed consent. Contraindications must be sought out. The nature of the procedure, risks, complications, and alternatives to the surgery must be understood by the patient. Consents should always include possible laparotomy. The patient must understand what circumstances would lead to laparotomy. If appropriate, contraceptive methods should be ascertained or elective surgery scheduled in the follicular phase of the patient's menstrual cycle. In some circumstances, such as anovulatory patients, elective surgery may be done in any nonmenstruating part of the cycle.

Preoperative checks
Laparoscopy should be performed with an empty bladder. This is usually done by asking the patient to void just prior to being taken to the operating room. If a long procedure (>1 hour) is anticipated, an indwelling Foley catheter should be placed in the operating room and removed immediately postoperatively, assuming there was no bladder disease or extensive dissection of the bladder. The use of broad-spectrum prophylactic antibiotics should be considered depending on the indication for surgery. Instances where antibiotics should be considered include suspected pelvic inflammatory disease, septic abortion, and infertility surgery with a history of sexually transmitted diseases. A potential undiagnosed pregnancy should again be reviewed.

Anesthesia
All diagnostic and operative laparoscopies require general anesthesia for good muscle relaxation. Both operative and diagnostic laparoscopy require careful inspection of the peritoneal cavity, which may require substantial time. Patients should be intubated with assisted ventilation as the pneumoperitoneum created and the Tredelenburg position may exacerbate hypercarbia. Exceptions include short procedures such as tubal sterilizations. In these situations, local anesthesia and intravenous sedation can be used in the well-motivated patient, with the availability of general anesthesia should complications arise.

Positioning
Positioning the patient correctly is of extreme importance. It facilitates the surgery and helps avoid complications of malpositioning, such as nerve palsies. After anesthesia is administered the patient's position is usually adjusted such that the patient's buttocks protrude slightly. This will allow sharp downward uterine manipulation with the cannula if needed. The patient is then placed in a dorsal lithotomy position. English or "candy-cane" stirrups may be used for short (<1 hour) procedures. Longer procedures require more supportive stirrups such as the Davies stirrups. The legs should be draped with cloth stockings, to help maintain body temperature and avoid skin abrasions. There should be padding around pressure points such as behind the knee, heel, or any part resting against metal. The hip should be flexed and abducted.

The arm of the patient, corresponding to the side the surgeon stands on, should be placed by the patient's side rather than on an extended side board. Attention should be given to the location of the hand placed at the side when the distal part of the table is lowered or raised.

Examination under anesthesia

An examination under anesthesia is a very important part of the surgery. As the patient's muscles are relaxed, this examination may yield important new information that could not be appreciated previously. Uterine size, position, and mobility as well as adnexal size should be noted. A uterine cannula is inserted under direct visualization. It is important to assess uterine position accurately to avoid perforation by the cannula. There are several kinds of cannulas available for uterine manipulation and chromotubation. The standard cannula is metal and known as a Cohen cannula. Humi and HUI plastic cannulas, which have an intrauterine balloon, are also available.

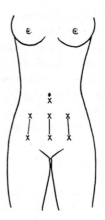

Fig. 68.1 Ancillary puncture sites. (From [1].)

Surgery

Prior to commencing, the surgeon should have reviewed the surgical instruments on the tray to insure that all the parts are available and in good working order. If intubation is difficult or gastric distention is suspected, a nasogastric tube should be placed to avoid gastric puncture. A pneumoperitoneum must first be established. A Verres or Tuohy needle is inserted, usually at the inferior rim of the umbilicus at approximately a 45° angle. Patients with previous surgical scars, abdominal mass, or morbid obesity may require selection of alternate sites. In the morbidly obese patients, placement of the needle through the center of the umbilicus should be done, as this is the thinnest area of the abdominal wall. In the extremely thin patient, the angle of force should be almost parallel to the abdominal wall to avoid aortic puncture. Ancillary puncture sites include cephalad to the umbilicus and beneath the costal margin at the lateral edge of the rectus muscle. It is important to assess liver size prior to placement on the right side. Ancillary puncture sites may be placed in the lower quadrants in the midline and laterally (Fig. 68.1). Insufflation through the posterior vaginal fornix should not be attempted in patients with suspected cul-de-sac disease.

The position of the Verres or Tuohy needle in the peritoneum can be checked three ways. Intraperitoneal pressures should not exceed 10 mmHg. There should also be variation of pressures with respiration. The syringe test consists of injecting 5 ml of sterile saline through the needle and aspirating. If the needle is correctly placed, the saline cannot be retrieved. If fluid returns, one may conclude that the needle tip is likely to be in the bladder, bowel or, most likely, the preperitoneal space. None of these measures assures placement in the correct space, but may increase its likelihood. Loss of hepatic dullness on abdominal percussion after 1 liter of carbon dioxide is reassuring.

After a pneumoperitoneum is obtained, a trocar and sleeve (5–12 mm) is inserted with the similar angle as the Verres or Tuohy needle. The laparoscope is inserted through the sleeve after the trocar has been removed. The surgeon should examine the abdomen to insure no inadvertent damage to bowel or omentum has occurred with trocar placement. The entire abdominal cavity should be inspected with attention to the liver edge (adhesions) and the appendix. The patient may be placed in the Trendelenburg position for pelvic visualization. Visualization may be obscured by omental adhesions. By moving the laparoscope laterally, it may be possible to bypass them. If not, the omentum can be either bluntly or sharply dissected to create a window for the laparoscope. If there are avascular filmy adhesions covering the pelvic floor, the laparoscope can be inserted through one of these areas. An ancillary puncture site is usually needed to inspect the pelvis adequately.

Open laparoscopy can be used when there is a high index of suspicion for abdominopelvic adhesive disease. The main difference is that, with open laparoscopy, there is no blind insertion of the laparoscope. The trocar and sleeve are usually larger (12–15 mm) and operating channels are usually not available. A subumbilical skin incision is made. Dissection continues down to the fascial layer. The fascia is then incised under direct visualization. The peritoneum is idenitified and incised in a clear transilluminated area. The trocar and sleeve can then be placed into the abdominal cavity. It is of utmost importance that the fascial incision should not be too large or there will be difficulty maintaining a pneumoperitoneum. A purse-string suture is placed in the fascia and attached to a special ring around the sleeve in an effort to maintain a tight seal.

A panoramic view gives a general impression of the state of the pelvis. A systematic inspection should then be performed. It is very important to establish a pattern and be meticulous during the inspection. One should not go directly to an area of pathology lest other areas with less obvious abnormalities be missed. The uterovesical reflection and anterior aspect of the uterus are examined by lowering the uterus. Evidence of endometriosis may be quite subtle. The uterus is then elevated and the posterior aspect as well as the shape and size of the uterus is noted. The right adnexa is then visualized. Using the ancillary probe to mobilize the ovary, its entire surface can be seen. One should note evidence of endometriosis, ovarian cysts, follicles, tumors, or corpus luteum. The ovary is a delicate structure and should be handled as such.

Complete visualization may require dissection. Mobilization of a densely adherent ovary requires operative laparoscopy and possible laparotomy and should not be undertaken during diagnostic laparoscopy unless the patient is fully consented and the surgeon has anticipated this situation. The fallopian tube in its entirety is then closely inspected. Its mobility, caliber, and size are noted. The presence of nodules on the proximal aspect of the fallopian tube may indicate the presence of salpingitis isthmica nodosa. The fimbriae must be carefully visualized and the presence or absence of phimosis or adhesions, which may prevent ovum pick-up, noted. Posteriorly, the broad ligament, uterosacral ligaments and the posterior cul-de-sac are inspected. Fluid in the posterior cul-de-sac may need to be aspirated for better visualization and, if appropriate, sent for cultures. Again the presence of endometriosis, adhesions or masses is noted. The other adnexa must be similarly examined.

Chromotubation

Chromotubation may be carried out at this time if appropriate. A dilute solution of saline and methylene blue can be injected through the uterine cannula and spill through the fimbriae of the fallopian tubes seen. If no dye or only passage through one side is seen,

this may be due to tubal spasm, tubal obstruction, or leakage from the cervix.

Ancillary puncture sites

Ancillary puncture sites may be required for manipulation and stabilization. In general, placement should be slightly anterior and to either side of the operative site for maximum ease. Each surgeon needs to tailor the site to the individual patient. The site of ancillary puncture should be indented with the operator's finger and this site should be visualized through the laparoscope. The room lights should be dimmed and, using the laparoscope light, the target site transilluminated to visualize any large vessels. The ancillary puncture should be placed under direct visualization to avoid any injury to the abdomino-pelvic cavity. The inferior epigastric arteries may cause major hemorrhage if lacerated and their course should be kept in mind.

Assistants

Assistants form an integral part of the operating team when operative laparoscopy is being performed. Usually an assistant will help stabilize ancillary instruments. Beam splitters, as seen in Figure 68.2, are available that allow the surgeon to look through the laparoscope while projecting the image on a video screen. This equipment has aided greatly in teaching as it allows the surgeon to look through the endoscope for nuances of color and depth, which is necessary, while still allowing assistants to follow the surgery. Diagnostic and operative laparoscopy is best learned with both options (direct visualization and videomonitor) available.

COMPLICATIONS

Although laparoscopy is an extremely safe procedure, there are several known major and minor complications. Even with meticulous adherence to proper technique, some complications may occur.

Blind insertion of the insufflation needle or the trocar accounts for a large number of complications. Extraperitoneal insufflation can occur when the Verres or Tuohy needle has been misplaced. As soon as this is recognized, the carbon dioxide should be allowed to escape and the needle reinserted. This complication can make it difficult to reinsert the Verres or Tuohy, as the depth of the preperitoneal space has been enlarged. In severe cases, mediastinal emphysema may occur and be first recognized by

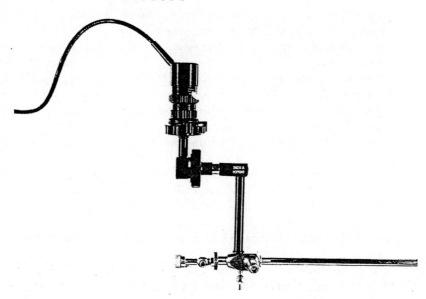

Fig. 68.2 Beam splitter and videocamera attachment.

the anesthesiologist. Close monitoring should then follow. Vessel or organ injury may occur with passage of the Verres needle or of the principal trocar. Most needle injuries do not require laparotomy; therefore, if perforation of a viscus is suspected the needle should be withdrawn and insufflation attempted at another site. Once the laparoscope is inserted, the suspected area should be meticulously evaluated. Close postoperative follow-up is required.

More serious complications tend to result from trocar penetration. These injuries usually require laparotomy for correction. If the lumen of the bowel or large vessel is entered, the laparoscope should be left in place and not removed. This limits possible bowel contamination or hemorrhage as well as identifying the area of damage quickly. Immediate laparotomy should follow. It is also possible to injure organs with the tip of the trocar and not the sleeve, so that when the laparoscope is placed, the area of injury may not be seen. This occurs infrequently but requires a high degree of suspicion. These types of injuries can be somewhat lessened by elevating the anterior abdominal wall when inserting the trocar and aiming toward the pelvis. This is especially important in the thin patient.

If damage occurs to small or medium-sized vessels, hemorrhage may be controlled through the laparoscope using a bipolar coagulator. This instrument should only be used by an experienced laparoscopist as electrocautery may be associated with complications as well. Operative laparoscopy is associated with all the above complications. In addition, complications

of additional instruments as well as those associated with electrocautery, thermocoagulation, and laser may be seen. Laparoscopy should only be done by or under the close supervision of an experienced laparoscopist. Instruments should only be used when the field of vision is complete. A 0.28% overall complication rate in 8943 laparoscopies was reported by Semm [2]. This series included both diagnostic and operative laparoscopy. There were 13 instances of vessel damage, nine cases of bowel or stomach puncture, two cases of cardiac arrest, and one case of ureteral damage. Ten laparotomies were performed and no deaths were reported. Of the reported cases, 6114 were operative laparoscopies.

EQUIPMENT

A gas insufflator is used to obtain a carbon dioxide pneumoperitoneum. The insufflators of laparoscopy and hysteroscopy are not interchangeable because the flow and volume required for these procedures are so different. It is imperative that a high-flow insufflator be available, especially if operative laparoscopy is done. Irrigation, aspiration, and multiple puncture sites all contribute to sources of gas leaks. The low flow of most insufflators produces 0.5−1.0 l/min while the high flow results in 4−6 l/min.

Two needle types are available for creation of the pneumoperitoneum: the Verres and the Tuohy needle. The Tuohy needle is readily available and inexpensive. It was originally intended for placement of epidural anesthesia. The Verres needle was designed to reduce the risk of viscus injury by having a spring that allows for retraction of the pointed tip once it encounters the decreased pressure past the abdominal wall.

There are two basic models of the trocar and sleeve: the flapper valve and the trumpet valve models. The flapper valve model markedly reduces the escape of gas from the pneumoperitoneum. A spring mechanism or safety shield may be found in the disposable trocars. These may increase safety as well as provide a sharp tip at all times. Laparoscopes come in a variety of sizes, as can be seen in Figure 68.3. The laparoscopes come in small- (5–7 mm) and large- (8–12 mm) bore calibers. The operating laparoscopes are usually large since they also contain an operating channel for ancillary instruments. There are three basic models of operating laparoscopes: a parallel, 45°, and 90° angle eyepiece. The Jacob–Palmer is the most commonly used operating laparoscope. The angle of view is offset by two right angles so the eyepiece is parallel and offset. The view is that of the straightforward laparoscope. The major disadvantage is that ancillary instruments are easily contaminated because they are held close to the operator's head. The 45° angle laparoscope offers a small increase in the operator's field but requires more experience and accommodation to use. The 90° angle laparoscope markedly decreases the chance of contamination of

ancillary instruments yet it can be quite confusing to use. The operating field is at right angles to the field of view.

Visualization depends on the adequacy of the lighting source. Fiberoptic technology has increased our ability to obtain a good image. Liquid light cables offer superior light with no known drawbacks, except the price. Xenon light is preferred if a video camera is used. Otherwise, metal halide is sufficient. It is important to check that broken fibers are not present, diminishing available light. The lighted end of the cable can be visualized. Any dark spots seen represent broken fibers that are not transmitting light. It is important not to turn on the cable light until it is ready to be placed on the laparoscope. The cable end becomes quite hot and, if left on, the drapes, may cause fire or burns.

Most manufactures produce an array of ancillary instruments, as seen in Figure 68.4. This myriad of instruments provides the surgeon with versatility. Ancillary instruments may be placed through an operating channel or through an ancillary puncture site depending on the surgeon's choice. Broad categories of instruments will be discussed. Probes are the most commonly used ancillary instruments for diagnostic laparoscopy. Almost all probes are blunt. They are used for stabilization and immobilization of structures. The probes may have ends

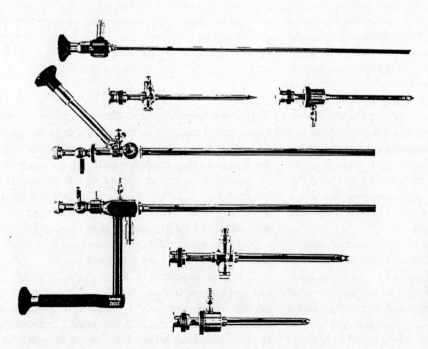

Fig. 68.3 Types of laparoscopes and trocars (from top to bottom). Straightfoward diagnostic laparoscope, small trocar sleeve with trumpet valve, small trocar sleeve with flapper valve, 45° angle operating laparoscope, Jacob–Palmer laparoscope, large trocar sleeve with trumpet valve, large trocar sleeve with flapper valve. All instruments made by Karl Storz Col Tuttlingen, FRG. (From [3].)

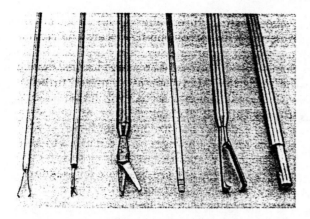

Fig. 68.4 Ancillary instruments. From left to right: atraumatic grasper, microscissors, large scissors, point thermocoagulator, traumatic forceps, morcellator. All instruments made by Wisap Co., Sauerlack, FRG. (From [1].)

marked in centimeters, allowing for more accurate measurements.

Forceps are another frequently used instrument. Grasping tongs and forceps can be used to stabilize a structure atraumatically. The forceps with springs must be used with caution so as not to cause trauma. Forceps with toothed edges as well as claws exist to work with uterine myomas or other tissue that is to be removed. Biopsy forceps may be used to sample the ovary or areas of peritoneal disease. There are a variety of scissors available for sharp dissection. These forceps as well as scissors must be kept sharp at all times to that tissue trauma does not arise from their use.

Aspirators consist of a hollow cannula with attached syringe for negative pressure or as an apparatus that is a combined aspriator and irrigator. These combined instruments are especially helpful if one encounters a hemoperitoneum. Needle aspirators can be used to puncture and drain cysts if necessary.

Large pieces of tissue may be removed in a variety of ways. Tissue may be grasped and removed with the laparoscope through the sleeve. A tissue morcellator can be used with the tissue being stored in the sheath of the morcellator. Finally, a small suprapubic incision may be made to remove the tissue. The need for pathologic diagnosis may influence the method of tissue removal.

Hemostasis may be achieved by a variety of methods such as unipolar or bipolar electrocautery, thermocoagulation, laser, and intraabdominal su-

turing. The surgeon should be familiar with a variety of these methods. Instrument availability and the location of bleeding usually determine the approach. Electrocautery uses electrical current to heat the tissue. The units are low-voltage, high-frequency solid-state units with insulated circuitry which can be used in unipolar or bipolar modes. The unipolar system passes the current from the generator through the instrument to a ground plate and then back to the generator. The ground plate must be in contact with the patient. Most units will emit a signal and stop if the ground plate is not in full contact. The bipolar system passes the current to and from the generator by insulated jaws, with the tissue between the jaws completing the circuit. Cutting and coagulating current can be used. The cutting current emits a constant high-energy waveform while the coagulating current emits an initial high-energy waveform which dissipates quickly. The current is usually activated by a foot pedal. It is essential that the current intensity be checked and adjusted properly. Even though the tip of the instrument is in view of the surgeon, the lateral spread of the current must be kept in mind as this is the most common cause of complications. With the unipolar unit, lateral spread can be up to 2–3 cm from the point of coagulation. This type of damage is markedly diminished with the use of the bipolar unit. Damage is usually limited to 1–2 cm from the point of coagulation. Many instruments, such as scissors, forceps, and probes, are available for use with electrocautery.

Thermocoagulation avoids direct electrical current and achieves hemostasis by heating the tissues to 100–140°C by heat convection. The denaturing of proteins and desiccation are thought to cause coagulation. Both the desired temperature and length of coagulation can be preselected. The heated mass of the instrument is small and does not release much heat. Although the "cool-down" is not immediate, penetrating burn injuries are unlikely. Superficial damage may occur and particular attention to this detail is important. Forceps and a jawed instrument are available for use with this unit. The most useful instrument is the point coagulator. It is particularly useful for ablation of endometriotic implants. However, the point is too large for fine coagulation.

Laser is another hemostatic device. It produces and amplifies light, creating intense, coherent electromagnetic energy. The lasers available currently include the carbon dioxide, argon, KTP (532 nm potassium–titanyl–phosphate) and Nd:YAG (neodymium:

yttrium aluminum garnet). Power density (W/cm^2) is the most important single factor in the effective operation of a laser. High power density (fine focusing) results in cutting, while low power density has co-agulating properties. The carbon dioxide laser is primarily used through laparoscopy for vaporization of tissue. The need to evacuate the plume of this laser can make it difficult to maintain a pneumo-peritoneum. The carbon dioxide laser can be used for coagulation of small vessels of 0.5–2.0 mm. The other three types of lasers have greater coagulative effect. They can be used as cutting instruments with the addition of a wave guide. The depth of penetra-tion of the argon and KTP lasers is 0.4–0.8 mm, much deeper than the carbon dioxide laser. The depth of penetration of the Nd:YAG laser is 0.6–4.2 mm. The KTP laser is most similar to the carbon dioxide laser. Because of the depth of penetration, the Nd:YAG laser is most often used in endometriosis and endo-metrial ablation.

Suturing has added to the armamentarium of the laparoscopist. The Roeder loop (modification of the rectal polyp snare) can be placed around struc-tures and tightened, thereby ligating the tissue and vessels. Depending on the amount of tissue, several loops may need to be placed. Suturing can also be accomplished with a straight needle placed through ancillary puncture sites. Intraabdominal instrument ties or an extracorporeal knot are used.

CONCLUSIONS

Diagnostic laparoscopy is an essential and invaluable tool for the gynecologist. However, both diagnostic and operative laparoscopy should not be attempted until adequate training in these techniques has been attained. Operative laparoscopy has recently received much deserved attention. The advantages of lapar-oscopy are numerous and include increased patient acceptance, decreased hospitalization time, and decreased cost.

REFERENCE

1 Murphy AA. Operative Laparoscopy. *Fertil Steril* 1987; 47: 1.
2 Semm K. *Endoscopic Intraabdominal Surgery*. Kiel: Christian-Albrechts-Universitat, 1984: p. 4.
3 Murphy AA. Diagnostic and operative laparoscopy. In: Thomson J, Rock J, eds. *TeLinde's Operative Gynecology*. Philadelphia: JB Lippincott, 1992.

FURTHER READING

Azziz R, Murphy AA, eds. *Practical Manual of Operative Laparoscopy and Hysteroscopy*. New York: Springer-Verlag, 1992.
Borten M. *Laparoscopic Complications — Prevention and Management*. Toronto: BC Decker, 1986.
Gomel V, Taylor PJ, Yuzpe AA, Rioux JE, eds. *Laparoscopy and Hysteroscopy in Gynecologic Practice*. Chicago: Year Book, 1986.
Murphy AA. Operative laparoscopy. *Fertil Steril* 1987; 47: 6.
Murphy AA. Diagnostic and operative laparoscopy. In: Thompson J, Rock J, eds. *TeLinde's Operative Gynecology*. Philadelphia: JB Lippincott (in press).
Sanfilippo JS, Levine RL, eds. *Operative Gynecologic Endoscopy*. New York: Springer-Verlag, 1989.

Laparoscopic complications

DAN C. MARTIN & BARBARA S. LEVY

Laparoscopic skills, awareness, and indications have reduced laparotomy, hospitalization days, and morbidity. While these changes are associated with an increased competence in and reliance on laparoscopic techniques, there is the worry that the rising numbers of laparoscopic procedures may reflect unnecessarily and inappropriately liberalized indications, surgical skills perhaps being exceeded, and facilities undoubtedly strained [1].

The use of laparoscopy has been accompanied by patients' belief that "band-aid" surgery is simple and without risks, particularly when they are able to return home on the same day. This simplified view of a complex procedure increases the vulnerability to litigious prodding if an untoward result occurs [2].

Although many of these procedures are performed on medically low-risk patients, others need extensive medical evaluation, electrocardiograms, chest X-rays, and biochemical profiles. The work-up and approach to a 35-year-old undergoing a tubal ligation are different than that for a 60-year-old having a cholecystectomy. The first safeguard against complication is an adequate history and physical examination (Fig. 69.1).

CONTRAINDICATIONS

As in all other areas of medicine, indications and contraindications must be considered. (The list of indications is much too long for a chapter of this scope. Contraindications are to some degree related to the surgeon's experience, though certain conditions will be covered here.)

Patients in hypovolemic shock with increased cardiovascular instability have a life-threatening condition. An approach must be taken which provides prompt and adequate hemostasis. Although a small group of physicians may develop adequate expertise to remove rapidly 2 units of clots from the pelvis and promptly to obtain hemostasis with a laparoscopic procedure, this carries with it the chance that the patient may be exposed to avoidable risks.

Patients with pulmonary and cardiovascular disease that can be decompensated by altered venous return, cardiac output, heart rate, and blood pressure may be much better served with a laparotomy than a laparoscopy. Early experience with laparoscopic cholecystectomies has suggested that these patients may be much better with a 45-min laparotomy than a 4-hour laparoscopy. When physicians are learning, patients in high-risk situations are not the optimal candidates for the educational process. This is particularly true with extensive operative laparoscopy in the pelvis, cholecystectomies, and other advanced operative procedures currently being investigated.

Although peritonitis had been considered a contraindication in the past, this may be an indication at present. The ability to provide an accurate diagnosis and to drain abscesses appears to be much more important than theoretic concerns regarding intra-abdominal spillage and systemic dissemination.

A large pelvic and abdominal mass, particularly a pregnant uterus, has an increased chance of perforation if closed insufflation and trocar techniques are used. If it is judged that these patients have more benefit than risk in performing a laparoscopy, the open insertion techniques suggested by Hasson should be considered [3].

Patients who have a history of previous abdominal laparotomies are at increased risk of bowel damage. These patients should be bowel-prepped. Preoperatively, both the patient and the surgeon should be ready for bowel surgery. This appears particularly true in patients who have previous exploratory laparotomies following motor vehicle accidents and blunt trauma to the abdomen, histories of abdominal cancer, and histories of previous diffuse peritonitis.

On rare occasion, plans need to be made for specific medical conditions. An example is avoiding electrosurgery in patients with pacemakers.

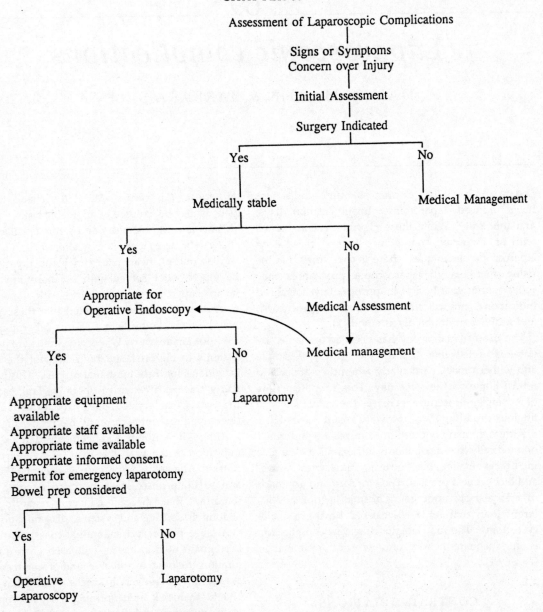

Fig. 69.1 Assessment of laparoscopic complications.

PREOPERATIVE COUNSELING

As rare complications can occur even in low-risk patients, all patients must be ready for emergency laparotomy [4]. Some attorneys also feel it prudent to warn patients about the possibility of paralysis, hysterectomy, colostomy, and death. Although these warnings have the potential for interfering with patient care, they can be followed by common-sense modifiers such as the observation that laparoscopy is safer than pregnancy or driving a car for 1 year. This approach has been used for several years and there have been no patients who have changed their mind about a laparoscopy on the basis of informed consent.

It is also prudent to inform patients that failures or complications can occur and the surgeon needs to be informed promptly of any abnormal symptoms. Prompt attention increases the chance of correcting the problem. Surgeons may need to modify their techniques in an attempt to prevent these complications from occurring in future patients.

INTRAOPERATIVE COMPLICATIONS

The increased use of laparoscopy for extensive pelvic surgery is associated with an increased chance of venous and arterial bleeding. Laparoscopists must be prepared with techniques of coagulation or mechanical occlusion in order to stop this bleeding. Furthermore, although major vessel damage is rare, the ability to perform emergency laparotomy and place digital pressure or vascular clamps is a requirement.

Needle insertion is checked by several techniques. A drop of saline at the hub of the needle will be pulled into the abdomen when negative pressure is created by pulling up on the lower abdomen. 10 ml of saline injected into the abdomen will disperse if the insertion is correct. If fluid, blood, or bowel contents are aspirated, a problem exists.

Although needle insertion into the bowel and stomach occurs, the major injuries are vascular. Open laparoscopy and safety trocars are said to decrease the chance of bowel entry, but this has occurred with all techniques. Even though this has occurred, open laparoscopy may be the best choice as the penetration may be recognized immediately and posterior bowel wall damage may be avoided. Although this is correct in theory, many surgeons have found that opening through a small incision increases the chance of bowel and bladder injury rather than decreasing it.

Percussion for liver dullness and stomach gas helps avoid these areas. If the trocar is inserted into the bowel or stomach, it should be left in place until the abdomen is opened. If it is removed, the entrance site may close and become difficult to find.

Thermal injury

Unipolar electrosurgical equipment, bipolar electrosurgical equipment, thermal coagulators, and lasers can produce thermal bowel injuries. Scissors have also been noted to cut holes in bowel. Of these, the most worrisome is inadvertent unipolar coagulation as the amount of damage may extend 2–5 cm past the apparent level of damage. Wide resection of the small bowel, usually 5 cm on either side, is thought to be prudent when unipolar coagulation occurs. Bipolar and laser devices produce a more discrete burn and a focal resection is possible.

One major point in avoiding damage to the bowel is to use electric and laser equipment through the second puncture. Some damage that has occurred is thought to have taken place in the blind spot created by using this equipment through a single-puncture laparoscope.

Cardiovascular

Gas embolism is a rare but potentially devastating complication. Problems related to this have been the source of a Food and Drug Administration alert regarding the use of air-cooled Nd:YAG laser tips at hysteroscopy. This alert is also concerned about this possibility at laparoscopy. The diagnosis is made on the basis of a "mill-wheel" murmur over the entire precordium. Treatment includes cessation of insufflation, turning the patient to the left lateral decubitus position, supportive measures, including resuscitation, and placement of a central venous catheter into the right ventricle to withdraw the gas [5].

Cardiac arrhythmias increase with inadequate ventilation and circulation. This is related to elevation of the diaphragm, absorption of carbon dioxide, Trendelenburg position, venous pooling, and vasovagal reflex. Monitoring of the electrocardiogram, use of atropine and similar medicines to suppress vasovagal reflex, and endotracheal intubation are of use in diagnosing and preventing this problem. Although anesthesiologists will generally be in charge of treatment, those surgeons who perform laparoscopy without anesthesia available must understand advanced cardiac life support and the medicines available for this.

Aspiration

Aspiration is infrequent but may occur because of pressure on the stomach from the pneumoperitoneum. A cuffed endotracheal tube is generally used and some surgeons consider use of a nasogastric tube. Percussion of the stomach for gas and observation of the stomach through the laparoscope may be useful in determining when a nasogastric tube is to be used.

Pneumothorax

In general the insufflation pressure of the abdomen is kept between 8 and 20 mmHg. This theoretically decreases the chance of pneumothorax. New gas insufflators that rapidly refill the abdomen decrease the pressure needed. This appears related to a better maintenance of a more constant operative field.

POSTOPERATIVE EMERGENCIES

One major concern about postoperative complications is the problem of who is available to care for the patient. If a surgeon turns cases over to a colleague not familiar with laparoscopic complications, this increases the risk of delayed diagnosis and increased morbidity. Physician coverage must be adequate to prevent delayed diagnosis. Postoperative complications can rapidly progress; evaluation must be immediate with laparoscopic complications treated as emergencies.

Preexisting pelvic inflammatory disease may be exacerbated and subclinical cervicitis or endometritis may be spread and turned into peritonitis or sepsis. Cultures taken preoperatively or antibiotics used in high-risk patients may be reasonable. If a fever develops, rapid assessment is needed to determine whether fever is from the pelvis, respiratory system, urinary system, or other site.

Increasing pain and fever may also be related to bowel, bladder, or ureteral injury. Careful abdominal examination may indicate the need for a diagnostic laparoscopy or exploratory laparotomy.

DELAYED COMPLICATIONS

Delayed bleeding can occur in any patient. Two specific areas of concern are tamponade of venous sources of bleeding by the pneumoperitoneum and temporary control of bleeding by Pitressin. To check for the possibility of tamponade, intraabdominal pressure is decreased and possible sites of bleeding are observed. This can generally be done under low pressure but completely releasing the pressure and reinsufflating the abdomen may sometimes be necessary. The possibility of rebound bleeding as Pitressin wears off and the possibility of other vessels opening after the surgery is finished can be monitored by placing a hemovac drain into the pelvis. Contemporary thoughts suggest that the first 2 hours are the most important. The hemovac should be left in during this time. Checking for orthostatic hypotension and performing serial hematocrits may also be useful.

Persistent ectopic pregnancies may follow conservative operations for tubal pregnancy or laparoscopic sterilizations performed at midcycle. Increasing pain 1—6 weeks following the initial procedure must be investigated. In patients with conservative operations for ectopic pregnancies, weekly or twice-weekly quantitative human chorionic gonadotropin (hCG) titers are mandatory until titers fall to zero. In patients who have had sterilization and who are late for their period or have signs of pregnancy, quantitative hCG needs to be performed.

Although life-threatening delayed complications such as pulmonary embolus can occur, these are very rare. More likely, but still uncommon, are delayed effects related to unrecognized damage to bowel, ureter, bladder, or vessels. When evaluating patients postoperatively with increasing abdominal pain, increasing distention, fever, or general malaise, these possibilities must be kept in mind.

Also of concern is the failure of the procedure. For sterilization, unintended pregnancies have resulted in legal action and judgments against physicians. Preoperative consent regarding this possibility and careful concern for the procedure itself help protect the patients and physicians from this possibility. Surgery for pain or infertility may fail to correct either of these. Plans for persistent infertility may include a more comprehensive evaluation or the use of assisted reproductive technologies. When pain persists, multiple surgical and nonsurgical modalities are available. Nonsurgical possibilities include pelvic diathermy, anesthetic blocks of sensate focal points, biofeedback, and desensitization. In addition, laparotomy may reveal lesions and problems that were not recognized at laparoscopy. Although laparoscopy appears to be an excellent tool for lesions which can be seen, many problems require palpation for adequate diagnosis.

CONCLUSIONS

The possibility and potential for complications demand the utmost caution at every step of preparation and performance of any medical procedure. Patient selection, equipment function, operating room personnel, and ongoing education are needed to develop and maintain excellence. Prompt diagnosis and therapy of complications will generally limit the amount of long-term damage.

REFERENCES

1 Borten M. *Laparoscopic Complications*. Philadephia: BC Decker, 1986.
2 Corson SL, Soderstrom RM, Levy BS. Emergencies and laparoscopy. In: Martin DC, Holtz GL, Levinson CJ, Soderstrom RM, eds. *Manual of Endoscopy*. Santa Fe Springs: American Association of Gynecologic Laparoscopists, 1990: 47—51.
3 Hasson HM. Open techniques for equipment insertion. In: Martin DC, Holtz GL, Levinson CJ, Soderstrom RM, eds. *Manual of Endoscopy*. Santa Fe Springs: American Association of Gynecologic Laparoscopists, 1990: 23—29.
4 Hulka JF, ed. *Textbook of Laparoscopy*. Orlando: Grune & Stratton, 1985.
5 Pentecost MP, Curtis EM. Laparoscopy. In: Ridley JH, ed. *Gynecologic Surgery: Errors, Safeguards, Salvage* 2nd edn. Baltimore: Williams & Wilkins, 1981: 135—158.

Diagnostic hysteroscopy

JILL T. FLOOD

INTRODUCTION

Hysteroscopy is the direct investigation of the interior of the uterine cavity and is possible with both panoramic and contact methods. Panoramic hysteroscopy involves distention of the uterine cavity with either liquid or gas. No distention is required for contact hysteroscopy; the objective lens of the hysteroscope is in contact with the structure to be viewed. The Hamou microcolpohysteroscope (Carl Storz, Tuttlingen, Germany), which permits observation in both panoramic and contact modes, is equipped with a lens system with magnification of 1× and 150×. This chapter will pertain primarily to diagnostic panoramic hysteroscopy.

INSTRUMENTATION

The panoramic hysteroscope is a modified cystoscope, usually a rigid telescope 2–6 mm in diameter, equipped with a lens system of 0–30°. Selection of angle is a matter of personal preference. For the beginner the 0° telescope is easier to use because orientation is similar to normal vision. A 4 mm telescope is the narrowest diameter that can provide an optically bright, clear, wide-angle view of an object. Rigid hysteroscopes are fixed-focus, but flexible and focusing endoscopes are also available. The care of hysteroscopes should follow the manufacturer's recommendations.

The endoscope is fitted to an external stainless steel sheath equipped with stopcock-controlled channels with leur-lock fittings through which distention medium is introduced. A 5 mm diagnostic sheath is necessary for clearance of a 4 mm endoscope, and its terminal end should fit flush with the end of the endoscope. Operative sheaths have additional channels for instrumentation, aspiration, and irrigation; they range from 7 to 8 mm in outer diameter. The operating channel must be fitted with a rubber nipple to prevent the loss of medium when instruments are introduced. Gaskets commonly slip off or leak when Hyskon is selected as the distending medium because of its slippery properties. Leak-proof operating gaskets (Cook, Spencer) that lock on to the leur-lock fittings provide a slip-proof fitting. Both flexible and semirigid instruments of 7 Fr caliber can be used through operative channels for intrauterine surgery. Grasping and biopsy forceps, scissors, electrodes, and laser fibers are available for use as experience permits. Specifically designed cannulas for hysteroscopic aspiration (Cook, Spencer) are banded at the terminal end with 1 ml space markings for measurement. In addition, these cannulas have side aspiration ports to make them more effective. Makeshift plastic tubing with an internal diameter of 1.6–1.7 mm and an outer diameter of 2.0–2.4 mm can be adapted for aspiration or irrigation through the operating channels.

Objects viewed within the endometrial cavity appear larger than they are because of the relative closeness of the lens to the object. Depth perception in human vision is the result of binocular vision; since endoscopes are monocular, depth perception is lost. However, interpretation of depth improves with practice.

LIGHT SOURCES

The simplest light generator provides 150 W of power, sufficient for direct-view hysteroscopy. The zenon generator provides 300 W, necessary for indirect video control and photographic hysteroscopy. Regardless of its source, the light which reaches the endoscope depends on the quality and maintenance of the fiberoptic cable. With one end of the cable held to an overhead light source, broken fibers can be seen at the other end as black dots. Additionally, if the light source is connected to the fiberoptic cable in a dark room broken fibers are detected as illuminated spots along the cable.

CHAPTER 70

DISTENTION MEDIA

The cavity of the uterus is potential rather than real. For a panoramic view, the cavity must first be distended. The media used most often are high molecular weight dextran (Hyskon), low-viscosity fluids such as D5W, saline, glycine, or sorbitol, and carbon dioxide (CO_2). A comparison of distention media is presented in Table 70.1.

High molecular weight dextran

High molecular weight dextran (Hyskon) has an average molecular weight of 70 000. It is electrolyte-free, nonconductive, and biodegradable. Its refractile index is 1.39, wheras that of CO_2 is 1.00. Therefore, higher magnification and a narrower field of view are obtained with Hyskon. It is particularly valuable in operative procedures because it does not mix with blood, is an excellent lubricant, and may facilitate dilatation of the cervix by dipping the external end of the hysteroscope before engaging the cervical os. Both laser and diathermy may be used with Hyskon

as the distending medium, but the volume must be carefully monitored. Dextran decreases the levels of fibrinogen, factors V, VII, and IX. Prolonged bleeding has been reported with volumes greater than or equal to 300 ml; the manufacturer's insert for Hyskon suggests a limit of less than 500 ml. Hyskon may be absorbed into the vascular spaces; noncardiogenic pulmonary edema has been reported, perhaps secondary to increased intravascular osmotic pressure, causing hypervolemia. Adult respiratory distress syndrome and vulvar edema have also been reported with Hyskon. These complications are rare and risk is increased with operative hysteroscopy. Dextran may also be associated with falsely elevated blood glucose levels, unreliable total protein and bilirubin assays, and imprecise blood cross-matching, although the latter has been a problem only with outdated enzyme methods of cross-matching procedures. Anaphylactic reaction has also been reported. Its incidence, estimated to be one in 10 000, is not associated with the volume of Hyskon.

The major disadvantage of high molecular weight

Table 70.1 Comparison of distending media

Distending media	Advantage	Disadvantages	Complications
Hyskon (dextran 70)	Immiscible with blood	Sticky	Anaphylaxis
	Can be used with laser and electrocautery	Messy	Pulmonary edema, noncardiogenic
		Expensive	Adult respiratory distress syndrome
	Biodegradable		Prolonged bleeding time/DIC
	Electrolyte-free		↑ Blood glucose, total protein and bilirubin, may affect blood cross-matches
			Vulvar edema
			Electrolyte disturbances
Low-viscosity fluids (D5W, saline, glycine, sorbitol)	Inexpensive	Miscible with blood	Water intoxication
	Physiological reabsorption	Electrolyte solutions	Electrolyte disturbances
	Can be used with laser	Contraindicated with electrocautery	
Carbon dioxide	Best-image transmission	Requires special insufflator	Carbon dioxide embolism
	Rapid absorption	Requires atraumatic technique	Acidosis
	Adaptable to office setting		Hypercarbia
	Inexpensive		Arrhythmia

DIC, disseminated intravascular coagulation.

dextran is its stickiness as it dries. Therefore, instruments must be thoroughly washed in warm water after each use and disassembled so that all stopcocks and other moving parts are thoroughly cleansed.

Hyskon can be used with a 50 mm leur-lock syringe connected directly to an intake channel or with a short piece of large-bore connecting tube placed between the syringe and the intake channel. Continued pressure on the syringe is necessary during viewing. Excess solution leaks slowly around the sheath, but some may enter the fallopian tubes and peritoneal cavity. In at least 50% of patients, Hyskon has been noted at laparoscopy to enter the cul-de-sac, with approximately 5% of the medium found in the peritoneal cavity.

Low-viscosity fluids

Although low-viscosity fluids such as D5W, saline, glycine, and sorbitol are miscible with blood, when administered by a pump with constant inflow and outflow they create a very clear view even for operative procedures. Large volumes are required, but most of the fluid escapes from the cervix or are removed by the pump. Flushing can be achieved by the introduction of a fine polythene catheter through the operative channel. Fluid may be delivered to the intake stopcock of the hysteroscope by a 50 ml syringe. Because a large volume of these fluids is usually necessary, a 1000 ml bag is hung from an intravenous pole with tubing connected to the intake stopcock of the hysteroscope sheath. A pneumatically inflated pressure bag, with the gauge at 100–110 mmHg, provides constant delivery for uterine distention and is the most effective.

Large quantities of D5W can be absorbed during prolonged hysteroscopy, exposing the patient to the risk of water intoxication. Other electrolyte abnormalities may also occur, but do so rarely. The advantages of these fluids are that they are inexpensive and physiologically reabsorbed. Disadvantages are that they cloud rapidly and are miscible with blood. Electrolyte solutions are contraindicated with electrocautery.

CO_2

The refractile index of CO_2 is 1.00, allowing a wider field of view and a lower magnification, and giving almost perfect image transmission as long as bleeding is not present. CO_2 is rapidly absorbed and easily adapted to the office setting, being less messy, but it requires a specialized CO_2 insufflator. Only insufflation equipment specifically designed for hysteroscopy should be used. The microhysteroflator is suitable for this purpose. (*Caution*: the insufflator designed for laparoscopy must *never* be used to perform hysteroscopy because it allows gas flow at a rate of up to 6 l/min rather than 100 ml/min. Deaths have occurred when 30–40 liters of CO_2 were insufflated. Pressures for hysteroscopy should not exceed 100 mmHg. At these pressures a flow rate of 40–60 ml/min is safe.) When CO_2 is used to distend the uterus, a gas-tight seal of the cervix is required. There is a 5% reported incidence of scapular pain with insufflation of CO_2, especially with local anesthesia. Intravasation of CO_2 during hysteroscopy theoretically can lead to arrhythmia, hypercarbia, and acidosis, although this is extremely rare in patients without cardiac disease. Recently, the Food and Drug Administration issued a warning of the risk of embolism during therapeutic intrauterine laser procedures when gas is used for cooling the laser fiber tip or for insufflation [1]. The emboli are presumably caused when the gas under pressure is forced into the vascular system. Deaths secondary to gas embolism have been reported. The alert does not apply to gas insufflation during diagnostic hysteroscopy or a short hysteroscopic operation when lasers are not used.

USES

The indications for hysteroscopy are listed in Table 70.2. Information gained from hysteroscopy is often adjunctive, collaborative, or confirmatory, and does not necessarily replace traditional methods of evaluation and treatment. In addition to diagnosis, hysteroscopy can be used to correct intrauterine adhesions; to resect leiomyomas, uterine polyps, and uterine septa; and to cannulate the tubal ostia or place material in it for sterilization (Table 70.3).

Abnormal uterine bleeding

Evaluation of pre- or postmenopausal abnormal bleeding is the most common indication for diagnostic hysteroscopy and constitutes 31–64% of indicated diagnostic hysteroscopies in various studies. Also 40–85% of patients undergoing hysteroscopy for abnormal bleeding have abnormal findings.

In a series of 768 hysteroscopies performed for abnormal uterine bleeding it was found that during reproductive years, submucous myoma, endometrial hyperplasia, and endometrial polyps were the most

Table 70.2 Indications for diagnostic hysteroscopy

Gynecology
  Abnormal uterine bleeding
  Lost IUD, foreign body
  Vaginoscopy in prepubertal females

Reproductive failure
  Evaluation of abnormal hysterosalpingogram
  Evaluation of recurrent abortion

Oncology
  Staging of endometrial carcinoma
  Cervical dysplasia — microcolpohysteroscopy

Obstetrics
  Retained placental tissue
  Embryoscopy
  Evaluation of uterine scars

IUD, intrauterine device.

Table 70.3 Operative hysteroscopy procedures

Lysis of adhesions
Resection of myoma
Resection of polyp
Resection of septum
Removal of foreign body
Endometrial ablation
Cannulation of the tubal ostia
Sterilization
Chorionic biopsy

common lesions detected, accounting for more than half of all lesions in the series. Pregnancy-related bleeding was the next most common diagnosis. In postmenopausal women, hyperplasia, polyps, and myomas were frequently found, as were endometrial atrophy and carcinoma. In some studies as much as 50% of postmenopausal bleeding was secondary to endometrial atrophy.

The traditional approach of dilatation and curettage (D&C) has been estimated to be inaccurate in 10–25% of patients, probably because many uterine abnormalities are focal and D&C samples only 50–60% of the endometrial cavity. Hysteroscopy, on the other hand, allows direct visualization of the entire endometrial cavity and directed biopsy of even the smallest focal lesions. In addition, it can be coupled with D&C so that after sampling of the endometrial cavity by curettage, the cavity can be reinspected with the hysteroscope to insure that

lesions have been removed. Solid lesions such as leiomyomas, which are often missed at D&C because they do not lend themselves well to curette biopsy, are easily seen with the hysteroscope. Atrophic endometrium, which often on traditional D&C yields little or no tissue, is easily identified by hysteroscopy. Placental polyps occur primarily in reproductive-age women and may present as menometrorrhagia. Occasionally, fetal remnants may be present along with trophoblastic tissue. A flow diagram for evaluation of abnormal uterine bleeding is presented in Figure. 70.1. Although hysteroscopic visualization of uterine abnormalities may suggest a discrete diagnosis, histologic sampling must also be performed to rule out neoplastic conditions.

Endometrial carcinoma

Endometrial carcinoma occurs most often in postmenopausal women but can occur at any age. Hysteroscopic evaluation and staging of endometrial adenocarcinoma, suggested by Joelsson in 1971 [2], is especially good at assessing the status of the lower uterine segment and cervix.

Peritoneal spillage of contrast medium from hysterosalpingography in patients with endometrial cancer suggests the passage of cancer cells into the pelvis. Intravasation of the same contrast medium appearing on film highlights the hazards of vascular dissemination. This danger is also found in curettage and panoramic hysteroscopy. Johnsson [3] compared two groups of patients examined for endometrial carcinoma, by curettage and hysterography or by curettage alone, and found no significant difference in the rate of metastasis. Therefore, the potential for spreading cancer is theoretic; nevertheless, contact hysteroscopy without distending medium may decrease the risk of cellular spread.

Location and retrieval of lost intrauterine devices (IUDs) or other foreign bodies

When the string of an IUD is not visible at the cervical os or when an IUD is possibly embedded in the uterine wall, a hysteroscopy can locate the IUD and facilitate retrieval, even of fragments. When no IUD is seen at hysteroscopy, a single flat-plate X-ray of the abdomen is necessary to rule out translocation of the IUD to the abdominal cavity. In one study of more than 300 patients evaluated for lost IUDs, only 6% required X-ray to rule out translocations. A flow diagram for localization of lost IUDs is presented in Figure 70.2.

HYSTEROSCOPY

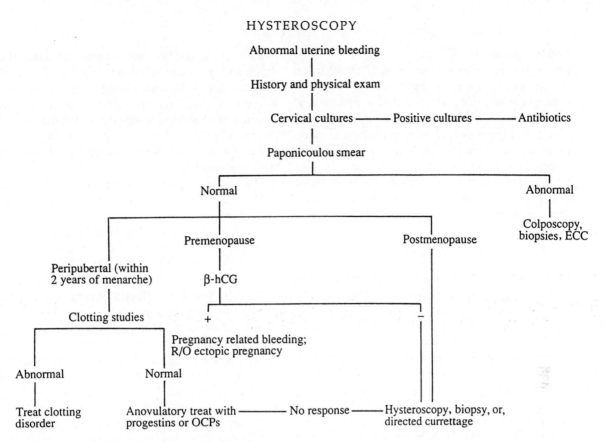

Fig. 70.1 Evaluation of abnormal uterine bleeding.

Evaluation of abnormal hysterosalpingograms and recurrent abortions

Hysteroscopy can locate abnormalities seen by hysterosalpingogram and can diagnose and treat intrauterine septa, which may be associated with reproductive failure. Large lesions on the posterior fundal wall are more likely to be associated with reproductive failure than are small lesions at other sites.

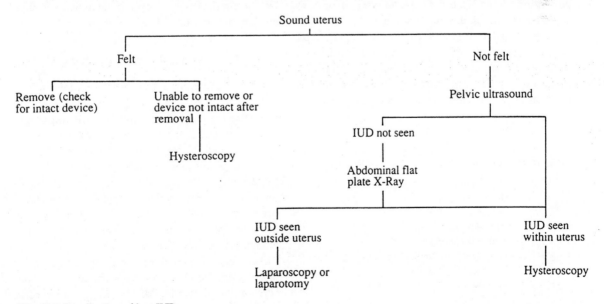

Fig. 70.2 Localization of lost IUDs.

Cervical dysplasia

Microcolpohysteroscopy allows full visualization of the squamocolumnar junction and transition zone under high magnification in the endocervical canal where visualization would be impossible with standard colposcopy and may preclude conization for inadequate visualization. It may also be helpful in pregnant patients where endocervical currettage or conization may be more difficult. Specialized training in the microcolpohysteroscopic appearance of the cervix is necessary.

COMPLICATIONS

Complications of diagnostic hysteroscopy are minimal; a complete list is in Table 70.4. Uterine perforation, the most significant complication, occurs in less than 0.1% of hysteroscopies and is usually associated with endometrial sounding, cervical dilatation, or blind manipulation of instruments. It is more common when the uterus is retroverted. Therefore, it is very important to determine the position of the uterus and to advance the hysteroscope under direct visualization.

Uterine perforation should be suspected if the sound or dilator passes a greater depth than is apparent by the size of the uterus on examination or if rapid flow of the distending liquid or very low distention pressure with CO_2 is noted when the telescope is introduced or passes through the uterine wall. In case of uterine perforation, the hysteroscope should be withdrawn and the patient observed. If profuse bleeding occurs or if injury to the bowel or other intraabdominal contents is suspected, laparoscopy or laparotomy should be performed immediately. Injury to the bowel and other organs can occur with electrocautery, and especially with extensive surgical procedures, which should be undertaken under direct laparoscopic examination.

Table 70.4 Complications of diagnostic hysteroscopy

Anesthesia-related
Cervical laceration
Distention media-related
Uterine perforation
Injury to intraabdominal contents
Rupture of hydrosalpinx
Infection
Hemorrhage

Infection is seldom encountered, but since the endoscope is passed from the vagina and cervical canal to the endometrial lining, bacteria may be introduced. Therefore, it is important to rule out any unusual cervical or vaginal bacteria. Because of the infrequency of infection, prophylactic antibiotics are unnecessary unless the patient has a history of mitral valve prolapse.

Medium-related complications are reviewed in Table 70.3. Other complications include anesthesia-related complications, rupture of hydrosalpinges and cervical laceration. The latter is probably the most frequent complication, although it is rarely reported and probably occurs when the tenaculum tears through the cervical stroma.

After hysteroscopy, a small amount of spotting may occur. Excessive bleeding is unusual except in cases of extensive manipulation. If excessive bleeding occurs, an intrauterine balloon distended to conform to the cavity is an excellent means of controlling and preventing postoperative bleeding. Balloon pressure can be released in several hours; if no bleeding occurs, it can be removed.

An adequate balloon can be formed by removing the tip of a Foley catheter immediately distal to the level of the balloon. The catheter is then inserted through the endocervical canal with the balloon deflated. The balloon is then inflated with 10–30 ml of sterile saline. Commercial balloons (Mentor, Goleta) conforming to the shape of the cavity can also be purchased. If a postoperative balloon or other IUD is left within the cavity, prophylactic antibiotics should be administered until its removal.

CONTRAINDICATIONS

A list of contraindications appears in Table 70.5. The only absolute contraindication to hysteroscopy is recent or existing pelvic infection. It is important to rule out infection and to be sure that it is completely resolved before considering hysteroscopy. Relative contraindications include pregnancy. Irregular bleeding can be secondary to ectopic pregnancy or abnormal intrauterine pregnancy. Therefore, a pregnancy test should be performed before examinations for any kind of abnormal bleeding in women of reproductive-age.

Bleeding is a contraindication only if it is profuse. It can often be overcome by a change of medium, Hyskon, or another liquid, or a change to the contact method.

Table 70.5 Contraindications of diagnostic hysteroscopy

Absolute
  Infection

Relative
  Pregnancy
  Cervical malignancy
  Examiner inexperience
  Profuse bleeding
  Marked cervical stenosis

Cervical malignancy is also a relative contra-indication because of the theoretic possibility of the spread of disease with manipulation. When the operator is unfamiliar with the appearance of the disease process or with instrumentation, hysteroscopy is contraindicated. Marked cervical stenosis not resolved by usual dilatation occurs in 1–2% of patients and may be overcome by the use of Premarin (2.5 mg) for 8 days preceding the procedure.

TECHNIQUE

The patient should receive a complete history and physical examination including pelvic examination, Pap smear, cervicovaginal smears and cultures to rule out infection, and negative pregnancy tests, when appropriate. The technique should then be explained in detail. Patients with a history of mitral valve prolapse should receive appropriate antibiotic prophylaxis prior to hysteroscopic examination.

The patient empties her bladder and is placed in the dorsal lithotomy position. The vulva and vagina are cleaned with antiseptic solution, which must be completely rinsed from the endocervical canal. This will prevent bubble formation, which may obstruct the view, particularly when CO_2 is the distending medium. Sterile drapes are placed. Following general or spinal anesthesia, if necessary, a pelvic examination is performed to determine the position of the uterus. If a paracervical block is to be performed, 5 ml of chloroprocaine hydrochloride 1% (Nesacaine) or 10 ml of 1% Xylocaine without epinephrine is injected superficially at the 4 and 8 o'clock position along the cervix at the juncture of the uterosacral ligaments. A small amount of anesthetic can also be placed in the anterior cervical lip where the tenaculum will be placed. (When general anesthesia is not used, administration of prostaglandin synthetase inhibitors, 30–60 min before the pro-

cedure, may decrease pain.) The anterior cervix is then grasped with a tenaculum. If CO_2 is used, the uterine cavity should not be sounded because of the possibility of bleeding. If another distention medium is used, uterine sounding may be performed to determine the depth and direction of the uterine cavity. The hysteroscope with distending medium is introduced into the external os under direct visualization and is advanced into the endocervical canal. The hysteroscope is gently pressed to the cervical os until it passes with minimal resistance. The endometrial cavity is then examined in a systematic fashion: the upper fundus is usually observed first, and then the tubal ostia. The scope is then withdrawn slowly, viewing the anterior, posterior, and lateral wall, finally the endocervical canal.

When the cervical os is too tight to allow passage of the endoscope under direct visualization, dilatation should be performed with Pratt dilators. Just enough dilatation should be obtained to allow passage of the sheath. (Since the diagnostic sheath in usually 5 mm wide, the cervix would be dilated to accommodate a number 17 Pratt dilator.) If the lens appears slightly cloudy, if bubbles are present, or if blood obscures the lens, it can be pressed to the top of the uterine fundus and then pulled back. This usually clears the view. When the cervix is patulous and allows leakage of the distention medium, a larger sheath (7 or 8 mm operating sheath), a shallow pursestring suture similar to a McDonald stitch, or a specially designed suction cup can be placed to insure a tight fit of the hysteroscope.

Diagnostic hysteroscopy is best performed after the patient has completed menstruation, when the endometrial lining is thin, the uterine cavity is relatively free of blood or debris, and little cervical mucus is present. The endometrium is highly vascularized and bleeds with a slight touch of the endoscope. Therefore, particularly with CO_2 as the distending medium, it is very important to use an atraumatic technique.

RECOGNITION OF ENDOMETRIAL PATHOLOGY

Recognition of the appearance of proliferative, secretory, and menstrual endometria requires practice. During the secretory phase the endometrium becomes velvety and reddish; it shows irregular, polyp-like patterns that protrude into the cavity. During this phase it may be more difficult to identify the tubal ostia, and the endometrium may bleed more easily when touched due to increased vascularization. Late secretory endometrium may be difficult to differentiate from hyperplastic endometrium because of its polypoid nature.

Close and careful examination of the endometrial cavity, particularly in the early follicular phase, can reveal small diverticular entrances into the myometrium, consistent with adenomyosis. Uterine leiomyomas may be sessile or pedunculated and polypoid. The endometrium overlying a leiomyoma may be atrophic, congested, ulcerated, or hemorrhagic. Typically, leiomyomas appear more whitish with vessels traversing their surface. Placental polyps appear pedunculated, firm or soft, mottled red or yellow necrotic tissue.

Endometrial polyps occur singly in 75% of cases. Although they may occur at any location in the endometrial cavity, they occur most often in the fundus, particularly in the cornual area, and may be broad-based or pedunculated. Most polyps are pink-grey to white with smooth, glistening surfaces beneath which small cysts may be visible. A variety of other lesions may have a polypoid configuration including carcinoma, sarcoma, carcinosarcoma, adenosarcoma, leiomyoma, and fragments of retained placenta, as well as secretory endometrium. It is therefore imperative that microscopic examination of any lesion be performed.

CONCLUSIONS

Hysteroscopy allows visualization of the uterine cavity which enhances diagnostic accuracy and in many cases may allow for definitive therapy. It is relatively safe and inexpensive, and often can be performed as an office procedure.

ACKNOWLEDGMENTS

The author wishes to thank Mrs Shirley Urich for her preparation of the manuscript, Ms Martha Wilson for her preparation of graphic materials, and Charlotte Schrader, PhD, for editorial assistance.

FURTHER READING

Alexander GP. Gas/air embolism associated with intra-uterine laser surgery. *FDA Drug Bull* 1990; 20: 6.

Baggish NS, Barbot J, Valle RF, eds. *Diagnostic and Operative Hysteroscopy: A Text and Atlas*. Chicago: Year Book Medical Publisher, 1989.

Jedeikin R, Olsfanger D, Kessler I. Disseminated intra-vascular coagulopathy and adult respiratory distress syndrome: life-threatening complications of hysteroscopy. *Am J Obstet Gynecol* 1990; 162: 44.

Mclucas B. Hyskon complications in hysteroscopic surgery. *Obstet Gynecol Surv* 1991; 46: 196.

Taylor PJ, Hamou JE. Hysteroscopy. *J Reprod Med* 1983; 28: 359.

Complications of hysteroscopy

JOHN S. HESLA

Faulty surgical techniques and inappropriate patient selection are the most frequent causes of adverse sequelae from hysteroscopy. The etiologies and therapies of the more common complications of hysteroscopy will be discussed in this chapter.

INFECTION

A careful history and pelvic examination are essential prior to the performance of hysteroscopy in order to identify an occult or overt infection. The surgical procedure should not be performed if the patient has a recent history of pelvic inflammatory disease or displays adnexal tenderness on bimanual examination. The gaseous or liquid medium used for distension of the uterine cavity predisposes such patients to the development of salpingitis or acute peritonitis. In addition, carbon dioxide insufflation of the endometrial cavity has been reported to cause rupture of a hydrosalpinx.

Infection can spread from the lower genital tract to the fallopian tubes by direct extension from the endometrium or by the lymphatic or vascular system. Bacteria are carried from the cervix into the uterine cavity by the tip of the hysteroscope; nevertheless, the incidence of clinical infection is extremely low — less than two in 1000 in one series [1]. The hysteroscopic equipment must be disinfected by an iodophor or glutaraldehyde solution that has the capability of killing all microorganisms, including Gram-positive and -negative bacteria, fungi, mycobacteria, and lipophilic and hydrophilic viruses. Sterilization is not essential. The instruments are rinsed completely after disinfection to remove chemicals that may irritate the epithelial surfaces of the genital tract [2].

If the patient develops a pelvic infection after hysteroscopy, broad-spectrum antibiotic therapy should be instituted as soon as possible. If the infection is minor and there are no peritoneal signs, outpatient therapy is acceptable. However, when acute peritonitis is present, parenteral antibiotics must be administered and other unusual causes of posthysteroscopy fever and pain should be strongly considered, such as an inadvertent uterine perforation with associated bowel injury or the development of an adnexal abscess.

BLEEDING

The endoscopic field of view may be obscured by bleeding that arises from cervical dilatation, minor endometrial trauma, or during a therapeutic hysteroscopic procedure. Observation should commence as the sheath and hysteroscope are inserted into the endocervical canal. The image may be clouded or reddened due to juxtaposition of the lens objective to the uterine wall, inadequate distention of the endometrial cavity, or adherence of blood or mucus to the lens. Because of possible increased bleeding or accidental injury to the uterine wall, the hysteroscopic instruments should not be advanced blindly. Heavy bleeding precludes a satisfactory examination, even when the visualizing medium used is 32% dextran 70 (Hyskon), a fluid immiscible with blood.

Mild uterine bleeding may commonly occur for several days following hysteroscopy, particularly when a therapeutic procedure has been performed. Clinically significant postoperative hemorrhage is rare but may develop following resection of a submucous myoma or a uterine septum. Insertion of a Silastic intrauterine balloon or an inflated no. 16 Foley catheter for 6–72 hours should tamponade the endometrium [2]. Electrocoagulation of bleeding uterine vessels is unnecessary and possibly hazardous.

Patients with clinically significant postoperative bleeding who did not undergo concurrent laparoscopy during the hysteroscopic procedure should be subjected to this diagnostic study (Fig. 71.1). Hemostasis of the perforation site may be achieved via laparoscopic cauterization or suture placement. If this is

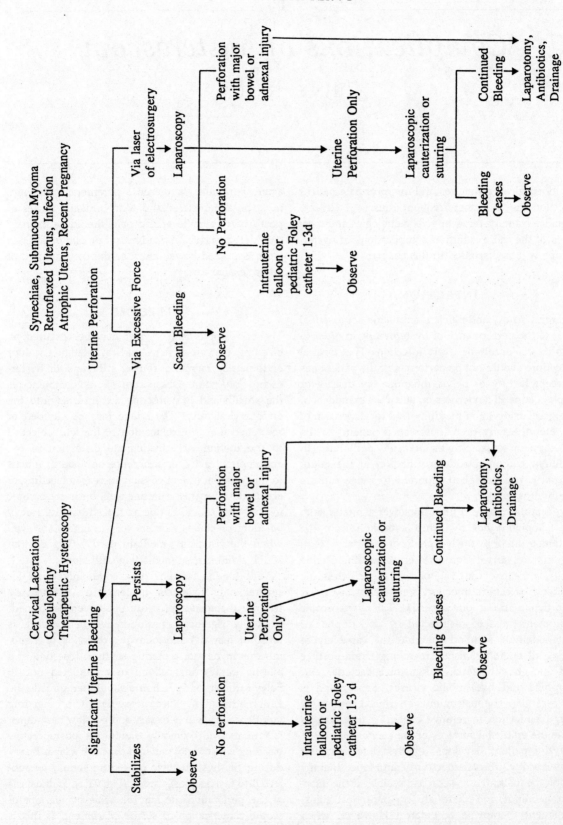

Fig. 71.1 Approach to hysteroscopic complications.

unsuccessful, a laparotomy should be performed.

An additional cause of postoperative uterine bleeding and hemoptysis is the coagulopathy that may arise from the vascular intravasation of dextran. Clotting studies should be performed in patients who manifest signs of a falling hematocrit.

Laser ablation of the endometrium by direct application of the fiberoptic guide to the tissue may cut into the myometrium and sever vessels anywhere within the uterus. Bleeding arises when the uterine distending medium no longer acts as a tamponade to the open vessels. With a nontouch technique, the lack of endometrial contact yields a greater degree of cauterization of bleeding vessel and less possibility of cutting into the myometrium [2]. Nevertheless, total amenorrhea is more often accomplished by the touch approach.

A hematometra may develop following hysteroscopic laser ablation of the endometrium. This rare occurrence may be prevented by sounding the uterus 1 month after the procedure to allow the egress of any retained fluid.

TRAUMA

Trauma to the genital tract may occur at any point during the hysteroscopic procedure. Excessive traction on the tenaculum results in a cervical laceration. Forceful dilation of the endocervical canal may cause bleeding, creation of a false passage, or perforation of the lower uterine segment [2].

The risk of uterine perforation is small except in those patients in whom the usual landmarks of the endocervical canal and uterine cavity are obscured. Synechiae or a large submucous myoma may predispose the patient to a greater chance of traumatic injury; in such circumstances the endoscope is more likely to be advanced without panoramic vision or with excessive force. Patients with a retroflexed uterus or atrophic cavity are also at greater risk. In addition, uterine perforations are more frequent during therapeutic procedures than diagnostic examinations. Lysis of severe intrauterine adhesions with scissors, laser, or the resectoscope, excision of a uterine septum or submucous myoma, and tubal cannulation may be effectively guided by concomitant laparoscopic monitoring of the uterine wall. To reiterate, the hysteroscope should be advanced inside the endometrial cavity only under direct visualization.

Uterine perforation does take place on occasion despite careful technique. Bleeding from these wounds is usually minimal. Lateral puncture wounds involving the uterine vasculature are rare. Withdrawal of the hysteroscope results in contraction and closure of the myometrial defect. Unless there is concern that a bowel injury has occurred, laparotomy is seldom required. The need for a laparoscopic examination varies depending upon the circumstances of the injury.

If the uterine perforation occurs during a hysteroscopic examination for retained placental tissue, uterine evacuation may be completed under laparoscopic guidance. Any injured patient should be observed for evidence of abdominal bleeding for several hours prior to discharge. She should be informed about the complication but reassured that the consequences are minimal. All tissue obtained during an operative hysteroscopic procedure should be reviewed by the pathologist, as unintentional bowel biopsy has been reported.

Energy-related injuries of the peritoneal cavity infrequently arise when the uterine wall is perforated during hysteroscopy. The laser fiber is relatively sharp and can easily penetrate the soft uterus, particularly if the laser is being fired while the fiber is being advanced. Electrocautery instruments also can be damaging. Intestinal injury is more likely when adhesions extend from the bowel to the fundus. In addition, the bowel may be draped over the uterus by chance, although the pneumoperitoneum created for laparoscopy usually displaces such a bowel loop. Thermal injury is possible during electrosurgical hysteroscopy even without perforation when a thin myometrial layer is inadequate to prevent heating of the uterine serosa. If laparoscopy reveals evidence of a superficial serosal burn of the bowel smaller than 1 cm in size, the patient may be observed for developing peritonitis while hospitalized for a 3–4-day period. Larger bowel burns as well as hysteroscopic puncture wounds must be repaired immediately. End-to-end anastomosis is usually required, although a small defect created by a puncture injury may only need to be oversewn. Drainage of pelvic and subdiaphragmatic areas and broad-spectrum antibiotic coverage are mandatory for cases of fecal contamination.

COMPLICATIONS FROM DISTENDING MEDIA

CO_2 is a safe distending medium for hysteroscopy. Arterial pH, partial pressure of CO_2 (Pco_2), and electrocardiograms are unchanged from baseline

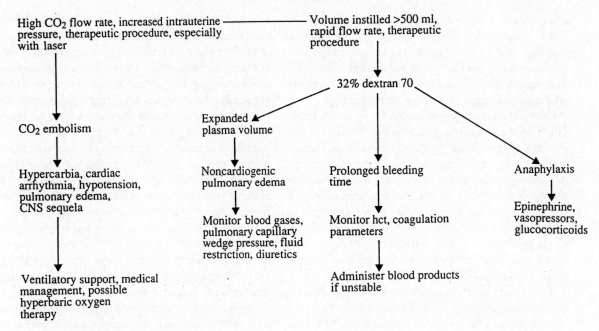

Fig. 71.2 Risk factors associated with distending media.

studies in patients undergoing CO_2 hysteroscopy [2]. However, intravasation is a potential risk (Fig. 71.2). Gas bubbles have been seen in the vessels of the infundibulopelvic kligaments in hysteroscopy patients undergoing simultaneous laparoscopy [3]. The total amount of gas insufflated is not the decisive factor, because CO_2 is readily transported in the blood and expired on the first passage through the lungs. Toxic complications are much more likely to occur when the flow rate is increased.

Rapid instillation of CO_2 may lead to hypercarbia and acidosis, cardiac arrhythmias, a fall in arterial blood pressure, superior vena cava syndrome, and death by pulmonary embolism [3]. Cardiovascular collapse following gas embolization results mainly from obstruction to right ventricular outflow, direct mechanical blockade by a bubble, or by the development of pulmonary hypertension in response to pulmonary embolization. A decrease in end-tidal CO_2 and sudden onset of collapse point to a massive embolism which initially obstructs blood flow proximal to the blood alveolar interface. Pulmonary edema is a well-described consequence of venous gas embolism.

The manifestations of cerebral gas embolism can be quite variable and include sudden death, coma, seizure, visual disturbance, confusion, personality change, aphasia, vertigo, headache, and focal sensory or motor deficits. Hyperbaric oxygen therapy is considered the treatment of choice for cerebral gas embolism.

Carbon dioxide or other gaseous media cannot be used when a sheathed fiber laser (e.g., Nd:YAG) is used to ablate the endometrial cavity. The disruption of the endometrium permits absorption of the gas through open venous sinuses and may lead to embolism. Only liquid should be instilled into the uterine cavity if the coaxial quartz fiber laser system is used.

The risk of pulmonary embolism is minimal using a controlled gas delivery system. The flow rate should be limited to 100 ml/min and the intrauterine pressure should not exceed 200 mmHg [3]. Hence, the insufflator that is used for laparoscopy cannot be used to distend the uterus during hysteroscopy because the uterus cannot tolerate the usual 1 to 2 l/min flow rate. If free CO_2 is present in the heart chambers during a contraction, a characteristic metallic heart sound may be auscultated. This may appropriately signal a temporary discontinuation of the procedure until the sound resolves.

The flow of gas through the fallopian tubes and into the peritoneal cavity can cause some diaphragmatic irritation. Mild shoulder pain is occasionally reported by the patient.

Hypercarbia is a potential side-effect of the use of nitrous oxide as the gaseous medium for uterine distention during hysteroscopy. This can lead to profound bradycardia; as a result, the use of nitrous oxide is contraindicated.

Dextrose 5% in water (D5W) can be used for some operative procedures, as this fluid permits clear visualization and avoids the stickiness of dextran around the operating instruments. However, the low viscosity of D5W results in rapid egress of the fluid through the cervix, which may obscure the operative field. In contrast with 32% dextran 70 (Hyskon), dextrose and normal saline readily mix with blood. Constant rinsing is necessary to prevent impairment of the view. The use of a hysteroscope with inflow and outflow channels allows the evacuation of mucus, clots, and debris from the endometrial cavity.

Besides that noted above, the low viscosity of D5W results in an increased intraperitoneal spillage via the fallopian tubes. Inappropriate perfusion of large quantities of D5W may produce water overload and electrolyte imbalance. Postoperative pleural effusions have been documented by chest radiographs in half of patients following intraperitoneal instillation of 400–500 ml of 10% dextran 40 [3]. This problem is easily prevented by limiting the quantity of the fluid used and by expediting the procedure.

High molecular weight dextran is optically clear, electrolyte-free, nonconductive, and biodegradable. Because it is immiscible with blood, it is the medium of choice for a therapeutic hysteroscopy procedure. Dextran manufactured for clinical use is not immunogenic, but sensitivity to dextran or bacterial contamination of commercial dextran has been associated with allergic reactions, including anaphylaxis [4]. The estimated incidence of anaphylactic reactions for all surgical procedures in which 32% dextran 70 is used is very low – only 1 per 10 000 cases [3]. Because of this remote albeit severe complication, it is advisable to have an intravenous line available when Hyskon is being used. Treatment of the anaphylactoid state includes the administration of epinephrine, vasopressors, and corticoids.

Prolongation of bleeding time is a recognized side-effect of vascular intravasation of large volumes of Hyskon during operative hysteroscopy. Open vascular channels that arise from endometrial dissection or ablation can increase absorption of 32% dextran 70. This causes expansion of the plasma volume and predisposes the patient to develop pulmonary edema. In addition, Hyskon may have a direct toxic effect on the pulmonary capillaries and promote interstitial pulmonary edema [5].

The inflow and outflow of 32% dextran 70 should be measured while performing hysteroscopy. If possible, the amount of medium instilled during operative hysteroscopy should be limited to 300 ml at an infusion pressure of less than 150 mmHg [4]. When greater than 500 ml of Hyskon is instilled, central venous pressure monitoring is recommended. If the patient manifests signs of cardiopulmonary compromise, a hypervolemic state must be differentiated from transient cardiogenic pulmonary edema. Temporarily decompensated valvular disease, arrhythmias, and bronchospasm must be ruled out. Measurement of blood gases and pulmonary capillary wedge pressure must be serially performed to monitor the patient's status. Fluid restriction may be necessary. Furosemide may be administered as indicated.

ADHESION FORMATION FOLLOWING HYSTEROSCOPIC SURGERY

Although the risks of estrogen therapy following hysteroscopic resection of a uterine septum are minor, the endogenous estrogen rise during follicular development should be adequate to stimulate endometrial growth and reepithelization of the retracted septal walls. An intrauterine device (IUD) placed following division of the uterine septum may cause excessive bleeding and increase the chance of both uterine and tubal infection. Hence, IUD insertion and hormonal therapy do not seem to be needed to prevent intrauterine adhesions after hysteroscopic metroplasty.

Most authorities are placing a number 8 or 10 pediatric indwelling catheter with a 3–3.5 ml balloon, a silicone rubber balloon stent, or an IUD inside the uterine cavity for 1 week following hysteroscopic lysis of moderate to severe adhesions. In addition, conjugated estrogens are frequently administered at a dose of 2.5 mg twice daily for 60 consecutive days. A progestin is given during the final 10 days of estrogen intake to promote endometrial sloughing. This regimen is followed in an effort to minimize the chance of adhesion reformation — a complication of this procedure.

CONCLUSIONS

The incidence of complications following hysteroscopic surgery is very low. Observance of proper surgical technique and appropriate patient selection

CHAPTER 71

will minimize the occurrence of adverse sequelae. The hysteroscope should never be advanced blindly into the endometrial cavity. Adequate clarity of the field of vision is essential for safety. Concomitant laparoscopic evaluation of the uterine serosa may guide the person who is performing a therapeutic hysteroscopic procedure. The surgeon must be familiar with the advantages and disadvantages of the various instruments and distending media available for hysteroscopy in order to make the appropriate choices for each individual case.

REFERENCES

1 Salat-Baroux J, Hamou JE, Maillard G, Chourqui A, Verges P. Complications from microhysteroscopy. In: Siegler AM, Lindemann HJ, eds. *Hysteroscopy: Principles and Practice*. Philadelphia: JB Lippincott, 1984: 112.
2 Siegler AM, Valle RF. Therapeutic hysteroscopic procedures. *Fertil Steril* 1988; 50: 685.
3 Pellicer A, Diamond MP. Distending media for hysteroscopy. *Obstet Gynecol Clin North Am* 1988; 15: 23.
4 Leake JF, Murphy AA, Zacur HA. Noncardiogenic pulmonary edema: a complication of operative hysteroscopy. *Fertil Steril* 1987; 48: 497.
5 Valle RF, Sciarra JJ. Intrauterine adhesions: hysteroscopic diagnosis, classification, treatment, and reproductive outcome. *Am J Obstet Gynecol* 1988; 158: 1459.

Conventional semen analysis

GRACE M. CENTOLA

A semen analysis is generally one of the first steps in the series of diagnostic tests performed to evaluate the male partner of an infertile couple. Although considered an important part of a comprehensive couple-based fertility examination, it is not a test of actual fertility, but perhaps of potential fertility. The semen analysis, as such, is an accurate measure of sperm production, and a rough estimate of the functional capability of the spermatozoa. A diagnosis of sterility is obvious in the complete absence of sperm (azoospermia), but a definitive diagnosis of male factor infertility cannot always be made as a result of reduced concentration and motility.

Nevertheless, the routine office- or laboratory-based semen analysis is an important initial examination providing important information which will, at the very least, determine the direction of further clinical evaluations and treatments. The routine semen analysis is also relatively inexpensive, and easy to perform in a timely manner. It is important that a minimum of three semen analyses be performed at 3–4-week intervals to eliminate any unexplained variations. The data from all three analyses must be considered carefully prior to instituting any treatment plan.

The results of the analysis must be interpreted carefully, particularly since semen parameters can be easily influenced by a number of factors, such as abstinence time and collection technique, as well as the accuracy and precision of those performing the analysis. As with any clinical laboratory, standardized protocols for specimen collection, analysis, and reporting of results, that is, quality assurance and quality control, should be established. This chapter will discuss the semen parameters obtained from a conventional, manual analysis, the interpretation of these results, and briefly include subsequent steps for the clinician in the management of the subfertile male.

SPECIMEN COLLECTION

The semen specimen should be collected into a clean plastic specimen container after 2–3 days of sexual abstinence. There have been suggested abstinence periods of 24 hours [1], 3–5 days [2], and 2–7 days [3]. The 2–3 days of abstinence is preferred since less than 1 or 2 days or greater than 3 days may affect both the sperm count and motility as well as the morphology and the presence of contaminating cells and debris. Furthermore, the 2–3-day timeframe is generally thought to be the "normal" interval in sexually active couples. It is important for each facility to establish a standard abstinence period since variability in this time period may increase the variability in the semen analysis results and make comparisons between ejaculates of individual patients virtually impossible. Semen analysis reports indicating abstinence times of greater than 4 days or less than 1 day should be taken with caution, particularly for those not demonstrating parameters within or close to the normal range. A prolonged abstinence may result in increased debris and white blood cells in the semen, as well as decreased motility. An abstinence period of less than 1 day may result in decreased volume and concentration.

The specimen is generally collected by masturbation without the use of lubricants [3]. A seminal collection condom (SCD; Milex, Chicago) may be used for those patients opposed to masturbation for religious or personal reasons. Zavos has shown that the use of these collection condoms optimizes semen collection, particularly for the oligospermic man [4].

The specimen should be delivered to the facility within 30–35 min of ejaculation, and not exposed to extremes of hot or cold temperatures. Analysis should begin upon specimen arrival at the facility, or at approximately 30 min postejaculation if collected on site. Although sperm motility may be maintained at an optimum level even at 1 hour postejaculation, it is not recommended that specimens be held for longer than 35 min prior to analysis. Diminished motility may then be attributed to prolonged exposure of the spermatozoa to seminal fluid and the lack of metabolic substrates for maintenance of motility. An incomplete specimen should be discarded since the results may be misleading.

INTERPRETATION OF THE SEMEN ANALYSIS RESULTS

Table 72.1 indicates the normal range of semen parameters. Each individual value should not be taken absolutely. Rather these parameters should be considered collectively to determine further evaluations or therapies.

Physical characteristics

Freshly ejaculated semen is a thick coagulum, which at 37°C, or even ambient temperature, liquefies within 5–30 min of ejaculation. The significance of non-liquefaction is unclear, particularly since human sperm can be found in the cervical mucus prior to semen liquefaction [1]. Increased viscosity, thickness, or consistency of the ejaculate is a different problem than nonliquefaction. Specimens with normal viscosity flow freely by drops from a pipette, while specimens with increased thickness do not flow freely, but remain as threads. Semen with hyperviscosity may inhibit sperm motility, and inhibit contact between the ejaculate and the cervix. Increased viscosity is often of unknown etiology, although a subclinical infection is occasionally implicated in this case. The significance of increased viscosity should be individually evaluated following assessment of sperm motility by both an examination of a prepared slide and, most importantly, by the postcoital examination. If the postcoital test reveals good sperm motility and

Table 72.1 Normal semen parameters obtained by conventional semen analysis. (From [3])

Parameter	Normal range
Semen volume	1.0–5.0 ml
pH	7.0–7.5
Sperm count	>20 million/ml
Total concentration	>40 million
Motility	>50%
Morphology	>50%
White blood cells	<1 million/ml

concentration in the mucus, then the increased viscosity is of no significance. However, if motility is reduced on the postcoital test, but normal on the visual examination of the semen, the female partner should be examined for cervical mucus incompatibility. If motility is reduced as a result of consistent hyperviscosity, sperm processing and intrauterine insemination (IUI) might be suggested. Supplementation of semen with nutrient medium and cervical artificial insemination might also be an option. α-Amylase suppositories inserted following intercourse have been recommended by some practitioners, with limited success. Increased liquid intake, as well as cough syrups with expectorant qualities, have also been suggested by some specialists for increased semen viscosity. However, the effectiveness of these therapies has not been scientifically proven and thus their efficacy remains questionable.

The volume of the ejaculate is normally 1–5 ml (Table 72.1). Reduced volume may be a significant cause of subfertility. Mattox and colleagues [5] showed that the fertilization rate and subsequent pregnancy rate in *in vitro* fertilization were reduced for hypovolemic semen specimens. Since 95% of the semen volume originates from the seminal vesicles and prostate [1,2], decreased ejaculate volume may suggest an abnormality of these organs. Men with congenital absence of the vas deferens and/or seminal vesicles may present with low semen volume, and this can be confirmed by analysis of the fructose content of the seminal fluid [3]. Reduced ejaculate volume may also be a sign of partial retrograde ejaculation. Examination of a postejaculatory urine should be done in all cases of low ejaculate volume. A few sperm may always be present from wash-out through the urethra. Significant numbers of spermatozoa in the urine may suggest dysfunction of the bladder neck. Urologic referral should be strongly considered in this case.

Hypervolemia, or increased ejaculate volume, is not as easily explained as its counterpart. Homologus artificial insemination of the entire ejaculate, or of the first portion of a split ejaculate, or withdrawal coitus, has been suggested for increased semen volume [1]. IUI of concentrated processed semen is also an option for these patients. Abstinence interval may affect the ejaculate volume and thus should be considered as a simple explanation. A repeat analysis may confirm or disprove increased or decreased volume parameters.

Routine semen analyses also measure ejaculate pH,

which should be in the range of 7.0–7.5. A pH significantly decreased or increased out of the normal range may signal infection or accessory gland dysfunction. If the pH remains out of the normal range on repeated analyses, complete urologic examination, with specific attention to the accessory glands (prostate, seminal vesicles) should be conducted before proceeding with further work-up or therapies.

Concentration and motility

The sperm concentration provides an accurate measure of a man's sperm production, while sperm motility is a rough measure of sperm functional capability. There is a wide fluctuation in the sperm count in any one individual [3]. Biweekly sperm concentrations in an individual demonstrated wide variations from oligospermic (<20 million/ml) to well within the normal range (>50 million/ml) [3]. Variations in the production of seminal plasma can affect sperm concentration. The time required for transport through the tubular system, 72–90 days, exposes spermatogenesis to environmental influences, such as injury, illness, and toxic exposure, which can ultimately affect concentration. Frequency of ejaculation and levels of stress or anxiety may also affect semen parameters.

The "normal" sperm count should be greater than 20 million per ml, with a total concentration, taking into account the ejaculate volume, of greater than 50 million. With the development of assisted reproductive techniques, as well as improved diagnostic tools to assess spermatozoa fertility, the low value of normal has been reduced over the past several years. Excessive sperm concentrations of greater than 150 million/ml should be of concern, particularly since motility might be compromised. In order to adequately assess the significance of the sperm count and concentration, one must consider all of the factors which might affect the count: abstinence period, semen volume, consistency or viscosity, for example. The viscosity might affect the reported concentration because of the inability of the laboratory to adequately sample the specimen for determining the count.

Generally, the sperm count should fall within the normal range on repeated analyses. A value within 5–7 million of the normal range (15 million versus 20 million, for example) is often received by the clinician and the patient with anxiety, but there is probably little difference between the two values. It is important to assess multiple ejaculates to determine

a pattern, and perhaps an average sperm count. A man with five normal semen analyses who has one abnormal semen analysis should not become alarmed. Likewise, a man with five abnormal analyses and one within the normal range should not be considered cured. Consistent low sperm count should be followed by assessment of serum follicle-stimulating hormone and luteinizing hormone, and plasma testosterone. If these are within normal limits, there is very little that can be done to stimulate increased sperm production. Clomiphene, tamoxifen, and halotestin treatment has been attempted by some clinicians with limited, if any, successful results. If the hormone levels are not within the normal range (i.e., elevated follicle-stimulating hormone, for example) a testicular biopsy to determine the activity of the germinal epithelium might be warranted. In these cases, referral to a urologist and/or medical endocrinologist specializing in reproductive disorders would be strongly suggested.

The percentage motility is an important parameter to consider in the semen analysis report. Recently, the sperm motility parameter has gained increasing importance in male fertility evaluations, perhaps even superseding sperm concentration in importance. The motile percentage should be 50% or greater, with an overall motility grade of 2 or better on a scale of 1 (lowest) to 4 (highest) for progressiveness. Once again, a motility on the order of 40% may not be of concern when one considers the sperm concentration. However, consistent motilities of less than 40% would be cause for further evaluations, and perhaps complete urologic examination. Ultimately, the postcoital test is a good measure of the efficiency of the spermatozoa. Both the sperm concentration and the motility must be sufficient to result in greater than 8–10 sperm with good progressive motility per high-power field on at least four separate fields.

When considering reduced sperm motility, the clinician initially may determine if the male frequents hot baths or hot tubs, or uses a waterbed. There is increasing evidence that sperm motility may be compromised by the increased temperature. A change in these recreational and sleeping habits may result in some improvement in sperm motility. Reduced motility is often accompanied by evidence of infection, such as agglutination and granular material in the seminal fluid coating the spermatozoa. Semen culture may confirm the evidence of infection. Appropriate treatment, which might include antibiotic therapy, might improve sperm motility.

Once again, reduced sperm motility must be considered relative to sperm concentration, abstinence period, and viscosity, all of which can affect the motility. Furthermore, the presence of antisperm antibodies — immunologic infertility — should be ruled out as a cause for consistently low motility. Immobilizing antibodies of the immunoglobulin G and A types have been found in seminal fluid bound to the spermatozoa tail and midpiece in approximately 8–10% of men presenting with reduced sperm motility [6].

The presence of a varicocele is a common cause of male subfertility in up to 41% of infertile men. The varicocele results from retrograde flow of blood into the internal spermatic vein, causing visible dilatation of the pampiniform venous plexus. It most commonly occurs on the left side (78%), but often affects both testes (20%) [7]. The pathophysiology and pathogenesis of the varicocele have yet to be clearly delineated and remain controversial. Theories include increased scrotal temperature and reflux of venous toxins. The presence of a clinical varicocele is often accompanied by decreased sperm count, and/or increased percentage of tapered sperm and immature sperm forms on morphologic assessment, as well as the reduced motility. Generally, in the absence of factors such as subclinical infection, waterbeds or hot tubs, and workplace hazards to account for the diminished motility and count, the patient should be examined for the presence of a varicocele, or referred to a urologist for complete urogenital examination. Compounding the controversy of the significance of the varicocele in infertility is the fact that not all men with a varicocele are deemed infertile. Fertile patients presenting for vasectomy often demonstrate varicoceles. Prior to consideration of the surgical repair of the varicocele, we often recommend assisted techniques such as IUI of washed concentrated sperm for six well-timed ovulation cycles. There is general consensus that in the case of a male partner demonstrating suboptimal semen quality and varicocele(s), and when the female partner has been thoroughly evaluated, a surgical repair should be seriously considered. Tinga and colleagues have shown a dramatic improvement in sperm count and motility following varicocele repair [8].

Treatment of low sperm count (oligospermia) and/or low motility (asthenospermia) in the absence of a varicocele or environmental factors has been variable, and perhaps empiric. Empiric antibiotic therapy, vitamin C, zinc, as well as clomiphene and vasodilators, have been used with questionable or limited success. Cervical artificial insemination has also been attempted. IUI of processed semen has recently been a common therapy for male factor. Semen-processing techniques are aimed at stimulating motility and concentrating the sperm count into a small volume prior to an IUI timed with the partner's ovulation. Success with IUI has also been variable, and in our program, has been 28% overall, with a monthly fecundibility of 12–14%. Ultimately, assisted reproductive technologies, such as *in vitro* fertilization, have been used, again with limited success for male factor patients [5].

Morphology

The morphologic assessment of the semen, examination of seminal cytology, is accomplished by microscopic examination of a stained slide by a well-trained technologist. The "normal" semen specimen should contain at least 50% normal sperm forms, with the remainder the so-called abnormal sperm forms, such as large, small, duplicate (tails or heads), amorphous, and immature forms. The morphologic assessment will also provide information on the presence of white blood cells, or white blood cell-like cells in the semen. Caution should be taken in this regard, since it is very difficult for even the experienced technologist to discern the immature or sperm precursor cell from a white blood cell, except for the most obvious cell types.

The morphologic analysis can give the clinician valuable information on the status of the germinal epithelium. If the normal forms consistently are less than 50%, or if there is a large percentage of particular forms, such as pin-head forms or spermatozoa with absence of acrosome caps, impairment in spermatogenesis and maturation is suspected. Hormone analysis, followed by testicular biopsy, would be strongly urged, and consultation with a reproductive specialist would be warranted.

CONCLUSIONS

Table 72.2 is a summary of the interpretation of the results obtained from the semen analysis. For each parameter out of the normal range, a possible explanation and therapy have been suggested. One must keep in mind that treatment should be individualized for each couple, and should take into consideration both female and male factors.

The conventional semen analysis can provide valuable information to the clinician during the work-up of the infertile couple. Multiple semen

Table 72.2 Summary of treatment for various problems with semen parameters

Problem	Treatment/consideration
Increased debris/white blood cells	Prolonged abstinence? Subclinical infection? Empiric antibiotics
Hyperviscosity	Subclinical infection? Empiric antibiotics, cough syrups, IUI Correlate with PCT
Hypovolemia	Retrograde ejaculation? Accessory gland dysfunction Urologic referral; AIH, IUI
Hypervolemia	Prolonged abstinence? AIH, withdrawal coitus, IUI
Decreased concentration; oligospermia	Injury, illness, toxic exposure; decreased abstinence; consider semen volume and viscosity Hormone replacement therapy Testicular biopsy; IUI, IVF
Decreased motility; asthenospermia	Analysis began >30 min postejaculation; exposure to cold; water bed, hot tub/baths Prolonged abstinence? Hyperviscosity? Subclinical infection? Antisperm antibodies? Varicocele? Correlate with PCT; AIH, IUI Empiric antibiotics, vitamins

Interpretation is based on a general summary of a minimum of three semen analyses performed at 3–4-week intervals. IUI, intrauterine insemination; PCT, postcoital test; AIH, artificial insemination by husband; IVF, *in vitro* fertilization.

analyses are needed to obtain accurate data on the semen parameters over time. The interpretation of the semen analysis report is critical. During the analysis of the results, multiple semen parameters constituting the entire analysis must be considered as a whole in order accurately to formulate a treatment plan. The results of the semen analysis should also be considered in light of the personal habits of the couple, as well as coital habits, and the postcoital test. The postcoital test results, considered with the results of the semen analyses, can provide important information to the clinician, which as a whole can determine the future course of evaluations and therapies.

REFERENCES

1 Howards SS. Semen analysis: routine techniques. *The Male Factor in Infertility: Pathophysiology, Evaluation and Treatment.* Postgraduate Course, 42nd Annual Clinical Meeting. The American Fertility Society, 1986.

2 Eliasson R. Semen analysis and laboratory workup. In: Cockett ATK, Urry R, eds. *Male Infertility, Workup, Treatment and Research.* New York: Grune & Stratton, 1976: 169–188.

3 World Health Organization. *WHO Laboratory Manual for the Examination of Human Semen and Semen–Cervical Mucus Interaction.* New York: Cambridge University Press, 1987.

4 Zavos PM. Seminal parameters of ejaculates collected from oligospermic and normospermic patients via masturbation and at intercourse with the use of silastic seminal fluid collection device. *Fertil Steril* 1985; 44: 517–520.

5 Mattox JH, Graham MC, Partridge AB, Marazzo DP. Impact of hypospermia on outcome in an IVF program. *J Androl* 1990; 11: 56.

6 Bronson R, Cooper G, Rosenfeld D. Sperm antibodies: their role in infertility. *Fertil Steril* 1984; 42: 171.

7 Lipshultz LL, Howards SS, eds. *Infertility in the Male.* New York: Churchill Livingstone, 1983.

8 Tinga DJ, Jager S, Bruijnen CLAH, Kremer J, Mensink HJ. Factors related to semen improvement and fertility after varicocele repair. *Fertil Steril* 1984; 41: 404.

73

Computer-assisted sperm movement analysis

KENNETH A. GINSBURG

INTRODUCTION

It has long been appreciated that the analysis of sperm motion is important in the study of sperm physiology and for the evaluation of known or suspected subfertile males. However, previous quantitative methods for this analysis — using such techniques as microcinematography, time-lapse photography, multiple-exposure photography, or manual image analysis — were quite cumbersome, labor-intensive, and costly. As a result, they found little clinical application and were used only in the research setting.

Over the last few years, self-contained, dedicated computerized sperm analysis systems have emerged as powerful tools for acquiring such motion data with unprecedented speed, ease, and efficiency. The systems now available commercially are capable of performing fine movement analysis on spermatozoa, reporting results for individual sperm cells and averaged measurements for an entire sperm population. These have already been extensively installed for use in both clinical and research settings, even as studies to evaluate this methodology and determine its diagnostic utility are in progress.

To provide the perspective necessary for the critical evaluation of videomicrographic computer-assisted sperm movement analysis (CASMA) systems by the clinician, this chapter will first discuss the principles and methods of operation, prior to a brief review of its validation, limitations, and clinical applications.

OPERATING PRINCIPLES AND METHODS

Central to an appreciation of computerized sperm analysis is an understanding of videomicrographic image digitization. Spermatozoa are observed under phase-contrast or dark-field microscopy with the image captured using a video camera and stored on video tape as appropriate (Fig. 73.1). Signals from the video camera (or video tape recorder) are then digitally processed in real time. The image processor maps each sperm head's position at an instant in time on a computerized representation of the microscope field, a process called digitization. This video page consists of a two-dimensional array of tiny picture elements (pixels), each with a unique address, which defines the pixel's location, and a state. The state of a pixel is a binary on or off condition corresponding to whether or not a portion of a sperm head overlies that location. Pixels are normally off unless turned on by the processor.

Instantaneous sequential video pages (Fig. 73.2) are obtained at a known frequency (the sampling frequency or framing rate) for a specified time interval. Current systems employ sampling frequencies of 15, 30, or 60 frames/second, and systems operating at 200 Hz are commercially available. Generally, sampling intervals of between 0.5 and 1 second are used. As the framing rate increases, more frames are captured per second and the time interval between successive video pages decreases. Hence more video images are taken of each sperm's track over the same sampling interval, and details of sperm motion can be recorded with higher resolution. On the other hand, higher sampling frequencies require more sophisticated optical systems, video cameras, digital processors, and computer hardware.

In a sense, the digitization process results in the creation and storage of a sequential series of computerized snapshots of the sample under the microscope, each one showing the instantaneous location of all sperm heads or other objects on the video page. When played back at the correct rate, this series of video pages would replay the paths of each sperm cell that moved through the microscope field over the sampling interval. Only the motion of sperm heads — not tails — is recorded for analysis.

The stored video pages are next analyzed by the computer system. Debris and cells other than sper-

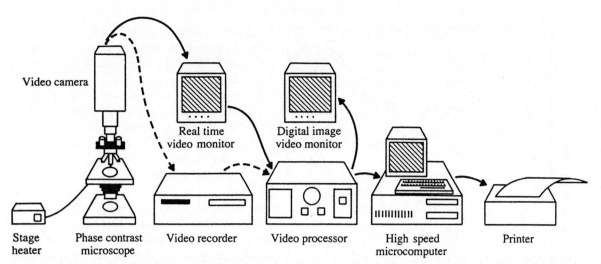

Fig. 73.1 Components of a generic computer-assisted sperm movement analysis system. The video signal (heavy line) passes from the camera to the video processor, in which digitization occurs. Alternatively, the signal can be recorded and the tape replayed later for analysis (dotted line). Both live and digital images are viewed on video monitors (in some systems these two images are superimposed on the same video screen). Digitized images are analyzed by the computer system, with results of the analysis stored on a computer database or printed.

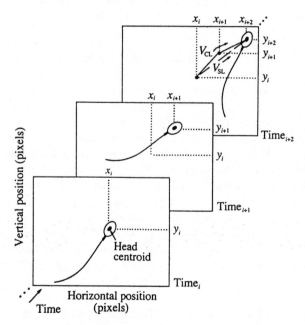

Fig. 73.2 Three sequential video pages tracking a single spermatozoan. The head centroid is mapped at pixel x_i, y_i on the first video page. An instant later at $time_{i+1}$ the sperm head centroid is located at pixel x_{i+1}, y_{i+1}; the time interval in seconds between video pages is 1/frame rate. On the last video page shown at $time_{i+2}$ the centroid has further advanced and is now located at pixel x_{i+2}, y_{i+2}. Linkage of centroids together by the path-finder algorithm defines sperm trajectories from which kinematic measurements are obtained, such as curvilinear (V_{CL}) and straight-line (V_{SL}) velocities shown.

matozoa are filtered out and ignored, based on their size and luminosity characteristics which differentiate them from sperm heads. Images of each sperm head are reduced to their digital outlines. The head centroid, a single pixel that defines the instantaneous "average" position of the sperm cell, is determined for each spermatozoa. The set of centroids denoting successive positions of a sperm head thus defines its swimming trajectory. The software links centroids and defines the path of each spermatozoon (whether motile or stationary) using proprietary path-finder algorithms. In addition to path definition, these algorithms must also sort out paths which cross and interpolate paths when centroids are lost by the digitization system. The details of these path-definition systems are complex and have been detailed elsewhere [1].

Once the path of each cell is defined, the system analyzes each sperm's translational (forward) and lateral motion. Trajectories of sperm cells are not straight, and with higher framing rates lateral deflections of the sperm heads around an average path are observed (Fig. 73.3), which are the consequence of flagellar beating. Various measured and derived kinematic parameters are obtained (Table 73.1). Measures of swimming speed include straight-line velocity (V_{SL}) and curvilinear velocity (V_{CL}). The ratio of straight-line to curvilinear velocity defines the linearity, or path straightness. A sperm cell that swims in a perfectly straight line with no deviation

439

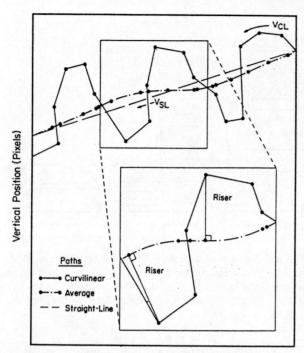

Paths

● — Curvilinear

● - ▪ - Average

— — — Straight-Line

Horizontal Position (Pixels)

Fig. 73.3 Diagrammatic representation of a digitized sperm trajectory and associated sperm paths. The spermatozoan enters the video image at upper right and is moving towards the left. Each dot along the curvilinear path denotes the location of a centroid from which the trajectory is defined. These centroid positions are also orthogonally projected onto the computer-derived average path. Each of the lines between centroids on the curvilinear and average path is termed a riser, as shown in the inset. These are used for calculation of maximum and mean amplitudes of lateral head displacement (see text).

from its straight-line path, i.e., $V_{SL} = V_{CL}$, will thus have a linearity of 1, while a sperm that has just completed an exact circle has an instantaneous linearity of 0. The distances (risers) between the actual path of the sperm head and a smoothed, average path are determined along each trajectory. Twice the maximum riser length in microns is the maximum amplitude of lateral head displacement, and twice the average riser length is the mean amplitude of lateral head displacement. The head beat frequency is the number of times the sperm head crosses the average path per second. Depending on the specific system used, these parameters may be reported as individual measurements for each cell identified, as averaged measurements for all motile cells, or both. Percentage motility is determined as the proportion of spermatozoa exceeding certain criteria which the user

minimally defines as a motile cell, e.g., V_{SL} greater than $10\,\mu$/second. Additionally, sperm concentration and motile cell concentration can be computed since the chamber volume is known.

In practice, the sample is analyzed shortly after liquefaction by loading a small aliquot (5 and $10\,\mu$l) into one of several calibrated chambers. It is maintained at 37°C during analysis using a microscope stage warmer. After digitization of the first microscope field, the stage is repositioned and the analysis repeated. In this way more sperm cells are analyzed than can be seen in one microscope field, and multiple fields can be examined to yield a cumulative CASMA analysis of several hundred cells. Either live or videotaped images can be analyzed; the latter allows tapes from distant sites to be analyzed centrally, reducing the need for duplicate instruments in large facilities and minimizing between-instrument variability.

SYSTEM VALIDATION AND LIMITATIONS

As new technologies are introduced first into research and then into clinical practice, method validation is necessary. Especially in implementing these bioassays of sperm function, the source and magnitude of errors in measurements must be determined before results should be interpreted. This requires recognition of the effects of varying testing conditions; determination of the within-sample reproducibility (coefficient of variation), which measures the precision of the system; and correlation of the results obtained with those of an accepted "gold standard," which relates to the accuracy of the system.

Beginning approximately 7 years ago, several groups have examined various aspects of videomicrographic CASMA system validation (Table 73.2). With a sufficient number of sperm cells sampled (at least 225) so that the results are statistically stable, the precision of CASMA instruments in measuring motion parameters has been shown to be acceptable. Notably, the precision of two different systems (CellSoft, CryoResources, New York, NY and Hamilton-Thorn HTM-2000, Hamilton-Thorn Research, Danvers, MA) for determination of motility, lateral head displacement, velocity and linearity has been found to agree closely [5,8]. Similar validation has been published for other instruments available commercially, such as the CellTrack/S system (Motion Analysis, Santa Rosa, CA).

However, these methods could be highly precise

Table 73.1 Measured and derived parameters of sperm motion derived by computer-assisted sperm movement analysis

Kinematic parameter	Explanation
Percentage motility	The proportion of all cells exceeding some minimal criterion set by the operator
Straight-line velocity	The distance in microns between the first and last centroid of a path divided by the sampling interval in seconds
Curvilinear velocity	The cumulative distance in microns between successive centroids of a path divided by the sampling interval in seconds
Average velocity	The distance in microns along the smoothed, average path defined by the computer divided by the sampling interval in seconds
Linearity	The ratio of straight-line to curvilinear velocity
Maximum amplitude of lateral head displacement	Twice the maximum riser distance in microns
Mean amplitude of lateral head displacement	Twice the mean riser distance in microns
Head beat frequency	The number of times the sperm head crosses the average path per second

yet possess significant systemic bias so as to affect the accuracy of measurements. To investigate accuracy, several studies have reported close agreement between computerized and manual determination of sperm concentration and motility, although one report [6] has documented differences between methods for which dilution of samples with seminal plasma was recommended. A recent publication [7] has demonstrated good correlation between CASMA and manual velocity and linearity measurements with one system in use. Similar studies with other instruments are needed to allow us to generalize from these encouraging results.

Limiting the widespread acceptance of this technology has been the early recognition by those active in its development that various problems, both technical and methodologic in nature, can significantly alter the quality of data generated. Digitized videomicrographic CASMA systems are influenced by variations in sample preparation (temperature, mixing, liquefaction); microscope magnification, optics and illumination [1]; chamber characteristics [9]; sampling frequency and interval [10]; and other aspects of

software design and set-up. For example, at low sperm densities one system was shown to overestimate sperm concentration by approximately 30%, probably because the nonsperm particles in semen were confused with spermatozoa by the imaging system [4]. As sperm densities increase and sampling intervals shorten, velocity measurements have been shown to be affected as well. Variation in CASMA measurements obtained from videotaped samples analyzed by different technicians has been reported [11].

It is thus apparent that while a body of data is beginning to accumulate which reassures us that these instruments can provide precise and reliable measurements, standardization of conditions for CASMA is critical. These standards must include determination of correct procedures for specimen handling and preparation, optical systems, digitization hardware, software algorithms for path definition and smoothing, and software settings of user-defined operating conditions. Optimal conditions will, in addition, vary depending on whether spermatozoa are studied in seminal plasma or in media after

Table 73.2 Representive early validation studies for various computer-assisted sperm movement analysis systems available commercially

Authors	Year reported	System studied	Conclusions
Katz et al. [1]	1985	CellTrack*	Phase-contrast illumination produced better images for digitization; errors in sperm centroid determination are associated with different edge detection algorithms; sampling frequency and magnification can influence results
Mathur et al. [2]	1986	CellSoft[†]	Good correlations between manual and computer-assisted sperm counts and motility; kinematic measurements obtained by different operator agreed closely
Knuth et al. [3]	1987	CellSoft	Kinematic measurements are infuenced by gray scale, number of frames analyzed and minimum number of frames analyzed for velocity measurements
Vantman et al. [4]	1988	CellSoft	Good correlations between manual and computer-assisted sperm counts and motility; acceptable precision for count and percentage motility; overestimation of count at low sperm density; velocity determinations influenced by sperm density and number of track points used to obtain trajectories.
Ginsburg et al. [5]	1988	CellSoft	A minimum of 225 sperm cells were needed for statistically stable kinematic results; analyzing four fields in triplicate yielded low intrasample coefficient of variation; instrument precision was acceptable for most kinematic measurements
Mortimer et al. [6]	1988	CellSoft	Nonsystematic differences were found between computerized and manual sperm concentration and motility determinations
Olds-Clarke et al. [7]	1990	Hamilton-Thorn[‡]	Percentage motility, linearity and curvilinear velocity measurements were highly correlated between manual and computerized determination systems

* CellTrack/S system, Motion Analysis, Santa Rosa, CA.
[†] CellSoft system, CryoResources, New York, NY.
[‡] Hamilton-Thorn motility analyzer, Hamilton-Thorn Research, Danvers, MA.

washing. Until such standards have been adopted, comparing computerized motion data between laboratories is impossible. In addition, statistically reliable normative data obtained from large fertile populations, or from homogeneous populations of infertile men with carefully defined problems, do not exist. Since normal values and ranges for these measurements are not yet defined, one must be cautious at present when utilizing these data for clinical infertility evaluation.

CLINICAL APPLICATIONS OF VIDEOMICROGRAPHIC SPERM MOTION ANALYSIS

The study of sperm motility has potential importance on a number of levels in science and medicine. To the cell biologist, disordered motility patterns may reflect changes in genomic organization, subcellular structure, or metabolism. The physiologist is concerned more with the effects of altered motility on sperm transport and sperm–oocyte interaction. Clinicians hope to use CASMA to confirm fertility or diagnose male infertility.

The nature of this relationship between movement and the functional competence of spermatozoa is unsettled at present. It is possible that movement patterns may be most important in determining whether the sperm can migrate to the site of fertilization. Alternatively, it may be that the disordered motility is reflective of a defect in spermatogenesis or epididymal maturation. This defect, in turn, would lead to the production of spermatozoa that are physiologically abnormal in other ways, and it is these other abnormalities that negatively impact upon the fertilization process.

Using manual recording and measuring methods, various studies have documented differences in motion parameters between fertile and infertile semen samples. To extend this earlier work, both these and new relationships are now being evaluated using videomicrographic CASMA technology. Several reports have documented differences in movement measurements between fertile and infertile sperm in semen. The presence of hyperactivated sperm motility — an apparent endpoint in the capacitation process that coincides with the capacity for acrosome reaction — has been identified using videomicrographic CASMA [12,13]. Altered sperm movement appears to be related to abnormalities in such diagnostic markers as mucus [14] or zona-free hamster oocyte penetration [15]. Similar relationships between sperm movement and human oocyte *in vitro* fertilization are currently under study. These instruments are also useful in the investigation of human and animal sperm movement under various physiologic, pathologic, and pharmacologic conditions in the laboratory; some have even used alterations in sperm movement as endpoints in systems for investigating possible toxic effects of drugs or environmental agents.

It is thus apparent that CASMA instruments provide the opportunity quantitatively to describe sperm movement in ways that were not possible a decade ago. The acquisition of these large volumes of data should provide insight into sperm physiology and function which will have meaningful clinical applications. After some of the problems detailed above have been addressed and standards developed, videomicrographic kinematic measurements will be recognized in the future as important diagnostic tests for the routine evaluation of male infertility.

REFERENCES

1 Katz DF, Davis RO, Delandmeter BA, Overstreet JW. Real-time analysis of sperm motion using automatic video image digitization. *Comp Method Prog Biomed* 1985; 21: 173.

2 Mathur S, Carlton M, Ziegler J, Rust PF, Williamson HO. A computerized sperm motion analysis. *Fertil Steril* 1986; 46: 484.

3 Knuth UA, Yeung C-H, Nieschlag E. Computerized semen analysis: objective measurement of sperm characteristics is biased by subjective parameter setting. *Fertil Steril* 1987; 48: 118.

4 Vantman D, Koukoulis G, Dennison L, Zinaman M, Sherins RJ. Computer-assisted semen analysis: evaluation of method and assessment of the influence of sperm concentration on linear velocity determination. *Fertil Steril* 1988; 49: 510.

5 Ginsburg KA, Moghissi KS, Abel EL. Computer-assisted human semen analysis sampling errors and reproducibility. *J Androl* 1988; 9: 82.

6 Mortimer D, Goel N, Shu MA. Evaluation of the CellSoft automated semen analysis system in a routine laboratory setting. *Fertil Steril* 1988; 50: 960.

7 Olds-Clarke P, Baer HM, Gerber WL. Human sperm motion analysis by automatic (Hamilton-Thorn Motility Analyzer) and manual (Image-80) digitization systems. *J Androl* 1990; 11: 52.

8 Pedigo NG, Vernon MW, Curry TE. Characterization of a computerized semen analysis system. *Fertil Steril* 1989; 52: 659.

9 Ginsburg KA, Armant DR. Influence of chamber characteristics on the reliability and sperm concentration and movement measurements obtained by manual and videomicrographic analysis. *Fertil Steril* 1990; 53: 882.

10 Mortimer D, Serres C, Mortimer ST, Jouannet P. Influence of image sampling frequency on the perceived movement characteristics of progressively motile human spermatozoa. *Gamete Res* 1988; 20: 313.

11 Levine RJ, Mathew RM, Brown MH *et al.* Computer-assisted semen analysis: results vary across technicians who prepare videotapes. *Fertil Steril* 1989; 52: 673.

12 Ginsburg KA, Sacco AG, Moghissi KS, Sorovetz S. Variation of movement characteristics with washing and capacitation of spermatozoa. I. Univariate statistical analysis and detection of sperm hyperactivation. *Fertil Steril* 1989; 51: 869.

13 Mack SO, Wolf DP, Tash JS. Quantitation of specific parameters of motility in large numbers of human sperm by digital image processing. *Biol Reprod* 1988; 38: 270.

14 Daru J, Williamson HO, Rust PF, Homm RJ, Mathur S. A computerized postcoital test of sperm motility: comparison with clinical postcoital test and correlations with sperm antibodies. *Arch Androl* 1988; 21: 189.

15 Ginsburg KA, Sacco AG, Ager JW, Moghissi KS. Variation of movement characteristics with washing and capacitation of spermatozoa. II. Multivariate statistical analysis and prediction of sperm penetrating ability. *Fertil Steril* 1990; 53: 704.

Part VIII

Treatment of the female

Ovulation induction: clomiphene

RICHARD J. WORLEY

Clomiphene citrate (CC) is a safe, effective, easily administered, and relatively inexpensive agent for use in treating ovulatory dysfunction. The drug was first synthesized in 1956, studied in clinical trials in 1961, and approved for clinical use in 1967. Its use in the treatment of infertility due to oligoanovulation is well within the purview of all experienced gynecologists. In addition, those particularly interested in and dedicated to the management of complicated ovulating regimens can now utilize luteinizing hormone (LH) detection kits, ultrasound, and steroid assays to develop and monitor highly modified CC regimens to produce ovulation and pregnancies in women for whom human menopausal gonadotropin (hMG) therapy would formerly have been required. Two preparations of CC with well-established records of efficacy are Clomid and Serophene.

INDICATIONS

After 30 years of use and study, the sites and mechanism of action whereby CC stimulates ovarian function are still unclear, but the vital consequence of its action is an increase in pituitary gonadotropin release. Hence, CC is able to generate follicular maturation and ovulation in those with estrogenic chronic anovulation, produce more timely ovulation in women with oligoovulation, correct luteal-phase inadequacy by enhancing follicular development, and produce intentional multiple follicle development when needed.

Chronic anovulation

In parlance this term refers not to all women who fail to ovulate, but specifically to those with normal or inappropriate gonadotropin release that produces ovarian steroidogenesis, but no ovulation. Hence, the gonadotropin release is acyclic and the follicular

response limited, but estrogen is generated. The term chronic anovulation therefore does not refer to women with either hyper- or hypogonadal ovarian failure. Many women with this disorder, the prototype of which is polycystic ovary syndrome, exhibit high serum concentrations of LH and suppressed concentrations of follicle-stimulating hormone (FSH). While the LH release that results from CC administration in such patients is not particularly welcome, in most instances enough FSH release also occurs to initiate follicle growth and culminate in maturation and ovulation.

The clinical features of women with chronic anovulation are typically oligoamenorrhea, highly estrogenized vaginal epithelium and cervical mucus, and predictable uterine withdrawal bleeding after progestin administration. A serum prolactin assay is in order, since a significant minority of such patients harbor a pituitary prolactinoma. If the prolactin concentration is elevated, a thyroid-stimulating hormone (TSH) assay is required to rule out hypothyroidism as a cause of the hyperprolactinemia. Some practitioners routinely obtain a TSH assay along with the initial prolactin measurement to rule out occult thyroid disease. If the patient exhibits androgen excess one should also obtain serum dehydroepiandrosterone sulfate (DHEAS) and testosterone assays. The androgen assays may point to an unsuspected underlying disorder, but more often serve to direct the later course of treatment if the patient is initially refractory to CC treatment. Gonadotropin assays are not required in the usual evaluation and management of women with estrogenic chronic anovulation.

Oligoovulation

It is reasonable to consider women with oligoovulation as exhibiting a variant of chronic anovulation syndrome. The clinical findings are similar and the laboratory evaluation is the same. Since such patients may have a prior history of normal ovarian function or fertility, it is important to search for intercurrent disease. Weight gain is a relatively common cause of oligoovulation. Treatment with CC produces monthly ovulation, and hence, more frequent and predictable opportunities to conceive. In women who require artificial insemination, CC is invaluable in achieving a predictable ovulatory pattern in those who are oligoovulatory.

Defective luteal phase

Since a large body of evidence is consistent with the view that most instances of defective luteal phase are the result of, in essence, a defective follicular phase, CC can effectively correct the problem by augmenting follicular development, producing greater preovulatory estradiol generation, and consequently, more abundant postovulatory progesterone secretion. The criteria required to establish a diagnosis of defective luteal phase are controversial. This is an uncommon cause of infertility or early pregnancy loss, and hence, it is best searched for after all other usual fertility studies have been found normal. The diagnosis is classically made with a late secretory endometrial biopsy which is inadequately developed relative to the subsequent menstrual cycle. However, some prefer to identify and monitor treatment of the disorder with serum progesterone (P_4) assays rather than endometrial biopsy. The P_4 concentrations that define defective luteal phase are also controversial. One may infer the diagnosis when the midluteal concentration is less than 10–12 ng/ml. For details, see the section on complex clomiphene protocol, below.

Multiple follicle development

Clomiphene may be useful, and a far cheaper alternative to hMG injections, to produce intentional multiple follicle development. One use for such regimens is *in vitro* fertilization and related technologies. Another is superovulation induction (SOI), the intentional ovulation of more than one ovum combined with artificial insemination of the husband's sperm in the treatment of unexplained infertility. While the utility of SOI for this indication is uncertain, CC regimens may be as effective as hMG regimens, and they are far cheaper and less cumbersome. The rationale for SOI in the treatment of unexplained infertility is simply to provide more opportunities for conception each month.

CONTRAINDICATIONS

Absence of an indication is one contraindication to CC administration. The agent should not be employed as a fertility elixir. Pregnancy is another contraindication. While there is no evidence that CC is teratogenic in humans, its administration to a pregnant woman is at least embarrassing. One should always rule out pregnancy in oligoamenorrheic women before prescribing CC. Ovarian cysts that are small in size and number do not contraindicate giving CC, but large, numerous, or functional cysts do. Pelvic or ultrasonic examination should precede each course of CC. If the ovaries are estimated to be 5 cm or greater in diameter by bimanual examination, an ultrasound study should be done. If several cysts in the range of 20 mm or greater are found, it is probably wise to skip the cycle and perhaps to suppress ovarian function with an oral contraceptive as well. If a single large cyst (e.g., 18–30 mm) is present, it is helpful to obtain a serum estradiol (E_2) concentration. A value greater than 100 pg/ml probably reflects lingering function that could interfere with the response to CC, and hence, warrant skipping the cycle.

RISKS AND SIDE-EFFECTS

The principal risks of CC administration are multiple gestation and ovarian hyperstimulation. The incidence of multiple gestation is probably 6% or less when the least amount of CC adequate to produce ovulation is used. Ovarian hyperstimulation requiring medical attention is rare when careful ovarian surveillance is provided each cycle. Common side-effects of CC administration are not dangerous, but they can be bothersome enough that the patient will decline to take the drug. Vasomotor symptoms and visual disturbances are the most common symptoms resulting from CC use. They are uncommon when low doses are used.

BASIC CLOMIPHENE PROTOCOL

For ovulation induction in anovulatory or oligo-ovulatory women, 50 mg of CC is given on days 5 through 9 of either a spontaneous or progestin-induced cycle (Fig. 74.1). The couple should be instructed to have intercourse about every other day from approximately the 13th through 17th days of the cycle, and the patient should either record basal

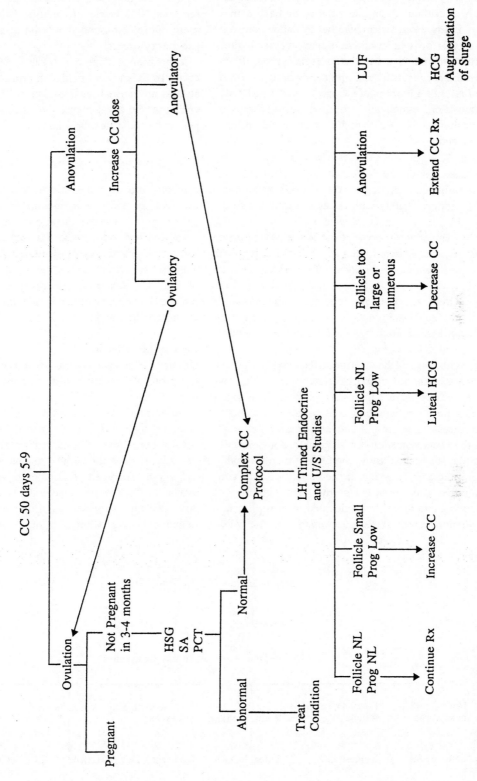

Fig. 74.1 Basic clomiphene protocol.

449

body temperature (BBT), be followed with ultrasound (with or without E_2 measurement), or have a mid-luteal P_4 assay to ascertain whether ovulation occurred. If the cycle is ovulatory and examination of the ovaries during menses is normal, the regimen should be repeated each month until pregnancy occurs. Within the first 3 or 4 months of CC treatment, a postcoital examination, semen analysis, and hysterosalpingo-gram should also be obtained, and abnormal findings addressed.

If the 50 mg dose of CC does not produce ovulation, the dose should be increased by 50 mg/day each cycle until ovulation occurs. While fertile cycles have been produced safely with doses as high as 250 mg/day, the yield using 200 mg or more is small. Hence, if ovulation does not occur at the 150 or 200 mg dose, it is wise to switch to the extended CC regimen (complex clomiphene protocol). If a postcoital exam-ination was normal at a lower but anovulatory dose of CC, the exam should be repeated at the ovulating dose. Postcoital examinations rendered abnormal by CC are best treated by intrauterine insemination (IUI) of washed sperm.

If ovulation still has not occurred, one maneuver that may enhance ovarian response to CC is low-dose dexamethasone suppression of adrenal androgen secretion. This is especially true in those with andro-gen excess. This simple and safe regimen consists of the administration of dexamethasone, 0.5 mg nightly, then reinstituting the CC regimen, probably beginning at 100 mg/day. If the patient's DEAS con-centration was measured at the outset because of hirsutism and found to be elevated, it is appropriate to demonstrate suitable suppression of the value

before resuming CC treatment. Such suppression requires 6–12 weeks of continuous low dose treat-ment. Dexamethasone should be discontinued once pregnancy occurs.

If pregnancy does not occur within four to six cycles of CC-induced ovulation and all other fertility studies are normal, or if ovulation has not occurred with the above regimens, the complex clomiphene protocol should next be followed.

COMPLEX CLOMIPHENE PROTOCOL

Women who do not conceive using the basic CC protocol, or those who require superovulation or treatment for defective luteal phase should undergo more detailed endocrine and biophysical study (Fig. 74.2). The principal components of this level of sur-veillance are urinary LH detection, ultrasonic studies of follicular maturation and collapse, and extended luteal-phase P_4 evaluation. Some would also perform an endometrial biopsy.

Urinary LH detection

Urinary LH detection is the key to accurate timing of the protocol. Ovulation occurs about 36 hours after onset of the LH surge. The inception of the surge is sleep-entrained in most women, but representative changes in urinary LH excretion do not occur until several hours later. Hence, testing at or after noon usually provides the earliest reliable evidence of an LH surge. There are a number of useful test kits available. To identify inception of the LH surge accurately, the patient should have at least 1 day of negative testing before the surge begins. If BBTs

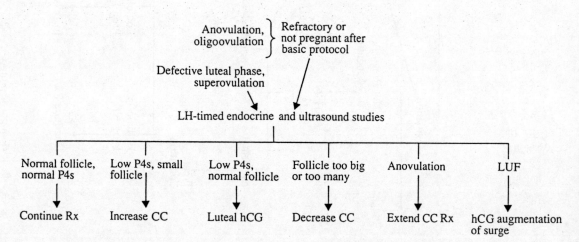

Fig. 74.2 Complex clomiphene protocol.

from ovulatory cycles are available, one can judge that the LH surge should begin about 48 hours before the temperature rise, and thus the patient should begin LH testing at least 1 day before that time. In general, however, it is suitable to ask patients using CC regimens to begin LH testing 3 days after their last day of medication. Testing before this time sometimes results in a false LH surge that reflects

Follicular monitoring

Ultrasonic measurement of follicle size at maturity followed by evidence of follicular collapse provides a basis for several therapeutic decisions in complicated cycles. In a cycle of good response to CC, an ultrasound study the day after inception of the LH surge should disclose one or more follicles 16–24 mm in diameter. If follicle size is at the low end or below this range, one should probably increase the dose of CC in the subsequent cycle. This is especially true if luteal-phase P_4 concentrations are less than optimal.

Two days after inception of the LH surge an ultrasound study should disclose collapse of one or more follicles. Ultrasonic studies of follicular collapse, however, may be inconclusive. Even when there is clear evidence of collapse, no technology can actually locate the ovum *in vivo*, so we are obliged to accept that all studies of ovulation and postovulatory function provide only secondary reflections of what we really want to know. While the diagnosis of luteinized unruptured follicle (LUF) syndrome is thus a difficult one to trust, when the follicle enlarges relentlessly after the LH surge without clouding of the fluid or crenation of the wall, LUF is probably a reasonable diagnosis to make. One can attempt to produce collapse in subsequent cycles by augmenting the LH surge with 10 000 IU of human chorionic gonadotropin (hCG), or 20 000 units if the lower dose is ineffective. If evidence of LUF persists, however, ovum retrieval for an assisted reproductive technology is warranted. Either gamete intrafallopian transfer (GIFT) or zygote intrafallopian transfer (ZIFT) should be considered.

The optimal window for fertility after CC treatment encompasses ovulation about 5–8 days after the last day of treatment. Hence, if the LH surge has not begun by the 6th day from the last tablet one should perform ultrasonic evaluation of follicular maturation the next day. If a follicle of clearly mature dimension is present, administer hCG 10 000 units intramuscularly and proceed with the rest of the protocol. In this way the patient will hopefully have timely and effective ovulation, and will know that ovulation is des-

tined each cycle to occur within a limited window of time. If follicle size is small 6 days after the last treatment, it is appropriate to discontinue the present cycle and increase the dose of CC in the next cycle.

Luteal-phase P_4 evaluation

A thorough discussion of the nature and importance of the luteal-phase defect is provided elsewhere. Some study beyond a single midluteal P_4 assay, however, is warranted at this juncture. Because of the expense, pain, and potential for misinterpretation of endometrial biopsy, one can consider using extended P_4 assays for the complex protocol, measuring them the 5th, 8th, and 11th days after inception of the LH surge. Although a midluteal P_4 of 10 ng/ml or greater is normal, the value in cycles of conception is closer to 15 ng/ml, and in such cycles the flanking values (post LH surge days 5 and 11) are usually about 8–10 ng/ml. Hence, these are the values sought in complex CC cycles.

USING THE COMPLEX PROTOCOL

Normal follicle, normal P_4s

If follicle size at maturation is normal, there is subsequent evidence of collapse, and luteal P_4 concentrations are normal, continue the effort to conceive.

Small follicle, low P_4s

In this circumstance, increase the dose of CC. There is a clear relationship between dose of CC, follicle size at maturity, and postovulatory P_4 concentration.

Normal follicle, low P_4s

Increasing the dose of CC in this patient will likely produce overly large or numerous follicles. The best treatment options are progesterone supplementation (25–50 mg vaginal suppositories b.i.d.), or luteal hCG injections given as 1000 IU intramuscularly every other day for five injections beginning 2 days after the LH surge begins.

Follicle too big or too many

Decrease the dose of CC to as little as 25 mg/day or as few as 3 days of treatment. In some patients, ultrasound evaluation before one anticipates a spontaneous surge may disclose that the follicle is already mature, and hence could be ovulated with a 10 000 IU injection of hCG.

Anovulation

The anovulatory woman who does not ovulate with traditional CC treatment should first have a serum FSH assay performed. If it is below the range of normal, question whether she has hypothalamic–pituitary disease, and evaluate as appropriate. If the FSH is near or above the upper range of normal, the patient may have early ovarian refractoriness or failure, and hence be less likely to have a successful response to any ovulating agent. Do not forget to try low-dose dexamethasone suppression for androgenized CC refractory women (see above). If none of the preceding applies, the patient is a candidate for extended CC therapy.

Extended CC therapy

Lengthening the course of CC may produce follicular maturation in patients for whom the 5 day course does not suffice. The regimen requires ultrasound studies and hormonal monitoring of both E_2 and LH. The E_2 result should optimally be available the same day the specimen is obtained, or the next day at the latest. LH can be measured either in serum or with a urine test kit, but if measured in serum the result must be available the day it is collected. It is helpful to obtain a baseline serum E_2 assay just before starting the extended regimen. The regimen consists of up to 150 mg CC days 3 through 9 of the cycle, followed by a serum E_2 assay on day 10. If the E_2 concentration differs little from the baseline value it may be worth continuing the same dose of CC 3 more days and repeating the E_2, but if still not higher the effort should probably be abandoned. If the day 10 E_2 is

higher than baseline but less than 300 pg/ml, continue CC at the same dose until the E_2 concentration reaches 300 pg/ml, then begin ultrasound monitoring next day. If there is a follicle approaching maturity, begin daily LH monitoring and proceed as appropriate when a surge occurs. Continue ultrasound monitoring, however, to insure that the follicle does not grow beyond about 22 mm without a spontaneous LH surge. If the follicle is mature but no surge has occurred, administer 10 000 IU of hCG and follow the remainder of the complex CC protocol.

Luteinized unruptured follicle

With the caveats expressed above about LUF in mind, if the diagnosis seems clear, the complex CC protocol is a good way to assess the response to hCG augmentation of the LH surge. If timely follicular collapse does not occur at the 10 000 IU dose, one may try 20 000 IU the next cycle. If collapse still does not occur, ovum retrieval for an assisted technology should be considered.

FURTHER READING

Speroff L, Glass RH, Kase NG. Anovulation, and Induction of ovulation. *Clinical Gynecologic Endocrinology and Infertility*. 4th edn. Baltimore: Williams & Williams, 1989: 213–231, 583–609.

Speroff L, Archer DF. Induction of ovulation. *Semin Reprod Endocrinol* 1986; 4: 223–312.

Speroff L, Yuen HB. New concepts in the induction of ovulation. *Semin Reprod Endocrinol* 1990; 8: 145–264.

Yee B. Ovulation induction. *Infertil Reprod Med Clin North Am* 1990; 1: 1–218.

75

Ovulation induction: gonadotropins

MARCELLE I. CEDARS

Human menopausal gonadotropins (hMG) become appropriate therapy when simpler modalities have failed to yield repetitive ovulatory cycles or pregnancy in the face of ovulation. Several basic principles must be kept in mind: (1) do no harm; (2) nothing replaces practical, hands-on experience; (3) there is always more than one approach; and (4) use of objective criteria is required for decision making.

PATIENT SELECTION AND EVALUATION

The primary indication for ovulation induction is the absence of spontaneous ovulation or its infrequent occurrence in a woman actively seeking pregnancy. Anovulation represents a dysfunction of the intricately synchronized hypothalamic−pituitary−ovarian axis. It may be due to an inappropriate balance between the functions of the hypothalamus, pituitary, and ovaries, or to the primary failure of any of these glands. Understanding of the normal ovulatory physiology and the specific pathology in the individual patient is necessary in order to optimize therapy for induction of ovulation with pharmacologic agents.

Gonadotropins act directly on the ovaries, thereby obviating the need for a functional pituitary or hypothalamus. They therefore can be utilized in women who have disruptions in the normal hypothalamic−pituitary−ovarian axis and fail simpler modalities, but remain the only option in the patient with panhypopituitarism or isolated gonadotropin deficiency. The only requirement for their use is responsive ovarian tissue.

Careful history and physical examination in all patients is required. Determination of estrogen status is essential. In all cases of hypoestrogenism, follicle-stimulating hormone (FSH) level must be assessed. For the purpose of this discussion, elevated FSH levels in the face of hypoestrogenism indicate ovarian

failure, and preclude the use of hMG. To complete the laboratory evaluation of the patient with anovulation, determination of thyroid-stimulating hormone (TSH), prolactin, and dehydroepiandrosterone sulfate (DHEAS) would be in order. Abnormalities in any of these hormonal parameters may affect therapeutic decision making.

The simplest therapeutic modality should be utilized once the diagnosis for anovulation has been made. Treatment with gonadotropins, which increases the patient's commitment of time as well as financial and emotional reserves, should be used only after adequate attempts have been made to achieve ovulation and pregnancy with less involved techniques. Patients with hypogonadotropic hypogonadism should be treated with pulsatile gonadotropin-releasing hormone (GnRH). Bromocriptine remains the first-line drug for patients with hyperprolactinemia. Low-dose clomiphene citrate (CC) may also be given a trial in both of these groups of women. Patients who are estrogenized, but fail to ovulate, should be treated with CC with or without adrenal suppression or the use of human chorionic gonadotropin (hCG) as appropriate. For the patient who ovulates using one of these modalities, a minimum of 6 months of documented ovulatory cycles, with optimization of other fertility parameters is necessary before making the decision to use hMG therapy.

While it may be appropriate to utilize a short course (3 months) of simpler ovulation-inducing techniques in the young, anovulatory patient without immediate evaluation of other infertility parameters, the use of gonadotropins should be preceded by complete and thorough evaluation of other infertility factors. This includes assessment of sperm parameters and the exclusion of tubal−peritoneal factors which would interfere with conception. Any detected abnormalities should be treated, or at least optimized, prior to induction of ovulation with gonadotropins.

GETTING STARTED

Before instituting gonadotropin therapy in an office setting, adequate facilities for careful monitoring of the stimulation cycle are required. Access to rapid serum estradiol measurement on a daily basis is necessary. The availability of progesterone, luteinizing hormone (LH), and follicle-stimulating hormone (FSH) assays may also be helpful in certain situations but is not required in all instances. Appropriate personnel and equipment for ultrasound monitoring of the stimulation cycle are required. The newer transvaginal ultrasound probes appear to be superior for ovarian measurement. It is helpful to have a designated nurse clinician who serves as an intermediary for the infertile couple and can help in the logistics of the stimulation cycle. The gynecologist who considers giving gonadotropins in his/her office should strongly consider a period of preceptorship during which stimulation cycles could be observed and direct patient management undertaken.

Currently used preparations of hMG are purified from the urine of postmenopausal women and are available as Pergonal (second laboratories), with a 1 : 1 ratio of FSH : LH in 75 and 150 IU ampules, or as Metrodin with 75 IU FSH and <1 IU LH. Cost for a single 75 IU ampule of gonadotropins is $45–60 so that drug cost alone may exceed $1500 for a single cycle. The medication is reconstituted with diluent and given as an intramuscular (I.M.) injection. One ml diluent may be used for 1–2 ampules; 2 ml of diluent should be used for 3–4 ampules. Typically, a dose of more than 4 ampules is split into two daily injections. It is most efficient for the patient if her partner can be instructed in intramuscular injection technique to decrease her need for frequent office visits.

Adequate monitoring for safety and efficacy requires the combined use of both ultrasound and serum estradiol measurement. The timing interval between hMG injection and subsequent blood sampling will affect the estradiol results obtained and should be kept constant. The peak estrogen level occurs approximately 8–10 hours after injection. It is usually recommended that the hMG injection be given between 7 and 9 p.m. with blood sampling at 8 a.m. This allows determination of the estradiol level and adjustment in dosage to be performed within a single day.

All patients should undergo baseline ultrasound scanning to document the absence of follicular activity prior to the institution of gonadotropin therapy. Stimulatory protocols and daily dosage regimes should be individualized.

For the patient who is estrogenized but fails to ovulate with CC alone or in combination with dexamethasone or hCG, a combination of CC and hMG may be utilized. These patients will often respond unpredictably to hMG alone. The use of CC for the initial FSH stimulation of the cycle may decrease the risk of hyperstimulation by decreasing the salvage of small follicles prior to the institution of exogenous gonadotropin therapy. The total dosage of hMG, and hence the cycle cost, are also reduced with this regimen. For the patient who ovulates but fails to conceive on CC, hMG alone may be more appropriate. hMG–hCG should also be utilized for the patient with hypoestrogenism not responsive to other treatment modalities. Patients with normal ovulation and a diagnosis of unexplained infertility, endometriosis, or male factor infertility may benefit from a trial of hMG prior to progressing to assisted reproductive techniques and should also be treated with hMG–hCG.

MONITORING

Different schools of thought exist as to the relative roles played by ultrasound and estradiol measurement. One's individual approach may be dependent upon available facilities and individual expertise. One may let the estrogen level dictate the initial adjustment of dosage and timing of the first ultrasound. This appears to be most appropriate as biochemical evidence of follicular development precedes physical evidence by ultrasound. In this case, if no estrogen rise is seen after 4 days of a given hMG dose, the dose is increased by 1 ampule at 3–4-day intervals until a doubling of the estradiol level is noted. Ultrasound monitoring is then begun and the dosage maintained. Once the estradiol rise has been established, a semilogarithmic pattern can be expected. It is often helpful to plot this rise in order to predict cycle parameters and to insure the estrogen level will not exceed safety levels prior to follicular maturation.

When ultrasound is used as the principal mode of management determination, scanning is performed after 5 days of therapy. If no measurable development (follicle size <10 mm) is noted and the estradiol level is <100 pg/ml, the dosage is increased by 1 ampule. Once follicular development has reached

GONADOTROPINS

the 12—14 mm stage, the dosage is maintained and daily ultrasound monitoring is begun. Follicle diameter increases at a rate of approximately 2 mm/day.

Whether using estradiol or ultrasound primarily, serum estradiol measurement is critical to safe, successful monitoring of superovulation. There is a narrow margin of safety between adequate stimulation for conception and risk for complication, particularly hyperstimulation and multiple gestation. The target estradiol is between 1000 and 1500 pg/ml. This value, however must be correlated with the ultrasound evaluation. Increased number of follicles salvaged by hMG therapy may increase the estradiol value to the target zone while the leading follicles (oocytes) may not yet have reached maturity. In this case, continued stimulation and reassay of the estradiol is necessary. hCG may be given with caution when the estradiol is above this zone.

Estradiol level on the day of hCG administration appears to be the best predictor of possible hyperstimulation [1]. A level above 2500 pg/ml would preclude the use of hCG and cancel the cycle. Again, this is based on an approximate 12-hour interval between injection and blood sampling. If the interval has been 24 hours, the upper limit for estradiol would be considerably lower — approximately 1000—1500 pg/ml.

Ultrasound evaluation is also required on the day of hCG administration. While fairly constant growth can be predicted, it should not be considered adequate monitoring to determine timing of hCG based on predicted follicle growth and number without actual measurement. Given normal sperm parameters, the finding of more than three mature-size follicles would cancel the cycle in order to decrease the risk of multiple pregnancy. It is imperative to remember, and to counsel patients accordingly, that follicles less than mature-size may ovulate and yield fertilizable oocytes.

Once adequate stimulation is achieved in any given patient, subsequent cycles tend to be repetitive in terms of required gonadotropin dose for initiating follicular growth. Day-to-day parameters and the number of follicles stimulated may differ, necessitating careful monitoring of each cycle. The variation in bioactivity between Pergonal lots also increases cycle-to-cycle variation. Baseline scanning is especially critical after a cycle of hMG when persistent cystic dilatation of the ovaries may be present, and would prohibit institution of gonadotropin therapy. Some have even suggested routinely by-

passing a cycle between each attempted ovulation with gonadotropins.

TREATMENT PROTOCOLS

In the combined CC—hMG stimulation, CC at a dose of 100 mg is begun on day 3 of either a spontaneous or induced bleed and continued for 5 days. hMG, at 75—150 IU, is then added beginning on day 8. Ultrasound monitoring is begun following 2—3 days of hMG therapy and continued as dictated by biochemical and physical parameters. Once the dominant follicle or follicles reach a diameter of approximately 12—14 mm, ultrasound monitoring continues on a daily basis until follicular maturity is attained at a mean follicular diameter of 18—20 mm. Measurement of serum estradiol may be performed daily at this time and is required on the day of anticipated hCG administration. If criteria for hCG administration are met with respect to estradiol level and follicle size and number, 5000 units of hCG are given intramuscularly, with intercourse on the day of hCG administration, and intercourse or insemination, timed approximately 36 hours after injection.

Treatment with hMG—hCG should be individualized but an acceptable starting dose would be 2 ampules or 150 IU FSH/LH beginning on day 2 of menses or a progestin withdrawal bleed. Average duration of therapy is 7—10 days with ultrasound monitoring beginning approximately day 5 of therapy. Monitoring specifics have already been discussed. Again, once the dominant follicle is 12—14 mm in diameter, constant growth can be anticipated. hMG only stimulated follicles appear to achieve maturation at a smaller mean diameter (15—17 mm) than follicles stimulated by CC. Once follicle maturity is detected by ultrasound, again assuming estrogen and ultrasound safety parameters are not exceeded, 10 000 units of hCG are given intramuscularly. A starting dose of 2 ampules may lead to excessive stimulation in some patients with chronic anovulation. Careful monitoring and a knowledgeable willingness to cancel the cycle are necessary.

SUCCESS RATES

One should be able to expect an ovulation rate approaching 100%. Pregnancy rates in estrogenized women who have failed simpler treatment modalities are approximately 15–20% per cycle. Hypoestrogenized patients may conceive at a rate up to 35% per cycle. Cumulative pregnancy rates would appear to justify a 4-month trial of hMG [2]. While some pregnancies do occur after this time period, their small number would not appear to justify universal application of longer treatment trials. This is especially true in the patient over the age of 35.

NEW ALTERNATIVES AND ADJUVANTS TO GONADOTROPIN THERAPY

Recent evidence has suggested that patients who fail to respond to gonadotropins given by the intramuscular route may respond to pulsatile intravenous or subcutaneous therapy [3]. For the present time, this therapy should be restricted to research centers.

For the patient with polycystic ovarian syndrome (PCOS), hMG therapy may not yield a successful pregnancy despite the presence of ovulation. If hMG therapy fails to induce adequate follicle development or when cycle parameters are not optimal, dexamethasone may be added [4]. Although Evron et al. made no reference to DHEAS levels in their article, 74% of patients who had failed to conceive on hMG–hCG conceived within two to four cycles when 0.5 mg of dexamethasone was taken nightly in addition to the standard hMG regime. This combined treatment also utilized significantly less gonadotropin for equivalent or greater response, thereby decreasing the cost for a given cycle.

The introduction of GnRH agonists to the clinical practice of gynecology has enhanced our ability to treat estrogen-dependent conditions such as endometriosis and leiomyomas. In addition to suppression of ovarian estrogen, these potent agonists eliminate excessive androgen secretion from the ovary. Again, in patients with PCOS, these elevated androgens may lead to suboptimal response during attempted ovulation induction and may cause lower pregnancy rates. The use of GnRH agonists to suppress androgen secretion prior to the initiation of gonadotropin therapy may improve ovulation and pregnancy rates over hMG-only therapy in some patients [5].

Preparations of "pure" FSH were introduced specifically for use in the PCOS patient with chronic elevations of LH. Preliminary studies seemed to suggest a more predictable response could be achieved with increased pregnancy rates. This has not been borne out in subsequent studies. While FSH may be useful

in some patients with PCOS, a clearly documented advantage should preclude its routine use in PCOS patients at this time.

COMPLICATIONS

The most significant complication of gonadotropin therapy is the syndrome of severe ovarian hyperstimulation. Deaths from this entity are still reported every year. Although clearly related to high ovarian estrogen production, hyperstimulation, except in rare instances, will not develop without the ovulating dose of hCG. The specific pathogenesis of this syndrome is still unknown. The main pathophysiologic event is massive enlargement of the ovaries with "third-spacing" of fluids. Fluid shifts can be large and occur suddenly. Massive ascites and hydrothorax are typical of the clinical picture. Much of the subsequent physical compromise is due to this fluid shift with hypovolemia leading to prerenal azotemia, oliguria, and electrolyte imbalance. There may also be hemoconcentration with increased risk of thromboembolic catastrophe. During the resolution phase, volume overload may develop.

Symptoms typically appear 3–7 days after hCG injection. In the absence of pregnancy, resolution can be expected within 4–5 days. Patients with high estradiol levels, especially in the face of numerous small follicles (<12 mm), should be considered at risk. These patients should be monitored with daily weights and measurement of abdominal girth. A weight gain of 4 lb (2 kg) or an increase in abdominal girth of 4 cm in a single day warrants careful evaluation and baseline measurement of electrolytes, hematocrit, serum osmolality, and creatinine.

A 20 lb (9 kg) weight gain, massive ascites, respiratory compromise, or evidence of hemoconcentration (hematocrit >50) or renal insufficiency necessitates hospitalization. Lesser findings still require careful follow-up and pelvic rest to minimize the chance for ovarian torsion or trauma. Once the patient is hospitalized, management is primarily supportive. Fluid and electrolyte balance must be maintained. Plasma volume expanders may be necessary. Paracentesis has recently been advocated in the compromised patient. If utilized, it should be performed under ultrasound guidance to avoid ovarian damage and hemorrhage. Animal studies have found an improvement is symptoms with antiprostaglandin treatment. This beneficial effect has not been borne out in clinical trials. The lack of sufficient data to support their use in the face of the theoretic risk during the early weeks of gestation would preclude the routine use of antiprostaglandins.

Ovarian hyperstimulation syndrome is four times more likely to occur in conception cycles. The duration of symptoms is also prolonged with an ongoing pregnancy due to the persistent elevation of hCG. Hyperstimulation syndrome is still a self-limited process and, with close monitoring and supportive management, prognosis is generally good.

The occurrence of multiple gestation is the second complication associated with the use of gonadotropins. While twins may seem an acceptable risk, it behooves us to remember patients come for a single healthy pregnancy. It is also important to remember, despite the availability of selective termination, we should not knowingly put our patients in the position of having to make this difficult decision. Having just made these statements, it is impossible to eliminate the risk of multiple births. Classically, 25–30% of pregnancies were complicated by multiple gestation. The use of ultrasound monitoring appears to decrease this risk to 10–15%. Of these multiples, 95% are twins, with 5% being triplets or more.

It is imperative that patients be appropriately counseled and precautions taken to decrease the risk of multiple gestation. As above, hCG is typically withheld with more than three mature-size follicles. Practical experience with *in vitro* fertilization has shown us that mature oocytes can be obtained from follicles of small diameters. Limiting the number of mature-sized follicles to any specific number must therefore take into account the number and size of the secondary follicles. In borderline cases, the patient should be included in the decision-making process in an informed manner. Couples with a significant male factor component to their infertility may continue through a cycle with four to five mature-sized follicles with less risk of multiple gestation.

There appears to be a slight increase in the risk of ectopic gestation with ovarian superovulation. This may be related to the increased estrogen levels as it is known both estrogen and progesterone affect tubal motility. This risk may be significant to the patient with known tubal damage but always warrants careful follow-up of pregnant patients and early documentation of intrauterine pregnancy. The small possibility of a heterotropic pregnancy should also be kept in mind.

CONCLUSIONS

In summary, gonadotropins can be successfully utilized in the office setting to enhance fertility in patients unresponsive to simpler modalities of ovulation induction or as an intermediary step prior to assisted reproduction in patients with unexplained infertility or male factor infertility. Their appropriate usage requires a careful, thoughtful approach with the availability of both ultrasound and serum estradiol monitoring. There is as much art as there is science in the appropriate use of these agents and nothing replaces practical experience.

REFERENCES

1 Haning RV, Boehnlein LM, Carlson IH, Kuzma DL, Zweibel WJ. Diagnosis-specific serum 17β-estradiol (E$_2$) upper limits for treatment with menotropins using a ^{125}I direct E$_2$ assay. *Fertil Steril* 1984; 42: 882.

2 Dor J, Itzkowic DJ, Mashiach S, Lunenfeld B, Serr DM. Cumulative conception rates following gonadotropin therapy. *Am J Obstet Gynecol* 1980; 136: 102.

3 Yuen BH, Pride SM, Callegari PB, Leroux A, Moon YS. Clinical and endocrine response to pulsatile intravenous gonadotropins in refractory anovulation. *Obstet Gynecol* 1989; 74: 763.

4 Evron S, Navot D, Laufer N, Diamant YZ. Induction of ovulation with combined human gonadotropins and dexamethasone in women with polycystic ovarian disease. *Fertil Steril* 1983; 40: 183.

5 Dodson WC, Hughes CL, Whitesides DB, Riley AF. The effect of leuprolide acetate on ovulation induction with human menopausal gonadotropins in polycystic ovary syndrome. *J Clin Endocrinol Metab* 1987; 65: 95.

Ovarian hyperstimulation syndrome

RAY V. HANING JR

The ovarian hyperstimulation syndrome (OHS) is a constellation of symptoms and physiologic changes which sometimes follows treatments administered to induce ovulation. OHS has been divided into mild, moderate, and severe forms:

1 *Mild hyperstimulation*: ovaries no larger than 5 × 5 cm with no marked weight gain.

2 *Moderate hyperstimulation*: ovaries enlarged up to 10 × 10 cm and weight gain up to 10 lb (4.54 kg).

3 *Severe hyperstimulation*: ovaries over 10 × 10 cm and weight gain over 20 lb (9 kg).

The mild form presents little clinical risk, occurs frequently, and requires no treatment. The moderate form requires only observation (weight, vital signs, hematocrit, blood urea nitrogen (BUN), electrolytes, and creatinine). In both mild and moderate hyperstimulation syndrome ovarian enlargement usually resolves by 12 weeks from the last menstrual period. Because it is the severe form of the hyperstimulation syndrome which is life-threatening, this chapter will concentrate mostly on the severe form of the condition.

PATHOPHYSIOLOGY

OHS has been observed to occur after stimulation of the ovaries with pregnant mare's serum gonadotropin (PMSG), human pituitary gonadotropins, clomiphene citrate, human menopausal gonadotropins (HMG), luteinizing-hormone releasing hormone (LHRH), or pure follicle-stimulating hormone (FSH). Follicular aspiration for oocyte recovery in *in vitro* fertilization has failed to protect against its occurrence [1]. The human chorionic gonadotropin (hCG) secreted by a pregnancy or administered for luteal-phase support increses both the likelihood of the occurrence of the syndrome as well as its duration and severity [2–4]. Spontaneous abortion leads to rapid resolution [3].

The exact pathophysiologic mechanisms of this condition remain poorly understood. In its severest form OHS is life-threatening, involving two primary processes: ovarian enlargement, and peritoneal, pleural, and pericardial fluid accumulation [2,3]. The extravascular shift of protein-containing fluid is known as third-spacing and results in a decreased total blood volume, hemoconcentration, and a rise in hematocrit. As a consequence, blood pressure and cardiac output fall unless the rate of sodium and fluid replacement by the oral or intravenous routes are sufficient to compensate for the rate of loss to the third space [2,3]. Compensatory mechanisms utilized by the body to maintain intravascular volume include vascular constriction and increases in heart rate, plasma renin, plasma aldosterone, and plasma antidiuretic hormone [3]. The combined effects of the elevations in aldosterone and antidiuretic hormone are to promote sodium and water retention. Oliguria and elevation of the serum BUN concentration result [2]. In severe cases, death or permanent injury have been reported. Although advances in medical knowledge have allowed a reduction in the incidence of this life-threatening condition, severe cases of ovarian hyperstimulation continue to occur, including occasional deaths.

AVOIDING THE HYPERSTIMULATION SYNDROME

Serum estradiol (E_2) assays have superseded urinary estrogen monitoring as the mainstay in avoiding the OHS. The concentration of serum or plasma estradiol determined on the day of hCG administration is now known to be the best predictor of the risk of severe OHS. It is important to realize that severe OHS almost never develops when ovulation does not occur (i.e., when hCG is withheld because the serum E_2 is too high and there is no spontaneous LH surge), and that at any given serum E_2 concentration a severe OHS is much more likely if pregnancy occurs. Indeed, pregnancy greatly increases the chance of a hyperstimulation syndrome, and pregnancy can result in a very prolonged severe OHS [2].

In monitoring the plasma E_2 concentration one must remember that the serum estrogen is maximal 8–10 hours after the prior gonadotropin injection. Therefore in our practice the serum E_2 is drawn at 8 a.m., and the patients have the gonadotropin injection at 5–8 p.m. It has been shown that an E_2 upper limit with such a protocol of 2417 pg/ml gives a 5% risk of a severe OHS in hypothalamic amenorrhea while in polycystic ovarian syndrome the equivalent level is 3778 pg/ml [5]. In *in vitro* fertilization (IVF) cycles we routinely downregulate the pituitary with 0.5 mg subcutaneous Lupron each day (TAP Pharmaceuticals, North Chicago, IL) and give 150 IU of FSH and 75 IU LH every 12 hours. Under these conditions we use an increased E_2 upper limit of 5000 pg/ml on the morning that hCG is to be given for all patients. However, although it has also been shown that the serum E_2 concentration is a good predictor of the OHS, it did not predict pregnancy. Therefore, we also use ultrasound for monitoring the number of follicles greater than 10 mm in average diameter, and this is a much better predictor of pregnancy but, conversely, not of the occurrence of OHS. Pregnancies begin to occur when the leading follicle reaches a diameter of 14 mm on the day that the hCG is given, but as a rule in hMG induction of ovulation, there is a spectrum of smaller follicles close behind the lead follicle. We aim to give the hCG when a reasonable number of follicles are 14 mm or greater but before the number of such follicles becomes unreasonably large, as the risk of a multiple gestation increases in such circumstances.

GUIDELINES FOR REDUCING THE CHANCE OF AN OHS

1 Do not give the hCG injection if the serum hCG exceeds the safe upper limit for the ovulation induction protocol you are using.

2 Avoid using an "ovulating" dose of hCG in excess of 10 000 IU.

3 Avoid using luteal-phase hCG support if the serum E_2 is near the upper limit for the protocol you are using or if there is evidence for an early presentation of a severe OHS.

4 Avoid using excessive doses of hCG for luteal-phase support.

TIMING OF THE CLINICAL PRESENTATION OF THE OHS

The OHS may occur in early or late forms. The late form usually presents just as the hCG from the implanting pregnancy starts to be detectable by radio-immunoassay. However, as the pre-hCG serum estradiol concentrations are driven higher and higher in IVF protocols, we have begun to see the early form of the syndrome presenting shortly after the first injection of hCG, which is the driving force in the early form rather than hCG secreted by a pregnancy. Usually in such cases the serum E_2 on the day the hCG was administered was very high. However, a single ovulating dose of hCG exceeding 10 000 IU or multiple doses of hCG for luteal-phase support also increase the likelihood of this early OHS.

We have seen two OHS cases in Lupron-down-regulated IVF patients whose serum E_2 was slightly over 5000 pg/ml when 10 000 IU of hCG was given 35 hours prior to egg retrieval and who became pregnant in the cycle of hyperstimulation. These patients received progesterone only for luteal-phase support at an intramuscular dose of 25–50 mg/day. In each case the hyperstimulation syndrome was manifested within days of the single hCG injection (abdominal pain, weight gain, and oliguria). The symptoms resolved after several days of observation, and severe ovarian hyperstimulation did not develop at the time of the hCG rise from the implanting pregnancy. If the serum E_2 had been considerably over 5000 pg/ml and/or luteal-phase support with hCG had been given, we feel the OHS would have been much worse and probably would have developed into the late form. The author has also seen, in consultation, examples of the early severe hyperstimulation syndrome produced by giving hCG to women with very high serum E_2s (over 6000 pg/ml) even when no pregnancy resulted, giving a second 10 000 IU injection of hCG 48 hours after the first (even without a resulting pregnancy), and giving hCG when the E_2 was very high; the OHS first appeared to resolve, and then developed into a protracted, severe, late syndrome driven by the rising serum hCG from the implanted pregnancy.

SYMPTOMS AND PHYSICAL FINDINGS IN SEVERE OHS

In addition to weight gain and oliguria, other early presenting symptoms of a severe OHS include nausea, vomiting, and pelvic pain. Physical findings include those associated with ascites, pleural effusion, pericardial effusion, bilateral ovarian enlargement, and peripheral dehydration. Note that in patients with severe vomiting weight gain may not occur due to inability to take in fluids. The physician should be alert for signs and symptoms of venous or arterial thrombosis or pulmonary embolism. Thrombosis and embolism are only indirectly associated with the OHS and should be treated in the usual manner.

LABORATORY FINDINGS IN SEVERE OHS

The combined effects of hypovolemia, decreased kidney perfusion, and secondary increases in the concentration of antidiuretic hormone and aldosterone result in increased concentrations of serum BUN, creatinine, and potassium, and decreased concentrations of serum sodium and chloride. The loss of plasma volume to the third space results in an increase in the hemoglobin and hematocrit. There is usually a marked increase in white blood cells as well with a shift to the left, but the etiology of this finding is unknown.

TREATMENT OF SEVERE OHS

Hospitalization is required in severe cases of OHS, and treatment should be problem-oriented (Fig. 76.1).

Ovarian enlargement
As long as ovarian rupture or torsion do not occur,

this problem can be handled using analgesics and expectant management. Abdominal examinations and pelvic examination should be avoided, as should surgery unless there is compelling evidence of torsion or intraabdominal hemorrhage.

Third-space sequestration of fluid
Sequestration of fluid can be tolerated as long as cardiovascular function and respiratory function are not compromised.

The acute phase
Establish baseline parameters: pulse, blood pressure, respirations, intake and hourly urinary output, weight, abdominal girth, extremity pitting edema, location of lung bases by examination and baseline chest X-ray, hemoglobin, hematocrit, white blood cells, and serum creatinine, BUN, sodium, chloride, carbon dioxide, hCG, E_2, and progesterone. So long as there is no loss of red cell mass, the hematocrit can be used to assess the loss in total blood volume and the decrease in the plasma volume (Table 76.1).

Correction with normal saline, with or without human serum albumin, should aim to maintain the hematocrit below an upper limit calculated to correspond to a 10–20% decrease in blood volume. Where the baseline hematocrit is not known, the aim is to return the hematocrit into the high normal range without rehydrating enough to provoke a marked increase in urinary output. Normal saline is chosen over Ringer's lactate due to the tendency toward hyperkalemia in these patients, and it is also more effective than human serum albumin for

Table 76.1 Absolute change in hematocrit and relative change in plasma volume corresponding to 10 and 20% changes in total blood volume

| Initial Hct (absolute value range) | 10% Decrease in total blood volume | | 20% Decrease in total blood volume | |
	Increase in Hct (absolute change)	Decrease in plasma volume (percent of baseline)	Increase in Hct (absolute change)	Decrease in plasma volume (percent of baseline)
30–31	3	13	8	30
32–34	4	16	8	30
35–38	4	16	9	31
39–40	4	16	10	33
41–42	5	18	10	33
43–46	5	18	11	36
47–49	5	18	12	38

Hct, hematocrit.

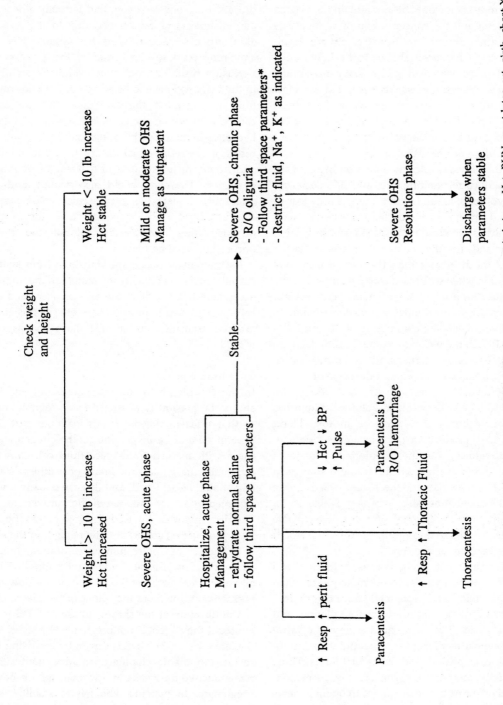

Fig. 76.1 Management of the ovarian hyperstimulation syndrome (OHS). *Third space parameters: vital signs, Hct, BUN, creat lytes, wt, girth, chest X-ray.

optimizing replacement of lost interstitial fluid, an advantage at initial presentation.

Human serum albumin has a high cost, and its only clear indication would be to maintain the plasma oncotic pressure if the concentration of endogenous serum albumin dropped to an extremely low level. Serum albumin has been shown to be better than crystalloid alone for treating the leaky membrane state which follows rattlesnake bites, but no trials of serum albumin versus normal saline have been performed in the OHS. A trial of human serum albumin should be considered if the patient cannot be stabilized on normal saline alone.

Table 76.1 provides calculated data on the increase in hematocrit corresponding to 10 and 20% decreases in blood volumes, assuming that there is only loss of plasma and that no change in the intravascular mass of red cells has occurred. Note that these changes are not linear and that the relative decrease in plasma volume is much greater than the decrease in total blood volume when expressed as a percentage of the initial value. With a premorbid hematocrit of 40%, a 10% decrease in total blood volume corresponds to an increase in hematocrit from 40 to 44% and a decrease of 16% in the plasma volume. A 20% decrease in total blood volume corresponds to an increase in hematocrit from 40 to 50% and a decrease of 33% in plasma volume. As a rule, healthy individuals can handle a 10% decrease in blood volume without too much trouble but a 20% decrease in total blood volume may produce major decompensation in some individuals. As the premorbid hematocrit increases, the magnitude of the absolute change in hematocrit corresponding to the 10 and 20% decrease in total blood volume also increases (Table 76.1). To prevent the development of a hypercoagulable state due to hemoconcentration, the hematocrit should be kept under about 50%.

Bear in mind that overgenerous hydration will come back to haunt you in the chronic phase when the sodium, fluids, and protein will have contributed to the accumulating volumes of ascitic, pleural, and pericardial fluid. The more fluid-replete the intravascular compartment is, the more rapid the accumulation of ascitic, pleural, and pericardial fluids. Thus, it is usually unwise to normalize the hematocrit completely. During the acute phase, frequent reviews of vital signs, hematocrit, white blood cells, BUN, sodium, potassium, chloride, and carbon dioxide should be performed with a program of providing the most minimal volumes of crystalloid and/or human serum albumin necessary to keep these parameters within the acceptable range. Hypotonic fluids should be avoided due to the elevated antidiuretic hormone secretion, and virtually all sodium administered will be retained due to the elevated aldosterone secretion. Serum potassium, BUN, and creatinine tend to climb due to the poor kidney perfusion resulting from hypovolemia. A small rise in the BUN will have to be accepted, but with careful fluid management the creatinine and potassium can be kept within the normal range in most cases. Diuretics should not be administered as they will result in *decreased* renal ability to eliminate BUN and other waste products in the face of poor renal perfusion. Diuretics would also acutely and preferentially deplete the intravascular volume rather than the third space, working against the program of supporting intravascular volume and further decreasing renal perfusion.

As the patient makes the transition from acute to chronic phase her ability to maintain the maximal acceptable hematocrit in the face of decreased fluid replacement will improve. Therefore, at this time a gradual transition to chronic-phase management is made.

The chronic phase

In the chronic phase sodium, potassium, and fluid should be maximally restricted in a program similar to that utilized in renal failure patients, but more protein should be given due to the pregnancy. In cases with marked third-space fluid collection and hyponatremia, a total fluid intake of as little as 400 ml/ day should be achieved, and this can usually only be achieved by discontinuation of the intravenous line. The diet should be low sodium, low potassium, and high protein (to support the pregnancy). In the event of a high serum potassium concentration, oral ion exchange resin can be used. Careful monitoring of all parameters with continued use of the flow chart is essential throughout the course of the severe OHS.

The duration of the chronic phase of OHS is self-limited if the patient is not pregnant. However, since the late form of the OHS is driven by the rising hCG secreted by the developing pregnancy, the OHS can remain active for weeks in a woman with a healthy pregnancy. In patients who fail to stabilize satisfactorily on fluid restriction and dietary management, the alternative approaches to management discussed below should be considered. As long as the patient can be stabilized on fluid restriction and dietary management, the prognosis is for ultimate spontaneous resolution.

The resolution phase

Resolution of the hyperstimulation syndrome will be signaled by onset of a spontaneous diuresis, weight loss, and normalization of all parameters. Ovarian enlargement usually resolves at about the 12th week from the last menstrual period in pregnant patients.

ALTERNATIVE APPROACHES TO MANAGEMENT OF THE SEVERE OHS

Antihistamines and indomethacin (and other prostaglandin inhibitors)

These medications have been advocated by some based on scanty studies in the rabbit model (which has a much less marked pathophysiology than the severe human syndrome) and anecdotal reports in the human, but there are few data to demonstrate effectiveness in the human and there are reports of lack of effectiveness of antihistamine [3] and prostaglandin inhibitors [4]. The fact that most hyperstimulated patients are pregnant should be borne in mind while selecting medications.

Thoracentesis, paracentesis, and pericardiocentesis

These procedures should only be performed if the amount of fluid accumulated in a given space is significantly interfering with respiration or cardiac function. While ultrasound guidance may increase safety, needle placement presents the risks of infection, bleeding, and pneumothorax, and removal of fluid ultimately increases the rate of fluid loss to the third space due to a drop in the pressure in the space from which fluid has been removed. Some physicians have advocated repeated tapping of fluid or the placement of a chronic drainage device in the abdominal cavity (such as that used in peritoneal dialysis). The decision to utilize any of these procedures must be based on a risk/benefit analysis.

Therapeutic abortion

Although no series of cases has been reported, clinical observations indicate that resolution of the severe OHS can be expected to begin within 24–48 hours of termination of pregnancy by either a spontaneous or a therapeutic abortion. This is due to the drop in serum hCG concentrations produced by elimination of the placental hCG secretion and a resultant decrease in hormonal stimulation of the ovary.

REFERENCES

1 Friedman CI, Schmidt GE, Chang FE, Kim MH. Severe ovarian hyperstimulation following follicular aspiration. *Am J Obstet Gynecol* 1984; 150: 436–437.
2 Schenker JG, Weinstein D. Ovarian hyperstimulation syndrome: a current survey. *Fertil Steril* 1978; 30: 255–268.
3 Haning RV, Strawn EY, Nolten WE. Pathophysiology of the ovarian hyperstimulation syndrome. *Obstet Gynecol* 1985; 66: 220–224.
4 Forman RG, Frydman R, Egan D, Ross C, Barlow DH. Severe ovarian hyperstimulation syndrome using agonists of gonadotropin-releasing hormone for in vitro fertilization: a European series and a proposal for prevention. *Fertil Steril* 1990; 53: 502–509.
5 Haning RV Jr, Boehnlein LM, Carlson IH, Kuzma DL, Zweibel WJ. Diagnosis specific serum 17β-estradiol (E$_2$) upper limits for treatment with menotropins using a ^{125}I direct E$_2$ assay. *Fertil Steril* 1984; 42: 882–889.

Infertility related to the cervix and its mucus

HOWARD D. McCLAMROCK

Abnormalities of the cervix and its mucus are thought to account for 5–10% of infertility problems [1]. The importance of sperm survival in the cervical mucus after intercourse has been recognized for over 100 years. The interaction of sperm and cervical mucus was first described by J. Marian Sims in the 1860s [2], expanded upon by Huhner in 1913 [3], and has since been known as the Sims–Huhner or postcoital test (PCT), a widely accepted tool in the diagnosis of infertility.

MULTIFACETED ROLE OF THE CERVIX

The cervix functions as a gate-keeper and as such acts as a biologic valve [1] preventing unwanted invasion by microbiologic invaders while allowing or denying entry of sperm into the uterus depending upon the time in the menstrual cycle and the quality of the sperm. The cervix must be able to mediate an immune response when faced with infectious organisms and stop this response when presented with foreign antigens in the form of spermatozoa.

The function of the cervix as a barrier to penetration is aided by the thick and tenacious mucus present during much of the menstrual cycle. During the peri-ovulatory period under the positive influence of estrogen, the cervical mucus increases in volume, becomes relatively acellular, and is thin and watery with the consistency of uncooked eggwhite. This watery mucus, rich in salts, mucin, and glycoproteins, develops an increased elasticity known as spinnbarkeit. When allowed to dry on a slide, the mucus develops arborization or ferning (Fig. 77.1). The cervical os and the endocervical canal are also thought to dilate slightly during this period. These changes in the cervical mucus act as a biologic marker for the periovulatory period. It is during this time that the mucus acts both as a facilitator for the passage of sperm into the upper reproductive tract and as a filter to stop the penetration of abnormal sperm.

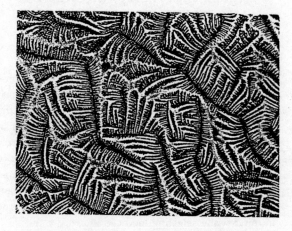

Fig. 77.1 Cervical mucus showing ferning pattern. (From [4].)

The cervical secretions which may also coat part of the upper vagina are more alkaline (pH = 8.5) than the normally acidic vagina (pH approximately 3–5). This, combined with the alkalinity of the seminal plasma, has a buffering effect on the vaginal acidity and allows sperm to live for hours to days in the cervical mucus. This favorable environment is also thought to allow the cervix to function as a reservoir which permits the continued passage of sperm from the cervix to the upper reproductive tract during the periovulatory period. In addition, the cervix may aid in sperm capacitation and provide supplemental energy to sperm traveling from the vagina to the distal fallopian tube [1]. Thus the cervix is not merely an opening through which sperm pass; rather it plays an important dynamic role in the events leading to fertilization.

EVALUATION OF THE CERVIX

The PCT

The interaction between sperm and cervical mucus is generally evaluated by using the PCT, otherwise known as the Sims–Huhner test. This test was first described over 100 years ago and is commonly performed early in the work-up of the infertile couple. In spite of its popularity and years of use, the test has never been standardized and there is disagreement as to how the results should be interpreted. The PCT may in fact lack validity as a test for infertility as there is no agreement on its diagnostic or prognostic value in predicting fertility (see below). Despite these concerns, the PCT remains the most frequently used test for diagnosing cervical factor-related infertility.

Timing

When planning a PCT, consideration must be given to both timing in the menstrual cycle as well as timing after intercourse [4]. The test must be performed during the periovulatory period when the sperm are expected to survive in the cervical canal. The previously mentioned estrogen-dependent changes in the cervical mucus begin on approximately the 9th day of a normal cycle and increase gradually until the time of ovulation. Within 2 days after ovulation, the penetrability of cervical mucus is usually impaired since progesterone is thought to inhibit the secretory activity of the cervical epithelial cells. For most women with a 28-day cycle, days 12–14 are the most appropriate days for postcoital testing. This period corresponds to the low point in the temperature chart together with 1 or 2 days surrounding that low point. However, because some women have a very narrow window for sperm penetrability of cervical mucus, and the time of ovulation may vary from month to month, it is sometimes difficult to choose the correct day for a PCT. Judgment and persistence may be necessary to insure that timing is correct. In some women, cycles are so irregular that use of clomiphene citrate has been suggested in an effort to regulate the menstrual cycle so as to avoid repeated office visits. Alternatively, urinary luteinizing hormone (LH) testing is sometimes of value in practices where the facilities allow daily postcoital testing on short notice.

The time between intercourse and postcoital testing remains controversial. Huhner stated that the test should be performed as soon as possible after coitus, but gave no reason [3]; other authors performed the test after 2 hours. There has been discussion of the standard test (6–10 hours), the delayed test (18–24 hours), and the early test (1–3 hours) – all perhaps providing different information [1]. However, because the cervix acts as a reservoir for sperm and the oocyte is thought to be fertilizable for less than 24 hours, the ability of sperm to survive in the cervical mucus and thus be in constant supply to the distal fallopian tube may be important to conception. For this reason, the couple should be instructed to have intercourse at bedtime the evening before the PCT or approximately 10–16 hours prior to testing. This allows evaluation of the cervical mucus as a reservoir and ascertains whether the sperm are living for an extended period of time after intercourse. In addition, it should be more convenient and less pressured for the couple involved.

Procedure

The PCT is done with the patient in the lithotomy position using an unlubricated bivalve speculum or one lubricated only with warm water. The mucus may be aspirated with a tuberculin syringe (without needle), a pipette, a large-gauge intravascular cathether, or mucus forceps. The PCT involves assessing both mucus and sperm. The mucus is evaluated for amount, viscosity, ferning, spinnbarkeit, cellularity, and pH. The amount is classified as scant, moderate, or profuse, or the volume is measured in tenths of milliliters. Noting the degree of clarity, the sample is tested for spinnbarkeit by placing the mucus sample on a microscope slide and covering it with a glass cover slip before slowly removing the cover slip and measuring the number of centimeters of mucus stretch. Six to 10 cm is thought to be consistent with impending ovulation. Under the microscope the degree of cellularity is noted by an estimate of the number of leukocytes and other cells per high-powered field (hpf) and the number of sperm is evaluated. The number of sperm/hpf required for a normal PCT has never been defined and the suggested number varies widely in the literature. Greater than 20 motile sperm/hpf probably represents normal cervical function and has been positively correlated with pregnancy. No sperm seen suggests poor coital technique, hostile cervical mucus, faulty sperm production in the male, or antisperm antibodies. One to 20 sperm/hpf is thought to be normal by some authors and abnormal by others. However, one study found that more than 30% of couples with no sperm seen on the PCT conceived within a 2-year period [5].

Sperm found shaking in place while not making progressive forward movement has been associated with immunologic infertility. After drying, the slide is evaluated for fern formation and graded 1–4, with 4 being best (Fig. 77.1).

Problems with the PCT

As mentioned above, lack of standardization and disagreement on how to interpret the PCT cause many people to question the reliability of the test. Some authors have suggested that it is so informative as to eliminate the need for semen analysis while others feel that it merely confirms the deposition of sperm in the vagina [5]. The number of sperm considered sufficient has never been identified and even sperm survival in the mucus has never been proven to have a bearing on conception rates. It will be impossible to establish the reproducibility of the PCT until the methodology is standardized.

Asch reported the recovery of sperm in the peritoneal aspirates obtained at laparoscopy in eight of 10 women in whom no sperm were present in the cervical mucus 3–8 hours after intercourse [6]. This information, along with other confirmatory studies, suggests that the PCT may not correlate with the presence of sperm in the ampulla of the fallopian tube, the site of fertilization. Griffith and Grimes reviewed the world's English literature on the PCT and calculated four indexes of validity for each study in which there was sufficient information [5]. These indexes included sensitivity, specificity, predictive value of abnormal, and predictive value of normal. In all areas the PCT seemed to suffer from poor validity. Many authorities acknowledge that one abnormal PCT has little clinical value, but the value of one normal or good test remains to be determined.

Additional tests

Fractional PCTs with samples taken at different levels of the endocervical canal have been described but have not been correlated with conception. Other studies [7] have shown a uniform sperm distribution throughout the canal, implying that fractional tests are not more reliable than the traditional PCT. When a well-timed PCT is poor in the face of a normal semen analysis, some authorities recommend cervical mucus penetration tests. Care must be taken to insure that the poor PCT was appropriately timed and that the mucus was periovulatory. This can be done by reviewing the temperature chart from the cycle

in which the test was performed. One method of cervical mucus penetration testing involves placing a semen sample adjacent to a cervical mucus sample on a microscope slide and covering it with a cover slip. After 3–4 hours the slide is evaluated and graded as 0, 1, or 2, such that 0 corresponds to sperm found only in the peripheral parts of the mucus, 1 to the majority of the sperm having invaded the periphery with some present in the center of the mucus, and 2 to sperm equally distributed throughout the mucus [4]. A second cervical mucus penetration test involves the use of a capillary tube. Mucus is taken from the cervix, placed on a slide, and aspirated into a capillary tube. Flat capillary tubes are easier to read than round ones. No air bubbles should be aspirated into the capillary tube. The capillary tube containing the mucus is then placed vertically into a test tube containing 1 ml of the partner's semen. At the end of 1 hour, the distance the spermatozoa have traveled upwards into the cervical mucus is measured [4]. It is important to compare sperm penetration of the patient's mucus to that of a donor mucus from another woman. Bovine cervical mucus is available in flat capillary tubes and may be substituted for donor human mucus. It may also be helpful to compare the male partner's semen to that of a donor's semen with known fertility. Normal migration occurs when motile sperm are seen throughout the 30 mm column of mucus. If no sperm, immotile sperm, or sperm shaking in place are seen in a well-timed PCT with abundant cervical mucus, sperm antibody testing is indicated.

Consideration should be given to cervical neoplasms, stenosis, lacerations and trauma, congenital anomalies, cervical incompetence, and ectropion in the patient with a poor PCT. Inflammatory diseases of the cervix should be ruled out. These may include *Chlamydia trachomatis*, *Neisseria gonorrhoeae*, mycoplasmas, and viral infections, as well as parasitic, granulomatous, and other bacterial infections. Appropriate testing and cultures may be indicated in an effort to make the appropriate diagnosis.

THERAPY

Patients with cervical inflammation and/or infection should be cultured and appropriately treated. Those with immune factors and male factor should be evaluated and treated in regard to these issues; however, a discussion of these problems is beyond the scope of this chapter. For the most part, treatment of cervical factor can be divided into two categories: treatment aimed at improving cervical mucus, and treatment aimed at bypassing cervical mucus.

Treatment aimed at improving cervical mucus

Certain patients may manifest poor cervical mucus as a result of inadequate follicular development. These patients may benefit from the use of clomiphene citrate which may improve cervical mucus by increasing preovulatory estrogen levels. On the other hand, clomiphene citrate may worsen the mucus production in some patients, acting via its antiestrogenic effect.

Sodium bicarbonate douching and potassium iodide drops have been used in patients with acidic cervical mucus and donor cervical mucus and guaifenesin have been used in an effort to augment poor cervical mucus; however, scientific evaluation of their effectiveness is lacking. Estrogen supplementation in the preovulatory portion of the menstrual cycle has been used to improve cervical mucus.

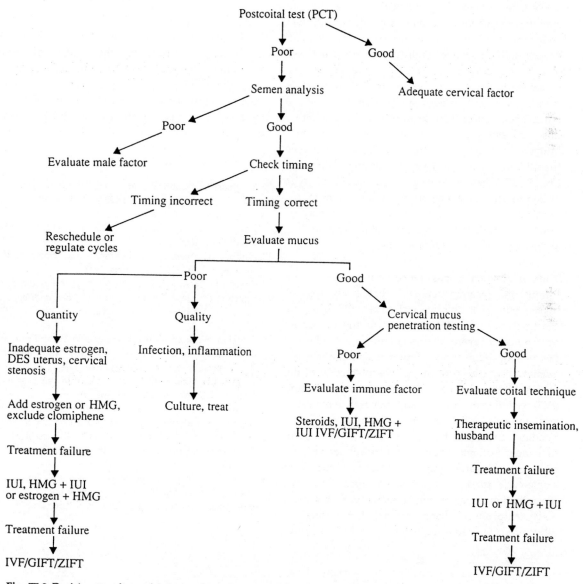

Fig. 77.2 Decision tree for evaluating and treating cervical factor. (Adapted from [5].)

CHAPTER 77

Estrogens which have been used include conjugated estrogens (Premarin), 0.3–1.25 mg/day; ethinylestradiol, 0.01–0.02 mg/day; and diethylstilbestrol, 0.1–0.2 mg/day on days 5 through 14 or for at least 4–5 days prior to ovulation. Estrogen supplementation may inhibit or delay ovulation and care must be taken when using higher dosages. In addition, human menopausal gonadotropins (hMG) have been used with some success in an effort to improve cervical mucus by raising endogenous estradiol levels. The need for exogenous estrogen may be questioned in the face of normal endogenous estrogen levels. The mechanism by which exogenous estrogen may improve cervical mucus to a greater extent than endogenous estrogen, if in fact such improvement does exist, has never been fully explained. One possibility is that exogenous estrogen allows a more sustained period of estrogen exposure. When estrogen supplementation fails adequately to improve cervical mucus, some success has been reported using higher doses of estrogen in conjunction with hMG and human chorionic gonadotropin (hCG) to overcome the inhibitory effect of the higher estrogen doses [8] (Fig. 77.2). When evaluating the success of this type of approach, consideration must be given to the possibility that improved pregnancy rates may be due to the production of multiple follicles rather than an improvement in cervical mucus.

Therapy aimed at bypassing cervical mucus

Intrauterine insemination (IUI) has been used to bypass poor or hostile cervical mucus. IUI of whole semen is not recommended due to the unwanted occurrence of severe uterine cramping secondary to the prostaglandins found in human semen, the introduction of foreign proteins, or overdistention of the uterus. Much has been learned in *in vitro* fertilization (IVF) regarding the washing and preparation of sperm, and protocols for IUI now call for washing and resuspending of sperm in buffer solutions. IUI does seem to benefit patients with pure cervical factor (Fig. 77.2). Success rates approach 60% over time, with single-cycle success rates ranging from 5 to 18%. Inseminations may be timed using previous basal body temperature charts, urinary LH testing, or ultrasound. Ovulation induction with hMG in com-

bination with IUI may be associated with pregnancy rates as high as 40% per cycle when done for pure cervical factor (Fig. 77.2). The success of IUI for male factor or immune factors is less clear.

It has been suggested that some IVF successes are due to bypassing the abnormal processing of sperm by the female reproductive tract. With this in mind, consideration may be given to IVF, gamete intrafallopian transfer (GIFT), or zygote intrafallopian transfer (ZIFT) as a last-resort treatment for cervical factor infertility (Fig. 77.2).

CONCLUSIONS

Cervical factors are thought to be causative of 5–10% of infertility. At this time, the primary diagnostic tools remain the PCT, and cervical mucus penetration tests, the validity of which are still in question. Treatment approaches aimed at improving or bypassing cervical mucus are often successful in patients with pure cervical factor.

REFERENCES

1 Moghissi KS. Cervical and uterine factors in infertility. *Obstet Gynecol Clin North Am* 1987; 14: 887–904.
2 Sims JM. *Clinical Notes on Uterine Surgery (with Special Reference to the Sterile Conditon)*. London: Robert Hardwicke, 1866.
3 Huhner M. Sterility in the male and female and its treatment. New York, Rebman, 1913.
4 Speroff L, Glass RH, Kase NG, eds. Investigation of the infertile couple. *Clinical Gynecologic Endocrinology and Infertility*, 3rd edn. Baltimore: Williams & Wilkins, 1983: 470.
5 Seibel M. Work up of the infertile couple. Part I: Evaluation of infertility. In: Seibel M, ed. *Infertility: A Comprehensive Text*. Norwalk: Appleton and Lange, 1990: 1–21.
6 Griffith CS, Grimes DA. The validity of the post coital test. *Am J Obstet Gynecol* 1990; 162: 615–620.
7 Asch RH. Sperm recovery in peritoneal aspirate after negative Sim–Huhner test. *Int J Fertil* 1978; 23: 57–60.
8 Drake TS, Tredway DR, Buchanan GL. A reassessment of the fractional post-coital test. *Am J Obstet Gynecol* 1979; 133: 382.
9 Check JH, Wu CH, Diettrich C, Louer CC, Liss J. The treatment of cervical factor with ethinyl estradiol in human menopausal gonadotropins. *Int J Fertil* 1986; 31: 148–152.

Distal tubal obstruction

WILLIAM D. SCHLAFF & JANETTE DURHAM

The fallopian tube is probably the most common site of permanent damage as a result of pelvic infection or inflammation. While the cervix, uterus, parametrial, and peritoneal tissues may be affected by an acute pelvic process, treatment with antibiotics commonly eliminates any permanent reproductive dysfunction. However, the fallopian tube and the important anatomic relationships of the tube to the ovary can be seriously and permanently adversely affected. In the classic study by Westrom, the investigators found a 13% incidence of tubal obstruction after a first episode of acute salpingitis, a 39% incidence after two episodes, and a 75% incidence after three episodes [1]. As the microbiologic pathogens causing acute pelvic infection seem to be shifting from gonorrhea to *Chlamydia* and others, the impression is that women may commonly have an anatomically destructive infection in the absence of clinically severe symptoms. This development is particularly worrisome when one considers the potential for tubal infertility.

Damage to the tube may take a variety of forms, but is most commonly associated with attenuation or destruction of the infundibulum and fimbria of the tube. Scanning electron microscopy has shown that inflammatory changes can severely damage the mucosa and can irreversibly destroy the cilia of the distal tube. Less severe infection may have a significant, though less profound effect on the mucosa or cilia of the distal tube. Tubal architecture may also be adversely affected by inflammatory damage resulting in dilatation and/or obstruction of the distal tube. Finally, the important anatomic relationships of the tube and ovary may be severely compromised by adhesions between these two structures as a result of an inflammatory process.

Surgical trauma can also have a profound effect on reproductive success by injury to the distal tube. Careless handling of the adnexa resulting in direct tissue injury, or failure to keep the adnexal structures wet during an operation can lead to tissue hypoxia, agglutination, and pelvic adhesions. Surgical injury is less likely to cause mucosal or ciliary damage, but can nevertheless result in significant reduction in the ability of the tube to perform its important role of ovum pick-up. This chapter will focus on strategies to make an accurate prospective diagnosis of distal tubal disease and will review alternative approaches to treatment.

DIAGNOSIS

Initial diagnostic steps should be directed by a careful patient history. At the time of an initial consultation, it is most important to review the patient's past gynecologic and surgical history in detail. A history of sexually transmitted disease, particularly when associated with previously diagnosed salpingitis, is clearly a major risk factor. On the other hand, patients will frequently relate a history of a tubal infection made on dubious grounds. It is most helpful specifically to ask and clarify whether the patient had had sexual exposure prior to the previous diagnosis of salpingitis, whether she had been febrile or had had a pelvic examination showing significant tenderness, or whether she had had appropriate blood tests to confirm the diagnosis. Furthermore, it is frequently instructive to ascertain whether the patient was treated as an outpatient or whether she was admitted for intravenous antibiotics. Second, a history of previous abdominal surgery, particularly on the adnexa, should be sought. Ovarian cystectomy or wedge resection are notorious initiators of adnexal adhesions which may adversely affect the tubal–ovarian relationship. Previous appendectomy, particularly if associated with perforation and drainage, can also be associated with severe pelvic injury. Such procedures should be considered major risk factors, and all operative records should be requested to review the potential impact of the previous clinical situation and surgical technique. Other significant risk factors for tubal damage include inflammatory bowel disease or surgery on the gastrointestinal tract. Finally, previous surgery on the tube itself, for instance an ectopic pregnancy, obviously can have significant implications as risk factors for tubal disease.

Pelvic examination should of course be performed in all routine infertile patients to search carefully for unsuspected pelvic abnormalities. Findings on examination that would suggest a tubal abnormality could include a relatively fixed, immobile uterus, or a clear and definable adnexal mass. More commonly, pelvic adhesions are associated with an indistinct, poorly definable adhesive complex that is frequently described as adnexal fullness. The sense on examination that multiple structures may be adherent to each other or that the mobility of the ovary or adnexa is reduced is frequently associated with significant pelvic pathology.

While many patients have clear risk factors for distal tubal disease on the basis of their history or physical examination, patients with neither of these findings may still have distal tubal disease. The initiation of diagnostic testing of anatomic factors in these patients may be deferred until a thorough review of medical, ovulatory, cervical, and male factors has been initiated, but should not be overlooked due to the absence of any known risk factor. The first major study one should obtain to evaluate the distal tube is a hysterosalpingogram (HSG). The HSG can be performed very easily in the outpatient setting and has minimum associated morbidity. The patient should be scheduled in the proliferative phase of her cycle after the menstrual flow has ceased but before ovulation. Patients with known risk factors by history or physical examination should be pretreated with oral antibiotics beginning 12 hours prior to the procedure. We recommend continuing treatment in these patients for 2 days following the HSG. In patients with no risk factors who prove to have HSG findings suggestive of previous infection, we recommend treatment with 3 days of oral antibiotics following the procedure.

Techniques of hysterosalpingography are critical in establishing a prognosis for the woman with distal tubal disease, and are reviewed in Chapter 67. To summarize, an injection apparatus which will provide a good seal at the level of the cervix is required. This is frequently accomplished with a tenaculum and a metal cannula with plastic or rubber acorn. We prefer a Wisap suction cannula which is applied to the cervix and held in place by wall suction.

The HSG should be performed with fluoroscopy, and will show the internal configuration of the uterus and fallopian tubes. The total volume of radiocontrast necessary to outline these areas is generally 5–10 ml. We use a 10 ml syringe and inject very slowly under fluoroscopic observation and take spot films to delineate four basic points of interest:

1 An early film of the uterine filling phase, generally after no more than 1 ml of injection, to exclude any intrauterine defect or congenital anomaly. During this phase, it is most important to put traction on the cannulation device to insure that the uterus is parallel to the X-ray plate so as to give a full view of the uterus.

2 A tubal filling film to insure that both tubes fill easily and that the radiocontrast can be seen all the way to the end of the tube. It is critical to assess the status of the distal tubal mucosa, as evidenced by the presence of rugal folds, and presence of distal tubal dilatation.

3 A film to assess fallopian tube patency (under fluoroscopic guidance) to insure that contrast is actually seen exiting the tube.

4 A film to insure free spill on contrast in the pelvis. We frequently change patient position on the X-ray table in an attempt to be certain that the contrast moves evenly throughout the pelvis. On occasion, peritubal loculation of contrast will herald tubal adhesions which otherwise would not be suspected. However, this latter observation tends to be rather nonspecific and will always require laparoscopic follow-up.

Details of the fallopian tube are much more easily seen on the spot films, though the dynamics of uterine and tubal mobility are more apparent during the fluoroscopic examination. Therefore, fluoroscopic evaluation alone is inadequate to provide all available information and the HSG films themselves should be carefully reviewed following the procedure. We use exclusively water-soluble contrast because the rugal folds of the distal tube are much more easily seen than they are with oil-soluble contrast. We have found this to be an important prognostic factor in assessing tubal abnormalities. Furthermore, in the presence of tubal obstruction (particularly proximal), excessive installation pressure can result in intravasation of the contrast and, at least theoretically, may result in embolism if oil-soluble contrast is used.

Hysterosalpingography is an extremely important prognostic test for evaluation of the fallopian tube. It cannot and should not be eschewed for a hysteroscopy and laparoscopy. The HSG gives extremely important information about the proximal fallopian tube which cannot be obtained in any other way. It also will allow the clear delineation of the normalcy of the distal tube, including mucosal status, which again cannot be seen at hysteroscopy or laparoscopy. Finally, it will allow the clinician to suspect tubal damage prior to general anesthesia and surgery. For all these reasons, it is extremely important that the gynecologist or reproductive surgeon either perform the hysterogram or, at the very least, review the films with the radiologist to reach agreement in the diagnosis.

Laparoscopy is the second critical step in thorough diagnosis of tubal abnormalities. Virtually all gynecologists are comfortable with performing laparoscopy, which should be seen initially as a diagnostic rather than as a therapeutic procedure. When laparoscopy is being performed for diagnosis alone, the clinician should try to have endoscopic video equipment available to make a permanent record of the procedure. In virtually all cases, an accessory trocar in the suprapubic area will be required, and in many cases a third or fourth puncture will be required. The diagnostic evaluation should very specifically assess all pelvic structures for normal mobility, presence of adhesions, and normal anatomic relationships, specifically those between the ovaries and tubes. The fimbria should specifically be visualized and patency should be tested by a transcervical injection of a dye, usually indigo carmine or methylene blue. Whether or not the procedure is videotaped, the operative report should specifically describe the above points with a detailed description of the state and anatomic relationships of the adnexal structures.

PROGNOSIS AND STAGE OF DISEASE

A number of descriptions of staging of distal tubal disease have been proposed. Table 78.1 shows a classification system derived by Rock and colleagues which has proved very useful in the prospective establishment of prognosis for patients [2]. The classification system rests on three basic factors — the presence of normal distal tubal architecture as evidenced by rugal folds; the extent of dilatation of the distal tube; and the presence of associated pelvic adhesions. It is notable that the first two parameters can easily be assessed at hysterosalpingography, long before the patient would be exposed to the risk of general anesthesia or a surgical procedure. Figure 78.1 depicts hysterographic findings suggestive of varying stages of disease.

Following the initial history and physical examination and hysterogram, the clinician should schedule a thorough discussion with the patient who is likely to have distal tubal disease. At this time the prognosis for anatomic repair should be reviewed along with the remainder of the orthodox preoperative evaluation including assessment of ovulation,

Table 78.1 Classification of the extent of tubal disease with distal fimbrial obstruction. (From [2])

Extent of disease	Findings
Mild	1 Absent or small hydrosalpinx <15 mm diameter 2 Inverted fimbria easily recognized when patency achieved 3 No significant peritubal or periovarian adhesions 4 Preoperative hysterogram reveals a rugal pattern
Moderate	1 Hydrosalpinx 15–30 mm diameter 2 Fragments of fimbria not readily identified 3 Periovarian and/or peritubular adhesions without fixation, minimal cul-de-sac adhesions 4 Absence of a rugal pattern on preoperative hysterogram
Severe	1 Large hydrosalpinx >30 mm diameter 2 No fimbria 3 Dense pelvic or adnexal adhesions with fixation of the ovary and tube to the broad ligament, pelvic side wall, omentum, and/or bowel 4 Obliteration of the cul-de-sac 5 Frozen pelvis (adhesion formation so dense that limits of organs are difficult to define)

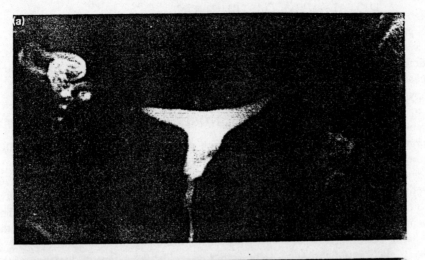

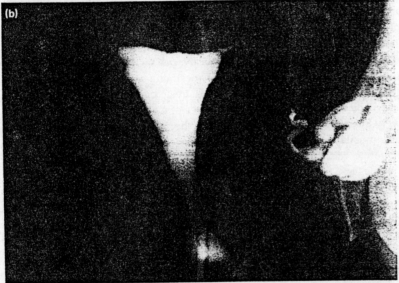

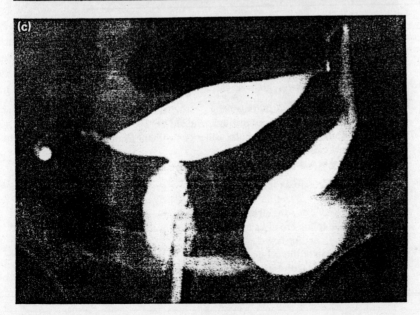

Fig. 78.1 Mild disease: (a) note normal tubal rugation and absence of tubal dilatation. (b) Moderate disease: note presence of some rugation associated with moderate distal dilatation. Patient has undergone previous contralateral salpingectomy. (c) Severe disease: note tubal absence of rugation ("bald tire") with profound dilatation of distal tube. Patient has undergone contralateral salpingectomy.

cervical factor, and male factor. Only at this point can the reproductive surgeon provide informed consent and can there be agreement with the patient as to the best surgical approach.

SURGERY FOR DISTAL TUBAL OBSTRUCTION

The classic approach to surgery for distal obstruction entails an initial laparoscopy for diagnostic purposes only followed by a postoperative discussion prior to definitive surgery. The traditional surgical approach most commonly performed would be to proceed to laparotomy with tubal repair using microsurgical technique. In certain cases, patients will prefer to have the definitive laparotomy at the same time as the laparoscopy to avoid a second anesthetic as long as full informed consent was provided. However, as techniques and instruments for endoscopic surgery develop, many reproductive surgeons will elect to perform definitive surgery by laparoscopy at the same time as the diagnostic procedure. Whether the procedure is performed by laparoscopy or laparotomy, or whether it is under the same anesthesia as the diagnostic procedure or at a different time, the reproductive surgeon must be certain to stay within the limits of his or her surgical training and skill and to seek consultation as appropriate.

The microsurgical approach to distal tubal disease has been well described in the literature. While many authors present individual variations, there are several important and consistent themes to the microsurgical approach. First, all tissue must be handled extremely delicately with minimal surgical trauma. Second, throughout the procedure, all tissues must be kept wet so as to avoid tissue drying, hypoxia, and subsequent adhesion formation. Third, careful hemostasis must be maintained throughout the procedure. Fourth, careful attention must be paid to normalization of anatomic relationships between fallopian tube and ovary. Finally, magnification is most helpful in allowing the surgeon to identify subtle tissue planes and to place minimally traumatic, small absorbable sutures when required.

The surgical approach to distal tubal disease first requires an initial assessment of anatomic distortion. Once this overview has been performed, it is easier to establish the desirable surgical goals during the case. First, adhesions between pelvic structures should be excised. Careful manipulation of pelvic organs by an experienced assistant is most helpful in putting all adhesions on stretch and thereby allowing excision of the adhesion from both origin and insertion rather than simply cutting the adhesions. A fine-tipped microcautery or surgical laser appears to be equally effective in removing adhesions. It is generally advisable to begin removing adhesions at the base of the pelvis, thereby allowing the adnexal structures and uterus to be brought anteriorly. Once this has been accomplished, a wet lap sponge can be placed in the posterior pelvis and used as a surgical table on which other structures may then be placed. It is important to keep the uterus and contralateral adnexa under wet packs while operating on the distal tube. In approaching the distal tubal obstruction, one must begin by attempting to normalize the relationship between tube and ovary. It is not enough simply to open the tube but, rather, one must make every effort to remove any adhesions between proximal tube and ovary or pelvic side wall and to recreate normal apposition of distal tube to ovary. Careful attention to identifying the fimbria ovarica, the most distal strand of tube and fimbria which connects the infundibulum to the ovary, is most helpful in recreating normal anatomic relationships between tube and ovary. This process can again be accomplished using either microtip cautery or a surgical laser. If one elects to use a laser, it is wise to use one which will have minimal tissue penetration, hence the carbon dioxide laser is likely preferable over other available instruments.

Once the distal tube has been isolated, one commonly finds the point of fimbrial agglutination by what appears to be a retracted whitish, sometimes stellate area of the distal tube. We commonly use an intrauterine catheter (either a small-gauge pediatric Foley or a HUMI catheter placed at the time of surgical preparation and inject methylene blue at this point. This will cause bulging of the distal tube and may allow the reproductive surgeon to have a better idea of the normal anatomic relationship. The distal tube is then opened using a cruciate incision and carrying the dissection along the fimbria ovarica to the ovary. The minimal number of sutures required to maintain the distal aperture should be placed. We recommend the use of 7−0 vicryl or similar suture for this procedure. Generally, no more than four sutures are required for this process. The use of accessory protective devices such as Mulligan hoods cannot presently be endorsed in the absence of any data which show them to produce better pregnancy rates and in light of the requisite second surgery to remove them. The procedure as described is outlined in Figure 78.2 [3].

Once opening of the tube has been accomplished, the adnexa should again be packed in wet lint-free packs and the contralateral tube should be approached in a similar manner. Uterine suspension may be considered in the case of severe uterine retroversion and posterior pelvic adhesions, though data do not support the routine use of uterine suspension as an operative adjunct. Antiadhesion barriers such as Interceed (Johnson & Johnson, New Brunswick) or Gore-Tex (W.L. Gore and Associates, Flagstaff) may be considered in cases where there has been significant adhesion of the ovary to the pelvic side wall. However, the use of either type of barrier to wrap the ovary or distal tube has not been studied, nor has it been approved by the Food and Drug Administration and therefore must be considered speculative at this point. Other antiadhesion adjuncts such as Hyskon can be considered and are discussed more thoroughly in Chapter 86.

We routinely administer preoperative antibiotics at least 1 hour before surgery. A broad-spectrum parenteral antibiotic such as cefoxitin or cefotetan is commonly used for one preoperative dose and for 24 hours, postoperatively. Because the incidence of perioperative infection is so low, no prospective trial has confirmed the effectiveness of this regimen. However, we feel the risk of routine antibiotic coverage is reasonable in light of the potentially catastrophic impact of a postoperative tubal infection. Routine use of postoperative hydrotubation using combinations of antibiotics and steroids has not

been shown to be effective and therefore we do not recommend this procedure after distal tubal operations [4].

Advanced endoscopic techniques may allow a laparoscopic procedure similar to that which is described to be performed with equally good success. Proper preparation of the patient and operating room is mandatory. We recommend the use of pre- and postoperative antibiotics as described above. The patient must be under general anesthesia for such an extensive procedure, and the operating room must be able to accommodate a three- or four-puncture approach with appropriate instrumentation to allow coagulation and precise incision of adhesions and of the fallopian tube. A more thorough discussion of general laparoscopic technique is included in Chapter 68. In order to perform the distal salpingostomy, the distal tube must be thoroughly isolated and precisely incised. Suturing back of the incised corners of the tube may or may not be required using this approach. The incision may be made by fine-tipped microcautery or by laser or cauterizing the tubal serosa. The commonly proposed technique of "flowering" of the distal tube by defocusing the laser has not been shown to have any effect on pregnancy outcome. It may be considered, but should not be construed to be a mandatory part of the surgical repair. Post-operative considerations are the same regardless of route of surgery.

A special comment regarding the use of lasers versus microcautery is in order. While there has been enthusiasm for the use of lasers for such procedures both in the medical literature and the lay press, there

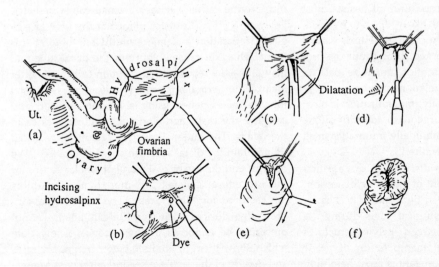

Fig. 78.2 Surgical approach to correction of distal tubal obstruction. (Reprinted with permission from Jones HW Jr, Rock JA. Surgery of the oviduct. In: *Reparative and Constructive Surgery of the Female Generative Tract*. Baltimore: Williams & Wilkins, 1983: 84.)

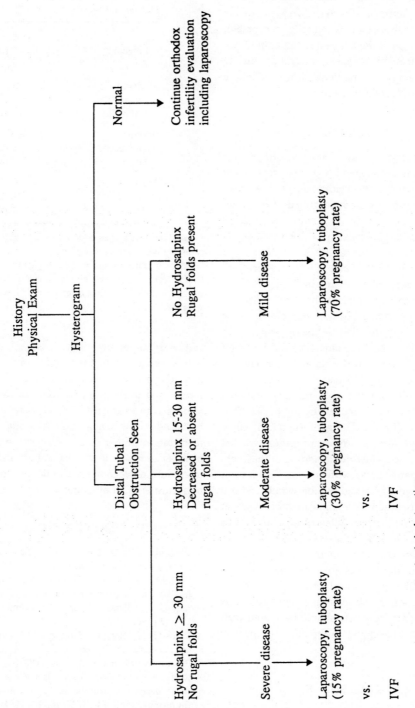

Fig. 78.3 Approach to distal tubal obstruction.

CHAPTER 78

are no data which show that lasers are more effective than more conventional techniques. To the contrary, in both animal and human studies, electro-microcautery and lasers have been shown to be equally effective, thus either tool is equally acceptable. Therefore, the focus of the surgical repair should not be on which instrument is chosen, but rather, on the delicacy and attention to fine detail of the technique used by the reproductive surgeon.

OUTCOME

The ultimate pregnancy rates following surgery for distal tubal obstruction depend to a very great extent on the condition of the tube prior to surgery. According to the classification system described earlier, only about 10% of patients with distal tubal obstruction have mild disease. Approximately 37% have moderate disease, and 60% have severe disease. Outcome can clearly be predicted on the basis of this classification, as shown in a recent study and in Table 78.2 [5]. While only a minority of patients have mild disease, it is clear that they can be told their outcome is likely to be very good. Unfortunately, at the opposite, more common extreme, only approximately 12% of women with distal tubal disease will ultimately conceive an intrauterine pregnancy. Of those who will ultimately conceive, 73% will do so within 12 months, and 96% by 24 months. The reproductive surgeon has an obligation to review all these data with the patient prior to deciding to perform a surgical procedure so that she may have an accurate understanding of the likely outcome. Pregnancy rates with *in vitro* fertilization have been shown to be highest for women whose indication for treatment is significant tubal disease. In many centers pregnancy rates as high as 30% or more per cycle have been observed in patients in this group. Therefore, in women with severe tubal disease in whom the ovaries are accessible to oocyte retrieval, careful consideration should be given to *in vitro* fertilization rather than the more orthodox surgical approach. These data should be shared with the patient prior to deciding on the most appropriate alternative.

CONCLUSIONS

Patients with distal tubal disease can be accurately staged by history, physical examination, hysterosalpingography, and laparoscopy. See Figure 78.3 for an outline of the approach to distal tubal obstruction.

Table 78.2 Pregnancy outcome by stage of disease. (Adapted from [5])

Degree of disease	Number
Mild	10
Pregnant*	7 (70)
Ectopic†	1 (10/14)
Moderate	29
Pregnant*	9 (31)
Ectopic†	4 (14/44)
Severe	56
Pregnant*	9 (16)
Ectopic†	2 (4/22)
Total	95
Pregnant*	26 (27)
Ectopic†	7 (7/27)

* Value in parentheses is percentage of patients in that category who become pregnant.
† Values in parentheses are percentage of total patients in that category with ectopic pregnancies/percentage of pregnant patients in that category who have ectopic pregnancies.

With careful preoperative assessment, one can establish a prognosis for successful outcome based on condition of the distal tube, degree of tubal dilatation, and presence of confounding adhesions. The approach to treatment of distal tubal disease should be based on the stage, and may optimally be *in vitro* fertilization rather than surgery in a significant number of cases. If surgery is indicated, meticulous microsurgical technique should be brought to bear to assure optimal outcome.

REFERENCES

1 Westrom L. Effect of acute pelvic inflammatory disease on fertility. *Am J Obstet Gynecol*, 1975; 121: 707.
2 Rock JA, Katayama P, Martin EJ, Woodruff JD, Jones HW Jr. Factors influencing the success of salpingostomy techniques for distal fimbrial obstruction. *Obstet Gynecol* 1978; 52: 591.
3 Jones HW Jr, Rock JA. Surgery of the oviduct. *Reparative and Constructive Surgery of the Female Generative Tract*. Baltimore: Williams & Wilkins, 1983: 84.
4 Rock JA, Siegler AM, Boer-Meisel M *et al*. The efficacy of post-operative hydrotubation: a randomized prospective multicenter clinical trial. *Fertil Steril* 1984; 42: 373.
5 Schlaff WD, Hassiakos DK, Damewood MD, Rock JA. Neosalpingostomy for distal tubal obstruction: prognostic factors and impact of surgical technique. *Fertil Steril* 1990; 54: 984.

Proximal tubal obstruction

MILES J. NOVY & AMY S. THURMOND

Although less common than distal fallopian tube disease, proximal obstruction of one or both fallopian tubes occurs in 10–20% of hysterosalpingograms (HSGs) performed to evaluate infertility [1]. As a result, visualization of the distal tube is prevented and there is concern that the proximal tubal obstruction (PTO) is contributing to the patient's infertility. PTO presents a significant diagnostic and therapeutic problem since underfilling of the tube, muscular spasm, and mechanical occlusion from a variety of pathologic causes are not easily differentiated from one another by conventional hysterosalpingography or even by laparoscopy. Evidence suggests that the proximal oviduct may also be functionally obstructed by amorphous material that can be dislodged by direct tubal flushing or probing [2].

Transcervical fallopian tube catheterization, using hysteroscopic or fluoroscopic guidance and a coaxial system of guidewires and catheters, has proven to be an effective method for evaluating cornual obstruction. In selected patients, fallopian tube catheterization techniques also have a therapeutic benefit by overcoming a reversible obstruction in the proximal tube. Proximal tubal occlusion which is not correctable by fluoroscopic or hysteroscopic catheterization methods may require resection and microsurgical anastomosis.

ANATOMY AND PATHOPHYSIOLOGY OF THE PROXIMAL TUBE

The length of the intramural tube varies between 8 and 14 mm. Its course is straight or slightly curved in 60% and convoluted in 40% of patients [3]. The intramural portion of the fallopian tube begins as a circular opening (0.5–1.5 mm in diameter) at the end of the endometrial funnel. The innermost portion consists of the tubal antrum, a bulge-like dilatation which tapers in the middle and outer third of the intramural tube to a diameter of 1.0 mm. Three muscle layers can be identified at the junction of the uterus with the proximal isthmus: the innermost longitudinal, the intermediate circular, and the outer spiral layer. The circular layer is the most prominent and is likely to influence the diameter of the tubal lumen.

The oviduct is supplied with both parasympathetic and sympathetic nerves and it is the circular muscle layer which is most heavily innervated. During the menstrual cycle, there are cyclic variations in the quantity and distribution of catecholamines, number of adrenergic receptors, steroid hormone receptors, and in epithelial morphology. Throughout the menstrual cycle, β-receptor activity generally predominates in isthmic circular muscle except around the time of ovulation when α-receptor activity is increased. Cyclic nucleotides and prostaglandins also modulate smooth muscle tone in the oviduct. Prostaglandin $F_{2\alpha}$ causes an increase in contractility of isthmic circular muscle while prostaglandin E_2 is generally inhibitory. Although many agents, including cyclic adenosine monophosphate, indomethacin, $\beta 2$-agonists, and α-adrenergic antagonists have been demonstrated to relax the circular muscle layer *in vitro*, their *in vivo* effects are variable or uncertain [4].

Ciliogenesis and secretory activity of the tubal epithelium are estrogen-dependent processes which are antagonized by progesterone. Scanning electron micrographs of human and monkey fallopian tube indicate that granular and membranous secretory products frequently pack the isthmic lumen to the point of occlusion and that an increase in lumen diameter is observed after ovulation in comparison with the preovulatory phase [4]. It is reasonable, therefore, that the passage of dye or contrast agents may be impeded by decreased compliance of the tubal wall or viscosity of the luminal contents, both of which are hormonally dependent.

PATHOLOGY OF PROXIMAL TUBAL OCCLUSION

Infection and subsequent inflammation or fibrosis are leading causes of proximal tubal occlusion and are frequently the consequence of chlamydial or gonococcal salpingitis or postpartum endometritis [5]. In proximal tubal segments resected at the time of surgery, obliterative fibrosis, salpingitis isthmica nodosa (SIN), and chronic inflammation together account for the vast majority of anatomic occlusions at the cornual–isthmic junction. Occasionally, the uterotubal ostium will be obscured by intrauterine adhesions (as in Asherman's syndrome), thereby simulating a complete intramural block on HSG. Such situations have yielded good results to hysteroscopic cannulation techniques or to a combination of microsurgery with tubal cannulation and hysteroscopic adhesiolysis [6]. Other causes of PTO include cornual polyps, fibroids, endometriosis, and parasitic infestations such as schistosomiasis and oxyuriasis (Table 79.1). Intraluminal endometriosis occurs in approximately 10% of tubes resected for PTO and may exist without relation to visible lesions elsewhere in the pelvis. Müllerian anomalies of the fallopian tube are rare but congenital atresia of the isthmus is known to occur. Fibrostenosis of the tubal lumen is sometimes marked by a prestenotic bulge or dilatation which is distinguished from the tapered lumen associated with other causes of tubal obstruction but these correlations are not exact. SIN begins with intermittent or partial obstruction of the proximal lumen but in time may progress to complete occlusion of the cornual–isthmic junction. It is characterized by the formation of diverticulae and tuboperitoneal fistulas visible on HSG. The associated muscular hypertrophy and isthmic nodularity can be appreciated at laparoscopy or laparotomy. Paradoxically,

Table 79.1 Conditions associated with proximal tubal obstruction or occlusion

Muscular spasm	Salpingitis isthmica nodosa
Stromal edema	Tuberculosis
Mucosal agglutination	Chronic salpingitis
Amorphous material	Fibrosis
Viscous secretions	Leiomyomas
Pinworm eggs	Endosalpingiosis
Schistosomiasis	Congenital atresia
Cornual polyps	Tubal sterilization
Endometriosis	

cornual occlusion is not correlated with the degree of diverticulosis on HSG.

Several authors have noted a lack of histologic confirmation of luminal occlusion in about 10–20% of patients, despite an apparent cornual block on repeated HSGs and even at laparoscopy. Recent data suggest that a substantial number of these cases of presumed spasm or pseudoobstruction may actually represent mechanical obstruction from a discrete plug of debris in the proximal portion of the tube [2]. In some tubes, these plugs coexist on a background of chronic inflammation. The prevalence of serum immunoglobulin G antibodies against *Chlamydia* is high (about 45%) in women with isolated reversible PTO, although it is significantly lower than in women with combined proximal and distal tubal disease [7]. The exact role of chlamydial infection in PTO is ambiguous because commercially available assays are not adequately serotype-specific for *Chlamydia trachomatis* but it is likely that an inflammatory component related to past infection is a factor in the etiology of proximal obstructions.

SELECTION OF PATIENTS

Before fallopian tube catheterization techniques were developed, the approach to managing patients with cornual obstruction was to repeat the HSG with an adjunctive spasmolytic agent prior to laparoscopy or reconstructive surgery. Only limited success was achieved with several smooth muscle relaxants, including glucagon, diazepam, and isoxsuprine [1]. Thus, pharmacologic methods have been supplanted by transcervical catheterization techniques to diagnose and confirm PTO.

The algorithm shown in Figure 79.1 summarizes our current strategy for evaluating the patient with cornual obstruction found on conventional HSG. If the HSG is done to establish postoperative patency or if the patient is otherwise not a candidate for laparoscopy (e.g., low suspicion for pelvic disease or previous laparoscopy with normal pelvic findings), fallopian tube catheterization is performed fluoroscopically. If cornual patency is not demonstrated by selective salpingography or fallopian tube recanalization, hysteroscopic catheterization at laparoscopy or laparotomy is a logical follow-up study.

If a history of pelvic inflammatory disease, endometriosis, or unexplained infertility is known or suspected to coexist with PTO, or if there is a uterine mass or filling defect on HSG (Fig. 79.2), PTO is

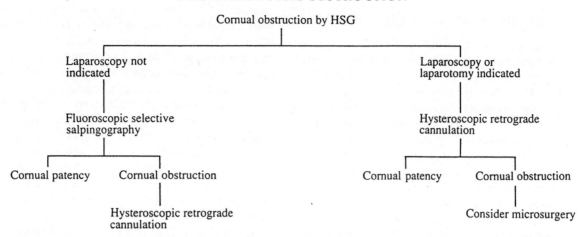

Fig. 79.1 Algorithm showing the recommended management of patients with proximal tubal obstruction. (From [11].)

initially investigated by hysteroscopic fallopian tube catheterization in conjunction with laparoscopy. It is useful to have the hysteroscopic cannulation set available in the operating room at infertility laparoscopy procedures so that an incidental finding of PTO

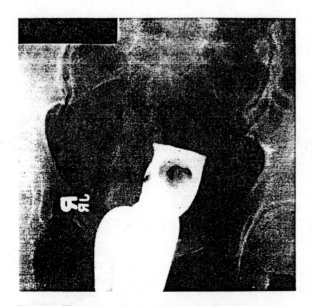

Fig. 79.2 This women had a history of infertility and menorrhagia. There is bilateral proximal tubal obstruction in the intramural portion and a large intrauterine filling defect on hysterosalpingogram. Bilateral cornual patency was established by hysteroscopic catheterization. Hysteroscopic resection of a submucous myoma was accomplished at the same sitting.

can be evaluated under the same anesthetic. Cornual obstruction due to muscular spasm or amorphous debris usually persists during laparoscopic chromotubation but with concurrent hysteroscopic catheterization one can resolve a false-positive finding in a cost-effective manner. Hysteroscopic fallopian tube catheterization can also be performed at the time of laparotomy (with the patient in modified lithotomy position in Allen stirrups) where it can be useful in directing surgical therapy as discussed below. Inevitably, the patient selection process for fluoroscopic or hysteroscopic catheterization will vary from one institution to another. It will depend in large part upon individual levels of expertise and the degree of cooperation between radiologists and gynecologists in a given practice setting.

Ideally, the patient is investigated in the early follicular phase or after suppression of endometrial growth by a gonadotropin-releasing hormone (GnRH) agonist or danocrine. The hypoestrogenic effects of ovarian suppression for 2 or more months have been seen to reverse some cases of PTO, presumably due to tubal secretions, intraluminal endometriosis (M.J. Novy and A.S. Thurmond, unpublished observations) or even cornual fibroids [8]. Because of the possible role of chlamydial infection in PTO, some authors have combined ovarian suppression with extended oral antibiotic therapy (doxycycline or clindamycin) before repeated HSG and/or tubal catheterization [9]. Prospective trials are under way to determine the place of GnRH agonists and broad-spectrum antibiotics in the management of PTO.

CATHETERIZATION TECHNIQUES

The instruments and techniques for fluoroscopic fallopian tube catheterization, selective salpingography, and recanalization have been described in detail [10]. The procedure is performed during the follicular phase of the menstrual cycle, utilizing sterile techniques and with antibiotic prophylaxis (usually doxycycline 100 mg orally b.i.d. is given before and for several days after the procedure). Small doses of midazolam and fentanyl citrate may be given intravenously during the procedure for sedation.

Briefly, the method consists of gaining access to the uterus with a vacuum cup hysterosalpingography device (Thurmond-Rösch Hysterocath; Cook, Bloomington, IN, or Cook Ob/Gyn, Spencer, IN). This provides a sterile conduit through which a series of coaxial catheters and guidewires can be introduced and allows traction on the uterus without the application of a tenaculum (Fig. 79.3). A conventional HSG with diluted water-soluble contrast medium is performed initially which localizes the uterine cornua without obscuring the catheters. A coaxial catheter system (9 Fr Teflon sheath and 5.5 Fr polyethylene catheter) is advanced over a 0.035-inch diameter (0.089 cm) J guidewire to the uterine cornu. The guidewire is removed and contrast agent is injected to visualize the tube (selective salpingography). If proximal tubal obstruction persists, a 0.015-inch diameter (0.038 cm) guidewire with a flexible platinum tip and 3 Fr Teflon catheter (Cook, Bloomington, IN) are advanced together into the fallopian tube and an attempt is made to recanalize the obstruction with probing movements of the guidewire. If there is an acute angulation in the tube at the site of the obstruction, a 3 Fr catheter tapered to 2.7 Fr at its tip, and a 0.016-inch guidewire tapered to 0.014 inch (Target Therapeutics, San Jose, CA) may be helpful. When the guidewire passes the obstruction, the catheter is advanced over the guidewire, the guidewire is removed, and contrast agent is injected through the 3 Fr catheter to delineate the distal tube. Alternatively, the smaller catheter is removed and contrast agent is injected through the 5.5 Fr catheter still wedged in the tubal ostium in order thoroughly to evaluate the tube. In the case of bilateral PTO, the procedure is repeated on the other side. A postcatheterization HSG is obtained to confirm tubal patency and to visualize the site of recanalization (Fig. 79.4).

The principles of transcervical fallopian tube catheterization by hysteroscopy are the same as for fluoroscopic catheterization but the catheter system is adapted to pass through the operating channel of a hysteroscope and to provide a gas-tight seal around the catheters and guidewires [11]. Carbon dioxide is the preferred distention medium for tubal catheterization but liquid distention media are also

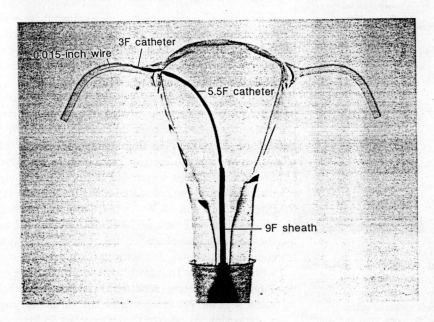

Fig. 79.3 Glass uterine model demonstrating the vacuum cup hysterosalpingography device used for fluoroscopic catheterization with 9 Fr sheath, the 5.5 Fr catheter in the cornua, and the 3 Fr catheter and guidewire in the proximal fallopian tube.

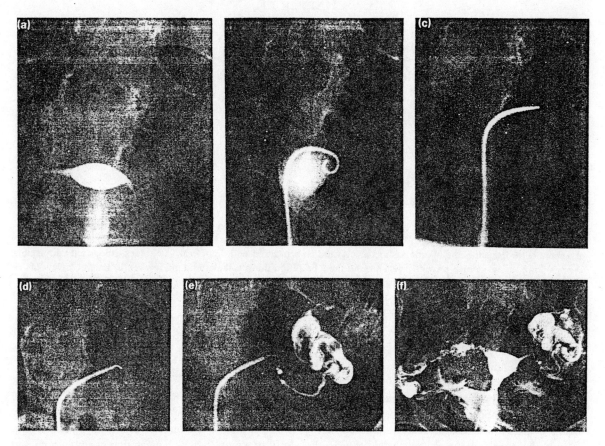

Fig. 79.4 Twenty-eight-year-old woman with 3 years of primary infertility. Prior to this examination, she had one hysterosalpingogram (HSG) and two laparoscopies which documented bilateral proximal tubal obstruction. During the most recent laparoscopy, she had bilateral fimbrioplasties but hysteroscopic fallopian tube catheterization was not performed. Fluoroscopic catheter recanalization of the proximal tubal obstructions was therefore requested. (a) Initial HSG confirms the bilateral proximal tubal obstruction. (b) The 5.5 Fr catheter (not visible) and 0.035-inch J guidewire (visible) are coaxially advanced through the Hysterocath and endocervical canal. Using fluoroscopic guidance, the catheter and wire are advanced into the left uterine cornu. (c) The catheter is wedged into the tubal ostium using a 0.035 inch straight guidewire (visible), and then the guidewire is removed. Full-strength contrast medium was directly injected into the left tube and obstruction was confirmed. (d) Because of the angulation in the tube just proximal to the site of obstruction, a soft, tapered catheter-guidewire system is used (Tracker-18 catheter and Taper guidewire, Target Therapeutics, San Jose, CA). With probing movements of the guidewire which extends approximately 5 mm beyond the tip of the catheter, the obstruction is recanalized. (Wire is visible; catheter tip is marked by a radiopaque bead.) (e) Injection through the 5.5 Fr catheter shows that the tube is now widely patent, and there are some nodules in the isthmic portion of the tube at the site of the prior obstruction consistent with salpingitis isthmica nodosa. Using a similar technique, the right proximal obstruction is probed. (f) Repeat conventional HSG at the conclusion of the procedure demonstrates bilateral tubal patency.

suitable. The tubal catheterization set consists of a 30 or 35 cm straight 5.5 Fr clear Teflon outer cannula (also available in polyethylene with a curved tip) which is fitted with a plastic Y-adapter that ends in Luer-lock hubs (Cook Ob/Gyn, Spencer, IN); (Fig. 79.5). The straight arm of the adapter is available for injection of contrast medium or indigo carmine dye into the tubal ostium; it is sealed with a screw cap when not in use. A 3 Fr Teflon inner catheter (tapered to 2.5 Fr) is passed through the outer arm of the Y-adapter which is fitted with an O-ring fitting that provides a seal around the catheter. A stainless

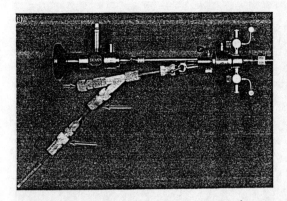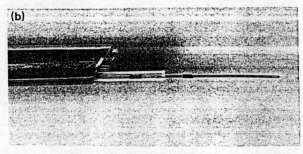

Fig. 79.5 Cornual cannulation set for hysteroscopic use. (a) 5.5 Fr clear Teflon outer cannula introduced through the operating channel of a Storz model 26163D hysteroscope. The Teflon cannula is fitted with a plastic Y-adapter consisting of a channel for irrigation and injection (short arrow) and an arm fitted with "stop-leak" Luer-lock fittings with adjustable O-rings (long arrows) which provide a seal around the 3 Fr Teflon inner catheter and guidewire. (b) Enlarged view of hysteroscope tip with 30° panoramic lens and coaxial catheter assembly. Operating channel contains 5.5 Fr clear Teflon outer cannula, 3 Fr Teflon inner catheter with 1 cm markings (tapered to 2.5 Fr in its distal 3 cm), and flexible stainless steel guidewire 0.018-inch (0.043 cm) in diameter with blunt tip.

steel guidewire of 0.018 inch (0.043 cm) diameter with flexible blunt tip completes the catheterization set. Guidewires of smaller diameter (0.015 inch) with platinum tips and greater flexibility are recommended as useful accessories. Modifications of the catheter assembly are available for flexible hysteroscopes.

After the tubal ostium is visualized, the 5.5 Fr outer catheter is wedged in the tubal antrum. We now recommend that selective chromotubation is first attempted using a 3 ml syringe with indigo carmine dye. It has been calculated that the force exerted by a column of fluid directed at the tubal ostium is several times greater than that which can be achieved by distending the uterine cavity during a conventional HSG. If patency is not achieved by selective tubal injection, the 3 Fr catheter and guidewire are then introduced coaxially, as in the fluoroscopic approach. Advancement of the guidewire through the uterotubal junction is observed by laparoscopy with video display of the guidewire movement in the isthmus. Upon entering the isthmus, the guidewire is withdrawn and indigo carmine is injected through the 3 Fr catheter to evaluate patency of the distal oviduct.

Hysteroscopic tubal cannulation with guidewires for PTO is not recommended in an office setting because it is difficult to distinguish between successful relief of an obstruction and tubal perforation. However, selective chromotubation can be undertaken in an outpatient setting for an assessment of proximal patency.

RESULTS OF TRANSCERVICAL CATHETERIZATION

We have performed transcervical catheterization of the fallopian tubes by fluoroscopy and hysteroscopy in more than 200 women without any clinically significant complications. Perforation of a tube occurs in about 5% of cases without apparent adverse sequelae. In our experience, fluoroscopic catheterization results in a radiation dose to the ovaries of 0.85 ± 0.56 rad, which is equivalent to estimated ovarian doses for a barium enema or excretory urogram [12].

Using similar equipment and techniques as described above, catheterization of the fallopian tubes has been successful in demonstrating patency in 75–92% of tubes attempted (Table 79.2). Wedging of the 5.5 Fr catheter in the cornu with subsequent flushing (ostial salpingography) results in patency of the fallopian tube in 20–40% of cases and no further diagnostic procedures are necessary [11].

About 30% of patients who undergo fluoroscopic transcervical catheterization for PTO demonstrate apparently normal tubal anatomy following the procedure. Another one-third also have normal tubes but the appearance of the peritoneal spill of contrast agent suggests peritubal adhesions. An additional 10% will have a distal occlusion or hydrosalpinx demonstrated. In the remaining patients, approximately 15% will have a small diverticulum at the site of recanalization or frank salpingitis isthmica nodosa and about 10% will have unsuccessful

Table 79.2 Results of transcervical fallopian tube catheterization for proximal tubal obstruction

Authors	Number of patients	Patency (%)	Intrauterine pregnancy rate (%)	Ectopic pregnancy rate (%)	Estimated 6-month patency (%)
Fluoroscopic catheterization					
Thurmond and Rösch (1990) [10]	100	86	33	6	75
Platia et al. (1989) [13]	21	76	38	13	75
Confino et al. (1990) [14]	77	92	35	1	82
Segars et al. (1990) [15]	19	73	20	10	71
Hysteroscopic catheterization					
Deaton et al. (1990) [16]	11	72	30	30	73
Novy (1991; unpublished data)	50	88	47	8	

attempts at recanalization [12]. The factors which contribute to unsuccessful fallopian tube catheterization are not always clear. However, recent data indicate that in skilled hands failure to successfully cannulate the proximal oviduct is usually due to intrinsic tubal disease rather than technical problems [16,17].

The therapeutic benefit of fallopian tube catheterization for PTO is more difficult to prove because infertility is often a multifactorial problem. In a clinically heterogeneous group of 100 women with PTO, many without prior laparoscopy, we observed a 33% intrauterine pregnancy rate and a 6% ectopic pregnancy rate (average follow-up 7 months) in those who had successful cannulations [10]. All of the patients with ectopic pregnancies had either laparoscopically proven peritubal adhesions or a history of tubal surgery and all ectopics were located in the ampulla of the tube. Similar pregnancy results have been reported by others using fluoroscopic or hysteroscopic techniques (Table 79.2).

Due to the patient selection process (Fig. 79.1), patients who undergo hysteroscopic tubal catheterization usually have a wider spectrum of pathologic findings in addition to PTO (e.g., adhesions, endometriosis, Asherman's syndrome, and more diffuse tubal disease). Therefore, evaluating the therapeutic benefit of transcervical catheterization is problematic in such patients because the reproductive outcome is also influenced by the ancillary surgical procedures [11]. Follow-up of a smaller group of carefully selected patients in whom PTO was judged to be the primary or sole cause of infertility (without evidence of other tubal disease) demonstrated that 58% of these women conceived within 1 year after fluor-

oscopic tubal catheterization and all pregnancies were intrauterine [10].

The tubal reocclusion rate is difficult to determine because, in part, it is time-dependent. In patients who do not conceive, it appears that approximately 50% of tubes reocclude by 6 months [12]. If we assume that the tubes are patent in the patients who conceive, this gives an approximate reocclusion rate of 25% (Table 79.2).

Some authors advocate using a balloon catheter over the guidewire which is wedged in the intramural tube, so-called balloon tuboplasty [14]. It is hypothesized that inflation of the balloon in the cornual region may result in improved long-term patency of the fallopian tube when compared to flushing or probing with a simple coaxial catheter. So far, however, recanalization rates, postprocedure pregnancy rates, and reocclusion rates are not different for the nonballoon techniques and the more expensive balloon techniques (Table 79.2).

MICROSURGICAL TUBOCORNUAL ANASTOMOSIS

Microsurgical tubocornual anastomosis is a well-established procedure and the preferred surgical option for women with occlusive disease in the proximal oviduct not opened by transcervical catheterization. Since the procedure was first described in 1977 by Gomel [18] and Winston [19], numerous reports have confirmed its effectiveness in treating cornual disease and its superiority to the tubouterine implantation method previously employed [20–22]. The advantages of tubocornual anastomosis over tubouterine implantation include: (1) preservation of an intramural portion of the fallopian tube; (2) creation of a longer oviduct; (3) decreased incidence of postoperative adhesions; (4) decreased risk of uterine rupture; (5) cesarean section not obligatory in subsequent pregnancy; and (6) it yields better overall pregnancy results (Table 79.3).

In a review of the literature comprising 187 patients, the mean intrauterine pregnancy rate after tubocornual anastomosis was 58%, with an ectopic pregnancy rate of 4% [25]. The results after uterotubal implantation are much more variable among surgeons, with a mean pregnancy rate of 27% and an ectopic pregnancy rate of 11% [5,26]. It is fair to conclude that tubal implantation is a less physiologic technique and has not stood the test of time in the hands of most reproductive surgeons.

Depending on the extent of disease in the intramural segment of the tube, the tubocornual anastomosis may be juxtamural, intramural, or juxtauterine (when most of the intramural segment requires excision and the anastomosis takes place at the level of the pretubal antrum) (Fig. 79.6). Fortunately, the deep transmural portion of the fallopian tube is spared in more than 80% of cases with proximal tubal occlusion [21,28]. Deep intramural anastomosis is facilitated by such modifications as seromuscular relaxing incisions in the cornu, the use of cutting needles with increased curvature, and the concurrent use of hysteroscopic catheterization with guidewires and a series of catheters at the time of microsurgery. According to the latter technique, the intramural segment of the tubal lumen is identified by hysteroscopic catheterization and a series of progressively larger catheters are placed coaxially over the guidewire, thereby dilating the intramural tube and facilitating a difficult anastomosis [6]. Various factors may adversely affect the outcome of tubocornual

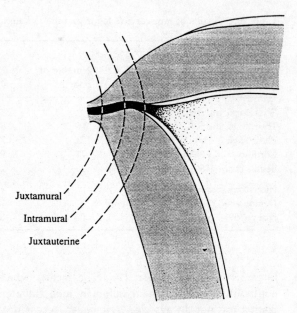

Juxtamural
Intramural
Juxtauterine

Fig. 79.6 Tubocornual anastomosis. Depending on the extent of disease of the intramural segment, tubocornual anastomosis may be juxtamural, intramural, or juxtauterine. (From [27].)

anastomosis, such as coexisting infertility factors, especially in the male, the presence of significant distal tubal disease, and technical difficulties encountered during surgery [24]. Some authors report that patients with chronic salpingitis or SIN have lower pregnancy rates than do patients with fibrostenosis [21]. Fertility after microsurgery for a coexisting proximal occlusion and distal hydrosalpinx (so-called bipolar occlusive disease) is poor, with pregnancy rates rarely above 10–15% and such patients are usually better served by *in vitro* fertilization [29,30]. However, if the proximal obstruction

Table 79.3 Results of tubocornual anastomosis for pathologic proximal occlusion of the oviduct

Authors	Number of patients	Conception rate (%)	Term pregnancy rate (%)	Ectopic pregnancy rate (%)
Gomel (1983) [23]	48	68	56	6
McComb (1986) [20]*	26		58	8
Donnez and Casanas-Roux (1986) [21]	82		44	7
Patton *et al.* (1987) [22]	27	69	53	11
Gillett and Herbison (1989) [24]	42	65		9

* The majority of patients had partial or complete intramural occlusion.

can be reversed by catheterization and if the condition of the endosalpinx or one or both fimbria is promising, then a microsurgical fimbrioplasty or neosalpingotomy may give superior results compared to *in vitro* fertilization. A unilateral tubocornual anastomosis for PTO (with reasonably normal fimbria on the same side) and a contralateral salpingostomy for distal occlusive disease alone yield similar fertility rates as tubocornual anastomosis for bilateral proximal occlusive disease alone [31]. This finding emphasizes that the prognosis after tubocornual anastomosis is influenced most by the extent of distal tubal disease.

FALLOPIAN TUBE CATHETERIZATION BY ULTRASOUND

Transcervical tubal catheterization guided by ultrasound or by tactile sensation alone has found its main application in the assisted reproductive technologies. In 1987, Jansen and Anderson demonstrated the feasibility of catheterizing the fallopian tube from the vagina with ultrasound and subsequently they reported the first pregnancy after intratubal embryo transfer by this technique [32,33]. The results of transcervical intratubal embryo transfer appear superior to the transfer of gametes, which probably reflects the difficulty of delivering gametes by this approach to the site of fertilization in the ampulla. This subject has been extensively reviewed by Balmaceda *et al.* [34], who quote an overall pregnancy rate of 20–25% after transcervical intratubal zygote or early embryo transfer. The efficiency of catheterizing the tubes blindly or with ultrasound imaging is similar (about 75%), which suggests that the use of ultrasound does not play a large role in guiding the catheter to the tubal ostium but that it may help to verify the catheter position once it is in the oviduct.

The obvious advantages of ultrasound imaging in comparison to other methods are the avoidance of radiation or anesthesia. Although ultrasound imaging of the small catheters and the flow of fluids in the fallopian tubes has been improved by color Doppler and increased resolution provided by the newer endovaginal probes, as well as by greater echogenicity of the catheters, it does not yet provide the accuracy of localization which is available with fluoroscopy or by endoscopic techniques. These limitations may be overcome in catheterizing normal tubes but may hinder successful recanalization of

potentially diseased tubes. Although preliminary reports suggest that transvaginal recanalization of proximally obstructed tubes with ultrasound guidance is feasible, the relatively poor visualization of the catheters and of the tubal anatomy limit this application in our opinion [35,36]. Additional studies are needed in larger numbers of patients with varying degrees of pathology in order to establish that efficacy is comparable to previously established fluoroscopic and hysteroscopic methods. Concerns remain about the inherent limitations of ultrasound in distinguishing between perforation and anatomic recanalization — nor does ultrasound provide adequate information about tubal anatomy at the site of recanalization or even distally.

FALLOPOSCOPY AND FUTURE APPLICATIONS

Transcervical access to the fallopian tube has paved the way for a variety of diagnostic and therapeutic procedures and has the potential to increase our understanding of tubal function. Hysteroscopic catheterization has been used in conjunction with advances in fiberoptics to permit visual observation of the tubal lumen by means of a flexible miniature falloposcope [37]. In some patients, the entire length of the fallopian tube is negotiable by catheters and fiberoptics introduced through the cervix. Although the diagnostic accuracy of falloposcopy needs to be validated by independent methods (i.e., biopsy and histology), it has the potential to identify and assess a variety of endotubal lesions. Clearly, the deficiency of cannulation techniques alone is that one cannot simply and uniformly differentiate between spasm, luminal debris, and obstruction by mild adhesions. Falloposcopy also has the potential to evaluate the efficacy of various endotubal manipulations such as guidewire cannulation or balloon dilatation. Prospective clinical evaluations must be performed to correlate falloposcopic findings with clinical outcome before the utility of falloposcopy can be determined objectively. At the moment, the practical usefulness of falloposcopy is limited and it remains a research technique. Nevertheless, extensive efforts are being made to improve and refine the optical capabilities of these very small-diameter endoscopes and to develop smaller stealth catheters (Target Therapeutics, San Jose, CA) and biopsy instruments that can safely negotiate the tubal lumen. A new ingenious linear eversion catheter is being developed for clinical trials in the human fallopian tube (Imagyn Medical, San Clemente, CA).

Another exciting future application of transcervical tubal catheterization may be the management of ectopic pregnancy in selected patients. Following selective salpingography, nonsurgical treatment of tubal gestation has been performed by injecting small doses of methotrexate through the tubal catheter [38]. At the other end of the reproductive spectrum, transcervical tubal catheterization with laser fiber ablation or silicone injection has been used to accomplish permanent or reversible tubal sterilization, respectively [39].

CONCLUSIONS

The diagnostic and therapeutic options for managing proximal tubal disease have been expanded by the development of transcervical fallopian tube catheterization techniques. Tubal catheterization, ostial injections (selective salpingography), and recanalization of PTO can be done in conjunction with other diagnostic infertility procedures such as hysterosalpingography, laparoscopy, and hysteroscopy. Hysteroscopic or fluoroscopic catheterization with selective salpingography and/or recanalization results in tubal visualization in at least 85% of patients with PTO. In addition to differentiating between true PTO and cornual spasm (and thus sparing the patient unnecessary tubal surgery), catheterization techniques can be used to open the obstructed tube when the blockage is presumably caused by filmy adhesions or intraluminal debris. It is quite clear that fallopian tube catheterization does allow some women with PTO to conceive but the therapeutic efficacy of fallopian tube recanalization is difficult to prove since the pathologic cause is usually not known. Microsurgical resection and tubal cornual anastomosis are recommended in the treatment of patients with persistent obstruction or true isolated proximal occlusion that is not amenable to recanalization. Fluoroscopic fallopian tube catheterization is useful in postoperatively evaluating patients who are apparent failures after microsurgical anastomosis. Again, selective catheterization will differentiate between postoperative fibrosis and cornual spasm or intraluminal debris. *In vitro* fertilization is a reasonable alternative in patients who have failed microsurgery.

REFERENCES

1 Thurmond AS, Novy M, Rösch J. Terbutaline in diagnosis of interstitial fallopian tube obstruction. *Invest Radiol* 1988; 23: 209–210.
2 Sulak PJ, Letterie GS, Coddington CC, Hayslip CC, Woodward JE, Klein TA. Histology of proximal tubal occlusion. *Fertil Steril* 1987; 48: 437–440.
3 Merchant RN, Prabhu SR, Chougale A. Uterotubal junction — morphology and clinical aspects. *Int J Fertil* 1983; 28: 199–205.
4 Jansen RPS. Endocrine response in the fallopian tube. *Endocr Rev* 1984; 5: 525–551.
5 Musich JR, Behrman SJ. Surgical management of tubal obstruction at the uterotubal junction. *Fertil Steril* 1983; 40: 423–441.
6 Novy MJ. Combined hysteroscopic and microsurgical approach to intrauterine synechiae with cornual occlusion. American Fertility Society Program and Abstracts, 45th Annual Meeting (San Francisco, CA, November 13–16, 1989): S8 (abstract O-018).
7 Hickok LR, Thurmond A, Patton PE, Novy MJ. The potential role of *Chlamydia* in the etiology of reversible proximal tubal obstruction. Pacific Coast Fertility Society Program and Abstracts, 39th Annual Meeting (Indian Wells, CA, April 10–14, 1991): A11 (abstract P-016).
8 Gardner RL, Shaw RW. Cornual fibroids: a conservative approach to restoring tubal patency using a gonadotropin-releasing hormone agonist (goserelin) with successful pregnancy. *Fertil Steril* 1989; 52: 332–334.
9 Martin DC, Sieger W. Therapeutic implications of diagnostic hysteroscopy for cornual occlusion. Presented at Third World Conference on Fallopian Tube in Health and Disease (Kiel, West Germany, July 3–6, 1990).
10 Thurmond AS, Rösch J. Nonsurgical fallopian tube recanalization for treatment of infertility. *Radiology* 1990; 174: 371–374.
11 Novy MJ, Thurmond AS, Patton P, Uchida BT, Rösch J. Diagnosis of cornual obstruction by transcervical fallopian tube cannulation. *Fertil Steril* 1988; 50: 434–440.
12 Thurmond AS. Selective salpingography and fallopian tube recanalization. *Am J Radiol* 1991; 156: 33–38.
13 Platia M, Chang R, Loriaux DL, Doppman JL. Therapeutic potential of transvaginal recanalization for proximal fallopian tube obstruction (PFTO). American Fertility Society Program and Abstracts: 45th Annual Meeting (San Francisco, CA, November 13–16, 1989): S24 (abstract O-056).
14 Confino E, Tur-Kaspa I, DeCherney A *et al.* Transcervical balloon tuboplasty: a multicenter study. *JAMA* 1990; 264: 2079–2082.
15 Segars JH, Herbert CM III, Moore DE, Hill GA, Wentz AC, Winfield AC. Selective fallopian tube cannulation: initial experience in an infertile population. *Fertil Steril* 1990; 53: 357–359.
16 Deaton JL, Gibson M, Riddick DH, Brumsted JR. Diagnosis and treatment of cornual obstruction using a flexible tip guidewire. *Fertil Steril* 1990; 53: 232–236.

17 Letterie GS, Sakas EL. The histology of proximal tubal obstruction in cases of unsuccessful tubal canalization. American Fertility Society Program and Abstracts, 47th Annual Meeting (Orlando, FL, October 21–24, 1991): S7 (abstract O-015).

18 Gomel V. Tubal reanastomosis by microsurgery. *Fertil Steril* 1977; 28: 59–65.

19 Winston RML. Microsurgical tubocornual anastomosis for reversal of sterilisation. *Lancet* 1977; 1: 284–285.

20 McComb P. Microsurgical tubocornual anastomosis for occlusive cornual disease: reproducible results without the need for tubouterine implantation. *Fertil Steril* 1986; 46: 571–577.

21 Donnez J, Casanas-Roux F. Prognostic factors influencing the pregnancy rate after microsurgical cornual anastomosis. *Fertil Steril* 1986; 46: 1089–1092.

22 Patton PE, Williams TJ, Coulam CB. Microsurgical reconstruction of the proximal oviduct. *Fertil Steril* 1987; 47: 35–39.

23 Gomel V. An odyssey through the oviduct. *Fertil Steril* 1983; 39: 144–156.

24 Gillett WR, Herbison GP. Tubocornual anastomosis: surgical considerations and coexistent infertility factors in determining the prognosis. *Fertil Steril* 1989; 51: 241–246.

25 Marana R, Quagliarello J. Proximal tubal occlusion: microsurgery versus IVF – a review. *Int J Fertil* 1988; 33: 338–340.

26 Haseltine FP, Von Arras JA. Current concepts in management of cornual disease of the uterus. *Semin Reprod Endocrinol* 1984; 2: 146–153.

27 Gomel V. Microsurgery in Female Infertility. Boston: Little, Brown and Company, 1983: 177.

28 Ehrler P. Anastomose intramurale de la trompe. *Bull Fed Soc Gynecol Obstet* 1965; 17: 866.

29 Frantzen C, Schlösser H-W. Microsurgery and postinfectious tubal infertility. *Fertil Steril* 1982; 38: 397–402.

30 McComb PF, Lee NH, Stephenson MD. Reproductive outcome after microsurgery for proximal and distal occlusions in the same fallopian tube. *Fertil Steril* 1991; 56: 134–135.

31 McComb PF, Lee NH, Stephenson MD. Reproductive outcome after unilateral tubocornual anastomosis and contralateral salpingostomy by microsurgery. *Fertil Steril* 1991; 55: 1011–1013.

32 Jansen RPS, Anderson JC. Catheterisation of the fallopian tubes from the vagina. *Lancet* 1987; 2: 309–310.

33 Jansen RPS, Anderson JC, Sutherland PD. Nonoperative embryo transfer to the fallopian tube. *N Engl J Med* 1988; 319: 288–291.

34 Balmaceda JP, Alam V, Borini A. Fallopian tube catheterization. In: Grunfeld L, ed. *Infertility and Reproductive Medicine Clinics of North America*, vol 2, no. 4. Philadelphia: WB Saunders 1991: 783–797.

35 Lisse K, Sydow P. Fallopian tube catheterization and recanalization under ultrasonic observation: a simplified technique to evaluate tubal patency and open proximally obstructed tubes. *Fertil Steril* 1991; 56: 198–201.

36 Stern JJ, Peters AJ, Coulam CB. Transcervical tuboplasty under ultrasonographic guidance: a pilot study. *Fertil Steril* 1991; 56: 359–360.

37 Kerin J, Daykhovsky L, Grundfest W, Surrey E. Falloposcopy: a microendoscopic transvaginal technique for diagnosing and treating endotubal disease incorporating guide wire cannulation and direct balloon tuboplasty. *J Reprod Med* 1990; 35: 606–612.

38 Risquez F, Mathieson J, Pariente D et al. Diagnosis and treatment of ectopic pregnancy by retrograde selective salpingography and intraluminal methotrexate injection: work in progress. *Hum Reprod* 1990; 5: 759–762.

39 Risquez F, Mathieson J, Zorn J-R. Tubal cannulation via the cervix: a passing fancy – or here to stay? *J In Vitro Fert Embryo Transf* 1990; 7: 301–303.

Management of endometriosis-associated infertility

NANCY A. KLEIN & DAVID L. OLIVE

INTRODUCTION

Endometriosis is found in 20–40% of patients under-going evaluation for infertility – a prevalence 10-fold greater than that found in the reproductive-age female population at large. Although a clear associ-ation exists between all stages of endometriosis and infertility, a causal relationship has not been established between infertility and mild or minimal disease. Nevertheless, a wide variety of treatment modalities have been utilized to remove, suppress, and prevent recurrence of endometriosis to improve subsequent fertility.

Infertility associated with moderate and severe endometriosis appears to be explained by anatomic distortion of the normal spatial relationships of the reproductive organs, resulting in decreased ovum recovery and transport. Less clear are the mechanisms responsible for the relative subfertility believed to exist with minimal and mild disease. This chapter will provide a brief overview of endometriosis, its relationship to infertility, and the therapeutic approaches available for treatment of the disease.

EPIDEMIOLOGY

Endometriosis is defined as the presence of endo-metrial tissue outside the endometrial cavity. The vast majority of patients with endometriosis have disease limited to the peritoneal surfaces of the pelvis or pelvic organs, although extrapelvic endometriosis occurs in a variety of locations. Most cases are diag-nosed in the third and fourth decades; however, endometriosis occurs even in teenagers. Patients with endometriosis under age 17 frequently have Müllerian anomalies with outflow obstruction. The disease is rarely seen outside the reproductive years. Other risk factors are not well defined, but there is an apparent increased incidence in nulliparous women and those of the upper socioeconomic classes. Further-

more, women with first-degree relatives with endo-metriosis are more likely to have endometriosis and tend to have more severe disease than do patients with no such family history.

PATHOGENESIS

The pathogenesis of endometriosis has not been proved; however, substantial scientific evidence supports either Sampson's theory of transplantation [1] or the related theory of induction of mesothelium as the mechanism for its development. Central to both theories is retrograde menstruation, a phenom-enon proved to occur in the majority of cycling women. Given this fact, however, the question remains as to what causes endometriosis in some, but not others, in the face of retrograde flow. Factors thought to be critical to the development of ectopic endometrial implantation and growth include the volume of retrograde menstruation, the capacity of the body to eliminate such peritoneal debris, and the presence of growth factors within the peritoneal environment. Studies to better define those con-ditions that promote the growth of ectopically located endometrial tissue are currently being conducted.

PRESENTATION AND DIAGNOSIS

The most common complaints of patients with endometriosis are pelvic pain and infertility. Pain is site-specific, usually taking the form of secondary dysmenorrhea 1–2 days prior to the onset of menses and continuing throughout the duration of menstrual flow. Patients may also complain of dyspareunia, low back pain, and noncyclic pelvic pain. Occasional patients will present with an acute abdomen sec-ondary to a ruptured endometrioma. Rarely, patients with extrapelvic endometriosis may present with organ-specific symptomatology such as hemoptysis or cyclic hematochezia. Interestingly, the severity of pelvic pain does not always correlate with the extent of disease. In fact, patients diagnosed with endometriosis in the course of a routine infertility evaluation are frequently asymptomatic.

Physical examination signs are limited. In cases of extensive disease, a pelvic mass or a retroverted, fixed uterus may be found. Other physical findings include cul-de-sac tenderness and nodularity of the uterosacral ligaments. There are no available serologic or radiographic tests that are sufficiently sensitive and specific to be of much value in the diagnosis of endometriosis, although in some experimental assay systems, patients may have elevated endometrial antibodies or an increase in serum levels of CA-125. The latter can be used to follow response to therapy and recurrence. Although ultrasound may reveal the characteristic appearance of endometriomas, these cannot be reliably differentiated from other cystic masses.

Diagnosis is made at laparoscopy and is confirmed by biopsy of implants, demonstrating the presence of glands and/or stroma, usually with hemorrhage or hemosiderin-laden macrophages. Both typical-appearing and atypical or nonpigmented endometriosis correlate well with histologic findings; however, failure to demonstrate endometriosis histologically in limited biopsies from a patient with characteristic laparoscopic findings does not rule out the disease. Diagnostic laparoscopy must include a systematic examination of the peritoneal surfaces for cysts and implants, which may be brown, red, blue, white, opacified, or a wide variety of additional appearances. The most frequent locations of implants are the ovaries and the dependent portions of the pelvis such as the cul-de-sac and uterosacral ligaments.

STAGING

In an attempt to standardize the classification of endometriosis for degree of severity and prognosis, several staging systems have been designed. The system most often used today is the revised American Fertility Society classification [2], which groups endometriosis into minimal, mild, moderate, and severe categories, in addition to assigning a numeric score. The main advantage of this system is that it provides a mechanism for uniform reporting and differentiates among a wide range of severity. Disadvantages are that the parameters for each stage are arbitrary, there is no clear correlation between stage and subsequent

fertility, and the accuracy and precision of the system are unknown. Currently, multicenter clinical trials are being conducted in the hope that a validated prognostic scale can be developed for clinical use.

TREATMENT OPTIONS

Treatment of endometriosis-associated infertility is difficult to assess secondary to the paucity of well-designed studies. Although many therapeutic trials and retrospective reviews have been reported, most are uncontrolled and poorly designed and are therefore difficult or impossible to interpret. For example, many studies do not report results according to severity of disease by utilizing a defined staging system. Also, selection bias is commonly introduced by including patients with multiple infertility factors. Ideally, patients should be matched to age and duration of infertility, two parameters known to affect fertility rates. Few studies compare a given treatment to the background, or treatment-independent, pregnancy rate by reporting a control group of patients managed expectantly. Finally, length of follow-up is variable and frequently not reported. The use of simple pregnancy rates is of little value without knowledge of the length of follow-up, as the two are directly related. Calculation of the monthly fecundity rate (MFR) controls for length of follow-up by expressing pregnancy rate as a function of follow-up time, although few studies report results in this manner. Comparative treatment trials are rare, and randomized, controlled trials are even less common. Thus, the data upon which to base treatment decisions are severely limited.

Treatment of endometriosis

Expectant management
It is clear that endometriosis is generally associated with a relative state of subfertility rather than sterility; therefore, many patients will ultimately achieve pregnancy in the absence of any treatment. It has been postulated that therapeutic effects of procedures commonly employed at diagnostic laparoscopy (including cervical dilatation, chromopertubation, and removal of peritoneal fluid) may be responsible for at least a portion of the pregnancies achieved without further therapy. As laparoscopy is required for diagnosis, any such therapeutic effect is of academic interest only.

In a review by Olive and Haney in 1986, 50.3% of

183 patients with expectant management of mild endometriosis became pregnant [3]. MFRs, when calculated, ranged from 5 to 11%. There is very little information in the literature regarding expectant management of moderate or severe disease; however, in a small number of patients with moderate and severe endometriosis, MFRs of 2.9 and 0% were reported, respectively [3].

Medical therapy

Danazol. Danazol is an isoxazole derivative of 17α-ethinyltestosterone (ethisterone) and has been used clinically to treat endometriosis since 1971. Hormonal profiles of patients treated with danazol indicate that it prevents the luteinizing hormone (LH) surge that usually results from low peripheral estrogen concentration, resulting in a chronic anovulatory state and atrophy of endometrial implants. It also has androgenic and progestational activity, decreases sex hormone-binding globulin, and inhibits several steroidogenic enzymes. An associated immunosuppressive effect may also contribute to the regression of endometriosis. Dosage regimens vary, but to cause regression of endometriosis, the dose must be sufficient to suppress ovulation. Serum levels may be adequate when the drug is administered twice a day, but they are best maintained with q.i.d. dosing. Although 80% of patients will be amenorrheic on 400 mg/day, some will require up to 800 mg/day. A 3–6-month course is usually given, with up to 9 months recommended for optimal suppression of severe disease. Side-effects (including weight gain, muscle cramps, decreased breast size, mood changes, acne, and hirsutism) occur in up to 85% of patients and are not necessarily dose-related. Hepatocellular damage can rarely occur, and adverse effects on lipid profiles have been demonstrated.

In uncontrolled studies of patients with mild endometriosis, the average pregnancy rate following danazol therapy is 32.6%, with MFRs up to 6% [3]. In a randomized, controlled study of patients with mild disease, pregnancy rates in patients treated with danazol were not significantly different from those in patients who were treated expectantly [4]. There are no controlled trials for the treatment of moderate and severe disease with danazol alone. Thus, no improvement in fertility has ever been demonstrated in patients with endometriosis treated with danazol.

Gonadotropin-releasing hormone (GnRH) agonists. Several agonists of GnRH have been utilized for the treatment of endometriosis. These drugs inhibit LH and follicle-stimulating hormone (FSH) release by downregulation at the pituitary, resulting in anovulation and hypoestrogenism. Estrogen levels often reach menopausal levels within 3–6 weeks. These agents must be administered parenterally (intravenously, nasally, or subcutaneously). To induce regression of endometriosis, doses must be sufficient to induce amenorrhea and hypoestrogenism. Studies in both animals and humans have shown marked regression of endometriotic implants, even with submaximal ovarian suppression [5]. Biopsies of sites of previous implants reveal glands and stroma to be atrophic but still present, despite a lack of visible evidence of disease. Side-effects are marked, including hot flushes, vaginal dryness, irritability and fatigue. Bone loss may occur acutely, but bone mineral content is recovered upon cessation of short-term therapy. Lipid profiles indicate no significant alteration in low or high density lipoprotein levels.

Efficacy in improving fertility with these agents has not been demonstrated. In a double-blind, randomized trial comparing the GnRH agonist nafarelin to danazol for the treatment of stage I–IV endometriosis, there was no difference in pregnancy rate between the two therapies [6]. As danazol has not been shown in controlled studies to enhance fertility in patients with mild disease [4], one can extrapolate these data to suggest that nafarelin may not be superior to expectant management. Thus, the value of GnRH agonists in the treatment of endometriosis-associated infertility remains unsubstantiated.

Progestogens. Treatment of endometriosis with continuous progestogens has been used with increased frequency in recent years. This treatment results in an initial decidualization of implants, followed eventually by atrophy. Both oral and parenteral forms exist; most commonly used is oral medroxyprogesterone acetate at doses of 30–100 mg/day for 3–6 months. Side-effects include breakthrough bleeding, nausea, breast tenderness, and depression. In small, uncontrolled clinical trials, pregnancy rates achieved were 46–55% with few side-effects reported [1]. However, a concurrent nonrandomized comparison of medroxyprogesterone, danazol, and expectant management showed no difference in fertility rates among the three treatments in women with minimal or mild disease [4]. Furthermore, in a randomized, controlled study, an identical rate of conception was seen in medroxyprogesterone-, danazol-, and placebo-treated women [8].

Combination estrogen—progestogens. These regimens have been used for many years in an attempt to mimic pharmacologically pregnancy and thus treat endometriosis. As with progestogens alone, initial decidualization and growth are followed by atrophy with long-term use. Oral contraceptives or a combination of progestogens (e.g., Delalutin (17-hydroxy-progesterone caproate), medroxyprogesterone acetate) and estrogens (e.g., Premarin, stilbestrol) have been used. There are few data regarding the use of combined therapy for infertility treatment, and there have been no randomized, controlled trials or comparative studies to evaluate its efficacy. The limited data that exist, however, are discouraging, as no studies suggest increased pregnancy rates over those of expectant management. Furthermore, there is a high rate of side-effects, including those encountered with progestogens as well as estrogen-related side-effects such as nausea, hypertension, and thrombophlebitis. New, lower-dose oral contraceptives are much better tolerated and may be useful in halting disease progression in women desiring future fertility, although few data are available to demonstrate this.

Summary of medical therapy. Medical therapy has not proved to increase fertility despite its success in the regression of active disease and in pain relief. A clear disadvantage to its use is the mandatory delay in attempting pregnancy for the duration of therapy. These agents are not without morbidity, and are associated with a significant incidence of side-effects. Furthermore, most effects of medical therapy are likely to be temporary, with a high frequency of recurrent symptoms after discontinuation of treatment. These agents may, however, be useful to prevent progression or recurrence of endometriosis, a theoretic but unproven use.

Conservative surgical therapy

Conservative surgery refers to any surgical procedure aimed at the treatment of endometriosis with the goal of preserving and/or enhancing fertility. The primary goal is to restore normal anatomy by eliminating adhesions and restoring the spatial relationships of the reproductive organs. Secondly, implants and endometriomas are removed as com-

pletely as possible to delay progression of disease and prevent formation of new adhesions. Finally, prevention of subsequent adhesion formation is essential for optimal results.

Conservative techniques include both exploratory laparotomy, with excision and fulguration of implants, lysis and excision of adhesions, and removal of endometriomas, and laparoscopy, with laser vaporization, fulguration, or excision of implants and adhesions. With improved techniques and instrumentation, far more extensive surgery can now be performed laparoscopically than was previously possible. Advantages of laparoscopic management include the possibility of diagnosis and treatment in a single procedure, as well as the possibility for outpatient management and decreased postoperative complications associated with major abdominal surgery. Disadvantages include a wide variation in operator experience and occasional suboptimal resection, especially in cases of bowel or urinary tract involvement. Use of the carbon dioxide laser with multiple specialized instruments available for operative laparoscopy has expanded the potential for laparoscopic management of even advanced disease. The added precision of this technique allows operation in more difficult locations and reduces the potential for adhesion formation.

Implants, when removed, should be eliminated as completely as possible with minimum trauma to the remaining tissues. This may be accomplished by excision, laser vaporization, or fulguration. For optimal results, microsurgical techniques may be superior to gross dissection. Reperitonealization is usually unnecessary and often increases adhesion formation unless one is careful to utilize microscopic suture materials and eliminate tension on the repair. Grafts have been advocated to close major defects; however, their use may actually be associated with increased adhesion formation. Adhesions should be excised in their entirety to avoid leaving devascularized tissue; also, implants often lie within the adhesions themselves. Studies in the pathogenesis of adhesion formation reveal that, in order to prevent adhesions, the surgeon should adhere to the following principles: (1) minimization of serosal trauma and drying; (2) meticulous hemostasis; (3) avoidance of tissue ischemia secondary to crush injury, tension and devascularization; and (4) prevention of peritonitis. Uterine suspension and partial omentectomy are further measures sometimes utilized to reduce adhesion formation.

In a review of conservative surgical treatment of endometriosis-associated infertility, Oliver and Haney cited a 52.7% overall pregnancy rate in 2094 reported cases [3]. Few of these studies were controlled, and none were randomized. Studies reporting fertility outcome in patients with mild endometriosis alone demonstrated a 60.7% overall pregnancy rate with MFRs of 2.2 and 3.9%. Those studies utilizing conservative surgery to treat patients with moderate and severe endometriosis revealed pregnancy rates of 50 and 39.2%, respectively. Despite the apparently lower pregnancy rates with increasing severity of disease, studies with calculable MFRs showed virtually no differences among the three stages [3]. Low MFR's may be partly due to the prolonged follow-up period reported in these studies. Although many patients who ultimately become pregnant conceive within 18 months of surgery, one report showed a rise in cumulative pregnancy rate from 33% at 12 months to 67% at 74 months [9]. Whether these delayed pregnancies are the result of surgical intervention cannot be determined without an appropriate control group.

In one comparative study, conservative surgery did not result in improved pregnancy rates over expectant management for either mild or moderate disease, whereas patients with severe disease had improved pregnancy rates with conservative surgery [3]. On the other hand, a controlled, randomized study revealed a 60.8% pregnancy rate in an 8-month follow-up period with laparoscopic fulguration of mild endometriosis in patients who had failed to conceive during an 8-month trial of expectant management, compared to 18.5% in those patients in whom the implants were left intact [10]. Clearly, data are inadequate for definitive conclusions, but it appears that surgical therapy improves pregnancy rates in patients with severe endometriosis and may also be of some benefit in selected subgroups of patients with milder disease.

Combined medical and surgical therapy

Many uncontrolled studies reported in the literature have utilized a combination of surgery and either pre- or postoperative medical therapy. Although many authors have advocated preoperative medical suppression of endometriosis to facilitate adequate surgical resection, no controlled studies have demonstrated enhancement of fertility with this approach. Comparative and uncontrolled studies show no benefit over surgery alone of pre- or postoperative danazol. For example, Chong and coworkers found no significant improvement in pregnancy rates with danazol therapy following laser vaporization of implants over laser therapy alone in patients with stage I endometriosis [11]. Therefore, limited data do not support use of adjuvant medical therapy to improve infertility.

Direct treatment of infertility — advanced reproductive technology

One approach to endometriosis-associated infertility is to direct the treatment toward the infertility itself, independently of the diagnosis of endometriosis. Empiric therapy includes superovulation followed by intrauterine insemination (SO/IUI), *in vitro* fertilization and embryo transfer (IVF/ET), or gamete intrafallopian transfer (GIFT). Use of these techniques provides information on ovulation, fertilization, and implantation rates in patients with endometriosis; they also result in conception in many patients where other therapy has failed. Improved overall pregnancy rates make these advanced techniques an alternative for many patients.

Although initial studies reporting fertilization rates in patients with endometriosis have revealed conflicting results, it now appears that ovarian stimulation and fertilization of oocytes are not impaired in these patients. Most studies of patients with endometriosis treated with IVF/ET report no significant differences in pregnancy rates between patients with tubal factor alone and those with endometriosis, regardless of stage. Egg recovery may be decreased in patients with severe disease, however, leading to a decreased number of embryos transferred. Damewood and coworkers reported a series of patients with at least 5 years of primary infertility and mild, moderate, or severe endometriosis, treated with IVF with concurrent extensive laparoscopic resection of endometriosis at the time of egg retrieval [12]. All patients had had prior conservative surgery in the 3 preceding years (with or without adjuvant danazol), with at least 1 year of persistent infertility. Of those patients not becoming pregnant during the IVF cycle (pregnancy rate 22% per cycle), 28% achieved pregnancy within the subsequent 10 months.

GIFT has been used successfully in patients having endometriosis but normal fallopian tubes. Preliminary results by some investigators suggest improved pregnancy rates in these selected patients over IVF/ET and SO/IUI, whereas others report higher pregnancy rates with IVF/ET. Conclusive results await further investigation with randomized clinical trials. Until then, each of these techniques remains a reasonable approach to the empiric treatment of endometriosis-associated infertility.

MANAGEMENT OF ENDOMETRIOSIS-ASSOCIATED INFERTILITY

When patients present with infertility, a full evaluation of both partners should be instituted. Multiple factors contributing to the couple's infertility are often present and should be addressed separately. Endometriosis may be an incidental finding in infertility patients, especially if it is mild or minimal, and may not be a causative factor. The presence of characteristic signs and symptoms of endometriosis should raise the index of suspicion.

Once other parameters have been assessed, diagnostic laparoscopy can then be performed to determine the presence of endometriosis and other peritoneal factors. When endometriosis is found, the extent of surgical treatment indicated is determined by the presence or absence of implants, adhesions, endometriomas, or gross anatomic distortion. Routine chromopertubation and removal of peritoneal fluid, although of unproven efficacy in enhancing fertility, can easily be accomplished as part of the procedure without added morbidity.

In patients found at diagnostic laparoscopy to have implants alone, it is reasonable to proceed with simple removal of implants by laparoscopic techniques, but only when easily accomplished, according to their location, skill of the laparoscopist, and available instrumentation. Laser vaporization is probably superior to fulguration, as it minimizes tissue destruction. Although surgical removal of implants is of no proven benefit in infertility treatment, possible advantages include improvement in endometriosis-associated pain and delay in disease progression.

When adnexal adhesions are also present, even in the absence of gross disturbances in spatial relationships, they should be excised as completely as possible at the initial laparoscopy to insure an optimal anatomic result. Unresectable adhesions and implants in the presence of otherwise normal anatomy do not warrant a major surgical procedure as primary therapy. Endometriomas should be removed, for they may enlarge if untreated and result in anatomic distortion, pain, or rupture. This can often be accomplished laparoscopically.

Endometriosis associated with severe distortion of anatomic spatial relationships deserves optimal surgical resection. The choice of laparoscopic versus open surgical techniques depends upon the surgeon's skill and instrumentation, as well as the extent and location of implants, adhesions, and endometriomas. Depending on the extent of disease, the patient's age, and the surgeon's assessment of the findings, optimal resection may be facilitated by preoperative medical suppression followed by laparoscopy or exploratory laparotomy. Although not of proven efficacy, preoperative medical suppression may decrease operative time, aid in achieving more complete resection, and increase the number of procedures amenable to laparoscopic, rather than open, techniques. Rapid, maximal suppression can be obtained with either danazol or GnRH agonists. Progestogens, although better tolerated and less expensive, are probably not associated with as rapid regression of endometriosis.

After initial laparoscopy, with or without surgical treatment, patients should be allowed a course of expectant management. This will be adequate therapy in at least 50% of patients with minimal or mild disease. An exception to this may be the older patient or one with long-standing infertility. Such a patient may benefit from proceeding directly to empiric therapy of infertility with advanced reproductive techniques, as discussed earlier. These techniques can also be offered to patients who fail to conceive with either expectant or surgical management. Choice of the technique should be individualized to the patient's needs, financial resources, and presence of other infertility factors. Superiority of one technique (e.g., SO/IUI versus IVF/ET versus GIFT) has not been established for this group of patients.

In the rare patient who also has signs or symptoms of extraperitoneal endometriosis, diagnosis should be confirmed by biopsy and specific therapy directed toward its location. Fortunately, extraperitoneal disease is rare and usually isolated, except when there is secondary involvement of the gastrointestinal and urinary tracts. Surgical removal is often necessary, due to issues unrelated to fertility enhancement.

Finally, it must be kept in mind that therapy should be individualized, and there are few strict guidelines that can be supported by the literature. Endometriosis may be associated with a subfertile state, but pregnancy can be achieved with all stages of disease. Patients should be counseled appropriately and offered a plan of management to suit their individual needs. Further information through controlled, randomized clinical trials is currently ongoing in an attempt to clarify the many issues involved in the treatment of endometriosis-associated infertility.

REFERENCES

1 Sampson JA. Peritoneal endometriosis, due to menstrual dissemination of endometrial tissue into the peritoneal cavity. *Am J Obstet Gynecol* 1927; 14: 422.

2 Revised American Fertility Society Classification of Endometriosis. *Fertil Steril* 1985; 43: 351.

3 Werlin LB, Hodgen GD. Gonadotropin-releasing hormone agonist suppresses ovulation, menses and endometriosis in monkeys: an individualized, intermittent regimen. *J Clin Endocrinol Metab* 1983; 56: 844.

4 Olive DL, Haney AF. Endometriosis-associated infertility: a critical review of therapeutic approaches. *Obstet Gynecol Surv* 1986; 41: 538.

5 Seibel MM, Berger MJ, Weinstein FG *et al.* The effectiveness of danazol on subsequent fertility in minimal endometriosis. *Fertil Steril* 1982; 38: 534.

6 Henzl MR, Corson SL, Moghissi K *et al.* Administration of nasal naferelin as compared with oral danazol for endometriosis. A multicenter, double-blind comparative clinical trial. *N Engl J Med* 1988; 318: 485.

7 Hull ME, Moghissi KS, Magyar DF *et al.* Comparison of different therapeutic modalities of endometriosis in infertile women. *Fertil Steril* 1987; 47: 40.

8 Telimaa S. Danazol and medroxyprogesterone acetate inefficacious in the treatment of infertility in endometriosis. *Fertil Steril* 1988; 50: 872.

9 Rock JA, Guzick DS, Sengos C *et al.* The conservative surgical treatment of endometriosis: evaluation of pregnancy success with respect to the extent of disease as categorized using contemporary classification systems. *Fertil Steril* 1981; 35: 131.

10 Nowroozi K, Chase JS, Check JH *et al.* The importance of laparoscopic coagulation of mild endometriosis in infertile women. *Int J Fertil* 1987; 32: 442.

11 Chong AP, Kenne ME, Thorton NL. Comparison of three modes of treatment for infertility patients with minimal pelvic endometriosis. *Fertil Steril* 1990; 53: 407.

12 Damewood MD, Rock JA. Treatment independent pregnancy with operative laparoscopy for endometriosis in an *in vitro* fertilization program. *Fertil Steril* 1988; 50: 463.

81

Management of endometriosis-associated pain

BRADLEY S. HURST

INTRODUCTION

Dysmenorrhea, pelvic pain, dyspareunia, and infertility are the classic symptoms associated with endometriosis. A patient with endometriosis may present with one or more of these symptoms. Endometriosis can be identified in approximately 50% of women with dysmenorrhea and 20% of those with chronic pelvic pain and dyspareunia.

The rate of endometriosis in the general population is difficult to determine. An autopsy series found endometriosis in 0.3% of women [1]. The true incidence of endometriosis may be much higher, however. Endometriosis has been identified by scanning electron microscopy in visually normal peritoneum [2]. Thus, the true incidence of endometriosis may be much higher than has been previously estimated both for patients with symptoms and in the asymptomatic general population.

The long-held theory that the extent of endometriosis is not directly correlated with the degree of pain was confirmed by Buttram in 1979 [3]. It remains a mystery why some patients with tiny endometriosis implants have severe pain, whereas others with extensive endometriosis have no pain whatsoever. Despite the considerable advances that have been made in our ability to diagnose and treat endometriosis, it remains a poorly understood disease process.

PATHOPHYSIOLOGY

Numerous mechanisms have been proposed to explain the occurrence of pain and dysmenorrhea with endometriosis. Pain may be due to an inflammatory response that occurs with endometriosis. Pelvic inflammation with increased macrophages, prostaglandins, or other inflammatory products may be caused directly by endometriosis implants or occur indirectly with reflex menstruation in endometriosis patients.

Increased prostaglandin concentrations are found in the endometrium and menstrual effluent in women with dysmenorrhea. Prostaglandins in peritoneal fluid may cause dysmenorrhea and pelvic pain as well. However, peritoneal fluid prostaglandins have been difficult to study. Prostaglandins are ubiquitous and have a very short half-life. If prostaglandin concentrations are changed with endometriosis, current analysis techniques are not sufficient to show conclusively the alterations.

Macrophages may contribute to pain associated with endometriosis. Macrophages comprise most of the white cells in peritoneal fluid, and many investigators have demonstrated an increase in macrophage number, concentration, and activation states with endometriosis. Macrophages produce prostaglandins, free radicals, enzymes, and lymphokines. These substances may irritate the peritoneum and cause pain or lead to formation of adhesions.

Mechanical alterations that occur with endometriosis may explain pain in some women. For example, ruptured or leaking endometriomas may cause peritoneal irritation and result in pain. Endometriosis may be associated with pelvic adhesions. Scarring or retraction of peritoneal surfaces may cause pain. A retroverted uterus and ovaries adherent in the cul-de-sac may cause dyspareunia because of compression of the structures or tension on the surrounding peritoneum. Uterosacral endometriosis may cause pain when touched because of stretching of the surrounding peritoneum. In addition, endometriosis involving the vulva or lower vagina may be painful when touched. Pain may be elicited by invasion of the urinary or gastrointestinal tracts.

DIAGNOSIS

Endometriosis should be considered in the differential diagnosis of all women who present with pelvic pain, dyspareunia, or dysmenorrhea (Fig. 81.1).

CHAPTER 81

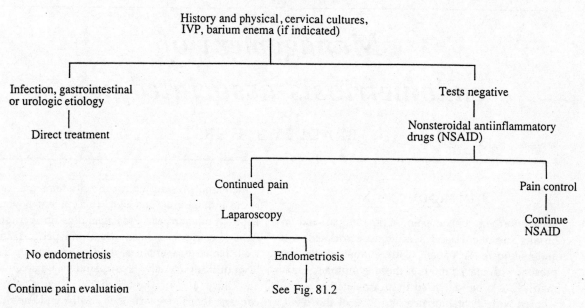

Fig. 81.1 Assessment of pelvic pain, dysmenorrhea, and dyspareunia.

A careful history should be taken, including details of the nature and character of the pain, exacerbating and relieving factors, and time of pain in the menstrual cycle. A careful sexual history should be taken to determine if dyspareunia is present. The review of systems should include a careful description of urinary or gastrointestinal symptoms, especially as they relate to the pain.

Acute pain may also be associated with endometriosis. Leaking endometriomas may cause an acute or subacute pain. Ovarian torsion due to an endometrioma causes an acute, intense, localized pain. Nausea, vomiting, and other symptoms commonly associated with an acute abdomen are expected with ovarian torsion.

The physical examination may be entirely normal with endometriosis. Positive findings on physical examination can raise suspicion that endometriosis is present, however. These findings include tender uterosacral nodularity, retroversion of the uterus, adnexal masses, and limited pelvic mobility. Tenderness may be diffuse or focal. Occasionally, with cervical or vaginal endometriosis, the endometriosis lesions may be directly visualized and biopsied to confirm the diagnosis.

The definitive diagnosis of endometriosis can only be made surgically. If pain is adequately relieved by medications and does not alter the patient's lifestyle, surgery is not appropriate. Pain that interferes with lifestyles or sexual activity should be surgically evaluated. Unless laparotomy is indicated, laparoscopy is the procedure of choice.

Laparoscopy should be performed in the follicular phase since it may be difficult to distinguish a corpus luteum cyst from an endometrioma. Preovulatory laparoscopy also prevents anesthesia exposure to an early pregnancy. In order to do adequate laparoscopy, the following procedures are recommended. A two-puncture technique is necessary to inspect carefully the cul-de-sac, ovarian fossae, and fallopian tubes. A rigid instrument should be placed on the cervix to allow for uterine manipulation and anteversion. The operating table should allow for steep Trendelenburg positioning to facilitate clearing the bowel from the pelvis. Peritoneal fluid should be aspirated to allow optimal visualization of the cul-de-sac. A careful systematic inspection of the pelvis should then be performed and lesions carefully described and recorded based on the American Fertility Society 1985 revised classification of endometriosis.

Endometriosis can take on a variety of appearances. Classic endometriosis appears as black "powder burn" lesions. These lesions may involve the peritoneum or the ovaries and may be diffuse or localized as nodules. Active endometriosis appears as reddish-blue proliferative endometriotic nodules. Less common forms of endometriosis can be encountered as well. Endometriosis implants that lack hemosiderin may present as white opaque peritoneal nodules. Superficial peritoneal ecchymotic areas or red raised peritoneal nodules may also be endometriosis. These lesions may be difficult to identify, since peritoneal trauma from rough tissue handling may give the same appearance. Scarring or retraction of the peritoneum in a stellate pattern surrounding lesions strongly suggests endometriosis. Peritoneal windows or defects are suggestive of endometriosis. In addition, adhesions that bind the ovary to the ovarian fossa are often a result of endometriosis.

Ovarian endometriosis may involve the surface or may be deep in the ovary. Endometriomas, or ovarian "chocolate cysts," are usually dark brown, black, or blue. Size can vary considerably. Endometriomas are usually thin-walled, and may be ruptured during laparoscopy. When the cysts are ruptured, a tarry-brown old blood is released in most cases, although a yellow·fluid can be seen in old endometriomas as blood is resorbed.

Suspicious pelvic lesions should be biopsied for pathologic confirmation when the diagnosis of endometriosis cannot be established by direct observation alone. The microscopic diagnosis of endometriosis may be difficult to confirm, however. Active endometriosis implants are composed of endometrial glands, endometrial stroma, fibrosis, and hemorrhage. Many pathologists consider the presence of hemosiderin and the presence of histiocytes with hemosiderin granules sufficient to make the diagnosis, however.

Although some magnification of the peritoneum is obtained with the laparoscope, not all implants are visible. Endometriosis is found in 25% of normal-appearing peritoneal biopsies in endometriosis patients when scanning electron microscopy is used [2]. Thus, normal findings on laparoscopy do not exclude the possibility of endometriosis. The clinical implications of microscopic endometriosis remain to be determined.

Other studies may be helpful to evaluate a patient with endometriosis. Ultrasonography, especially with a vaginal probe, aids in the identification of ovarian endometriomas. A marbling pattern of internal echoes is typically seen within the endometrioma cyst. However, no ultrasonographic pattern can be used to diagnose or exclude the diagnosis of endometriosis. Magnetic resonance imaging and computed tomography are used by some, but these techniques are expensive and lack the specificity needed to diagnose endometriosis.

CA-125 levels are elevated in patients with advanced stages of endometriosis. A patient with an adnexal mass and an elevated CA-125 may have endometriosis, but also may have ovarian carcinoma. Neither radiographic studies nor markers that can be measured in blood have the sensitivity or specificity to diagnose endometriosis.

THERAPY

Many therapeutic options are available for patients with endometriosis (Fig. 81.2). Options include expectant management, laparoscopic surgery, hormonal therapy, advanced reproductive technologies, laparotomy with pelvic reconstruction, and removal of the reproductive organs. In order to determine the appropriate approach, the patient's symptoms, age, extent of disease, and desire for future reproductive capacity must be considered.

Infertility

Patients with endometriosis and infertility should be treated to maximize the patient's chances for pregnancy. Expectant management is as effective as medical therapy or surgery for infertile patients with early endometriosis. Approximately 50% of patients with mild disease conceive in the first year with expectant management. Medical therapies including danocrine, progestins, and gonadotropin-releasing hormone (GnRH) analogs require considerable time, expense, and provide no better success for pregnancy.

Pregnancy rates for minimal and mild endometriosis are comparable when expectant management is compared with surgical therapies including laparoscopic coagulation, carbon dioxide laser laparoscopy, and conservative resection. Considering expense to the patient and potential morbidity associated with surgery, expectant management is preferable for infertile patients with mild endometriosis. Surgery is recommended when adnexal anatomy is altered with advanced endometriosis.

Assisted reproductive technologies appear significantly to increase fecundity and may be appropriate for a patient who has failed to achieve a pregnancy with traditional therapy. Patients with stage I and II endometriosis undergoing superovulation with intrauterine insemination can expect fecundity rates of 0.15–0.20. Gamete intrafallopian transfer provides a clinical pregnancy rate of approximately 25% per transfer for patients with endometriosis. In vitro fertilization provides a clinical pregnancy rate of approximately 15% per embryo transfer [4].

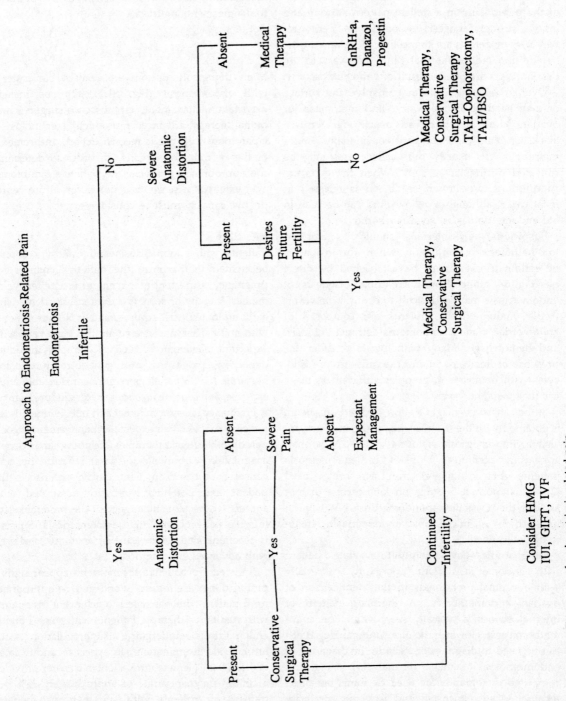

Fig. 81.2 Treatment of endometriosis-related pain.

Pain and infertility

Expectant management and fertility-enhancing therapies may be a consideration for a patient with mild pain and infertility. When pain is considerable, however, expectant management and the use of assisted reproductive technologies may not be reasonable choices. Therapy should be directed to relieve pain and maximize fertility. Surgery may relieve pain without significantly delaying conception attempts. Laparoscopic surgery and laparotomy with conservative resection each offers distinct advantages.

Endometriosis may be coagulated by laparoscopic electrocautery, thermal endocoagulation, or by laser. Endometriomas less than 5 cm may be removed by an experienced laparoscopic surgeon. Removal of the entire cyst wall is necessary to prevent reformation of the endometrioma. Avoid leaving large areas of denuded peritoneum, which may be a nidus for adhesion formation. Medical therapy or laparotomy with conservative resection and microscopic reconstruction are preferable to laparoscopic surgery when extensive raw surfaces would be caused by laparoscopy.

There is no evidence that any one type of laparoscopic surgery is superior to another. Data evaluating relief of pain, dyspareunia, and dysmenorrhea with laparoscopic surgery are limited. Approximately 60–90% of patients treated laparoscopically experience some pain relief [5]. Laparoscopic surgery does not improve fertility compared to medical therapy or expectant management.

Conservative surgery remains the procedure of choice for patients with extensive adhesions, large endometriomas, and patients with severe midline dysmenorrhea. Complete resection of visible disease with preservation of adnexal structures is the goal of conservative surgery. Microsurgical techniques are essential to reduce adhesion formation. Adhesion barriers such as Interceed for pelvic side wall adhesions or Gore-Tex surgical membrane for any exposed peritoneal membranes can be used to reduce further adhesion formation.

Presacral neurectomy is advisable during conservative resection for patients with midline dysmenorrhea or pain. Presacral neurectomy effectively relieves midline pain in 90% of properly selected patients [6]. Complications associated with presacral neurectomy include postoperative adhesion formation, significant blood loss, urinary bladder dysfunction, and chronic constipation. Bowel and bladder dysfunction are rarely severe following presacral neurectomy, however.

Uterosacral ligament ablation is performed by some physicians at the time of laparotomy or laparoscopy to treat pain associated with endometriosis. Bleeding and bowel injury are potential complications of this procedure. The risks could be justified if this procedure was of proven benefit. However reports to date are little more than anecdotal experiences with limited patient numbers. Well-designed prospective studies are needed to define the risks and benefits of this procedure.

The overall pregnancy rate following conservative surgery is 50–60% for all stages of endometriosis [7]. Conservative surgery is the procedure of choice for those with continued pain after medical therapy and for patients with significant anatomic distortion when preservation of fertility is desired.

Pain

Medical therapy is ideal for patients with endometriosis and pain who wish to preserve their reproductive capacity but wish to delay child-bearing. Most hormonal therapies involve treatment for 6 months to allow for regression of endometriosis. No hormonal therapy will improve adhesive disease, nor is hormonal therapy effective for large endometriomas. Of the hormonal therapies available, GnRH analogs, danazol, progestins, and oral contraceptives are the most widely used.

GnRH analogs recently have been approved for patients with endometriosis and are rapidly becoming the medical therapy of choice. GnRH analogs cause a downregulation of pituitary GnRH receptors and desensitization, resulting in a hypogonadal state in 2–6 weeks. Glandular involution and stromal atrophy of endometriotic implants occur in a hypoestrogenic environment. Side-effects of GnRH analogs are those expected from castrate levels of estrogen and include hot flushes, headaches, irritability, insomnia, and depression. Vaginal dryness may be experienced. Osteopenia may occur, but does not appear to be significant during a 6-month treatment period. Treatment beyond 6 months is not advised due to risks associated with osteopenia.

Relief of pain and dysmenorrhea is excellent with GnRH analog therapy. Seventy to 90% of patients experience considerable improvement of pain. These response rates are comparable to those reported with the use of danazol.

Currently, there are two GnRH analogs available

in the USA. Nafarelin (Synarel) and leuprolide acetate (Lupron) have been approved by the Food and Drug Administration (FDA) for the management of endometriosis-related pain. The standard dose of nafarelin is 200 µg intranasally twice a day for 6 months. The standard dose of leuprolide is 1 mg/day injected subcutaneously. A monthly injectable depot formulation of leuprolide is available which calls for a dose of 3.75 mg i.m. Other GnRH analogs are likely to be approved. There is no evidence that one GnRH analog is superior to another for symptomatic relief of endometriosis.

Until GnRH analogs were available, danazol was the only agent approved by the FDA for treatment of endometriosis. A derivative of 17-ethinyl testosterone, danazol works at several sites to treat endometriosis. Danazol reduces serum estradiol by inhibiting follicle-stimulating hormone and luteinizing hormone. In addition, danazol directly inhibits the enzymes responsible for ovarian steroidogenesis. An additional effect is produced at the endometriosis implant. Danazol binds to estrogen and progesterone receptors and inhibits normal response of these receptors.

The standard dose of danazol is 800 mg daily in divided doses for 6 months. Side-effects include weight gain, muscle cramps, reduced breast size, nausea, headaches, dizziness, and oily skin. A dose-dependent male-pattern hair growth and deepening of the voice may occasionally occur. Preliminary results suggest that the androgenic symptoms of danazol may be reduced with intense exercise.

Danazol is effective in improving pain, dyspareunia, and dysmenorrhea in approximately 90% of patients. Studies directly comparing danazol and GnRH analogs have shown similar pain relief. Approximately 33% of women have recurrent symptoms after treatment with danazol.

Progestogens cause decidualization and atrophy of endometrial tissue. The most common regimen to treat endometriosis calls for medroxyprogesterone acetate 30 mg/day for 6 months. Depot forms of medroxyprogesterone acetate and other progestins including megestrol acetate at a dose of 40 mg/day have been used. Side-effects include breakthrough bleeding in approximately 50% of patients treated with progestogens. Significant depression has been reported. Other reversible side-effects include weight gain, fluid retention, and nausea.

The therapeutic results for progestogen therapy are difficult to interpret because of the wide selection of agents studied and the varying doses of drug and duration of therapy. Progestogens do not improve posttherapy pregnancy rates. However, excellent relief from pain and dysmenorrhea is reported in most studies [8]. Pain relief appears to be comparable to danazol and GnRH analog therapy.

Continuous oral contraceptives have been used to treat endometriosis. Progestationally dominant oral contraceptives are believed to produce decidualization and atrophy of endometriosis implants. Side-effects, indications, and contraindications are the same as those described for oral contraceptives.

Pregnancy rates are not improved after treatment with oral contraceptives. Improvement of pain is noted in 75–90% of patients. Oral contraceptives may be useful for patients with endometriosis-associated pain who wish to delay child-bearing after completing other therapeutic measures.

Radical surgery may be indicated after conservative therapies have failed. When fertility is no longer desired, total abdominal hysterectomy with bilateral salpingo-oophorectomy may be considered. Hysterectomy and oophorectomy often are advised for a climacteric patient. Estrogen replacement therapy is initiated 6–8 weeks after surgery. Recurrence of endometriosis with estrogen replacement therapy after bilateral oophorectomy is rare [9].

Ovarian conservation may be elected for younger patients who desire hysterectomy. However, 15–85% of these patients have recurrent symptoms.

CONCLUSIONS

Endometriosis is common in women with chronic pelvic pain, dysmenorrhea, or deep dyspareunia. Endometriosis is diagnosed only by direct observation of endometriosis lesions. A wide variety of treatment modalities are available for women with endometriosis-associated pain. Treatment plans should consider the patient's symptoms, desire for reproduction, extent of disease, age, and associated pelvic pathology. When all of these factors are taken into consideration, a rational treatment regimen may be made.

REFERENCES

1 Dreyfuss ML. Pathologic and clinical aspects of adenomyosis and endometriosis: a survey of 224 cases. *Am J Obstet Gynecol* 1940; 39: 95.
2 Murphy AA, Green R, De La Cruz I, Rock JA. Unsuspected

endometriosis documented by scanning electron microscopy in visually normal peritoneum. *Fertil Steril* 1986; 46: 522.

3 Buttram VC. Conservative surgery for endometriosis in the infertile female: a study of 206 cases with implications for both medical and surgical therapy. *Fertil Steril* 1979; 36: 751.

4 Medical Research International and the Society for Assisted Reproductive Technology, The American Fertility Society. *In vitro* fertilization-embryo transfer in the United States: 1988 results from the IVF-ET Registry. *Fertil Steril* 1990; 53: 13.

5 Schenken RS, ed. *Endometriosis: Contemporary Concepts in Clinical Management*. Philadelphia: JB Lippincott, 1989.

6 Tjaden BL, Schlaff WD, Kimball A, Rock JA. The efficacy of presacral neurectomy for the relief of midline dysmenorrhea. *Obstet Gynecol* 1990; 76: 89.

7 Rock JA, Guzick DS, Sengos C, Schweditsch M, Sapp KC, Jones HW Jr. The conservative surgical treatment of endometriosis: evaluation of pregnancy success with respect to the extent of disease as categorized using contemporary classification systems. *Fertil Steril* 1981; 35: 131.

8 Schlaff WD, Dugoff L, Damewood MD, Rock JA. Megestrol acetate for the treatment of endometriosis. *Obstet Gynecol* 1990; 75: 646.

9 Hammond CB, Rock JA, Parker RT. Conservative treatment of endometriosis: the effects of limited surgery and hormonal pseudopregnancy. *Fertil Steril* 1976; 27: 756.

82

Ruptured ovarian cyst

WENDY J. SCHERZER & EUGENE KATZ

The ruptured ovarian cyst is an important differential in the female patient of reproductive age with lower abdominal pain, as the potential development of hemoperitoneum can be massive, causing shock.

Multiple histologic ovarian cysts types have been described in the ovary. A discussion of the consequences of the rupture of malignant cysts is beyond the scope of this chapter. Moreover, the rupture of benign nonhemorrhagic cysts, i.e., follicular cysts and cystadenomas, is of no consequence and does not require immediate attention. In addition, the rupture of endometriomas, although potentially harmful, does not require emergency treatment. The rupture of a benign ovarian teratoma (dermoid) results in oozing of the sebaceous material from the cyst producing a severe chemical peritonitis and requiring immediate operative treatment. Rupture occurs in only 0.7–4.6% of dermoids and occurs more frequently during pregnancy. Copious irrigation and a cystectomy or oophorectomy should be performed. This chapter will focus on the rupture of corpora lutea cysts causing hemoperitoneum.

INCIDENCE

Ruptured cysts represented the fourth most common gynecologic admission diagnosis between 1962 and 1979 in England and Wales [1]. The incidence of rupture appears to have declined over time despite increased detection of asymptomatic cysts due to an increase in routine screening, ultrasound use, and laparoscopic procedures. Furthermore, the use of oral contraceptives may have played a role in this phenomenon. For instance, a study from the Center for Disease Control, has shown that users of oral contraceptives containing 80 µg of estrogen display a relative risk of functional ovarian cyst formation of 0.07 of nonusers [2].

Since pregnancy is associated with the formation of corpus luteum cysts, there is an increased incidence of rupture during pregnancy.

PATHOPHYSIOLOGY

Novak and Woodruff described four stages of the development of the corpus luteum from the mature graafian follicle [3]. The first stage, ovulation, is characterized by proliferation and luteinization of granulosa and theca cells in the collapsed follicle. Bleeding is rare in this stage. The second stage occurs 2–4 days later and is characterized by vascularizaton. Thin-walled capillaries invade the granulosa cells, leading to spontaneous bleeding into the central cavity. Most often this is self-limiting and the blood in the central cavity is organized into a fibrinous clot. The clot is reabsorbed leaving a cystic space. During the third stage, 4–10 days postovulation, there continues to be vascularization of the theca interna. If pregnancy does not occur, regression (stage 4) begins 10 days postovulation.

While in general the corpus luteum measures 2 cm in diameter, corpus luteum cysts usually exceed 3 cm and their formation predisposes to rupture. Although there is no difference in hemorrhagic cyst formation or size of cyst between the right and left ovary, there is a 66% dextro-preponderance for rupture [4]. Whether this is due to increased pressure in the venous plexus which drains the right ovary, compared to the pressures in the single vein which drains the left ovary, is a matter of speculation.

Patients with bleeding disorders or on anticoagulation therapy, i.e., dialysis patients, prosthetic valve patients, and patients with deep vein thrombosis, are at increased risk [5]. Thus, while recurrences are rare in the general population, the reported recurrence rate among patients with bleeding disorders is 31%.

CLINICAL PRESENTATION

The patient is most often in her reproductive years. However, 16% occur in women older than 40 years of age. Furthermore, 12% occur during the second decade of life. Only one in 200 patients is on oral contraceptives [6]. Corpus luteum cysts rupture without any obvious extrinsic factors in the majority of cases but rupture may occasionally follow exercise, trauma, defecation, or pelvic examinations. Intercourse appears to be a common antecedent but its relevance is difficult to determine. Menses are delayed in 43−63% of the patients but one-third of them are pregnant.

In 60% of the patients, the pain is characterized as sudden, severe, and located in the lower abdomen [7]. Interestingly, the site of pain may not reflect the site of rupture. A third of the patients have dull, aching unilateral abdominal pain 1−2 weeks before rupture. This is due to ovarian capsule distention from the hemorrhagic cyst prior to rupture. In such cases, the presence of a corpus luteum cyst previously documented by ultrasound increases the suspicion of a ruptured ovarian cyst. For instance, Hallatt and coworkers [6] reported that 79% of the patients with ovarian rupture had a known corpus luteum cyst. Nausea, vomiting, and diarrhea secondary to chemical irritation from the hemoperitoneum are present in one-third of the patients. A palpable mass is present in a third of the cases. A low-grade fever occurs in 25% of the patients. Leukocytosis in excess of $12\,000/mm^2$ occurs in 20% of the patients. The hematocrit is variable and depends on the severity of the intraperitoneal hemorrhage. The average hematocrit on admission is 37% and only 7% present with an hematocrit of less than 30%. A large hemoperitoneum may cause peritoneal signs such as rebound and cervical motion tenderness. Abdominal distention rigidity and hypotensive shock may be found in rare cases — approximately 1%. The amount of hemorrhage is variable. Half of the patients present an estimated 100−500 ml of hemoperitoneum while approximately 25% have less than 100 ml of hemoperitoneum. The remaining 25% display greater than 500 ml of hemoperitoneum.

DIFFERENTIAL DIAGNOSIS

The key to the diagnosis is early suspicion. In fact, the accuracy of preoperative diagnosis is only 18%. The major differential diagnosis includes pelvic inflammatory disease (PID), appendicitis, ovarian torsion, and ectopic pregnancies (Fig. 82.1). Patients affected with PID are more likely to present during or just following menses. Fever and leukocytosis are more pronounced. Nausea, vomiting, and diarrhea are common and peritoneal signs such as rebound and cervical motion tenderness are more pronounced. A pelvic mass consistent with a tubal ovarian abscess may also be found. If an abscess is present, it is more likely to be bilateral than unilateral unless the patient presents with a history of use of an intrauterine device. Ultrasound may show free fluid but the finding is nonspecific since it may represent purulent as well as hemorrhagic material.

Appendicitis classically begins as diffuse periumbilical pain which then focuses at McBurney's point. Anorexia and nausea are prominent symptoms. Occasionally, there is a right-sided palpable abdominal mass. There is severe pain with a rectal examination. Peritoneal signs including rebound and cervical motion tenderness may be present. White blood cell count is rarely greater than $16\,000/mm^2$.

Ovarian torsion also causes sudden, sharp, severe abdominal pain. Its occurrence is unrelated to the phase of the menstrual cycle. It occurs more frequently with ovarian enlargement due to any type of cyst formation (i.e., dermoid, endometrioma, or corpus luteum). The patient is afebrile with a normal white blood count. Ultrasound may reveal a unilateral pelvic mass.

Other intraabdominal pathology must also be considered such as mesenteric lymphadenitis, regional enteritis, urinary tract infection, ureteral or renal calculi, intestinal obstruction, perforation or infection. Systemic diseases which should be considered are Henoch−Schönlein purpura, sickle cell crisis, porphyria, and thrombocytopenic thrombotic purpura.

An ectopic pregnancy is assumed to be present unless proven otherwise. A negative serum pregnancy test is reassuring. A positive test strongly suggests an ectopic pregnancy. However, 13−15.6% of the patients with ruptured ovarian cysts are pregnant. In a large series of ectopic pregnancies, 9% of corpora lutea were cystic. Usually there is less hemorrhage with a corpus luteum than with an ectopic pregnancy since the bleeding is more often nonrecurrent and self-limiting. Vaginal bleeding is more common with an ectopic pregnancy than with a ruptured corpus luteum. Interestingly, of 27 patients with a positive pregnancy test and a ruptured ovarian cyst, seven were found to harbor an unruptured

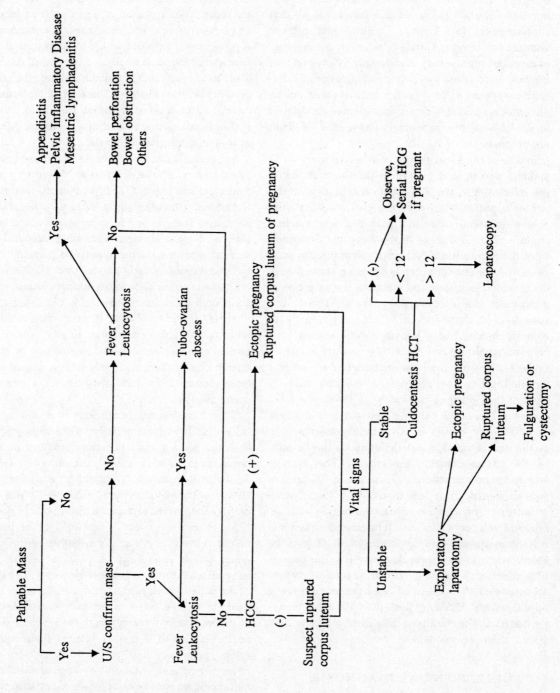

Fig. 82.1 Diagnosis and treatment of lower abdominal pain.

ectopic pregnancy — an incidence 20 times greater than expected. Hibbard studied 200 consecutive cases which were operated on for corpus luteum cysts [2]. One hundred and sixty-six of these were ruptured. Of these, 26 patients were pregnant and, not surprisingly, 22 of the 26 patients underwent surgery with the presumptive diagnosis of an ectopic pregnancy. All patients were in the first trimester and two-thirds were less than 8 weeks pregnant.

In the patient presenting with acute onset of lower abdominal pain, the absence of a clear adnexal mass on clinical or sonographic examination does not rule out a ruptured corpus luteum cyst, an ectopic pregnancy, or torsion of the adnexa (Fig. 82.1). In a febrile patient, the most probable diagnosis is PID or appendicitis. In this circumstance, the presence of a mass suggests a tuboovarian abscess.

A sensitive serum pregnancy test must be obtained in all cases of acute lower abdominal pain. A positive result must direct the attention toward early intervention, allowing conservative treatment of ectopic pregnancy. A culdocentesis may be of help, particularly if free fluid is observed on pelvic ultrasound. In Hibbard's study [7], three of 165 patients who had a culdocentesis for possible cyst rupture had false-negative results. These patients only had minimal hemoperitoneums at surgery. Four of 23 patients had false positives, of which three had a hematocrit of the fluid obtained from a culdocentesis of less than 6%. There was a rough correlation between culdocentesis hematocrits and volume of hemoperitoneum found at surgery but there were notable exceptions to this rule. When serosanguineous blood with a hematocrit of less than 12% is obtained, the patient may be observed without surgical intervention. The blood obtained at culdocentesis may or may not clot depending upon how long it has been present in the abdomen.

If the patient is pregnant, stable, and culdocentesis fails to reveal hemorrhage, serial β human chorionic gonadotropin determinations are mandatory. Titers that are not rising adequately strongly suggest tubal pregnancy. In the hemodynamically stable patient, a positive culdocentesis with a hematocrit higher than 12% or intractable pain prompts surgical intervention. Given the proper equipment and depending on the experience of the operator, ectopic pregnancies as well as ruptured corpora lutea and adnexal torsions can be managed through the laparoscope. It is not uncommon to find, at laparoscopy, ruptured hemorrhagic cyst in which active hemorrhage has subsided.

MANAGEMENT

The management for all ruptured ovarian cysts initially involves support care, including intravenous access, hydration, and transfusions as needed. When surgery is performed, ovarian conservation is the rule. If the patient is stable, laparoscopy should be performed. Cautery or laser vaporization can be used to stop bleeding and obliterate the cyst wall. Cystectomy may also be performed via the laparoscope. If bleeding cannot be adequately controlled via the laparoscope, one should proceed with an exploratory laparotomy.

In the hemodynamically unstable patient, blood transfusion and exploratory laparotomy must be performed as soon as possible. Fulguration, laser vaporization, or cystectomy should be performed as indicated. Oophorectomy should be avoided unless absolutely necessary.

The pregnant woman with a hemorrhagic corpus luteum that must be excised at surgery should be given exogenous progesterone to support the pregnancy until 8–10 weeks of gestation.

The use of oral contraceptives is advised to prevent recurrences in patients with bleeding disorders or who are on anticoagulation therapy.

REFERENCES

1 Westhoff CL. Patterns of ovarian cyst hospital discharge rates in England and Wales, 1962–79. *Br Med J* 1984; 289: 1348–1349.

2 Ory IT. Functional ovarian cysts and oral contraceptives. *JAMA* 1974; 228(1): 68–69.

3 Novaker, Woodwff JD. *Gynecologic and Obstetric Pathology*, 7th edn. Philadelphia: WB Saunders Co: 334–340.

4 Tang L, Cho HKM, Chan SYM, Wong VCW. Dextropreponderance of corpus luteum rupture: a clinical study. *J Reprod Med* 1985; 30: 764.

5 Peters WA, Thiagarajah S, Thornton WN. Ovarian hemorrhage in patients receiving anticoagulant therapy. *J Reprod Med* 1979; 22: 82.

6 Hallatt JG, Steele CH, Snyder M. Ruptured corpus luteum with hemoperitoneum: a study of 173 surgical cases. *Am J Obstet Gynecol* 1984; 149: 5.

7 Hibbard L. Corpus luteum surgery. *Am J Obstet Gynecol* 1979; 135: 666.

83

Unexplained infertility

EDWARD E. WALLACH

To complete an evaluation for infertility and fail to identify the causative factor(s) is frustrating for both patient and physician. The term unexplained infertility has been applied to such a situation. This designation is preferable to idiopathic infertility or the normal infertile couple with which it has been used interchangeably. Unexplained infertility implies that a diagnostic evaluation has been thorough but has failed to reveal any specific etiologic factor.

No explanation can be identified in approximately 15% of infertile couples. The incidence of unexplained infertility varies among the several reported studies. The thoroughness of the evaluation varies among different centers and is related to the expertise of the physician, availability of laboratory facilities, and perseverance of the patients concerned. The

more detailed the diagnostic evaluation, the greater is the probability of uncovering factors responsible for infertility.

The infertility evaluation needs to begin with a detailed interview consisting of medical, surgical, and family history, past use of contraceptive techniques, exposure to pregnancy and time of occurrence, and outcome of any previous pregnancies (Fig. 83.1). The physician should not be reluctant to raise pertinent leading questions regarding sexual habits, coital frequency, status of the marital relationship, emotional stability, and motivation. A history should include possible exposure to toxic agents and drugs, such as chemotherapy or radiation treatment, which may influence either male or female fertility. A thorough physical examination as well as pelvic

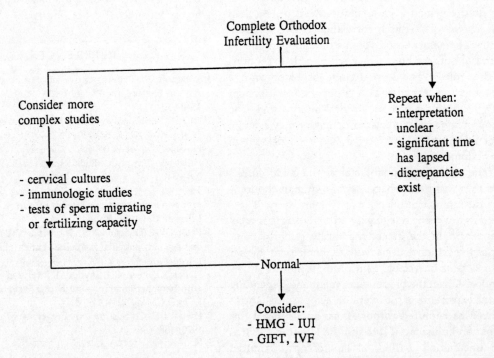

Fig. 83.1 Approach to unexplained infertility.

examination should focus on detecting signs of systemic disease and reproductive tract disorders. The occurrence and regularity of ovulation and the quality of the postovulatory phase must be assessed. The appraisal should consider not only semen characteristics as judged by semen analysis, but also adequacy and timing of sperm deposition at the cervix and sperm–cervical mucus interaction. The uterine cavity and endometrium must be examined for abnormalities which may adversely influence the intrauterine environment (e.g., neoplasia, infection, anomalous development) and impair implantation. The adnexa should be observed directly to appraise the anatomic relationship of fallopian tube and ovary on each side, detect evidence of endometriosis and periadnexal adhesions, and determine oviductal patency. Basic studies must include: investigation of the male factor; evaluation of cervical, uterine, tubal, peritoneal, ovarian, and immunologic factors; and assessment of coital techniques and patterns.

The following studies should be incorporated in the basic infertility evaluation:
1 Basal body temperature recordings.
2 Postcoital test, performed in the immediate preovulatory phase.
3 Semen analysis.
4 Hysterosalpingography.
5 Laparoscopy and tubal lavage.
6 Late postovulatory phase endometrial biopsy.

If these studies have already been previously performed by another physician, the endometrial biopsy slides and the basal body temperature record during the cycle in which it was obtained, the hysterosalpingogram and the operative note from a laparoscopy should be reviewed personally. It is advisable to repeat a postcoital test since the observations are usually highly subjective.

Other studies which may be performed when the basic evaluation is negative include:
1 Cervical culture for *Ureaplasma urealyticum* and *Chlamydia*.
2 Immunologic studies in the male and/or female.
3 Tests of fertilizing capacity of spermatozoa.
4 Tests of migrating capacity of spermatozoa, e.g., using bovine cervical mucus (Penetrak).

Assuming the couple fulfills the criteria for unexplained infertility, a postcoital test should have been previously performed and considered normal. Since postcoital testing is simple, inexpensive, and provides significant information, it can easily be repeated, especially under the following circumstances:

1 Whenever the results of the previous postcoital test are imprecisely reported. For example, if the report states "many sperm seen," commentary is lacking as to their location, the percentage and quality of motility, and the characteristics of the cervical mucus.
2 Whenever the results of the previous test suggest borderline concentration, morphology, or motility of spermatozoa.
3 Whenever the interpretation of the previous observer is in doubt.
4 Whenever significant time has elapsed since the previous postcoital examination.
5 Whenever a marked discrepancy exists between semen analysis findings and postcoital observations.

Since examination of endometrial histology provides a cumulative demonstration of the sequential effects of estradiol and progesterone on the endometrial tissue, a biopsy conveys considerable insight into the degree and duration of corpus luteum function as well as the ability of the endometrium to respond appropriately. For the optimum interpretation it should be ideally carried out as late as possible in the postovulatory phase.

Laparoscopic examination is invaluable in identifying the fallopian tubes and ovaries and revealing adnexal relationships. Concomitant tubal lavage helps to determine tubal patency. Subtle lesions may impair tubal transport of gametes (including periadnexal adhesions, endometriosis, and hydatid cysts). These can also often be treated endoscopically at the time of diagnostic laparoscopy. Assuming that laparoscopy has been previously performed, a repeat procedure should be considered under the following circumstances:

1 When interpretation by the previous laparoscopist is in question or if the previous laparoscopist lacks experience in identification of subtle disturbances associated with infertility.
2 Whenever the previous laparoscopist identified peritubal or periovarian pathology, but did not at the time consider the lesions to be significant.
3 If the patient has experienced some relevant pelvic disorder in the interval between previous laparoscopy and the current evaluation (e.g., salpingitis, pelvic surgery, recent onset of pelvic pain, possible disruption of an ovarian cyst).
4 If the patient has a condition which is associated with a high likelihood of progression (e.g., endometriosis).
5 Following reconstructive adnexal surgery if pregnancy has not occurred after an interval of

approximately 2 years (e.g., second-look laparoscopy) to determine the efficacy of the previous surgery in restoring patency and/or recreating normal anatomic relationships.

6 After a course of danazol for minimal endometriosis if pregnancy has not occurred within 12 months of attempt following medical therapy.

Ureaplasma urealyticum has been associated with both infertility and repeated spontaneous abortion. In males, the organism may be associated with decreased sperm motility or abnormal morphology. Although conception rates of 17–46% have been observed in couples with unexplained infertility following treatment [1], double-blind studies using doxycycline, placebo, and no medication failed to demonstrate any significant differences in pregnancy establishment among these three groups [2]. As controversial as the subject may seem at present, *Ureaplasma* cultures should be obtained in both partners with unexplained infertility, and if positive in either, a course of treatment is indicated for both. Antimicrobials of choice include tetracycline (500 mg four times daily for 10 days) or doxycycline (100 mg twice a day for 10 days). Culture-positive evidence is strongly urged before initiating antimicrobial therapy. However, exceptions to this general principle are reasonable for couples with long-standing unexplained infertility in communities in which the specific culture capability is unavailable. The presence of numerous pus cells in the cervical mucus of women or in the male's ejaculate should also prompt culture and/or appropriate antibiotic therapy. Tetracycline 500 mg four times per day for 10–14 days is usually adequate therapy for salpingitis.

Antigenicity of spermatozoa and other components of the ejaculate has been recognized for many years. Under certain circumstances, including trauma to the male ductal system (e.g., following vas ligation), males may produce autoantibodies against seminal components. Such antibodies may result in impairment of sperm motility through the female reproductive tract. In the presence of antibodies to seminal components in the female, penetration of cervical mucus or transport through the uterine cavity and fallopian tubes may be compromised. Experimental evidence also points to the possibility of antibodies to the zona pellucida, the gelatinous layer surrounding the oocyte. Immunologic phenomena at this level could interfere with sperm penetration of the zona pellucida, thus preventing fertilization. The role of autoantibodies to the zona in human infertility has not yet been elucidated.

Because of controversial data regarding antisperm antibodies, studies need not be carried out routinely in every infertile couple. Immunologic evaluation is helpful specifically in the following instances:

1 Study of the male with previous vas ligation prior to reversal or following reversal if infertility persists.
2 Study of the female if postcoital testing and post-artificial insemination testing consistently demonstrate immotile spermatozoa despite normal motility in the freshly ejaculated specimen.
3 The consistent appearance of a shaking movement rather than forward motion of spermatozoa in the endocervical canal at the time of postcoital testing.
4 Investigation of any couple in whom no factor has been uncovered to explain infertility despite normal semen analysis and postcoital testing. The yield of positives, however, in such cases will be small.

There is a reasonably high correlation between long-standing unexplained infertility and sperm antibodies in sera and/or reproductive tract fluid. Prolonged duration of unexplained infertility correlates fairly well with the presence of sperm antibodies. Immunobead binding is currently the most widely used test available for determining the presence of antisperm antibodies [3]. It utilizes micron-sized plastic spheres which adhere to antibodies on the surface of spermatozoa. The test can be used to detect antibodies on the sperm surface or in husband's or wife's serum. Three options are available for treatment of couples with antisperm antibodies: (1) corticosteroids; (2) sperm washing and intrauterine insemination; and (3) *in vitro* fertilization.

The functional capacity of spermatozoa takes into consideration their ability to exist in the female reproductive tract and their fertilizability. Transportation of gametes to the site of fertilization can only be surmised indirectly. Assessment of ovum transfer to the lumen of the fallopian tube cannot be carried out using currently available technology. Most tests of sperm behavior in the female genital tract are based upon *in vivo* or *in vitro* observations of the interaction of spermatozoa and cervical mucus. The ability of such tests to predict the ability of sperm to reach the site of fertilization is limited. However, sperm recovery from the pelvis by laparoscopy immediately following artificial placement of husband's sperm at the cervix or after coitus during the immediate preovulatory interval has been advocated to assess sperm migration.

Tests for the fertilizing capacity of spermatozoa have been sought by numerous investigators for many years. In 1976 Yanagimachi *et al.* [4] demonstrated that human spermatozoa can penetrate zona-free hamster ova and thereby established the basis for potential development of a standardized test for assessing the fertilizing capacity of human spermatozoa. The virtue of this approach is that it raises the possibility of detecting defective sperm function in the face of normal semen parameters using conventional standards for semen analysis, especially in evaluating couples with unexplained infertility.

Although the significance of this sperm penetration assay (SPA) is still incompletely understood, further data attempting to correlate ability of sperm to penetrate zona-free hamster eggs with standard parameters for semen analysis, immunologic studies, and fertility status of the couple, are bound to clarify the ultimate role of this procedure in an infertility evaluation. Advantages of the SPA are listed below:

1 Sperm must undergo the acrosome reaction to allow fusion with the hamster egg plasma membrane.
2 The SPA tests fusion/decondensation, thus pronuclear formation.
3 Multiple penetrations permit use of a sperm penetration index.
4 The SPA tests sperm chromosomal complement.
5 The test is relatively simple.
6 Hamster eggs are readily available.

Potential problems associated with this procedure are obvious when one considers interspecies tests. There are other specific drawbacks to the SPA: (1) natural inducers of the acrosome reaction are removed; and (2) test results can vary greatly depending upon specific conditions under which the assay is conducted.

Additional approaches to study sperm fertilizing ability are rarely used, but some of them show some promise. These include:

1 Ultrastructure of spermatozoa.
2 Penetration of homologous zona-intact oocytes (oocytes matured either *in vivo* or *in vitro* and stored nonviable zonae)
  (a) matured *in vivo*;
  (b) matured *in vitro*;
  (c) stored, nonviable.
3 A hemi-zona assay, which uses control and the unknown sperm.
4 Competitive mixed insemination penetration assay.
5 Measurement of sperm acrosin concentration.

The term luteal-phase defect (LPD) refers to abnormal ovarian function leading to inadequate progesterone production during the postovulatory phase of the cycle. LPD has been associated with both infertility and recurrent early pregnancy loss. The diagnosis of LPD may be established by utilizing several parameters of corpus luteum function, including basal body temperature recordings and patterns, endometrial histology, and serum progesterone levels. Correlation among these parameters is essential. The simplest and most accurate diagnostic method is through interpretation of endometrial histology correlated with the point of rise in basal body temperature or with luteinizing hormone assays at midcycle [5]. The biopsy should be obtained as close to the onset of the next menstrual period as possible in order to assess the cumulative affect of corpus luteum secretions on the endometrium.

Basal body temperature recordings tempt overinterpretation. Although an abbreviated thermal shift is highly suggestive of defective luteal function, the physician should resist reliance on temperature patterns alone and utilize endometrial biopsy, possibly supplemented by serum progesterone levels. Three approaches are available for treatment of LPD: (1) ovulation-inducing agents such as clomiphene citrate or human gonadotropins in an attempt to create a better follicle; (2) postovulatory endometrial support using exogenous progesterone; and (3) stimulation of the corpus luteum with human chorionic gonadotropin (hCG).

In summary, the physician should reevaluate the work-up to insure that no essential diagnostic studies have been omitted and that those already performed have been properly interpreted. Occasionally, studies will have to be repeated if validity of the previous interpretation is in doubt or if significant time has elapsed since performance of the original study. Consideration should be given to immunologic studies and tests of gamete transport and fertilizing capacity of spermatozoa, possibly using the SPA. Bacteriologic studies should be conducted, especially for *Ureaplasma urealyticum*, which appears to have a possible etiologic relationship to infertility and *Chlamydia*. The luteal phase needs to be thoroughly investigated. Additional studies which may be conducted thus include follicle tracking by ultrasound and cul-de-sac aspiration for spermatozoa.

From a therapeutic standpoint, a specific diagnosis is essential prior to initiation of any specific treatment. Empiric treatment of the couple with unexplained infertility is usually considered inappropriate and may be intrinsically dangerous or even emotionally damaging by raising expectations of the couple without logical or scientific basis. Although thyroid medications, bromocriptine, danazol, and mucolytic agents have in the past have been suggested as

CHAPTER 83

efficacious in unexplained infertility, their effectiveness is still unproved and their empiric use should be avoided and discouraged. Likewise, there is little rationale for the administration of ovulation-inducing agents such as clomiphene citrate or gonadotropic substances in the normally ovulating woman with a normal postovulatory phase. However, Dodson and coworkers have associated washed intrauterine insemination and human menopausal/chorionic gonadotropin (hMG/hCG) superovulation in patients with "refractory infertility," reporting a 16% pregnancy rate during four cycles of treatment in women prior to entering an *in vitro* fertilization (IVF) program [6]. Corsan and colleagues have also reviewed applications for the use of gonadotropins in couples with ovulatory infertility [7].

Likewise Welner *et al.* carried out empiric hMG/hCG therapy in patients with long-standing infertility of unknown etiology while awaiting IVF. Twelve conceptions (12.4%) and eight (8.2%) term births occurred in their study group, as compared to 1% in controls [8]. On this basis the authors suggest a 4-month empiric trial of hMG/hCG in patients with unexplained infertility. This approach is still considered controversial. Resorting to artificial donor insemination in unexplained infertility is also highly controversial and should only be preceded by substantial evidence of immunologic interference with gamete transport or of a defect in the fertilizing capacity of the male partner's spermatozoa. In the latter instances, it appears possible that IVF may offer a reasonable approach to treatment. In Lopata's review of indications for IVF during 1981, 32 of 229 patients underwent IVF-ET (embryo transfer) with an indication of unexplained infertility [9]. The gamete intrafallopian (GIFT) procedure has also been used successfully in patients with unexplained infertility. Finally, one should realize that many of the processes responsible for fertility are currently beyond our diagnostic reach and defy direct evaluation. This concept must be shared with the couple in whom that basis for infertility cannot be determined.

FINAL CONSIDERATIONS

To put the problem of unexplained infertility into perspective, Collins *et al.* [10] suggested that of 597 infertile couples, 41% conceived following medical and/or surgical therapy. In contrast, 191 of 548 untreated controls (35%) became pregnant. Seventy-five additional patients conceived 6 months or more

Table 83.1 Investigations in 57 couples. (Adapted from [12])

Modality	Diagnosis	Patients	
		Number	%
Ultrasound	LUF	3	5
Sperm	Antibodies present	11	5
SPA	Penetration	11	11
HLA	HLA homozygosity	21	37

LUF, luteinized unruptured follicle; SPA, sperm penetration assay; HLA, human leukocyte antigen.

after surgical therapy or at least 3 months after cessation of medical treatment. In addition, Miller *et al.* [11] reported on 197 patients during 623 cycles in which 152 pregnancies occurred. Of these, 43% (64) resulted in pregnancy loss. Only 14 of the 64 losses were recognized as spontaneous abortions; the other 50 had only positive urinary hCG levels, but no other evidence of pregnancy. Finally, Coulam and her coworkers have amplified on yield for investigations for unexplained infertility [12]. Table 83.1 summarizes their yield.

REFERENCES

1 Friberg J. Mycoplasmas and ureaplasmas in infertility and abortion. *Fertil Steril* 1980; 33: 351.
2 Harrison RF, Blades M, DeLouvois J, Hurley R. Doxycycline treatment and human infertility. *Lancet* 1975; 1: 605.
3 Bronson R, Cooper G, Rosenfeld D. Sperm antibodies: their role in infertility. *Fertil Steril* 1984, 42: 171.
4 Yanagimachi R, Yanagimachi H, Rogers BJ. The use of zona-free animal ova as a test system for the assessment of fertilizing capacity of human spermatozoa. *Biol Reprod* 1976; 15: 471.
5 Li T-C, Rogers AW, Lenton EA, Dockery P, Cooke I. A comparison between two methods of chronological dating of human endometrial biopsies during the luteal phase, and their correlation with histological dating. *Fertil Steril* 1987; 48: 928.
6 Dodson WC, Whitesides DB, Hughes CL, Easley HA, Haney AF. Superovulation with intrauterine insemination in the treatment of infertility: a possible alternative to gamete intrafallopian transfer and in vitro fertilization. *Fertil Steril* 1987; 48: 441.
7 Corsan GH, Ghazi D, Kemmann E. Home urinary luteinizing hormone immunoassays: clinical application. *Fertil Steril* 1990; 53: 591–601.
8 Welner S, DeCherney AH, Polan ML. Human menopausal gonadotropins: a justifiable therapy in ovulatory

women with long-standing idiopathic infertility. *Am J Obstet Gynecol* 1988; 158: 111.

9 Lopata A. Concepts in human *in vitro* fertilization and embryo transfer. *Fertil Steril* 1983; 40: 289.

10 Collins JA, Wrixon W, Janes LB, Wilson EH. Treatment independent pregnancy among infertile couples. *N Eng J Med* 1983; 309: 1201.

11 Miller JF, Williamson E, Glue J, Gordon YB, Gmudzinskas JG, Sykes A. Fetal loss after implantation. *Lancet* 1988; 2: 54.

12 Coulam CB, Moore SB, O'Fallon W. Investigating unexplained infertility. *Am J Obstet Gynecol* 1988; 158: 1374.

84

Infections and infertility

RONALD S. GIBBS

Pelvic infections are an important cause of infertility, primarily as a result of tubal damage. In this chapter, we will discuss those infections related to infertility, notably gonorrhea, chlamydial infections, and pelvic inflammatory disease (PID). An outline of the approach to pelvic infections is shown in Figure 84.1.

GONORRHEA INFECTIONS

Within the past 5 years, several important changes have occurred in the area of gonorrheal disease, making an update on its diagnosis and management important.

Recent data from the Centers for Disease Control (CDC) have indicated a marked decrease in the prevalence of gonorrhea [1]. In the late 1970s, reported rates of gonorrhea peaked at approximately 450 per 100 000 population. Over the last decade, there has been a marked decrease in this rate, to approximately 275 per 100 000 in 1990. Although all of the factors influencing this decrease in gonorrhea are not clear, it is likely that the acquired immune deficiency syndrome (AIDS) epidemic with subsequent institution of safe sex practices may have influenced this rate favorably.

In women, the endocervix is the most common site of gonococcal infections. The majority of these are asymptomatic. Untreated gonococcal cervicitis can result in serious complications, including disseminated gonococcal disease and acute salpingitis. Salpingitis occurs in approximately 15% of women with gonococcal cervicitis if untreated. Of all patients with PID, *Neisseria gonorrhoeae* is isolated in a highly varying percentage from the endocervix — from 20 to 80% depending upon the clinical setting. *N. gonorrhoeae* is isolated in a much smaller proportion of tubal aspirates from patients with PID.

Disseminated gonococcal infection includes common manifestations of tenosynovitis, arthralgia, arthritis, and rash. Pharyngeal gonococcal infection may occur in individuals who had oral sexual relations and is usually asymptomatic. A pharyngeal infection may be more difficult to eradicate than genital or anal gonococcal infection.

Until 1987, penicillin had been the antibiotic of choice in the treatment of gonorrhea. Since then, however, treatment guidelines from the CDC have been revised in view of the rising incidence of penicillinase-producing *N. gonorrhoeae*. Penicillinase-producing *N. gonorrhoeae* (PPNG) first appeared in the USA 1976. By 1986, there were over 16 000 cases of PPNG reported.

The standard for diagnosis of gonorrhea is a culture. Although there are rapid diagnostic tests available, the culture remains both practical and reliable. The CDC recommends that all gonorrhea cases should be diagnosed or confirmed by culture to facilitate antibiotic susceptibiliy testing. Since the susceptibility of *N. gonorrhoeae* to antibiotics may change over time in any location, gonorrhea control programs should include a system of regular antibiotic susceptibility testing for surveillance of PPNG. Accordingly, for patients with uncomplicated urethral, endocervical, or rectal infections, the current recommended regimen is as follows: ceftriaxone (Rocephin) 250 mg i.m. once plus doxycycline 100 mg orally twice a day for 7 days. The purpose of the doxycycline regimen is for presumptive treatment of *Chlamydia trachomatis*, which may occur in 40–50% of patients with genital tract gonorrhea. For patients who cannot take ceftriaxone, the preferred alternative is spectinomycin 2 g i.m. in a single dose, also followed by doxycycline. In 1989 the CDC also suggested that there may be other alternatives, although the experience with these regimens is less extensive [2]. These regimens may include ciprofloxacin 500 mg orally once, norfloxacin 800 mg orally once, cefuroxime axetil 1 g orally once with probenecid 1 g, cefotaxime 1 g i.m. once and

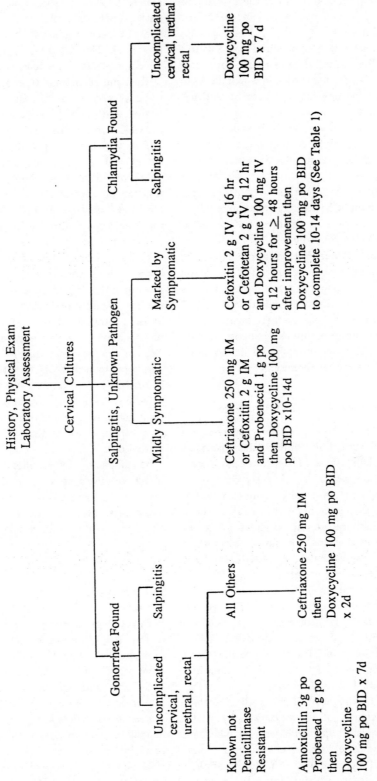

Fig. 84.1 Approach to pelvic infections.

ceftizoxime 500 mg i.m. once. All of these regimens should also be followed by doxycycline as in the cefotetan regimen.

If these infections have been acquired from a source known not to be penicillinase-resistant gonorrhea then a penicillin such as amoxicillin 3 g orally with probenecid (1 g) may be used for treatment and followed by doxycycline.

For patients who cannot take tetracycline, erythromycin may be substituted. As with other regimens, these should include presumptive treatment for C. trachomatis.

Patients exposed to gonorrhea within the preceding 30 days should be treated presumptively. In addition, cultures should be obtained, but treatment should not await culture results.

Because treatment failure following ceftriaxone and doxycycline therapy is rare, a follow-up culture is not essential. CDC recommends a more cost-effective strategy [3] — maybe reexamination with culture 1–2 months after treatment. Because there has been less experience with other regimens, patients treated with these alternative regimen should have follow-up cultures 4–7 days after therapy.

CHLAMYDIAL INFECTIONS

During the past 15 years, there has been a marked rise in the rate of chlamydial infections so that Chlamydia is now approximately three to four times more common than N. gonorrhoeae.

Chlamydial cervicitis is usually asymptomatic but clinical findings may include cervical edema, and a mucopurulent discharge. As noted above, N. gonorrhoeae and Chlamydia are commonly coinfecting organisms with approximately 20–40% of patients with Chlamydia having no gonorrhea.

In women, most chlamydial infections are limited to the cervix and urethra, but acute salpingitis and the Fitz-Hugh–Curtis syndrome are not unusual.

Overall, the incidence of a chlamydial infection varies widely from 2 to 25% of pregnant women and in a higher percentage in patients attending sexually transmitted disease clinics.

The standard for diagnosis of chlamydial infection remains the isolation of C. trachomatis by tissue culture. Recently rapid diagnostic tests have become commercially available and these include a monoclonal antibody (Microtrack) and the enzyme-linked immunosorbent assay (Chlamydiazyme). In populations with moderate to high rates of C (approxi-

mately 9–20%), these rapid diagnostic techniques have acceptable reliability. However, their reliability has not been evaluated thoroughly in patients of lower risk. The Pap smear is an unreliable technique for diagnosis of C. trachomatis infection.

The drug of choice in treating chlamydial infections is doxycycline or tetracycline. For treatment in uncomplicated urethral, endocervical or rectal infections, the CDC currently recommends a regimen as follows [2]: doxycycline 100 mg orally twice a day for 7 days. An alternative is tetracycline 500 mg orally four times a day for 7 days. Some clinics prefer to use the latter regimen because of a lower cost, but this potential advantage may be offset by poor compliance since this regimen requires a four-times-a-day dosing, whereas the doxycycline requires dosing twice a day. For patients who cannot take either doxycycline or tetracycline, such as patients who are pregnant, the recommended regimen is erythromycin, either as the base, 500 mg orally four times a day for 7 days, or erythromycin ethylsuccinate, 800 mg orally four times a day for 7 days. Because some patients cannot tolerate erythromycin due to side-effects, an alternative regimen that may be effective is sulfisoxazole, 500 mg orally four times a day for 10 days.

Because antibiotic resistance of C. trachomatis to these above recommendations has not been observed, it is not recommended that test of cure cultures be carried out.

Sexual partners of patients who have C. trachomatis infection should be tested and treated for C. trachomatis if the contact was within 30 days of onset of symptoms. If testing is not available, sexual partners should be treated with an appropriate regimen.

PID

PID is also known as acute salpingitis. This infection is usually ascending infection and often polymicrobial in etiology. In recent studies in the USA, approximately 20–50% cases of acute PID have occurred in association with C. trachomatis, and 20–80% in association with N. gonorrhoeae [3,4]. Mixed cultures of aerobes and anaerobes may be obtained from the tubal or peritoneal fluid in 20–70% of cases. Actinomyces israelii is rarely isolated; when it is, it is usually in conjunction with a foreign body such as an intrauterine device.

As seen with N. gonorrhoeae, the rate of PID has undergone a marked decrease in the last decade. Data from the Centers for Disease Control indicated that the rate was 850 per 100 000 women in the late 1970s [1]. There has been a gradual decrease in the USA since then, with an estimated rate of cases of approximately 550 per 100 000 women for 1990. Again, it is suggested that this decrease may have been brought about by more widespread use of safe sex practices.

The diagnosis of PID remains largely a clinical diagnosis. Hager and colleagues [5] recommended the following diagnostic criteria for acute PID — all of the following must be present: (1) abdominal tenderness; (2) cervical motion and uterine tenderness; and (3) adnexal tenderness. In addition, at least one of the following must be present: (1) a cervical Gram stain positive for Gram-negative intracellular diplococci; (2) temperature greater than 38°C; (3) white blood count greater than 10 000/mm^3; (4) presence of a pelvic mass on examination or sonography; and (5) purulent material in the cul-de-sac on culdocentesis or at laparoscopy. The role of sonography in the diagnosis is mainly in excluding other conditions such as an accident to an ovarian cyst or ectopic pregnancy. Laparoscopy may be used to make the diagnosis, particularly in cases where the diagnosis is not clear or the patient has not responded well.

Patients who have PID should have cultures of the endocervix for *N. gonorrhoeae* and *C. trachomatis*. In markedly symptomatic patients, blood cultures may be obtained but these are infrequently positive. The role of culdocentesis in the diagnosis may be helpful to rule out intraperitoneal hemorrhage as well as to collect specimens for Gram stain and culture.

Diagnostic accuracy of clinical findings in patients with PID has varied widely (as low as 65% up to 90%).

Within the past few years, there has been an increasing emphasis on hospitalization of patients with PID. Particularly hospitalization is suggested in any of the following conditions: (1) if the diagnosis is uncertain; (2) when surgical emergencies including appendicitis and ectopic pregnancy cannot be ruled out; (3) if pelvic abscesses are suspected for the patient who is pregnant; (4) if the patient is an adolescent (because adolescent patients may be less compliant and because long-term sequelae may be particularly severe in adolescents); (5) if severe symptomatology precludes successful outpatient management; (6) with an unreliable patient who cannot follow the outpatient regimen; and (7) in cases of poor response to previous outpatient therapy or when follow-up within 72 hours cannot be arranged.

Table 84.1 Treatment schedule for acute salpingitis

Setting	Regime
Ambulatory	Ceftriaxone 250 mg i.m. or cefoxitin 2 g i.m. plus probenecid 1 g orally concurrently plus doxycycline 100 mg p.o. b.i.d. × 10–14 days
Inpatient	Cefoxitin 2 g i.v. q 6 hours or cefotetan 2 g i.v. every 12 hours plus doxycycline 100 mg i.v. b.i.d. for ≥48 hours after improvement, then doxycycline 100 mg p.o. b.i.d. to complete 10–14 days or Clindamycin 900 mg i.v. q 8 hours in same solution with gentamicin, 2 mg/kg then 1.5 mg/kg i.v. q 8 hours for 48 hours after improvement; then doxycycline 100 mg b.i.d. for 10–14 days total or clindamycin 450 mg p.o. q.i.d. or equivalent cepholosprin to complete 10–14 days of therapy

In 1989, the Centers for Disease Control recommended revised treatment regimens for patients with acute salpingitis [2]. These are shown in Table 84.1.

Sexual partners with PID should also be evaluated for sexually transmitted diseases. These sexual partners should then be empirically treated with regimens effective against both *N. gonorrhoeae* and *C. trachomatis*.

Several clinical evaluations have been carried out to compare the efficacy of the two CDC recommended inpatient regimens for PID [3,4]. These have found no statistically significant difference in efficacy, although in each there has been a small, but not significant, advantage in favor of the cefoxitin–doxycycline regimen.

Approximately 5% of patients will not respond to antibiotic therapy often because of tuboovarian abscess. Surgical drainage may be obtained by colpotomy if appropriately fixed and pointing in the cul-de-sac, but in most cases laparotomy is used. In cases of women desiring future fertility, surgery may be limited to unilateral salpingo-oophorectomy, particularly if adnexa side has an essentially normal anatomy.

Long-term sequelae of PID include involuntary,

ectopic pregnancy, and recurrent disease. In classic works carried out in Scandinavia over 20 years ago, it was recognized that the incidence of involuntary sterility due to tubal occlusion increased geometrically with the number of episodes of salpingitis. After one episode, 13% of women had involuntary sterility due to tubal occlusion. After two episodes, this rate rose to 35%, and after three or more episodes, the rate rose to 75% [6]. A risk for ectopic pregnancy also correlates with previous chlamydial infection, as evidenced by serum antichlamydial antibodies. Women with ectopic pregnanies are more likely to have higher antichlamydial antibodies than matched pregnant control women [7]. This observation strongly suggests that previous chlamydial infection (presumably on the tube) predisposes to ectopic pregnancy.

Because these genital tract infections may adversely affect fertility, it is important for physicians caring for women to provide the most appropriate care in diagnosing and treating these common disorders.

REFERENCES

1 Progress toward achieving the 1990 objectives for the nation for sexually transmitted diseases. *MMWR* 1990; 39: 53–57.
2 Sexually Transmitted Disease Treatment Guideline. *MMWR* 1989; 38: 1–43.
3 Walters MD, Gibbs RS. A randomized comparison of gentamicin-clindamycin and cefoxitin-doxycycline in the treatment of acute pelvic inflammatory disease. *Obstet Gynecol* 1990; 75: 867.
4 Wasserheit JN, Bell TA, Koviat NB *et al*. Microbial causes of proven pelvic inflammatory disease and efficacy of clindamycin and tobomycin. *Ann Intern Med* 1986; 104: 87–93.
5 Hager WD, Eschenbach DA, Spence MR, Sweet RL. Criteria for diagnosis and grading of salpingitis. *Obstet Gynecol* 1983; 61: 113–114.
6 Westrom L. Effect of acute pelvic inflammatory disease on fertility. *Am J Obstet Gynecol* 1975; 122: 876.
7 Walters ML, Eddy CA, Gibbs RS *et al*. Antibodies to *Chlamydia trachomatis* and risk for tubal pregnancy. *Am J Obstet Gynecol* 1988; 159: 942–946.

Referral for assisted reproduction

DAVID S. GUZICK

Assisted reproduction, including *in vitro* fertilization (IVF), gamete intrafallopian transfer (GIFT), and related procedures, has become an important method of infertility treatment. Over the past decade, assisted reproduction has progressed from a set of procedures that were viewed with skepticism to ones that are being successfully performed on a large number of infertility patients at many centers across the country. During 1990, the last year in which complete national data are available, 16 405 cycles of IVF and 3750 cycles of GIFT were initiated by centers reporting to the US IVF registry [1]. The clinical pregnancy rates per egg-retrieval cycle during 1990 were 19% for IVF and 29% for GIFT.

For all but a small number of patients, such as those with absent fallopian tubes or premature ovarian failure, assisted reproduction should only be performed after a thorough infertility evaluation has been completed and conventional medical and surgical treatments have been attempted. The purpose of this chapter is to assist clinicians in answering the question "Should my patient be referred for assisted reproduction?"

CONCEPTUAL OVERVIEW

A conceptual overview of assisted reproduction evaluation is shown in Figure 85.1. Infertility patients should undergo a standard evaluation consisting of semen analysis, hysterosalpingogram, postcoital test, timed endometrial biopsy, and laparoscopy. A good overview of this evaluation is available from the American Fertility Society [2]. If any of these tests are abnormal, appropriate medical and/or surgical treatment should be initiated. While a complete discussion of these treatments is beyond the scope of this chapter, certain conditions and their treatment that have particular relevance for assisted reproduction will be considered below. If no conception occurs after a suitable duration of conventional

infertility treatment, the patient should be referred for assisted reproduction.

If all infertility tests are normal, then the couple is said to have unexplained infertility. Couples with unexplained infertility who are followed without treatment have a cumulative pregnancy rate of 35–50% after 2 years of follow-up, and 60–70% after 3 years of follow-up. Thus, depending on age and duration of infertility, a period of expectant management (i.e., timed intercourse) is indicated. Alternatively, or following expectant management, superovulation (with or without intrauterine insemination (IUI)) has been advocated as a means of enhancing the likelihood of pregnancy in couples with unexplained infertility. Such an approach is less invasive and costly than assisted reproduction and therefore deserves consideration prior to referral. If expectant management and/or superovulation fails to result in pregnancy, the couple become candidates for assisted reproduction.

The potential importance of assisted reproduction as a treatment for infertility is suggested by the data in Table 85.1. Estimates of the distribution of causes of infertility, according to available cohort studies, are shown. Assuming that 2 years of treatment and

Table 85.1 Causes of infertility and pregnancy outcome after treatment

Infertility factor	Percentage of infertile couples	Percentage pregnant by 2 years	Precentage of couples remaining infertile
Male	30	40	18
Tubal	20	40	12
Endometriosis	15	65	5
Ovulatory	15	65	5
Unexplained	20	50	10
Total	100		50

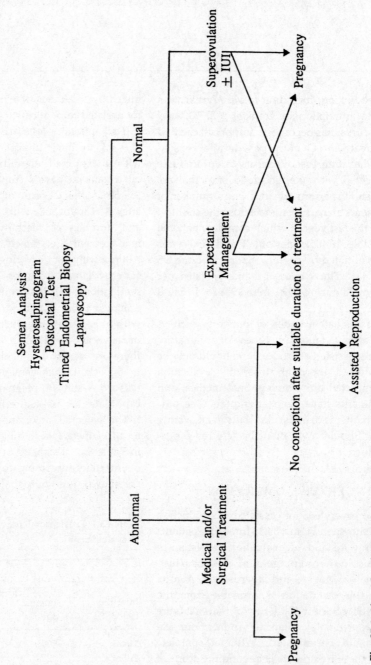

Semen Analysis
Hysterosalpingogram
Postcoital Test
Timed Endometrial Biopsy
Laparoscopy

Normal

Abnormal

Superovulation
± IUI

Expectant
Management

Pregnancy

Medical and/or
Surgical Treatment

No conception after suitable duration of treatment

Assisted Reproduction

Pregnancy

Fig. 85.1 Algorithm for referral for assisted reproduction.

follow-up is considered an appropriate interval for attempts at conventional medical and surgical treatment, the proportion of couples in each infertility category who do not become pregnant by 2 years can be calculated by applying the expected pregnancy rates of treatment in each category. Thus for example, a 65% pregnancy rate after 2 years of follow-up following treatment of the 15% of infertile women with endometriosis would imply that 5% remain infertile after 2 years. Summation across categories indicates that, after 2 years of follow-up, half of the initial infertile group would not have conceived. Since approximately 2.5 million couples in the reproductive age group in the USA are infertile, it is clear that the potential need for assisted reproduction (apart from the issues of access and affordability) is quite large.

REFERRAL FOR ASSISTED REPRODUCTION AFTER CONVENTIONAL TREATMENT HAS FAILED

Given the above conceptual framework, we now pass to a consideration of individual clinical conditions in which assisted reproduction may be appropriate after conventional treatment has failed.

Tubal factor
Tubal factor can be considered under several categories as follows.

Previous tubal ligation
Reversal of a previous tubal ligation is the most successful form of tubal surgery and is recommended as a first treatment instead of assisted reproduction. In experienced hands, cumulative pregnancy rates from tubal reanastomosis range from 40 to 50% for electrocautery sterilizations, to 60–70% for modified Pomeroy sterilizations, to 80–90% for Silastic bands or clips. A hysterosalpingogram should be obtained if there is no pregnancy 6 months after surgery to confirm tubal patency. If there is no pregnancy 2 years after tubal reanastomosis, consideration should be given to referral for assisted reproduction, especially in women ≥35 years years of age. For women in their late 30s or beyond, consideration might be given to referral for assisted reproduction after only 1 year of follow-up.

Peritubal adhesions
Peritubal adhesions may result from a previous history of appendicitis or pelvic surgery. In such cases, there may be no intrinsic damage to the fallopian tubes but peritubal adhesions may interfere with egg pick-up. Mild inflammatory disease or endometriosis may result in a similar picture. In the absence of intrinsic tubal disease, cumulative pregnancy rates following lysis of adhesions is in the 50–70% range. Therefore, surgery is warranted before IVF, especially if it can be accomplished laparoscopically. The same considerations with respect to duration of follow-up and age that were discussed in relation to tubal reanastomosis apply here as well.

Proximal tubal obstruction
If there is proximal tubal obstruction without a history of tubal ligation, fluoroscopic tubal cannulation should be attempted prior to consideration for assisted reproduction. If tubal cannulation is unsuccessful, then the X-ray study should be examined with respect to the amount of interstitial tube present. If it is thought that sufficient interstitial tube is present to perform a tubocornual anastomosis, then such an approach should be considered prior to referral for assisted reproduction, as it is associated, in experienced hands, with a pregnancy rate of 40–50%. If the intersitial tube is virtually or completely absent, then surgical correction would involve tubal implantation. Such an approach has been associated with variable success, and also carries the risk of uterine rupture during pregnancy or labor. In such cases, it would appear prudent to refer the patient directly for IVF.

Distal tubal disease
Distal tubal disease associated with bilateral hydrosalpinges is the most common type of tubal factor, and the most difficult to treat. Occasionally, the hydrosalpinx may be of small diameter, with a few, filmy adhesions, and, when opened, the tubal wall is thin and the fimbria are found to be healthy. In these cases, a cuff salpingostomy performed by way of laparoscopy or laparotomy carries an expectation of pregnancy sufficiently high to warrant surgery prior to consideration for IVF referral. In the vast majority of cases, however, the tubal disease is more severe in nature. In such cases, surgery for distal tubal disease results in cumulative pregnancy rates of only 15–30%. Moreover, among those who con-

ceive, the probability of an ectopic pregnancy is quite high — as much as 10—20%. In counseling such patients, these results must be compared with those of IVF. If an IVF program has a clinical pregnancy rate of 15% per cycle, then the expectation of pregnancy after three cycles is 39%. Moreover, the likelihood of ectopic pregnancy is low, perhaps 5%. In these situations, recommendations for surgery versus IVF must be tailored to the individual patient, and also to the results of the tubal surgeons and IVF programs in the clinician's locality. In our practice, we recommend IVF for women with moderate to severe distal tubal disease who are ≥35 years old. We generally recommend an attempt at tubal surgery before considering IVF for women less than 30 years old. For women 30—35 years old, the extent of disease, the likelihood of being able to perform the surgery laparoscopically, and the patient's wishes after being presented with pertinent outcome data are all important components of the counseling process.

In general, repeat tubal surgery does not confer any benefit with respect to the likelihood of pregnancy, especially in the case of distal tubal disease. While some pregnancies occasionally occur after a second or third attempt at tubal surgery, there are no data to suggest that this occurs any more often than do pregnancies from continued follow-up after the first surgery. Thus, if pregnancy has not occurred 2 or more years after tubal surgery, the patient should be counseled that, if additional treatment is desired, IVF is recommended rather than repeat tubal surgery.

Endometriosis

There are numerous lines of epidemiologic and experimental evidence that endometriosis and infertility are associated. Minimal or mild endometriosis can be excised or ablated laparoscopically at the time of diagnosis. Medical treatment with danazol or a gonadotropin-releasing hormone (GnRH) analog may be effective in treating subclinical foci of endometriosis. However, medical and surgical treatment of minimal and mild endometriosis has not been shown to enhance pregnancy rates beyond that of controls who are managed expectantly. Moderate or severe endometriosis generally requires surgical intervention (laparoscopy or laparotomy), as discussed in Chapter 80. If there is no pregnancy after 2 years of follow-up, referral for assisted reproduction should be considered. Many studies of endometriosis treatment have shown that pregnancies occur in a

consistent manner beyond 2 years of follow-up; nonetheless, a large majority of pregnancies that occur following treatment do so within 2 years, and the timing of referral for assisted reproduction must take into account the patient's age and the extent of disease. Advanced endometriosis with tubal involvement generally requires IVF if conventional treatment fails. If the tubes are uninvolved and appear to be normal throughout their length, then GIFT may be preferred, as it is generally associated with a higher pregnancy rate than IVF. The decision concerning whether to perform GIFT or IVF in these situations depends on the experience of the particular assisted reproduction center to which the patient is referred.

Ovulatory dysfunction

Although ovulatory function (either spontaneous or in response to ovarian stimulation) is necessary for assisted reproduction, ovulatory dysfunction alone should not be an indication for referral. Effective treatment is available for women who are anovulatory (see Chapters 74, 75). If pregnancy does not occur despite an adequate number of documented ovulatory cycles with appropriately timed intercourse, then it is likely that there is another cause for the infertility than anovulation. A similar argument can be made for treatment of luteal-phase deficiency. Thus, if treatment of ovulatory dysfunction does not result in pregnancy, a thorough review of all other possible cause of infertility should be conducted, including a laparoscopy if one has not been performed. If no other etiology for infertility is found, then the patient can be considered to have unexplained infertility and be treated as such (see below).

Male factor

A semen analysis should be performed to obtain information on sperm density, motility, and morphology, and on evidence of infection. An abnormal number of leukocytes in the semen should be further evaluated and treated with antibiotics. If repeated semen analyses show abnormal sperm parameters, a physical examination should be performed and serum concentrations of testosterone and follicle-stimulating hormone should be obtained. Appropriate surgical or medical treatment should be performed for any anatomic abnormalities that are identified. If such treatment fails to result in a pregnancy or, as is most often the case, there is no identified etiology for the abnormal semen parameters, a screening sperm wash should be obtained. If more than 1 million motile sperm can be recovered from the sperm wash, IUI of washed sperm may be of benefit and should be attempted prior to referral for assisted reproduction. If fewer than 1 million motile sperm can be obtained from a sperm wash, especially if they do not maintain their motility in culture, it is highly unlikely that IUI will result in a pregnancy. If IUI fails, or if the number of sperm that can be recovered is too low to consider IUI, then appropriate counseling for such couples would involve discussion of donor insemination versus assisted reproduction. Many couples are not accepting donor insemination before attempting at least one cycle of IVF, as IVF would serve a diagnostic as well as therapeutic role in such cases. That is, if mature preovulatory eggs are obtained but fail to fertilize, this implies a fundamental problem and the couple can then turn to donor insemination as a last resort. On the other hand, if fertilization occurs, then there is at least the possibility of pregnancy from assisted reproduction. Such couples should be counseled that, since fertilization rates may be lower than in couples with normal semen parameters, fewer embryos may be produced and more cycles may be necessary to achieve a given expectation of pregnancy from IVF. If fertilization is documented and the fallopian tubes are normal, such couples are candidates for GIFT, which may be recommended by some centers in mild to moderate cases of male factor infertility after conventional treatment has failed.

When donor insemination has been performed for 12−18 cycles without a pregnancy, this may signify that a female infertility factor is present. Evaluation for possible female etiologies should be reviewed in a comprehensive manner and any positive findings should be appropriately treated. Couples in this circumstance who fail to achieve a pregnancy through donor insemination represent a special category of patients who have a particularly high pregnancy rate from assisted reproduction.

Cervical factor
Because the results of a postcoital test are highly dependent on the day of the cycle in which it is performed, an abnormal postcoital test should be repeated during the preovulatory phase. If the results are consistently abnormal despite good cervical mucus, information from an antisperm antibody test may provide a clue as to the reason for the abnormality.

There is controversy concerning the association between an abnormal postcoital test and infertility. Doubters believe that, in the absence of any other infertility factor, couples with an abnormal postcoital test are no different from those with unexplained infertility. Until there is a prospective, cohort comparison of fertile and infertile couples to resolve this question, however, a reasonable approach would be to try several cycles of IUI, as there are some studies to support such treatment in cervical factor. Failing this, the couple would become a candidate for assisted reproduction.

Uterine factor
All couples referred for assisted reproduction should have evaluation of the uterine cavity with a hysterosalpingogram or hysteroscopy. Unsuspected lesions in the uterine cavity that may interfere with implantation could thus be identified. Depending on the reproductive history, it may be recommended that some lesions, such as a uterine septum or intrauterine adhesions, be surgically treated prior to assisted reproduction. In other cases such as uterine malformation associated with *in utero* diethylstilbestrol exposure, there may not be any treatment available, but the couple could be counseled appropriately with respect to reduced pregnancy rates from assisted reproduction and an increased likelihood of premature labor if pregnancy does occur.

Unexplained infertility
Unexplained infertility occurs in 10−20% of all couples who undergo evaluation. Such a diagnosis is particularly frustrating for both patient and physician. Some reassurance can be found in the knowledge that such couples have a 35−50% chance of pregnancy after 2 years of follow-up and 60−70% after 3 years. As duration of infertility or age of the female partner increases, however, the likelihood of pregnancy from expectant management is reduced.

Records pertaining to previous infertility evaluations should be reviewed to determine whether any part of the evaluation has been overlooked, inappropriately performed, or misinterpreted. If the diagnosis of unexplained infertility is confirmed, several treatment options, including superovulation, IUI, or a combination of superovulation and IUI, might enhance the likelihood of pregnancy during a given treatment cycle among couples who have no absolute barrier to pregnancy and who might eventually conceive on their own. However, a large, randomized clinical trial investigating the relative efficacy of these various treatment options has not been performed. Pregnancy rates of approximately 10% per cycle can be expected.

If superovulation, with or without IUI, has not resulted in pregnancy after three to six cycles, the couple become a candidate for assisted reproduction. GIFT may offer a higher pregnancy rate than IVF, but may not provide important information on fertilization unless there are sufficient residual eggs beyond those used for gamete transfer. The decision as to which type of assisted reproduction technique will be used depends on the experience of the center to which the patient is referred.

REFERRAL FOR ASSISTED REPRODUCTION IN SPECIAL SITUATIONS

In some cases, conventional infertility treatment is not possible or appropriate. When both fallopian tubes are absent, IVF provides the only realistic chance for pregnancy. After documenting adequate sperm and ovulatory function, such patients can be referred directly for IVF. Direct referral for assisted reproduction is also indicated in cases of absent ovarian function, whether because of oophorectomy, gonadal dysgenesis, or, most commonly, premature ovarian failure. In such cases, ovarian hormones can be replaced to mimic a normal menstrual cycle, and donor oocytes can be used with the husband's sperm in the context of GIFT or IVF. Pregnancy rates are comparable to those of standard GIFT or IVF. Assisted reproduction with donor oocytes may also be considered in women with a poor response to ovarian stimulation. The sources and anonymity of donor oocytes vary from program to program and represent important questions that should be investigated by referring physicians and their patients.

When the sperm parameters are so poor that less than 1 million motile sperm are obtained from a standard swim-up procedure, direct referral for IVF should also be considered. The likelihood of pregnancy in such situations is remote, and IVF would provide important diagnostic information on whether fertilization can occur, in addition to offering the possibility of successful treatment. In the absence of fertilization despite several mature oocytes, the couple can be referred for IVF in conjunction with gamete micromanipulation. These techniques are still in the developmental stage, however, and have resulted in a relatively small number of live births.

CONCLUSIONS

During the past decade, assisted reproduction has progressed from a technology that was performed with limited success at only a few centers around the world to one in which most large cities (and some smaller ones) contain at least one program that consistently produces pregnancies. Thus, physicians with infertility practices should develop a working relationship with a successful program in their area. Appropriate evaluation prior to referral and ongoing communication between referring physicians and the assisted reproductive center foster consistent success.

REFERENCES

1 Medical Research International and the Society for Assisted Reproductive Technology. *In vitro* fertilization-embryo transfer results in the United States. 1990 results from the IVF-ET Registry. *Fertil Steril* 1992; 57: 15–24.
2 American Fertility Society Practice Committee. *Investigation of the Infertile Couple*. Birmingham: American Fertility Society, 1991.

Adhesion prevention after reproductive surgery

FAYEK SHAMMA & MICHAEL P. DIAMOND

Adhesions are noted to develop after most gynecologic and reproductive surgeries despite intricate efforts undertaken to prevent their development. The adhesions can represent reformation of previously lysed adhesions and/or *de novo* adhesion formation. The significance of adhesions lies in the potentially major impact that they have on the reproductive capacity of the female, presumably secondary to interference with tubal ovum pick-up. Additionally, adhesions can cause long-term morbidity in terms of pelvic pain and disturbance of gastrointestinal function.

This chapter will attempt to describe the pathogenesis of pelvic adhesions and evaluate the role of various surgical approaches and adjuvants used in their prevention.

PATHOGENESIS OF ADHESIONS

Adhesions result secondary to deviations from the normal healing processes. The mechanisms of normal peritoneal healing were first described by Rafferty in 1979. Peritoneal healing is thought to occur within a short period of time, probably 5 days. This repair occurs by metaplasia of the underlying mesothelium rather than from the defect margins, as occurs in skin.

As part of the response to peritoneal trauma, there is exudation of a proteinaceous serosanguineous fluid. In normal healing processes this fluid is resorbed as a consequence of peritoneal fibrinolytic activity, with the result that the mesothelial lining is healed without scarring. However, as a result of ischemia or foreign bodies (such as glove talc or suture material), there is a decrease in the natural endogenous fibrinolytic activity, namely plasminogen activator. Consequently, the serosanguineous coagulum is not absorbed, and is later invaded by polymorphonuclear and mononuclear cells followed by fibroblasts. The result is scar build-up, e.g., adhesion development. Individuals, however, demonstrate considerable variability pertaining to scar formation. The reasons for this interindividual variation are not known.

Ryan has shown the importance of whole blood in potentiating adhesion formation even in the absence of tissue trauma. He also showed that in the presence of ischemia, infection, and trauma, the extent of adhesion formation is increased. However, such an adverse role of whole blood could not be demonstrated by others.

SURGICAL APPROACHES IN ADHESION PREVENTION

Several surgical techniques exist, and are being used in an attempt to decrease adhesion formation. Of foremost importance is the application of microsurgical technique. Microsurgical principles include gentler tissue handling, meticulous hemostasis, use of magnification as appropriate, precise approximation of tissue planes, and careful attention to sterile techniques. The purpose of the above is to decrease tissue ischemia, avoid raw surfaces and eliminate intraperitoneal whole blood. The magnifying capacity, where appropriate, allows closer inspection and differentiation between normal and abnormal tissue, coagulation at bleeding points, and allows the use of smaller-caliber suture material (hence resulting in lesser foreign body reaction).

Keeping the tissue moist, to prevent tissue desiccation, is important. It has been suggested that this should be achieved with Ringer's lactate, being a more physiologic solution when compared with normal saline; however, data to support this hypothesis are not well delineated. Irrigation is better than sponging, the latter being sometimes associated with persistence of foreign materials, traumatization of the peritoneal surface, and therefore an increased potential for adhesion development. The use of an untraumatic technique cannot be overemphasized. This reduces tissue injury, abrasion, and bleeding. The use of microcoagulation (or its equivalent) is important in cutting and also in achieving hemostasis from small vessels. As mentioned above, the least reactive — namely small-caliber — sutures, should be utilized. Additionally longer operating times predispose to tissue drying and ischemia; thus, operating room time should be minimized whenever possible.

Despite advocating the use of microsurgical techniques, it is difficult to compare microsurgery with conventional macrosurgery, as patient selection plays a major role in any data analysis. Outcomes should not only be limited to pregnancy but also to the presence or absence of adhesions (since so many factors other than adhesions *per se* can impact upon pregnancy outcome). Most of the available studies favor the use of the microsurgical technique [2].

Recently, operative laparoscopy has been suggested as a replacement for laparotomy in managing many aspects of gynecologic and reproductive surgery, as it is associated with less patient morbidity, hospital time, hospital charges, and time to return to full activity. However, as far as adhesion reformation is concerned, gross differences between operative laparoscopy and laparotomy with the use of microsurgical techniques are not apparent from current studies.

In addition, the use of the laser has been touted for reconstructive and pelvic surgery. The laser's capacity in making precise incisions with little adjacent tissue injury and the suggestion of shorter operating time were thought to enhance its adhesion prevention properties. However, many of these claims of the benefits of lasers have not been substantiated, and a reduction in postoperative adhesion development was not noticed when compared with conventional microsurgical nonlaser surgery. On the other hand, at least one report describes an improvement and maintenance of tubal patency when the laser was used in comparison with conventional nonlaser surgery. A translation to an increased pregnancy rate is yet to be proven.

Despite the use of the above techniques, adhesions were noted to develop in 55–95% of patients undergoing reproductive pelvic surgery when second-look laparoscopy was utilized to evaluate the presence of the adhesions. There adhesions take the form of either *de novo* adhesion formation or adhesion reformation. Second-look laparoscopy has been utilized not only diagnostically, but also to lyse the newly

formed adhesions [3]. The ability of this technique to cause an ultimate decrease in adhesion formation has been suggested, but the ability to enhance the occurrence of pregnancy is yet to be proven.

ADJUVANTS AND MATERIALS USED IN ADHESION PREVENTION

Various adjuvants have been used as part of the armamentarium in adhesion prevention. Most have failed to be proven effective. Classes of surgical adjuvants used in an attempt to minimize the occurrence of postoperative adhesions include fibrinolytic agents, anticoagulants, antiinflammatory agents, antibiotics, and finally mechanical separation by the use of intraabdominal instillates, or endogenous or exogenous barriers.

Various antiinflammatory agents have been utilized. Corticosteroids have been given intravenously for 48 hours perioperatively. Their theoretic ability to decrease vascular permeability and enhance lysosomal stabilization has not been manifested in efficacious results in adhesion prevention in larger animals or humans.

Antihistamines, including intravenously administered promethazine, have been used extensively based on their ability to decrease vascular permeability and fibroblast proliferation. However, their solo use in adhesion prevention has not been examined. Prostaglandin inhibitors including ibuprofen have also been used. Most animal studies have failed to demonstrate their efficacy.

Anticoagulants including low-dose heparin (5 μg/ml) have been used as intraabdominal irrigants, but have not been demonstrated to be effective. In addition, high doses of heparin were also used systematically for adhesion prevention. The latter use, however, was associated with a high incidence of hemorrhagic complications and hence is not recommended.

Antibiotics are used perioperatively, and hence prophylactically to reduce the incidence of infection that could have detrimental effects on any type of reconstructive surgery. Vibramycin is being used more frequently because of the identification of *Chlamydia* as a potential pathogen in tuboperitoneal adhesive disease.

Various new adjuvants are being investigated, including calcium channel blockers and plasminogen activators [4]. The use of calcium channel blockers is based on a variety of characteristics, including their ability to decrease tissue ischemia, limit prostaglandin release, reduce adenosine triphosphate-dependent platelet aggregation, and reduce prostacyclin vasodilation. Their systemic use in hamsters was associated with a decrease in adhesion formation and absence of marked side-effects. Their use has not yet progressed to human studies.

The use of plasminogen activators in adhesion prevention is also still limited to animal studies [4]. The use is based on the activity of plasminogen activators to act locally at the site of the fibrin clots, activating plasminogen to plasmin and hence, accelerating fibrinolysis. Plasminogen activators also induce collagenases and other proteases. In animal studies the use of plasminogen activators in the form of a gel has resulted in a decrease in adhesion formation without significant side-effects.

Mechanical separation has been utilized in adhesion prevention in the form of either intraabdominal instillates or endogenous and exogenous barriers. The most widely used instillate is 32% dextran 70 (Hyskon). The mechanism of action is probably related to its hydroflotation action on raw surfaces, its siliconizing effect, and its mild fibrinolytic activity. Its use has been evaluated in various animal models and in a randomized human clinical trial. The use of 200 ml of Hyskon was noticed to cause limited ascites for approximately 7 days. It seems to be well tolerated for routine use as an antiadhesion adjuvant; side-effects are mostly limited to spontaneous leakage from the incision, bilateral labial swelling, abdominal bloating, weight gain, transient increase in liver function tests, and an increase in central venous pressure. The results of human clinical

trials, however, have been mixed. Two large human trials suggested a beneficial action, while two others were unable to substantiate this claim.

Barriers to adhesion formation have included various endogenous and exogenous materials. Some of the endogenous materials, including omental or peritoneal grafts, have been associated with a decrease in fibrinolytic activity and an increase rather than a decrease in adhesion formation. Hence, their use has been largely abandoned.

It has been noted that the use of oxidized regenerated cellulose (Surgicel), a hemostatic agent, is associated in some studies with a decrease in adhesion formation and an antibacterial effect against staphylococcus and *Pseudomonas*. Recently Surgicel has been modified to produce a new product with different porosity, oxidation, and density, TC-7. Interceed (TC-7) has been identified to be efficacious in animal models for adhesion prevention. An early human report has shown beneficial effects of TC-7 in reducing the incidence, extent, and severity of postsurgical pelvic adhesions [5]. Another barrier, Gore-Tex surgical membrane, has been shown to be effective in one of two animal studies and is undergoing clinical evaluation.

An algorithm below provides a decision making tree in adhesion reduction (Fig. 86.1).

CONCLUSIONS

Adhesions continue to be an important cause of infertility and pelvic pain. Adhesion prevention should be a major focus of every reproductive surgeon. The use of various adjuvants has limited efficacy and

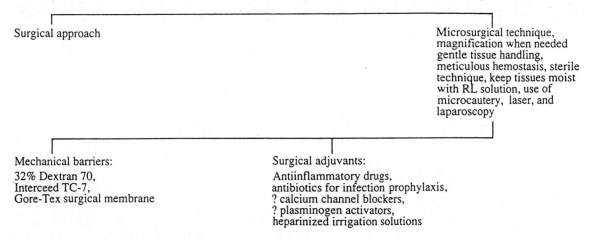

Fig. 86.1 Prevention of postoperative adhesions. RL, Ringer's lactate.

should complement, not substitute for, the use of microsurgical technique in adhesion prevention. Research should continue to evaluate and study the available techniques and adjuvants in appropriately designed clinical trials, and to identify new adjuvants and barrier materials.

REFERENCES

1 Diamond MP, DeCherney AH. Pathogenesis of adhesion formation/reformation: application to reproductive pelvic surgery. *Microsurgery* 1987; 8: 103−107.

2 Gomel V. The impact of microsurgery in gynecology. *Clin Obstet Gynecol* 1980; 23: 1031−1310.

3 Jansen RP. Early laparoscopy after pelvic operations to prevent adhesions: safety, efficacy. *Fertil Steril* 1988; 49: 26−31.

4 Meyer WR, DeCherney AH, Diamond MP. How good are the new adhesion-reduction adjuvants? *Contemp Obstet Gynecol* 1990; 35: 81−84.

5 Interceed Adhesion Study Group. Prevention of post-surgical adhesions by Interceed (TC-7), an absorbable adhesion prevention barrier: a prospective randomized multicenter clinical study. *Fertil Steril* 1989; 51: 933−938.

87

Gamete and embryo tubal transfer

PASQUALE PATRIZIO & RICARDO H. ASCH

INTRODUCTION

During the past decade, there has been an extraordinary growth and development of assisted reproductive technologies (ARTs) aimed to treat human infertility. In this chapter, two of these techniques are presented: gamete intrafallopian transfer (GIFT) and tubal embryo transfer (TET).

GIFT was pioneered in 1984 [1] and was first used as a form of therapy for unexplained or idiopathic infertility.

After preliminary work in monkeys [2], TET was reported in 1986 [3,4] as a successful treatment for infertility due to immunologic or severe male factor infertility.

The presence of at least one accessible, patent, and anatomically normal fallopian tube represents a necessary prerequisite shared in common by these two procedures.

In essence, GIFT involves the direct deposition of both gametes, preovulatory oocytes and washed sperm, in the ampullary portion of the fallopian tube(s), overcoming any potential defect in the gamete transport mechanisms, thus allowing fertilization to occur *in vivo*, as for a spontaneous human conception.

With TET, fertilization of the oocytes takes place *in vitro* (IVF), and the resulting fertilized eggs, or cleaving embryos, are replaced in the ampullary tract of the fallopian tube(s), as opposed to the uterus as in conventional IVF-embryo transfer (IVF-ET) [5]. The rationale behind transferring embryos in the tubes instead of the uterus relies on the hypothesis that the secretions of the fallopian tubes could have nurturing and embryotropic properties, and additionally, the arrival of the embryos in the uterine cavity is more physiologic and better timed.

The overall pregnancy rate for GIFT is around 40%, while TET is 32% per cycle, and 50% per transfer; both are higher than those generally reported for IVF and uterine embryo transfer [6].

INDICATIONS

The correct identification of the cause of the couple's infertility and the correct selection of one of the available ARTs, represent a key factor for successful treatment.

For the GIFT procedure the main indications are:
1 Unexplained or idiopathic infertility.
2 Mild to moderate endometriosis.
3 Periadnexal, not firm, adhesions.
4 Failure of previous cycles of artificial insemination either by husband (AIH), or by donor (AID).
5 Borderline male factor infertility.
6 Cervical factors (stenosis, hostile mucus, etc.)
7 Premature ovarian failure using donor oocytes.

For the TET procedure the indications are:
1 Severe male factor infertility.
2 Borderline male factor infertility with previous GIFT failure.
3 Immunologic infertility (presence of antisperm antibodies in the female).
4 Unexplained infertility with previous GIFT failure.
5 Premature ovarian failure with concomitant male factor.
6 Obstructive azoospermia when microsurgical epididymal sperm aspiration (MESA) is indicated.

Male factor infertility represents the most common indication for the TET procedure. By definition, male factor is present when semen analysis parameters do not fulfill the criteria set forth by the World Health Organization manual [7]. Our definition of severe male factor infertility, however, involves a sample that, after being prepared (wash and swim-up or other procedure), contains a total number of motile sperm less than 1.5 million, with less than 30% normal forms and with progression not greater than 2, on a scale of 1–4 [8].

Obstructive azoospermia, mainly due to congenital absence of the vas deferens, represents a recent indication for TET [9]. Other indications for this novel technique are represented by obstruction of the excurrent pathways due to inflammatory or infective causes (tuberculosis, or gonorrhea, etc.), or for failure of vasectomy reversal. In such cases, TET is part of a combined treatment involving the microsurgical aspiration of sperm from the epididymis, and their use for IVF of the oocytes. The resulting embryos are then transferred preferentially to the fallopian tube.

PREPARATION OF THE PATIENT

Intratubal gamete and embryo transfer have identical preliminary steps for the preparation of the female partner. The starting point is represented by the controlled ovarian hyperstimulation phase, where the main goal is to achieve multiple follicular development by using a combined sequence of clomiphene citrate (CC), human menopausal gonadotropin (hMG), follicle-stimulating hormone (FSH), and gonadotropin-releasing hormone (GnRH) analog. Additionally, another hormone, human chorionic gonadotropin (hCG) is used to mimic the luteinizing hormone (LH) preovulatory peak.

These drugs are arranged in different combinations or protocols.

The three protocols mostly used in our center are:
1 CC administered from day 3 to 7 of the menstrual cycle; hMG added from day 5 on, and hCG 36 hours before oocyte retrieval.
2 GnRH analog is started in the last 4–5 days of the luteal phase of the previous menstrual cycle, followed by hMG and FSH, from day 2 to 4, and then only hMG, until the time of hCG administration.
3 Same as above, the only difference being that GnRH analog is started in the follicular phase of the menstrual cycle (day 1).

While the action of FSH and hMG is stimulatory for the induction of multiple follicular growth, that of the GnRH analog, after an initial short period of a stimulatory effect on the pituitary enhancing the release of the storage of FSH and hMG, is of inhibition (down-regulation-desensitization), thus preventing the risk of a spontaneous premature LH surge.

The follicular development is monitored by serial vaginal ultrasounds and by serum estradiol radio-immunoassays.

When two or three follicles have a mean diameter of at least 18 mm, and correspondingly, the level of estradiol is greater than 250 pg/ml for each follicle, then hCG is administered. Oocyte retrieval is then scheduled 34–36 hours from the time of hCG injection. Almost all the retrievals are now performed using a transvaginal ultrasound approach (Fig. 87.1); however, there are some cases, for example, ovaries dislodged high in the pelvis, where the best choice for the aspiration is still by laparoscopy.

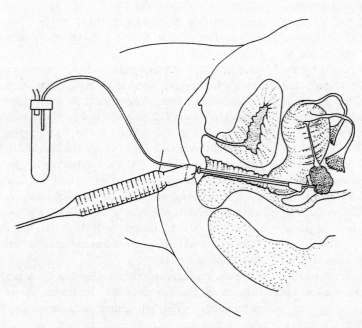

Fig. 87.1 Oocyte retrieval.

ROLE OF THE LABORATORY

The retrieved oocytes are identified and graded for maturity in the laboratory adjacent to the operating room. The most mature, preovulatory ones are those featuring a radiating cumulus–corona complex and a visible polar body. For the purpose of GIFT, it is advisable to have at least three to four mature oocytes that will be transferred to the fallopian tubes. If, instead, the plan is TET, then the oocytes will be inseminated *in vitro* according to classical IVF techniques.

The preparation of the sperm for GIFT is carried out 2 hours before the oocyte retrieval. Basically, the sperm sample is washed with culture medium, centrifuged, and the resulting pellet is overlaid with fresh medium in order to allow the most motile sperm to swim up from the pellet in a time frame of 30–45 min. For GIFT in nonmale factor, 100 000–300 000 motile sperm per fallopian tube are sufficient for the transfer; in cases of borderline male factor it is preferable to increase the number of sperm to 500 000 or more per tube. At the time of transfer, oocytes and sperm are loaded in a special catheter, with bubbles of air separating the two sets of gametes.

For TET, fertilization takes place *in vitro* and the resulting embryos, preferentially two to four of good quality, are also transferred in the ampullary portion of the fallopian tube (Fig. 87.2). However, the transfer can be performed either at the pronuclear stage, 15–20 hours after insemination, or at the two to four cell stage, which is 40–48 hours postinsemination.

There are currently three possible routes for the transfer: by laparoscopy, by minilaparotomy, or by ultrasound-guided catheterization of the fallopian tubes through a nonstenotic cervix. The transfer by laparoscopy requires three entry sites. Once the fallopian tube is stabilized and correctly positioned by using holding forceps, the catheter, loaded with gametes or embryos, is then inserted approximately 3 cm in the ampullary portion of the tube(s) and the contents carefully expelled. Transfer by minilaparotomy (a 4 cm transverse incision) allows direct manipulation and access to the fallopian tubes. Transcervical nonsurgical transfer uses a specially designed catheter that under transvaginal ultrasound guidance is directed towards the tubal ostium and is inserted 4–5 cm into the distal isthmic region of the fallopian tube.

The last phase of the procedure is that of luteal support. Essentially, this consists of administration of progesterone, starting 2 days after the GIFT procedure and 1 day after TET. If pregnancy ensues, then progesterone is continued for another 8 weeks.

RESULTS

The overall pregnancy rate per GIFT cycle is around 40%, while TET is 32% and 50% respectively for egg retrieval and for transfer. Table 87.1 summarizes the results of these two techniques according to the etiology of infertility. It is apparent that the main indications for GIFT, unexplained infertility or mild to moderate endometriosis, have the highest pregnancy rate (36%), while the male factor infertility treated by GIFT has a lower success rate (17%). For these cases, TET represents the treatment of choice, yielding a pregnancy rate of 30% per cycle and 51%

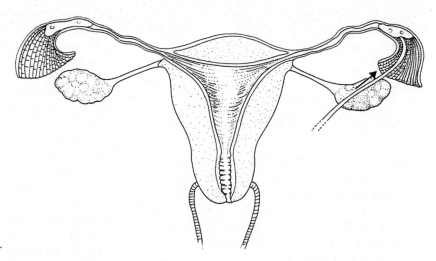

Fig. 87.2 Tubal embryo transfer.

Table 87.1 Results of gamete intrafallopian transfer (GIFT) and tubal embryo transfer (TET) by etiology

Etiology	GIFT		TET		A%*	B%†
	Cases	Pregnancy (%)	Cases	Pregnancy		
Unexplained	84	30 (36)	27	7	26	35
Male Factor	40	11 (17)	104	31	30	51
Endometriosis	30	11 (37)				
Failed AID	6	2 (33)	9	5	55	62
POF	15	8 (53)	5	4	80	80
Cervical factor	4	2 (50)				
Total	179	64 (36)	145	47	32	50

* Pregnancy rate/cycle.
† Pregnancy rate/transfer.
AID, artificial insemination by donor; POF, premature ovarian failure.

Table 87.2 Results of tubal embryo transfer (TET) and gamete intrafallopian transfer (GIFT) in male factor infertility

	TET	GIFT
Follicular aspiration	104	50
Transfers	61	50
Pregnancies	31	8
Pregnancies/aspiration	30%*	16%*
Pregnancy rates/Transfers	51%†	16%†

* Not significant.
† P < 0.001.

Table 87.3 Comparison of *in vitro* fertilization (IVF) and tubal embryo transfer (TET)

	IVF	TET
Transfers	93	94
Embryos transferred	401	354
Embryo/transfer	4	3.7
Pregnancy	21*	47*
Gestational sacs	30	66
Implantation rate†	7%*	19%*

* Difference statistically significant (P < 0.001).
† Implantation rate = gestational sacs/embryos transferred.

per transfer (Table 87.2). Compared to overall IVF (Table 87.3), TET shows a much higher pregnancy and implantation rate, both statistically significant.

The abortion rate after GIFT is 20% and it is the same for TET. However, the abortion rate seems to be increased for both procedures when a patient's age is over 40 years.

The risk of ectopic pregnancy is about 3–4%, while the incidence of multiple pregnancy is approximately 25–28% when up to four oocytes or four embryos are transferred.

CONCLUSIONS AND FUTURE

It is clearly demonstrated and recognized worldwide that cases of nontubal infertility benefit from gamete or embryo transfer to the fallopian tubes. The higher pregnancy rates with GIFT for unexplained infertility or mild endometriosis could be related to the fact that direct deposition of both gametes in the ampullary portion of the tube might overcome mechanical defects in the transport mechanism of the female genital tract.

TET, on the other hand, represents the first choice of treatment for severe male factor infertility. With TET in such cases, it is possible to document fertilization, and to decide if the numbers and the quality of the resulting embryos warrant a surgical transfer procedure. The transfer of embryos in the fallopian tube(s) is associated with a higher implantation rate, compared to IVF and uterine transfer for the same etiology. We can theorize that the tubal environment is superior to that of the uterus for preimplantation embryos, or that the embryos arrive in the uterus at a more appropriate stage of development; additionally, the mechanical problems and trauma associated with transcervical transfers are avoided.

A decision making plan is detailed that should facilitate the diagnostic work-up for infertile couples, and indicate which of the ARTs are the more appropriate for each individual case (Fig. 87.3).

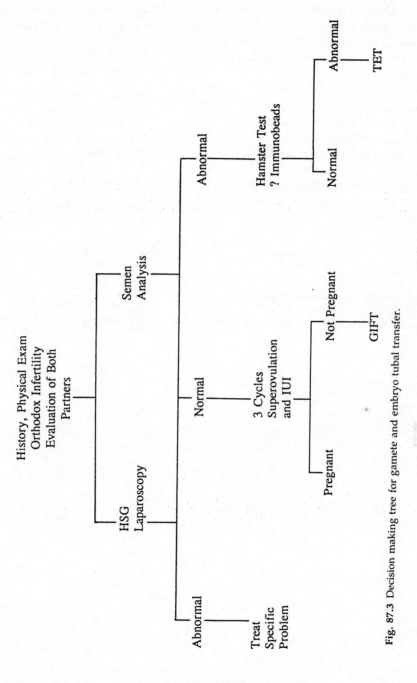

Fig. 87.3 Decision making tree for gamete and embryo tubal transfer.

There are several new research lines in human reproductive technology that are growing rapidly, directed towards a better refinement of the nonsurgical intratubal gamete or embryo transfer through the cervix, by using an ultrasound-guided catheter, or a flexible hysteroscope, or by selective tubal cannulization via falloposcopy. Pregnancies have been confirmed with the use of an ultrasound-guided transfer [10].

Another new area of research involves the use of a micromanipulator to perform zona pellucida dissection, or microinjection of sperm into the perivitelline space of the oocytes in order to obtain fertilization in extreme cases of male factor infertility.

In the very near future, one can easily predict that these new technologies will be incorporated in the list of routine procedures available for the treatment of infertile couples.

REFERENCES

1 Asch RH, Ellsworth LR, Balmaceda JP, Wong PC. Pregnancy following translaparoscopic gamete intrafallopian transfer (GIFT). *Lancet* 1984; 2: 1034.

2 Balmaceda JP, Pool TB, Arana JB, Heitman TS. Successful *in vitro* fertilization and embryo transfer in cynomolgus monkeys. *Fertil Steril* 1984; 42: 79.

3 DeVroey P, Braermans P, Smitz J. Pregnancy after translaparoscopic zygote intrafallopian transfer in a patient with sperm antibodies. *Lancet* 1986; 1: 1329.

4 Yovich JL, Blackledge DG, Richardson PA, Matson PL, Turner JR, Draper R. Pregnancies following pronuclear stage tubal transfer. *Fertil Steril* 1984; 48: 851.

5 Edwards RG, Steptoe PC. Current status of *in vitro* fertilization and implantation of human embryos. *Lancet* 1983; 2: 1265.

6 Johnston I, McBain J, Baker G, DuPlessis Y, Odawara Y: *In vitro* fertilization and embryo transfer. In: Asch RH, Balmaceda JP, Johnston I, eds. *Gamete Physiology*. Norwell: Serono Symposia, 1990: 273.

7 World Health Organization. *Laboratory Manual for the Examination of Human Semen and Sperm Cervical Mucus Interaction*. Singapore: Press Concern, 1980.

8 Patrizio P, Asch RH. Intratubal gamete and embryo transfer in male infertility. In: Rajfer J, ed. *Common Problems in Infertility and Impotence*. Chicago: Year Book, 1990: 137.

9 Silber S, Ord T, Balmaceda JP, Patrizio P, Asch RH. Congenital absence of the vas deferens: studies on the fertilizing capacity of human epididymal sperm. *N Engl J Med* 1990; 323: 1788–1792.

10 Guidetti R, Balmaceda JP, Ord T, Asch RH. Non surgical tubal embryo transfer *Hum Reprod* 1990; 5: 221.

In vitro fertilization

DAVID R. MELDRUM

In the dozen years since the first *in vitro* fertilization (IVF) birth, this procedure has progressively developed from one which was rarely successful, to where the most successful clinics are achieving a delivery in one-quarter to one third of egg retrievals. It is estimated that over 200 clinics provide this service in the USA alone.

One of the most striking features of this procedure continues to be the wide variation of success rates, due to the complex nature of the technique and consequently the numerous variables which may impact on success. Unfortunately, only a few determinants of success are agreed upon, resulting in a myriad of variations in the small but probably crucial details making up the procedure.

This chapter will review the various components of the IVF procedure, emphasizing the variations of technique, but also pointing out evidence supporting certain preferred methods. Finally, some guidelines will be given to aid the practitioner in choosing an appropriate IVF program for patient referrals.

PATIENT SELECTION AND PREPARATION

The most common indication has been for women with tubal disease after failed surgery, or when IVF is felt to be a better alternative. However, it is now recognized that IVF is an effective treatment for women with endometriosis, unexplained infertility, sperm antibodies, male factor, and anovulation. Essentially, every infertile couple can benefit from IVF when other treatments fail, unless there are problems with the uterus or implantation, or unless the semen is at a very low level.

Age

IVF success decreases progressively with age. In the 1988 US Registry results [1], the delivery rate per retrieval was 4% in women over age 40, compared with 12% overall. There is accumulating evidence that within the group over 40, women with a normal day 3 serum level of follicle-stimulating hormone (FSH) will have a better prognosis, whereas in those with a distinctly elevated FSH (over 20 mIU/ml), IVF is probably not worthwhile. In addition some younger women needing IVF have a high day 3 FSH, indicating ovarian dysfunction and a reduced prognosis.

Endometriosis

Severe or extensive endometriosis is associated with a markedly reduced chance of success [2]. IVF following adequate treatment carries a normal prognosis. Furthermore, since pregnancy is unlikely to eradicate extensive disease, treatment is likely to be required at some point. We have therefore always advised full thereapy before embarking on IVF. If a gonadotropin-releasing homone agonist (GnRHa) is used, it is possible to move directly into stimulation with human menopausal gonadotropins (hMG).

Chlamydia and *ureaplasma*

These sexually transmitted organisms are not uncommon in the IVF population and may interfere with pregnancy or lead to fetal loss. Multiple studies have shown lower rates of IVF success in women with serologic evidence of *Chlamydia*, presumably through active disease. Other studies have shown that endometrial cultures can be positive with negative cervical cultures. We currently treat all IVF couples with a 10-day course of doxycycline as a routine before starting IVF.

Uterine abnormalities

The uterine cavity may be assessed by either hysterosalpingogram or hysteroscopy. Significant defects should be corrected before IVF. Women with diethylstilbestrol exposure should persist with methods short of IVF for as long as possible to limit the risk of multiple pregnancy and to establish success with a treatment which is more readily repeatable if the pregnancy is not carried to viability.

Male factor

Various findings may signal the increased chance of fertilization failure: density under 5 million/ml, motility under 20%, strict morphology under 5%, lack of zona-free hamster egg penetration, or swim-up retrieval of fewer than 1.5 million sperm. Evidence is accumulating that sperm capacitation can be improved with a variety of techniques: test-yolk buffer, Percoll, follicular fluid. If failure of fertilization has occurred in a previous cycle, fertilization can be improved by removing the cumulus and corona with hyaluronidase or by micromanipulation (partial zona dissection or subzonal insertion of sperm). If antisperm antibodies are detected, fertilization will generally be normal if enough unbound sperm are added, which can be calculated on the immunobead test results.

OVARIAN STIMULATION

Currently the most common regimen involves the use of GnRHa/hMG given as a long protocol [3]. The GnRHa is started either in the midluteal or very early follicular phase. The latter is more problematic regarding the formation of follicle cysts, even if the GnRHa is given more than once daily. Following ovarian suppression, hMG is then begun. GnRHa and hMG have also been given at approximately the same time in the early follicular phase. This regimen takes advantage of the agonist rise of gonadotropins (flare-up) and requires less time and hMG. Success with these short protocols appears to be lower, perhaps due in part to stimulation of progesterone, which may inhibit endometrial development. Use of GnRHa improves ovarian response and reduces the number of cycles cancelled (generally to about 10%) due to poor response or a premature luteinizing hormone (LH) surge. Its principal advantage may be the avoidance of premature luteinization by keeping LH levels low late in follicular maturation. We have found that even with GnRHa suppression of LH, prognosis is best if the stimulation is not carried too long. Excessive luteinization of the leading follicles can still occur and can compromise the outcome.

Alternative means of stimulation are clomiphene citrate (CC) combined with hMG, or hMG alone. With both, the rates of cycle cancellation can be as high as 30% or more. Many pieces of information suggest the CC can inhibit endometrial development. In some CC/hMG cycles there may be delayed or absent secretory change at the time of embryo transfer, and endometrial progesterone receptors are significantly lower than with normal cycles. In some CC/hMG cycles, the endometrial thickness is reduced based on vaginal ultrasound, with a lower prognosis in those women. Although CC/hMG cycles are less costly, the lower success rate and higher cancellation rate have led to its gradual disappearance as a component of IVF stimulations.

Stimulation can rarely lead to hospitalization for hyperstimulation (about 0.3% of cycles). Thorough aspiration of all follicles seems to limit this risk. We have also kept the starting hMG dose at a moderate level and the level of estradiol (E_2) on the day of hCG under 3500 pg/ml. Administration of hCG 1–2 days early in very high responders will decrease the number of follicles capable of responding to hCG, but has not compromised the success rate. The lower rate of fertilization may be counterbalanced by limiting the inhibiting effect of E_2 on the endometrium.

Stimulation is monitored by E_2 and vaginal ultrasound scanning to assess maturity of developing follicles, and serum progesterone to indicate premature luteinization. All indices are indirect indications of the status of egg maturity. The proper timing of human chorionic gonadotropin (hCG) can be refined as experience is gained with a particular protocol and is probably one of the more important aspects influencing results. When the proper time is reached, an injection of hCG is given to induce resumption of meiosis to prepare the oocyte for fertilization.

OOCYTE RETRIEVAL

Over the last 3 years there has been an almost complete shift from laparoscopic to transvaginal ultrasound-directed follicle aspiration. This avoids incisions and in most individuals, the aspiration can be done under intravenous sedation. With careful monitoring by a pulse oximeter, this procedure can be done in an office setting. Because of the rare occurrence of intra-abdominal bleeding, it is ideally carried out with very close access to an operating room. The procedure is usually scheduled 34–36 hours after hCG. Many programs administer a prophylactic antibiotic to limit the risk of ovarian infection. We prefer to avoid the use of local lidocaine, which has embryotoxicity. If anesthesia is required, 1.5% enfluorane, oxygen, and air or a regional block appear to be the most free of toxic effects on the oocyte. Nitrous oxide combined with isofluorane is the most toxic and less so combined with narcotic.

Rare complications of egg retrieval are bleeding with remote chance of laparotomy, infection, and a very remote chance of bowel injury. Discomfort is usually easily tolerated, with women often stating it is less than starting an intravenous line, having a hysterosalpingogram, or even less than menstrual cramps.

LABORATORY

Probably the single most important variable in IVF success is the embryo laboratory. Conditions must approach as closely as possible those in the body.

Embryotoxicity

Oocytes and embryos are extremely sensitive cells. Everything contacting them must be as free as possible from any substance injurious to their normal function. Various bioassays are used to screen for embryotoxicity. In order of sensitivity (high to low): hamster sperm motility or zona-free two-cell mouse embryos; one-cell mouse embryos', two-cell mouse embryos, and human sperm motility. Examples of potential sources of embryotoxicity are: water, media solutes, purified proteins, some maternal or fetal cord sera, some culture ware, incubator gases, new incubators, aspirating needles (particularly reused), coupling gels, Foley catheters, some streptomycin preparations, lidocaine, Betadine, cul-de-sac fluid, fluorescent light (and light in general), glove powder, some plastic syringes, and rubber-topped blood collection tubes. Endotoxin, which can be present in water from even minor bacterial growth, is embryotoxic but is not picked up by routine mouse embryo culture. Water sources should be tested for this with a simple kit. Osmolarity of media should be 280–285 mosmol/kg; pH should be 7.35–7.45. Media should contain at least 5 mmol potassium.

Environmental

Embryo lab air should be HEPA-filtered to remove bacteria and particles which could be embryotoxic. Mixing of media and all manipulation of gametes and embryos should take place in a low level of incandescent light. Incubator gases should be checked by mouse embryo culture before human use. Incubator temperature should be kept at 37.0–37.5°C and checked regularly with a highly accurate thermometer. Incubator carbon dioxide level (4.5–5.5%) should be checked regularly by some independent method and by assuring that media pH is appropriate. Openings of the incubator should be kept to an absolute minimum. Handling of oocytes or embryos outside of the incubator must be very rapid or done in a temperature- and carbon dioxide-controlled atmosphere. Other alternatives are to use an oil overlay technique to limit carbon dioxide loss or to transfer to media designed to maintain proper pH at ambient conditions.

INSEMINATION

Following retrieval of the eggs, generally 5–8 hours is allowed in culture medium before insemination. During this time, the percentage of eggs reaching metaphase II increases. This can be detected by examination for a polar body under the inverted phase-contrast microscope and some laboratories inseminate earlier based on this finding. However, cytoplasmic maturation is also occurring and cannot be confirmed. We prefer to avoid disturbing the oocytes and to allow 7–8 hours for these events to occur.

The most common method of sperm preparation has been a double-wash and swim-up. This does not retrieve a very high percentage of the motile sperm and may not capacitate the sperm adequately in some men. Percoll, a graded-density centrifugation, harvests a much higher percentage. In some cases, Percoll, test-yolk buffer (a sperm-freezing medium), or follicular fluid from a mature follicle will aid capacitation. In men who have failed to fertilize, removal of the cumulus and corona with hyaluronidase will improve fertilization. In some cases, an opening is made in the zona by micromanipulation (partial zona dissection), or sperm may be inserted under the zona with a micropipette.

EMBRYO TRANSFER

The uterine cavity is a potential space between two thickened walls of endometrium, presumably with a very low capacity. Most successful IVF programs transfer the embryos in less than 50 µl. A wide variety of transfer catheters is used. The critical factor is probably that the transfer be gentle and atraumatic, regardless of the catheter used. Any minor irritation could cause cramping and any blood or serum could displace the embryos [4]. After transfer a variable period of rest is suggested, to promote retention of the embryos.

LUTEAL-PHASE SUPPORT

The higher levels of E_2 accompanying ovarian stimulation may inhibit implantation, as demonstrated in animal models. According to those same studies, supplementary progesterone helps to overcome this effect. A number of reports have shown that higher early luteal progesterone levels are associated with a greater chance of pregnancy but this could simply be a reflection of better follicle development. The only prospective randomized studies which have shown a higher pregnancy rate with luteal support were with hCG-supplemented cycles with a long GnRHa/hMG protocol [5]. Whether progesterone or hCG is better or whether they are additive is not known.

A study of serial hCG levels and E_2 and progesterone levels in the late luteal phase has revealed that in some cases there is a normal early rise of hCG is association with inadequate levels of progesterone, followed by a subsequent fall-off of hCG. The authors suggested that some IVF pregnancies may be lost due to an inadequate duration of the luteal phase and that a follow-up dose of hCG may rescue these otherwise normal implantations.

The mean rate of spontaneous abortion has been about 25% with IVF pregnancies. This increase of 5–10% over the normal rate may be due to greater ascertainment because of close observation, or due to multiple implantation, or in some cases, luteal insufficiency.

Ectopic pregnancy occurs in about 5% of IVF pregnancies, due to flux of fluids following transfer [1]. They occur almost entirely in women with abnormal tubes and can occur in tubes which are densely adherent and would otherwise not ever develop an ectopic. Even if an intrauterine pregnancy is present, a thorough assessment of the adnexa should be done with the vaginal ultrasound, since a coexisting ectopic is not rare. If there is no intrauterine sac and β-hCG levels are stable or rising, an ectopic pregnancy must be excluded. If curettage shows no villae or ultrasound is conclusive for an adnexal sac, methotrexate may be ideal for a simple solution. This is particularly true if the adnexae are known to be densely adherent, since laparoscopic management may not be possible.

CHOOSING AN IVF PROGRAM FOR REFERRAL

In March of 1989 a Congressional committee report was published of hearings into consumer concerns regarding IVF clinics, due to marked variability of results and the feeling that patients were not receiving full disclosure of actual rates of success in individual clinics. As a result, a survey was carried out and published giving data on cycles done in 1987 and 1988. A copy of the report can be obtained by writing to the Subcommittee on Regulation, Business Opportunities and Energy, Room B363 RHOB, Washington, DC, 20515. These rates are also reprinted in a lay book on assisted reproductive technology [6]. Discounting rates calculated on very small numbers, the delivery rates for 1987 varied from 0 to 25%. The 1988 data are incomplete since the data were due in December and also suffer from major errors due to ambiguity in the questionnaire. As a result, the 1988 delivery rates for some programs are overestimated. Data for 1989 and 1990 are available for programs which are members of the Society for Assisted Reproductive Technology (SART). These results may be obtained from the American Fertility Society, 2140 Eleventh Ave South, Suite 200, Birmingham, AL 35205–2800.

In general all well-qualified programs should be members of SART. Membership assures compliance with minimum standards regarding personnel and a minimum level of success is required for membership. All SART members are required to submit data for release to the public.

Travel may be very worthwhile for patients to have care at one of the more established and highly successful clinics, although in general it is best not to add the difficulties of travel to an already arduous procedure.

It is best to refer patients to a clinic which gives individual attention and personalized care. IVF is an emotion-charged procedure and requires personal attention to those aspects. A psychologist should be available to patients having difficulty coping with the inherent stresses involved in IVF. Patients who have already gone through a particular program can best bear witness to these important aspects of IVF care.

Cost is generally $6000–10 000 per cycle including medications. Although cost is a consideration, the success rate is an overriding consideration. The tighter quality control and individual care which produce good results do make the procedure more costly.

CONCLUSIONS

The referring physician has a responsibility in referring patients for IVF to be familiar with results of various clinics or to direct the patient to appropriate resources described above. With objective information, the patient can then make a logical decision on the provider for this vital service.

REFERENCES

1 *In vitro* fertilization — embryo transfer in the United States: 1988 results from the IVF-ET Registry. *Fertil Steril* 1990; 53: 13.

2 Chillik CF, Acosta AA, Garcia JE *et al*. The role of *in vitro* fertilization in infertile patients with endometriosis. *Fertil Steril* 1985; 44: 56.

3 Meldrum DR, Wisot A, Hamilton F, Gutlay AL, Kempton W, Huynh D. Routine pituitary suppression with leuprolide before ovarian stimulation for oocyte retrieval. *Fertil Steril* 1989; 51: 455.

4 Englert Y, Puissant F, Camus M, Van Hoek J, Leroy F. Clinical study on embryo transfer after human *in vitro* fertilization. *J In Vitro Fert Embryo Transf* 1986; 3: 243.

5 Smith EM, Anthony FW, Gadd SC, Masson GM. Trial of support treatment with human chorionic gonadotropin in the luteal phase after treatment with buserelin and human menopausal gonadotropin in women taking part in an *in vitro* fertilisation programme. *Br Med J* 1989; 298: 1483.

6 Wisot A, Meldrum DR. *New Options for Fertility: A Guide to in vitro Fertilization and other Assisted Reproduction Methods*. New York: Pharos Books, 1990.

Part IX
Diagnosis and treatment of the male

Hypogonadotropic hypogonadism in men

DANIEL I. SPRATT

INTRODUCTION

Hypogonadotropic hypogonadism in men refers to decreased testosterone secretion by the testes secondary to hypothalamic or pituitary dysfunction. This disorder most frequently presents as delayed puberty in boys or as decreased libido and/or potency in men, but may occasionally present as infertility or gynecomastia. The principal laboratory finding is a low testosterone level (usually <2 ng/ml or 200 ng/dl) accompanied by serum luteinizing hormone (LH) and follicle-stimulating hormone (FSH) levels below or within the normal range (in contrast to primary hypogonadism in which LH and FSH levels are elevated). Other situations may be confused with hypogonadotropism. In elderly men, a decline in serum testosterone levels normally occurs without a rise in gonadotropins above the normal range. In addition, transient suppression of LH, FSH, and testosterone frequently occurs in serious illnesses.

Hypogonadotropic hypogonadism is important to recognize because it is usually easily treatable and because it may be a sign of a hypothalamic or pituitary tumor. However, in our culture, self-consciousness in the patient and, at times, the physician regarding sexual issues often leads to overlooked diagnoses. The purposes of this chapter are to: (1) outline the normal physiology of the male reproductive axis as a background to evaluation of abnormalities; (2) present the clinical situations in which hypogonadotropic hypogonadism should be suspected; and (3) provide schemes for evaluation and options for therapy.

NORMAL PHYSIOLOGY

The reproductive axis is driven by small pulses of gonadotropin-releasing hormone (GnRH) secreted from the hypothalamus at approximately 2-hour intervals in men [1]. Pulsatile GnRH stimulation of the anterior pituitary is necessary for normal secretion of LH and FSH. LH in turn stimulates the Leydig cells of the testes to synthesize and secrete testosterone while FSH, with testosterone, stimulates sperm production.

From early infancy until puberty, the reproductive axis remains essentially quiescent. Male puberty is normally initiated between the ages of 9 and 13 or 14 by increased hypothalamic secretion of GnRH. The consequent increases in circulating FSH and LH levels stimulate increases in testicular size and serum testosterone levels, resulting in the appearance of secondary sexual characteristics. In early puberty, increases in gonadotropin and testosterone secretion occur at night and early morning, so that serum levels obtained in the afternoon may appear prepubertal. Following completion of puberty, normal serum testosterone levels are usually between about 3 and 11 ng/ml (300 and 1100 ng/dl). However, in healthy men, serum testosterone levels may briefly fall below the normal range during the day [1]. At about age 50, serum free testosterone levels normally begin to decline, followed by a decline in serum total testosterone levels beginning at about age 60–70 [2].

If the hypothalamus and pituitary are functioning normally, the pituitary senses circulating levels of testosterone through negative feedback (Fig. 89.1). Prolonged decreases in serum testosterone levels below normal (>2 days) result in rises of serum FSH and LH levels above the normal range. Thus, serum gonadotropin levels within or below the normal range in the presence of consistently low serum testosterone levels suggest hypothalamic or pituitary dysfunction.

ABSENT OR DELAYED PUBERTY

Delayed puberty refers to a delay in activation of the hypothalamic–pituitary–testicular axis until after the age of 13 or 14. Absent puberty results from hypothalamic–pituitary damage (e.g., tumor, radiation therapy, etc.) or from failure of the GnRH

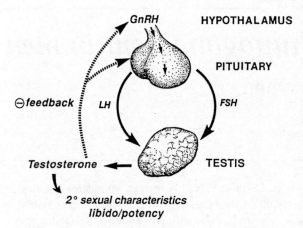

Fig. 89.1 Circulating levels of testosterone exert negative feedback through the hypothalamus and pituitary.

neurons in the hypothalamus to develop properly so that GnRH is never secreted in sufficient amounts to initiate puberty [3]. The latter developmental deficiency of GnRH is referred to as idiopathic hypogonadotropic hypogonadism (IHH), or, if anosmia is also present, Kallmann's syndrome. "Fertile eunuch" syndrome refers to a variant of IHH with normal serum FSH levels (stimulating testicular growth) but low LH levels (resulting in low serum testosterone and eunuchoid features). Table 89.1 lists the differential diagnosis of delayed puberty.

When puberty has not begun by age 13 or 14, several signs and symptoms may suggest potential etiologies. Anosmia or hyposmia suggests the diagnosis of Kallmann's syndrome, while unusual headaches, visual changes, or signs and symptoms of

Table 89.1 Differential diagnosis: delayed puberty

"Constitutional" delay of puberty

Idiopathic hypogonadotropism
  Intact sense of smell (IHH)
  Anosmia/hyposmia (Kallmann's syndrome)
  Predominant LH deficiency ("fertile eunuch" syndrome)

Hypothalamic or pituitary tumor

Other
  Nutritional (malnutrition, bulimia, anorexia, etc.)
  Hyperprolactinemia (rare in children)
  Rare genetic syndromes (e.g., Prader–Labhart–Willi)

IHH, idiopathic hypogonadotropic hypogonadism; LH, luteinizing hormone.

other pituitary dysfunction suggest hypothalamic–pituitary disease. These signs and symptoms include nocturia, decreased growth velocity, hypothyroidism, and hypoadrenalism. On the other hand, the earliest signs of puberty (testicular enlargement, pubertal hair, or breast budding) or a family history of late puberty suggest delayed puberty. Otherwise, no tests have been demonstrated to distinguish reliably between delayed puberty and IHH. Diagnosis of IHH is often delayed by several years due to the patients' self-consciousness regarding lack of sexual development. Patients may present in their 20s during routine physical examination or after prompting from relatives or friends who have noted the lack of secondary sexual characteristics (e.g., beard growth, voice change).

Initial evaluation of the boy with delayed puberty should consist of a history regarding headaches, sense of smell, other symptoms of hypothalamic–pituitary dysfunction, and any delayed puberty in close relatives. A physical examination should include accurate sizing of testes, Tanner staging of pubic hair development, and examination for pubertal gynecomastia. If there is no reason to suspect hypothalamic–pituitary disease and no physical evidence of early puberty, 8 a.m. levels of LH, FSH, and testosterone should be obtained. In the early stages of puberty, an early morning rise in serum testosterone with a predominant rise in FSH compared to LH is evident. Even with a thorough evaluation, it may not be possible to determine if the boy has delayed puberty or IHH. Computed tomography (CT) or magnetic resonance imaging (MRI) of the hypothalamic–pituitary region should be undertaken if hypothalamic–pituitary tumors are suspected by signs or symptoms or if puberty is delayed past the age of 16.

After serious etiologies have been reasonably ruled out, the initial treatment of delayed puberty or IHH is the same. Its primary goal is initiation of secondary sexual development to ease socialization. The contribution to adult bone density is currently being evaluated. Testosterone enanthate or cypionate is injected at a dose of 50–100 mg i.m. at 4–8-week intervals. This dose has been demonstrated to advance sexual development without accelerating bone age so that ultimate adult height may be preserved [4]. If delayed puberty is suspected, therapy is interrupted every 3–6 months to determine, by physical examination and 8 a.m. serum testosterone level, if spontaneous puberty has begun.

Table 89.2 Differential diagnosis: postpubertal onset of hypogonadism.

Hypothalamic or pituitary tumor*

Damage from CNS surgery or radiation*

Adult-onset IHH

Infiltrative
  Hemachromatosis (pituitary)
  Sarcoidosis, histiocytosis X (hypothalamus)*

Other
  Nutritional
  Renal or hepatic failure
  Major illness (transient)
  Cranial trauma*
  Poorly controlled diabetes

---

* May involve other endocrine deficiencies.
CNS, central nervous system; IHH, idiopathic hypogonadotropic hypogonadism.

POSTPUBERTAL HYPOGONADOTROPIC HYPOGONADISM

Hypogonadism occurring after the completion of puberty usually presents as decreased libido and/or potency. As mentioned above, it may occasionally present as gynecomastia or infertility. Evaluation of impotency and decreased libido must consider other causes including drugs and neurologic, vascular, and psychologic causes. The persistence of spontaneous early morning erections often suggests a nonorganic or psychologic cause. Because sexual symptoms are often concealed by the patient, the first evidence of hypogonadism may be decreased testicular size on physical examination. Since hypogonadism is a common disorder, sexual histories and genital examinations should be performed during initial evaluations and routine reassessments of male patients.

Table 89.2 lists the differential diagnosis of hypogonadotropic hypogonadism. A suggested scheme for evaluation of suspected hypogonadism is provided in Figure 89.2. Serum testosterone levels consistently below the normal range with serum LH and FSH levels within or below the normal range are consistent with hypogonadotropic hypogonadism (as described above). GnRH stimulation testing is not generally useful because of the broad overlap of responses in normal men and men with hypogonadotropic hypogonadism.

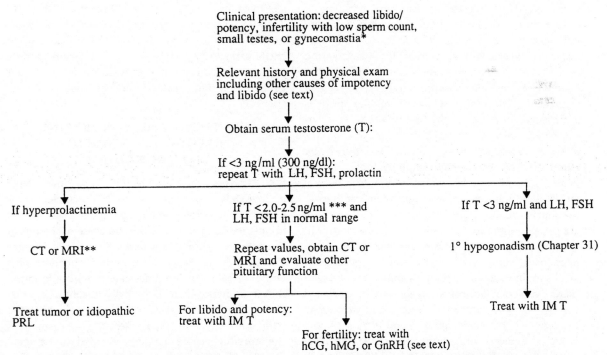

Fig. 89.2 Suggested scheme for evaluation of hypogonadotropic hypogonadism in men. * Unusual presentation of hypogonadotropic hypogonadism: requires measurement of serum estrogen levels. ** Level of prolactin which justifies a CT or MRI scan is somewhat controversial. *** See text for special considerations of transient or borderline hypogonadotropic hypogonadism or evaluation in elderly patients.

Because adult onset of IHH is rare [3], detailed histories and physical examinations should be undertaken in men with postpubertal onset of hypogonadotropic hypogonadism for evidence of other hypothalamic—pituitary dysfunction or tumor. Hyperprolactinemia in men also presents as decreased libido and/or potency or, occasionally, as decreased sperm count or gynecomastia. Measurement of prolactin levels should be undertaken in all men with hypogonadotropic hypogonadism. Since hypothalamic or pituitary tumors may cause adult onset of hypogonadotropic hypogonadism, CT or MRI of the hypothalamus and pituitary should be obtained in men when hyperprolactinemia or hypogonadotropic hypogonadism are confirmed biochemically.

Treatment of IHH, once any serious etiology has been ruled out, is determined by the desire for fertility and the degree of previous sexual development. For secondary sexual development and treatment of impotence or decreased libido, injections of testosterone enanthate or cypionate are sufficient. This treatment, like estrogen replacement therapy in women with ovarian failure, also appears beneficial for preserving bone density. The prostate should be examined before and during testosterone therapy to ensure that nodules or significant hypertrophy are not present. Doses range from 200 to 400 mg i.m. every 2—4 weeks, with an average dose being 300 mg every 3 weeks. An initial dose is usually 200—300 mg every 3—4 weeks unless profound hypogonadism is present (testosterone <1 ng/ml) and priapism is anticipated. In this case, the first two to three doses can be administered as 50—100 mg i.m. at a 4-week interval. Adequacy of dosing is determined by persistence of symptomatic improvement over the dosing interval and by trough serum testosterone levels. A trough testosterone is obtained just prior to the fourth or fifth dose. Trough levels of 2—6 ng/ml are usually appropriate. Higher levels may result in increasing hematocrits. After the dose is stabilized, hematocrit, serum AST, and a trough testosterone level should be monitored on an annual basis. Treatment with oral androgen agents (with 17α-alkyl substitutions) is not used because of the small incidence of cholestatic jaundice and hepatic tumors (which is avoided with parenteral formulations).

If fertility is desired, then hCG, hMG (Pergonal), or GnRH (Lutrepulse) is required for treatment of hypogonadotropic hypogonadism [5]. Both LH and FSH are required for initial development of spermatogenesis. However, if hypogonadotropism occurs after the onset of puberty, or if "fertile eunuch" syndrome is evident, then, in many men, human chorionic gonadotropin (hCG; structurally homologous with LH) may be successful by itself in reestablishing spermatogenesis. hCG therapy is simpler and much less expensive than human menopausal gonadotropin (hMG) or GnRH therapy and is generally the initial therapy of choice if testicular size is >6 ml. It is usually administered at a dose of 1000—2000 IU subcutaneously or intramuscularly Monday, Wednesday, and Friday. Semen analyses are repeated 3 and 6 months after initiation of therapy and hMG is added or GnRH substituted if progress is inadequate. hMG is given at a dose of 75 IU ampules intramuscularly Monday, Wednesday, and Friday. Alternatively, GnRH is administered at a dose of 5—20 μg subcutaneously every 2 hours via automatic infusion pump (Pulsamat, Ferrina, Inc.). Progress is monitored by serum testosterone levels and semen analyses at 2—3-month intervals. If a response is to occur, good sperm counts are usually evident in 6—12 months in men with evidence of previous puberty. Often 1—3 years of therapy are required to produce fertility in men with no previous puberty. If no clear improvement in sperm count is evident after 6—12 months of therapy, a testicular biopsy may be considered to assess further potential of this therapy. Clomiphene citrate elicits variable hypothalamic and pituitary responses in hypogonadotropic hypogonadal men and is not generally used for treatment of these men.

TRANSIENT AND BORDERLINE HYPOGONADOTROPIC HYPOGONADISM

Both transient and borderline hypogonadotropic hypogonadism present diagnostic difficulties. Transient hypogonadotropic hypogonadism often occurs in hospitalized patients without disease of the reproductive axis. Serum testosterone levels may fall into the prepubertal range with serum gonadotropins within or below the normal range. We have reported that this hypogonadism usually resolves by discharge, but may persist for several weeks after the patient leaves the hospital. Therefore, assessment of the reproductive axis should be avoided during acute illness and recovery. In addition, serum testosterone levels may briefly fall below the normal range occasionally in healthy young men with serum LH and FSH levels remaining within the normal range [1].

Thus, a single abnormal testosterone level does not necessarily confirm a diagnosis of hypogonadism and should be repeated (with LH and FSH levels as in Fig. 89.1). Pooled serum specimens are not recommended because normal ranges are determined from single samples and because pooled samples cannot detect day-to-day variations in serum testosterone levels.

Borderline hypogonadotropic hypogonadism may also be encountered in men being evaluated for sexual dysfunction. Serum testosterone levels may consistently lie at or slightly below the normal range with serum LH and FSH within the normal range. It is usually difficult to determine the relationship between these mild abnormalities and the clinical symptoms. CT or MRI of the hypothalamic–pituitary region rarely yield positive findings and are usually not performed unless hypogonadotropic hypogonadism is clearly evident. A 3-month diagnostic and therapeutic trial of testosterone is justified in patients in whom the diagnosis of hypogonadotropic hypogonadism is equivocal if prostate examination and blood pressure are normal, and fluid retention is not a problem. Testosterone enanthate or cypionate can be administered intramuscularly in a dose of 300 mg at 3-week intervals. If symptomatic improvement is observed, therapy is continued.

HYPOGONADISM IN ELDERLY MEN

Testosterone levels in healthy elderly men are lower than in healthy young men [2]. Whereas a normal range of about 3–11 ng/ml is usually appropriate for young and middle-aged men, the range is slightly lower in men over age 60–70. Serum levels of LH and FSH tend to rise slightly with age in healthy men but usually remain within the normal range [2]. The incidence of nonendocrine-related impotency and decreased libido also increases with age [2]. Since changes in sexual function and serum testosterone levels commonly occur independently in the elderly, the relationship between the two may be difficult to assess. In general, if serum testosterone levels are consistently below 2 ng/ml and LH and FSH are in the mid to low normal range or low, the diagnosis of hypogonadotropic hypogonadism should be considered and evidence for other hypothalamic–pituitary dysfunction should be evaluated. Hormone testing and hypothalamic–pituitary imaging should be obtained.

Borderline hypogonadotropic hypogonadism is common in elderly men and should be evaluated and treated as discussed above. Since it may be impossible to discern normal changes in the aging reproductive axis from mild hypogonadotropic hypogonadism in elderly patients, a brief diagnostic and therapeutic trial of testosterone is warranted if the laboratory evaluation is equivocal and the prostate examination is not worrisome. Testosterone therapy should be approached with caution in men with congestive heart failure or hypertension which is resistant to treatment.

REFERENCES

1 Spratt DI, O'Dea LStL, Schoenfeld D, Butler JP, Crowley WF. The neuroendocrine–gonadal axis in men: frequent sampling of LH, FSH and testosterone. *Am J Physiol* 1988; 254: E648.

2 Korenman SG, Morley JE, Mooradian AD *et al*. Secondary hypogonadism in older men: its relation to impotence. *J Clin Endocrinol Metab* 1990; 71: 963–969.

3 Spratt DI, Carr DB, Merriam GR, Scully RE, Rao PN, Crowley WF. The spectrum of abnormal patterns of gonadotropin-releasing hormone secretion in men with idiopathic hypogonadotropic hypogonadism: clinical and laboratory correlations. *J Clin Endocrinol Metab* 1987; 64: 283.

4 Moorthy B, Papadopolou M, Shaw DG, Grant DB. Depot testosterone in boys with anorchia or gonadotrophin deficiency: effect on growth rate and adult height. *Arch Dis Child* 1991; 66: 197–199.

5 Spratt DI, Hoffman A, Crowley WF. Hypogonadotropic hypogonadism and its treatment. In: Santen R, Swerdloff R, eds. *Male Reproductive Dysfunction: Diagnosis and Management of Hypogonadism, Infertility, and Impotence.* New York: Marcel Decker, 1986: 227–249.

90

Azoospermia

JONATHAN P. JAROW

INTRODUCTION

Traditionally, a semen analysis has been used as the primary screening test to determine the presence or absence of a male factor in an infertile couple. However, experience has revealed the pitfalls of basing a man's fertility status upon this single examination. For instance, patients with hypogonadotropic hypogonadism can be fertile with extremely low sperm counts (less than 1 million/ml), suggesting that the quality of sperm rather than quantity is the most important factor. Conversely, recent studies have shown that seminal parameters within the normal range are not predictive of fertility. In contrast, complete absence of sperm within the ejaculate (azoospermia) is an absolute predictor of sterility. Unless a couple is willing to explore the alternatives of donor insemination or adoption, a pregnancy will not occur without therapy of the male partner. Although many of the causes of azoospermia are untreatable, there are several treatable causes which mandate andrologic evaluation of all azoospermic patients. In addition, the association of upper urinary tract anomalies with some of the causes of azoospermia mandates urologic evaluation of some of these patients.

Azoospermia is present in approximately 2% of men in the general population and its incidence has ranged from 10 to 20% of men attending infertility clinics. The different causes of azoospermia can be divided into pretesticular, testicular, and posttesticular factors (Table 90.1). Pretesticular factors include the endocrinopathies which result in secondary hypogonadism. These include hypogonadotropic hypogonadism caused by Kallmann's syndrome, prolactin-secreting pituitary adenomas, pituitary trauma or surgery, and anabolic steroid abuse. These are relatively rare but treatable causes of azoospermia.

Primary testicular failure is the most common cause of azoospermia, accounting for approximately

Table 90.1 Causes of azoospermia

Pretesticular
  Hypogonadotropic hypogonadism (idiopathic)
  Prolactin-secreting pituitary tumor
  Kallmann's syndrome
  Pituitary trauma
  Anabolic steroid abuse
  Nonfunctional pituitary tumor

Testicular
  Anorchia
  Cryptorchidism
  Mumps orchitis
  Testicular torsion (bilateral)
  Gonadotoxin exposure
  Varicocele
  Chromosomal
  Idiopathic

Posttesticular
  Vasal agenesis
  Epididymal atresia
  Epididymitis
  Ejaculatory duct obstruction
  Young's syndrome
  Ejaculatory dysfunction
  Iatrogenic

60% of these patients. The various causes include but are not restricted to chromosomal abnormalities, gonadotoxin exposure, cryptorchidism, mumps orchitis and varicoceles. Testicular biopsy of these patients will reveal abnormalities in spermatogenesis ranging from maturation arrest to complete germinal cell aplasia (Sertoli cell only syndrome).

Experience has shown that long-term obstruction of the testicular excurrent ductal system does not preclude fertility and that most patients will have a normal testicular biopsy. Therefore, all posttesticular causes of azoospermia are potentially treatable. One of the more common causes of obstruction is bilateral congenital absence of the vas. Other etiologies include epididymal atresia, epididymitis, ejaculatory duct obstruction, Young's syndrome, and iatrogenic.

EVALUATION

The evaluation of an azoospermic patient should be performed with the goal of obtaining a rapid determination as to whether a patient has a treatable, potentially treatable, or irreversible cause of azoospermia with a minimum of cost and invasiveness. More specifically, this means differentiating between patients with pre- or posttesticular causes, which are usually treatable, from those patients with primary testicular failure. In addition, patients with congenital anomalies should be evaluated for associated abnormalities of the urinary tract. Considering recent technologic advances, this goal can now be accomplished in many cases within a single office visit. The features most important in differentiating testicular failure from treatable causes of azoospermia include testis size, serum follicle-stimulating hormone (FSH) levels, and ejaculate volume (Fig. 90.1).

As with every patient, the evaluation begins with a thorough history and physical examination (Table 90.2). Risk factors for testicular failure and obstruction should be identified. A history of prior fertility will usually rule out a congenital disorder. A history of delayed sexual development and anosmia will suggest the diagnosis of Kallmann's syndrome. Patients with a history of sinusitis and chronic bronchitis may have Young's syndrome. Conversely, patients with a history of cryptorchidism, mumps orchitis, and prior radiation or chemotherapy most likely have testicular failure.

Physical examination is the next step in the evaluation. A general physical examination including inspection of secondary sex characteristics is important. However, both testicular size and location as well as the presence of the vasa deferentia and epididymides are the most critical factors. Although there is some variation with race, normal testis size is greater than 19 ml. Bilateral testicular atrophy is consistent with either primary or secondary testicular failure. Measurement of serum FSH and testosterone can differentiate between these two disorders (Fig. 90.1). Bilateral absence of the vasa is an obstructive cause of azoospermia and the evaluation can stop at that point unless epididymal aspiration is being considered. Other important physical factors include the consistency of the epididymides and fullness of the seminal vesicles and prostate upon rectal examin-

ation. Both of these findings are suggestive but not diagnostic of obstruction.

Semen analysis is usually the first laboratory study available. Azoospermia is based upon the complete absence of sperm within a centrifuged specimen. However, severely oligospermic patients — sperm count of less than 1 million — are evaluated in a similar fashion. The next most important parameter is the ejaculate volume. Decreased ejaculate volume (less than 1.5 ml) is consistent with ejaculatory dysfunction, ejaculatory duct obstruction, or hypogonadism. Hypogonadism can be ruled out on the basis of testis size and the results of hormonal testing. In the past, serum fructose was used to identify absence or obstruction of the seminal vesicles and ejaculatory ducts. However, the standard fructose test used is qualitative rather than quantitative and the results may be misleading in cases of incomplete obstruction or hypoplasia.

In patients with low ejaculate volume the next test

Table 90.2 Evaluation of the patient with azoospermia

History
  Prior fertility
  Cryptorchidism
  Torsion
  Orchitis
  Gonadotoxin exposure
  Epididymitis
  Sinusitis
  Anosmia
  Sexual development

Physical
  Testicular size and consistency
  Vas
  Epididymis
  Rectal examination
  Neurologic

Semen analysis
  Volume
  Fructose
  Postejaculatory urinalysis

Laboratory
  Follicle-stimulating hormone
  Testosterone
  Prolactin

Radiologic
  Transrectal ultrasound
  Renal ultrasound
  Vasography

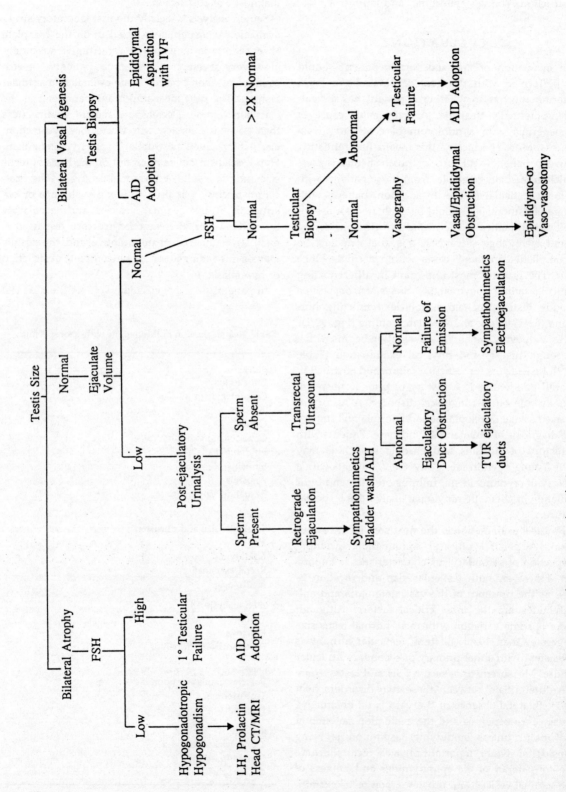

Fig. 90.1 Evaluation and treatment of an azoospermic patient.

performed is a postejaculatory urinalysis. Presence of sperm within the bladder is consistent with retrograde ejaculation. However, patients without sperm in the bladder may still have ejaculatory dysfunction due to failure of emission. These patients usually have a history of spinal cord injury or prior retroperitoneal surgery. Transrectal ultrasound evaluation of the seminal vesicles will differentiate these patients from those with ejaculatory duct obstruction.

Serum FSH is used to differentiate between the treatable and untreatable causes of azoospermia (Fig. 90.1). Patients with bilateral testicular atrophy and a low FSH most likely have secondary hypogonadism. Their evaluation should include a full endocrine panel to rule out panhypopituitarism and radiologic imaging of the sella turcica to rule out a pituitary tumor. A serum FSH greater than twice the upper limits of normal is diagnostic of primary testicular failure, regardless of testis size. However, a normal serum FSH level does not rule out testicular failure. Patients with normal-sized testes and relatively normal FSH require testicular biopsy to rule out primary testicular failure.

Testicular biopsy should be performed through a small scrotal incision using a window technique to prevent development of adhesions which may make later reconstructive surgery more difficult. Since frozen sections of testicular biopsies may be difficult to interpret, it is better to stage the reconstructive repair. Histologic findings consistent with testicular failure include germinal cell aplasia (Sertoli cell only), maturation arrest, and hypospermatogenesis. A late maturation arrest can sometimes be difficult to distinguish from an obstructive pattern. Therefore, a testicular touch imprint can be obtained to look for mature spermatozoa which are frequently lost from permanent sections due to processing. Normal spermatogenesis is consistent with obstructive azoospermia and these patients are candidates for reconstructive surgery.

A scrotal exploration is performed in order to identify and treat the cause of obstruction. A large scrotal incision is used to deliver the testis and spermatic cord. A partial-thickness transverse incision is made through the scrotal portion of the vas just above the convoluted portion. Vasal contents are aspirated after massaging the epididymis, and then examined microscopically. Presence of sperm confirms proximal patency. Vasography is performed through injection of contrast into the distal vas to confirm distal patency. Contrast should not be injected into the proximal vas deferens or epididymis. Alternatively, colored dye may be injected into the distal vas and the subsequent bladder catheter drainage inspected for a change in color. The drawback of this method is that the site of obstruction is not identified.

Patients with congenital anomalies of the male reproductive tract frequently have abnormalities of the urinary system because of their related embryologic origin. Patients with seminal vesicle cyst or unilateral vasal agenesis have a greater than 50% incidence of ipsilateral renal agenesis, whereas patients with bilateral vasal agenesis have a 10–20% incidence of renal agenesis. Therefore, evaluation of the upper urinary tract is mandatory in patients with azoospermia due to congenital anomalies. Ultrasound is the preferred screening technique for this clinical setting.

TREATMENT

Hypogonadotropic hypogonadism

Patients with bilateral atrophic testes and low basal serum FSH and luteinizing hormone (LH) have a treatable endocrinologic cause of infertility. The most common cause is a prolactin-secreting pituitary adenoma which can be identified by obtaining a serum prolactin level. Levels below 50 ng/ml are usually due to functional causes (medication, stress, etc.), while levels above 100 ng/ml are consistent with tumor. The next step is radiogically to assess the pituitary with either computed tomography or magnetic resonance imaging. Most functional tumors can be treated satisfactorily with bromocriptine alone. Tumors that do not respond to medical therapy should be treated with either radiation or surgery. Idiopathic hypogonadotropic hypogonadism or those associated with midline defects such as anosmia (Kallmann's syndrome) can be successfully treated with exogenous hormone replacement. Initial therapy begins with human chorionic gonadotropin (hCG) alone. Human menopausal gonadotropin (hMG) should be added in those patients who do not respond to hCG alone. Alternatively, patients can be treated with gonadotropin-releasing hormone (GnRH). However this therapy is very cumbersome because of the need for continuous, pulsatile administration, requiring use of a pump. In addition, the success rate of this type of treatment does not appear to be significantly better than the combination of hCG and hMG. Interestingly, these patients can be fertile with extremely low sperm counts which would usually be considered in the subfertile range.

Ejaculatory dysfunction

Patients with low ejaculate volume or aspermia have either failure of emission or retrograde ejaculation. These disorders are initially treated with sympathomimetic medications in an effort to increase vasal peristalsis and stimulate bladder neck closure. Pseudoephedrine and imipramine are the most commonly used agents starting at a dose of 60 mg q.i.d. and 25 mg t.i.d., respectively. Imipramine appears to work best in diabetic patients. Tachyphylaxis is frequently observed with these medications. Therefore, they should not be administered for periods of greater than 2 weeks at a time.

Bladder wash procedure combined with artificial insemination is reserved for patients with retrograde ejaculation who fail medical therapy. The urine should be alkalinized and the patient well hydrated so that urine pH is around 7 and osmolality is 300 mosmol. The bladder is catheterized and rinsed with a physiologic buffer leaving approximately 50 ml behind. The patient is then asked to obtain a semen specimen and immediately voids or is catheterized to obtain the entire bladder contents. The specimen is centrifuged at 600 g and then brought up to a volume of 1 ml for artificial insemination.

Patients with failure of emission who do not respond to medical therapy can be treated with electro-ejaculation. Rectal probe electrostimulation of the pelvic organs and nerves has been successfully used to recover semen from spinal cord-injured patients and men who have undergone retroperitoneal surgery. This semen is then processed for artificial insemination in the spouse. Premedication with a calcium channel blocker is used to prevent autonomic dysreflexia in those patients at risk. Patients who are insensate can be done without anesthesia, whereas those with intact sensation will require a general anesthetic.

Ejaculatory duct obstruction

Patients found to have low ejaculate volume and gross dilatation of the seminal vesicles by transrectal ultrasonography have ejaculatory duct obstruction. Treatment consists of transurethral resection of the ejaculatory ducts. Massaging the prostate during this procedure will help determine when the ducts have been satisfactorily opened by the presence of milky discharge within the prostatic urethra. Follow-up semen analysis should be performed to document the result. Timed sexual intercourse should be performed if all parameters have normalized. Repeat transrectal ultrasonography should be performed if ejaculate volume is persistently low. Some patients with ejaculatory duct obstruction will develop a secondary obstruction of the epididymis due to a pressure-induced blowout. This patient will have persistent azoospermia despite normalization of ejaculate volume postresection of the ejaculatory ducts. Scrotal exploration should then be performed as described below.

Vasal epididymal obstruction

Azoospermic men with at least one normal-sized testis and a relatively normal FSH level should undergo testicular biopsy to rule out ductal obstruction. A normal testicular biopsy in the presence of azoospermia is pathognomonic of obstruction. This patient should then undergo scrotal exploration with vasography anticipating microsurgical repair. A partial-thickness transverse incision is made through the scrotal portion of the vas and vasal contents are aspirated. Presence of intravasal sperm confirms proximal patency of the epididymis and vas, whereas intravasal azoospermia is consistent with a more proximal obstruction.

Vasography is performed by injecting dilute contrast into the vas toward the prostate end. Performing a simultaneous pneumocystogram is helpful in delineating the vasal ampulla and seminal vesicles. The results of the vasogram and microscopic examination of vasal fluid will determine the need for vasovasostomy versus epididymovasostomy. Unfortunately, some patients with a vasal obstruction will develop a secondary epididymal obstruction due to the back-pressure effect, thus requiring both vasovasostomy and epididymovasostomy on the same side. The success rates of these operations are lower than for patients undergoing vasectomy reversals in whom the obstructive interval is of a much shorter duration.

Vasal agenesis

Most patients with bilateral vasal agenesis are discovered upon initial physical examination. Previous attempts at treatment by reconstructing the excurrent ducts or replacing them with an artificial reservoir were very dissappointing. Although a successful connection can be achieved between the epididymal remnant and an artificial spermatocele, the quality of the sperm obtained was poor, such that pregnancies rarely occurred. The treatment fell into disfavor and patients with vasal agenesis were offered the theraputic options of donor insemination or adoption only.

More recently, a technique of epididymal aspiration combined with *in vitro* fertilization has shown some promise. In contrast to the previously held belief that sperm quality improved as they progressed through the epididymis, the best-quality sperm are found in proximal epididymis of patients with vasal agenesis. Pregnancies have been reported using a protocol which combines microscopic aspiration of sperm from the epididymis with *in vitro* techniques for fertilization. The best results have been obtained in couples where more than 10 eggs are retrieved. This technique is still under evaluation and should not be considered the standard of care at this time.

Primary testicular failure

Unfortunately, there is very little to offer patients with primary testicular failure. Most of these patients are offered the therapeutic alternatives of donor insemination or adoption. Varicocelectomy might be considered if the FSH is less than three times normal and testicular biopsy reveals maturation arrest rather than germinal cell aplasia. There have been several reports of pregnancies using empiric medical therapy in azoospermic men with primary testicular failure. However, regardless of therapy used, the overall prognosis for obtaining a biologic child is poor for this subset of patients.

CONCLUSIONS

Azoospermia represents a relatively infrequent but absolute cause of male factor infertility. Every azoospermic patient should be evaluated, even though many of the causes are untreatable. Some etiologies, such as hypogonadotropic hypogonadism, have a high success rate with treatment, whereas other treatable causes such as vasal agenesis have a low pregnancy rate. However, every couple deserves an accurate assessment of their chances of having a biologic offspring before considering therapeutic alternatives. In addition, many of these patients should be evaluated for coexisting urologic disorders. In most cases, this evaluation can be completed in a minimal amount of time with relatively low cost and invasiveness.

FURTHER READING

Coburn M, Wheeler T, Lipshultz LI. Testicular biopsy: its use and limitations. *Urol Clin North Am* 1987; 14: 551.

deKretser DM, Burger HG, Hudson B. The relationship between germinal cells and serum FSH levels in males with infertility. *J Clin Endocrinol Metab* 1974; 38: 787.

Jarow JP. Transrectal ultrasonography in the evaluation of male infertility. In: Resnick MI, ed. *Prostatic Ultrasonography*. Philadelphia: BC Decker, 1990: 153.

Jarow JP, Espeland MA, Lipshultz LI. Evaluation of the azoospermic patient. *J Urol* 1989; 142: 62.

Stanwell-Smith RE, Hendry WE. The prognosis of male subfertility: a survey of 1025 men referred to a fertility clinic. *Br J Urol* 1984; 56: 422.

Diagnosis and treatment
of oligospermia

GABOR B. HUSZAR

INTRODUCTION

Oligospermia and asthenospermia are usually discovered when a semen analysis is ordered within the infertility work-up of a couple. The basic semen analysis results include semen volume, sperm concentration and motility, and sperm morphology. In most laboratories the motility values are also supplemented with parameters that arise from computer-assisted analysis including sperm curvilinear velocity, linearity, amplitude of lateral head displacement, and tail beat/cross frequency. The clinical value of these measurements is not yet apparent.

In the case of couples with at least a 1-year history of unsuccessful attempts for pregnancy the question arises: When to order a semen analysis? The answer is easy: in *each* infertility work-up, and at least two semen analyses 2−3 weeks apart to make the results representative considering the physiologic fluctuation in sperm concentrations. This should be the rule even if the husband had a normal semen analysis in another laboratory or physician's office. Another important point is the abstinence period which should be standard in the population studied by a laboratory. We recommend 2 days of abstinence; shorter abstinence may result in lower sperm concentrations, and after longer than 5 days of abstinence sperm motility usually declines due to the effects of epididymal storage. The abstinence question is particularly relevant in oligospermic men who tend to "collect up" prior to a semen analysis.

OLIGOSPERMIA

Oligospermia, according to the World Health Organization classification, means that the sperm concentrations in a specimen are <20 million sperm/ml [1]. This number has changed historically; earlier the normal sperm concentrations were thought to be at least 40 or 60 million sperm/ml. Also, now we understand better than sperm concentrations in men are changing from day to day or month to month; indeed some investigators believe that there are seasonal variations. It has also been well documented that sperm concentrations decline with age in men over 45−50 years old.

To document oligospermia it is important that the semen analysis should be repeated, and if the sperm concentrations are controversial, a third semen analysis should follow. Obviously, sperm concentrations alone will not adequately and accurately define the quality of the semen. Associated factors of sperm motility, velocity, sperm survival, and morphology are also important. All of these are well reflected by the values of the motile sperm yield — the measure of the number of sperm "in play" — from the specimen. In our laboratory at Yale this parameter is measured by the sperm migration test according to our published method [2]. We report the motile sperm yield as a percentage value derived from the number of motile sperm in the migrated (or swim-up) fraction over the total motile sperm in the specimen.

At the outset, there are three points that must be emphasized regarding oligospermia:

1 Lower sperm concentrations or abnormal sperm morphology are not related directly to the loss of fertility — they are merely signs of diminished testicular function.

2 Beyond the parameters of sperm concentration, motility and morphology, the volume of the semen has also to be considered. From the point of view of the efficacy in fertilization, one has to consider the sum of motile sperm with normal morphology in the specimen. Although each case has to be individually evaluated, one can offer a rule of thumb that if over 8 million of such sperm are present in the ejaculate it is a promising finding, although, as will be discussed later, the concentrations of sperm in the semen are

not necessarily related to the biochemical maturity of the sperm, neither do they confirm fertility.

3 Because oligospermia or asthenospermia is not automatically associated with diminished fertility, the prompt, thorough, and vigorous work-up of the female partner should not be neglected.

PATHOGENESIS OF OLIGOSPERMIA

Oligospermia may be caused by either lower sperm production or increased sperm destruction and it can have extratesticular or testicular causes. Extratesticular pathogenesis due to deficiency in pituitary hormone production occurs very rarely. An experimental model that mimics this mechanism has been developed recently by the use of gonadotropin-releasing hormone (GnRH) analogs for male contraception.

Common examples of testicular causes of reduced sperm production are as follows:

1 Physiologic variations in sperm concentrations. It is well established that such fluctuations occur: however, fertilizing potential, as measured by the zona-free hamster oocyte penetration assay or by sperm creatine kinase measurements, remains unchanged. This group would also include aging men in whom a premature decline in male reproductive function could result in lower sperm production.

2 Recent exposure to heat, whether it is high fever, frequent baths in very hot tubs, visits to steam rooms or extended sunbathing during tropical vacations, etc.

3 Chronic heat exposure at the work place, i.e., iron workers, truck drivers, pizza bakers, etc.

4 Radiation damage in workers at nuclear power stations, X-ray technicians or those in research laboratories utilizing radioisotopes.

5 Elevated intratesticular temperatures due to varicocele. Varicocele is somewhat of an enigma of male infertility. It is true that varicocele, which is associated with lower blood flow in the testicle, may cause higher intratesticular temperatures that are detrimental to spermatogenesis and sperm survival. However, it is well established that the incidence of varicocele in the populations of fertile and infertile men is not very different. The other unclear question about varicocele is the possible relationship between varicocele and abnormalities in testicular function as corollary events, both originating in congenital or developmental factors. In any case, varicocele should be evaluated by a urologist who has an interest in

male infertility: varicocele repair may bring an improvement in sperm concentrations or motility, although this is not always true.

6 Examples of conditions that cause intratesticular destruction of sperm (in light of normal sperm production) are damage to the epididymal epithelium (causing lower secretion of carnitine and similar agents that inhibit sperm metabolism and motility prior to ejaculation) which usually follows infections of the male genital urinary tract or occurs in men who had vasovasostomy reconstruction following a vasectomy. Another frequent cause of sperm destruction or lower sperm motility is the presence of antisperm antibodies.

WORK-UP OF THE OLIGOSPERMIC MAN

It cannot be emphasized enough that the World Health Organization standards of 20 million sperm/ml of semen classfying men as oligospermic or normospermic should not be interpreted strictly or accepted as a predictor of male fertilizing potential. Indeed, in cases of couples with oligospermic husbands who were treated with intrauterine insemination the sperm concentrations were indistinguishable in those who did or did not achieve pregnancies. As we will discuss later, we discovered that sperm creatine kinase, a biochemical sperm parameter, predicts fertility among oligospermic men who otherwise are indistinguishable in sperm concentrations. Our serial studies of sperm creatine kinase activity (an objective biochemical measure of sperm development and fertilizing potential: see later) and sperm concentrations in men of our intrauterine insemination population indicated that the group of men with between 20 and 30 million sperm/ml concentrations in the repeat samples very often show sperm concentrations in the <20 million or the >30 million sperm/ml range, thus men in the 20–30 million sperm/ml concentration range should be further investigated and scrutinized similarly to that of oligospermic men. We call these men variable-spermic, indicating the fact that about 50% of these men are oligospermic, and occasionally produce a normospermic sample. The sperm biochemical properties also showed this 50–50% distribution in variable-spermic men between the creatine kinase parameters specific for low and high likelihood for fertilization ranges.

In the work-up of oligospermic men it is very important to take a good history with respect to the profession of the man, previous recent and childhood illnesses (high fever, pneumonia, viral diseases, mumps, congenital hernias or hernia operations, accidents, late-descending or undescended testes, etc.). Subsequently, a physical examination should be carried out, at least looking at the size and the consistency of the testes (Fig. 91.1). In general, men with oligospermia may not necessarily show gross adverse physical findings. In the endocrine profile of these patients the first-line studies would include serum follicle-stimulating hormone (FSH) and luteinizing hormone (LH) levels which, when elevated, indicate pituitary compensation to the inadequate testicular response by the Sertoli and Leydig cells. Testosterone levels — particularly free testosterone which is the physiologically important factor — are usually normal because the diminished function by the Sertoli and Leydig cells at most times is confined to germ cell production. In men younger than 50 years old the decline in semen parameters is not usually coupled with lower testosterone levels or loss of virility.

If there are any questions with respect to varicocele or testicular size, it is a good idea to refer the patient to a urologist who has an interest in male infertility. The urologist with the newly available visualization techniques — Doppler ultrasound stethoscopy, transrectal ultrasonography, scrotal thermography, venography, radioisotopic angiography, computed tomography scanning and with magnetic resonance imaging — is able to evaluate the male reproductive tract.

If extratesticular and epididymal origin of oligospermia or azoospermia are excluded, spermatogenesis or its defects may be further probed with a testicular biopsy. The most commonly found pathologic tissue diagnoses associated with infertility are hypospermatogenesis, maturation arrest, and germinal cell aplasia (Sertoli cell only syndrome) which may occur with the total lack of or with focal spermatogenesis.

AZOOSPERMIA

In a case of very low sperm concentrations or of azoospermia, the total lack of sperm in the semen, one has to establish that the man has not missed the cup in making the masturbated sample (about 70% of the sperm are contained by the first burst in the ejaculate). The semen analysis has to be repeated along with a thorough physical examination including the size and consistency of the testicles and serum hormone levels of FSH, LH, and testosterone. Chemical analysis of the seminal fluid is also diagnostic as it indicates the presence of an obstruction in the system. The presence or absence of fructose will signify communication to the seminal vesicles and accessory glands. Zinc, arginine, and citric acid originates in the prostate gland and carnitine signifies the presence of epididymal fluids. Thus, detection of these compounds in semen suggests that the man has a genuine azoospermia due to the lack of sperm production rather than related to blockage or anatomic factors. The lack of spermatogenesis may be confirmed with testicular biopsy.

Unless there is a posttesticular defect, in which case there are recent advances in achieving pregnancy following epididymal sperm retrieval and *in vitro* fertilization, azoospermia may lead to the decision about donor insemination. In this situation it is the responsibility of the infertility specialist to present the facts to the couple in a gentle, factual, but firm manner, *always* in the presence of both wife and husband. This approach will minimize the natural response of denial and facilitate the further communication between wife and husband which is essential for the timely decision making that is particularly important if the wife is in her mid or late 30s.

ADVANCED LABORATORY TECHNIQUES

In addition to the conventional and computer-assisted semen analysis parameters, there are a host of tests used with more or less success to establish the fertility of oligospermic men. As mentioned, in our Sperm Physiology Laboratory at Yale we establish the motile sperm yield from the specimen. The motile sperm yield depends not only on sperm motility, but on the velocity and linearity of the sperm and it also reflects the survival or short-term decline in sperm motility. These are very important questions toward establishing the therapeutic utility of the sperm in insemination treatments into cervical mucus, the uterus, or into the fallopian tube, or if *in vitro* fertilization is contemplated.

In case of unexplained infertility or if in the semen sperm aggregation "clumping," and/or low motility is reported the couple should be investigated for antisperm antibodies. Antisperm antibodies may be directed to the tail or to the head of sperm or to both. Tail antibodies may cause a loss of sperm motility: on the other hand the head-directed antibodies

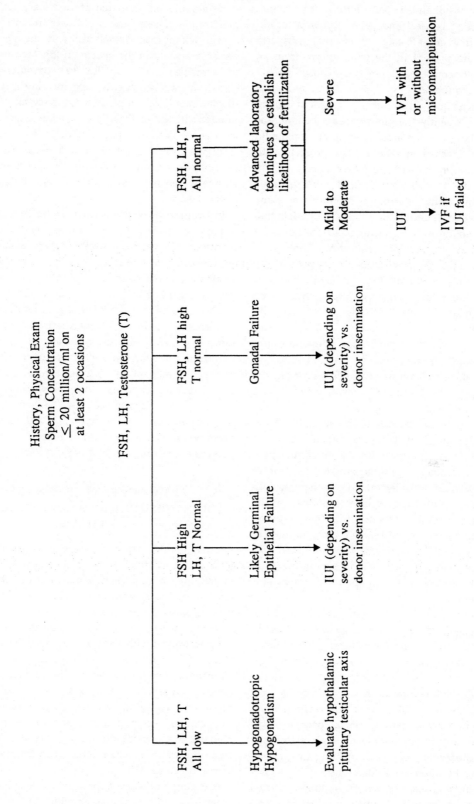

Fig. 91.1 Approach to oligospermia (findings, likely diagnosis, therapy).

may or may not diminish sperm fertilizing potential. Because testing cervical and pelvic fluids is technically difficult, in order to establish whether antisperm antibodies are present in the wife, sperm from an antisperm antibody-free donor are exposed to her serum prior to the test.

Several techniques are available to test for antisperm antibodies. Presently the immunobead technique is most popular, in which antihuman immunoglobulin antibody is attached to a bead. One problem with this technique is that for the correct interpretation the sperm has to swim by the bead with vigorous motility. Thus, samples with low motility may show a false-negative result. However, due to the fact that the motile sperm may be anchored to the beads by the head or tail, the regional localization of antisperm antibodies on the sperm is possible. Also, because the beads are available with different kinds of antihuman immunogobulins, one can now detect whether the sperm antibodies arise from the immunogobulin G, M, or A types.

Removal of antisperm antibodies from the sperm is not possible, although separating sperm subpopulations to which antisperm antibodies did or did not attach is possible. Ejaculating into sperm-washing buffers to minimize antibody binding to sperm did not prove to be successful. If the motility of the sperm is not impaired it is very difficult to assess the impact of antisperm antibodies in diminishing fertilizing potential. Taking a pragmatic point of view, one should consider that the antisperm antibodies cover up functionally important sites on the sperm, thus sperm populations which were exposed to antisperm antibodies will have a reduced number of fertile sperm. The degree of this reduction may change from time to time in a man depending upon the titer of the antibodies and sperm concentrations in the semen.

Other tests thought to reflect sperm functional integrity include sperm morphology with respect to the size and shape of the sperm head. Studies using the strict criteria developed recently indicate that abnormal sperm should be present in an incidence of up to 90–95% before the fertilization rates were significantly reduced in *in vitro* fertilization. From the point of view of fertility the acrosomal status is a particularly important morphologic factor that may be tested with differential staining in light microscopy or by fluorescent microscopy using lectins or acrosome-directed antibodies. Another related biochemical approach is the measurement of sperm

acrosine, the enzyme that is necessary for oocyte penetration. These studies evaluate the incidence of sperm without acrosomal cap and the per sperm acrosine activity in the specimen [3]. Measurements of acrosine levels, similar to computer-assisted measurements of sperm velocity, linearity, head displacement, or beat/cross frequency all carry the inherent handicap that they provide a mean value for the whole sperm population. This is a problem from the clinical point of view because the results do not allow the identification of sperm subpopulations which may have more or less advantageous properties.

In conjunction with sperm morphology, methods are also available to probe the integrity of the sperm membrane in the head of the sperm with various supravital stains and in the tail by the hypoosmotic swelling test. We found that sperm membrane integrity in the head and the tail show about an 85% correlation and that diminished membrane integrity is associated with the loss of sperm motility in the sample. Other sperm functions that are relevant to fertilization are the binding of sperm to the oocyte and penetration of the oocyte, which are studied in the recently developed human sperm hemizona binding assay and with the zona-free hamster oocyte penetration assay, respectively. The description of these two tests and the evaluation of their diagnostic potential are dealt with in other chapters.

SPERM CREATINE KINASE: A BIOCHEMICAL MEASURE OF SPERM FERTILITY

Because semen parameters are not predictive for fertilization potential, the key management question in treating an oligospermic man is to establish the fertility of the spermatozoa, which until now has been an unsolved problem due to the lack of adequate tests for the assessment of sperm fertility. Indeed, in couples treated with intrauterine insemination there were no differences in semen parameters among oligospermic men who did or did not achieve pregnancies. Other available assays reviewed above that prove selected sperm function, e.g. acrosine activity, hypoosmotic sperm tail swelling or the zona-free hamster ova penetration assay, have all failed thus far to show a reliable correlation with the results of *in vitro* fertilization [3].

Pursuing a different approach, we searched for an objective biochemical marker which is a constituent of spermatozoa, reflects functional integrity of sperm, and thus would predict the fertilizing potential. We have identified such a marker in sperm — the enzyme creatine kinase. In a study conducted on our intrauterine insemination population we have compared the sperm creatine kinase activities of oligospermic men who achieved pregnancies versus infertile oligospermic men, and found highly significant differences. The predictive value of sperm creatine kinase activities was further supported by a logistic regression analysis of the 160 study samples, which gave evidence that sperm creatine kinase activities were significantly related to fertilizing potential, whereas sperm concentrations provided no predictive power [4].

In connection with the differences in per sperm creatine kinase activity, which we believe are a consequence of a defect in cytoplasmic extrusion during terminal spermatogenesis, we also discovered developmental changes in the constituent creatine kinase isoforms in sperm. The B-type creatine kinase (CK-B) is being replaced by the more differentiated M-type of CK (CK-M), a switch which apparently signifies sperm cellular maturation and indicates that synthesis of "new" proteins occurs during spermatogenesis as the sperm attain fertility. Analyzing 159 samples we found that the CK-M concentrations (expressed as %M/M + B) in the normospermic samples was about five times higher than that in oligospermic specimens (26.2 ± 2.1 versus $6.7 \pm 0.9\%$; $P < 0.001$). Indeed, some samples of infertile men contained none of the sperm CK-M isoform [5].

The value of CK-M concentrations in predicting fertilizing potential was tested in a recent blind study of couples who were treated with *in vitro* fertilization. We classified the samples based on their sperm CK-M concentrations (without receiving any information on semen parameters, the number of sperm in the pellets analyzed, reproductive history of the couples, or the outcome of the IVF cycles) into low likelihood (<10% CK-M) and high likelihood (>10% CK-M) for fertilization groups. The CK-M values in the two groups predicted the rate of oocyte fertilization, the failure of fertilization of any oocyte in couples, and the pregnancies that have occurred independently from the sperm concentration in the ejaculates [6].

SPERM FUNCTION TEST

Using the recent advances of our laboratory we have developed a three-part sperm function test. The first part provides the semen analysis and migration test, including the measurement of motile sperm yield. In the second part of the test we use a combination of hypoosmotic swelling test (HOS) and supravital staining with the Hoechst-32183 fluorescent supravital stain to establish the integrity of the sperm membrane in the tail and the head of the spermatozoa. The third part of the test probes the biochemical maturity of the sperm by the measurement of creatine kinase activity and the concentrations of the sperm CK-M isoform. These three studies together give us good information with respect to the motility and survival properties of the sperm and a fairly good indication how the sperm will travel through the female reproductive tract. The membrane integrity parameters in the sperm head and sperm tail test for possible damage to the spermatozoa in the male genital tract, which may be a consequence of epididymal damage or exposure to sperm antibodies. Finally, the sperm creatine kinase parameters tell about the biochemical maturity and the fertilization potential of the spermatozoa.

THERAPEUTIC CONSIDERATIONS

Following the principle that oligospermia does not necessarily signify a lack of male fertility, it is very important to avoid the trap of overlooking female infertility factors. Indeed, the majority of oligospermic men never find out that their sperm count is low or see a fertility specialist. In most cases low sperm concentrations may only cause a delay in the occurrence of pregnancy, provided that the wife is of sound reproductive health and younger than the mid 30s, when age starts to become a subfertility factor. A good demonstration of this point is a study by Silber and Cohen [7] in which wives of oligospermic men were treated arbitrarily with Clomid. Indeed, in the patient population of 30 couples, within 1 year 10 reported pregnancies. It is of interest from the point of mild versus severe oligospermia that among the couples who became pregnant, the men with sperm concentrations over 5 million sperm/ml had a 43% pregnancy rate (9 of 21), whereas in those who had less than 5 million sperm/ml, and thus had severe oligospermia, the pregnancy rates were only 10% (1 of 10).

If the CK-M criteria indicate that the oligo-/asthenospermic man is fertile, we can offer therapy based on a more efficient utilization of the sperm by intrauterine [8] or intratubal insemination or, in the case of severe oligo-/asthenospermia, *in vitro* fertilization. In addition to artificial insemination or *in vitro* fertilization, there are two other methods of assisted reproduction directed to male factor infertility in current development. One of them is the partial removal of the zona or creation of a window on the zona which allows the sperm to fertilize by getting into the perivitelline area of the oocyte. The other approach is micromanipulation, or sperm injection, in which the immotile but fertile sperm may be injected under the zona or into the cytoplasm of the oocyte to initiate fertilization. However, these methods at the present time are strictly experimental, particularly the micromanipulation, because the conditions in which the sperm injection does not harm the oocyte are not yet understood. Also, the cellular processes of capacitation, acrosomal reaction, and oocyte activation that occur as a sequential interplay between sperm and egg, contributing to the fertilization process, are not understood. Finally, it is not yet established how the oocyte could be stabilized so that the mechanical damage associated with the sperm injection will not eliminate its capacity for fertilization.

Once the micromanipulation techniques are further developed, biochemical markers of sperm fertilization potential, such as the CK-M isoform, which may allow the identification of single fertile sperm, will be important.

CONCLUSIONS

In this brief overview the author has summarized the practical information which is necessary for the work-up and interpretation of diagnostic data as well as for the management of men with oligospermia. The essential concepts of male factor subfertility/infertility and the steps of the work-up are presented in Table 91.1:

1 The suspicion of male factor subfertility may be based on reduced total number of sperm which are not of short-term motility and abnormal morphology. A good cut-off value is below 8 million such sperm in the ejaculate. However, sperm concentrations have only an advisory role and they do not necessarily reflect the man's fertility.

2 Men with sperm concentrations in the 20–30 sperm/ml range (variable-spermic men) should be viewed and managed as potentially subfertile men.

3 In men with suspicion of subfertility the semen

values should be confirmed by repeat semen analysis and by monitoring of the total motile sperm with normal morphology.

4 It is important that in the light of suspected male subfertility, the possible presence of a female factor is also thoroughly investigated and documented. The paradigm of postcoital test has little clinical value: sperm–cervical mucus interaction should be tested on a glass slide by direct observation.

5 In case of confirmed subfertility an attempt should be made to elicit all correctable underlying conditions. This should start with a comprehensive medical history, including diseases, lifestyle, and factors related to endocrine conditions, genitourinary infections, and exposure to other harmful environmental factors, etc.

6 The first line of specific tests is focused upon physiologic functions: sperm migration test and motile sperm yield, survival of motility, and linear velocity. The sperm motility parameters derived from computer-assisted sperm analysis can only detect gross abnormalities, as they provide average values for all sperm in the specimen rather than values derived from identifiable sperm subpopulations.

7 The second line of sperm tests is those probing for specific functions, including testicular biopsy to assess spermatogenesis, antisperm antibodies in the husband and wife, extended sperm morphology and visualization of the acrosomal cap, acrosine activity, supravital staining tests to probe membrane integrity in the head and tail of sperm, oocyte binding, and the human sperm–hamster zona-free oocyte penetration assay.

8 We have discovered a new approach in testing fertilizing potential of spermatozoa by the measurement of sperm creatine kinase activity and CK-M isoform concentrations. It is unlikely that the presence or absence of CK-M isoform directly affects fertilizing potential; rather we believe that the appearance of the CK-M signifies sperm cellular maturation and the synthesis of various new proteins that are necessary for the sperm in order to attain fertilizing capacity. The data so far indicate that semen samples with <10% sperm CK-M (expressed as %CK-M/CK-M + CK-B) are associated with a low likelihood for fertility independently from the sperm concentrations [6]. Thus, the sperm CK-M concentration measurements for the first time also provide an approach to detect unexplained male infertility.

9 Because historically the medical or surgical treatment of subfertile/infertile men has not been successful

Table 91.1 Male factor subfertility

Overt male factor: normal volume−low sperm concentration, low volume−normal sperm concentrations.

Suspicion of male factor: reduced but steady sperm motility, sperm concentrations in the 20−30 million/ml range (variable-spermic).

Unexplained male infertilty: incidence (role of sperm CK-M determinations).

Presently limited therapeutic reach: asthenospermia (or short survival of sperm motility), nonendocrine azoospermia.

How to approach the problem? Men doctor or sperm doctor?

Confirm	Other diagnostic factors	Tests of physiologic and medical significance	Targeted tests	Treatment
Repeat SA (2−3 weeks later); abstinence time; not only concentration but also volume and motility Total motile, normal sperm in the ejaculate	Medical history: age Reproductive history; (pregnancy caused); Occupation: (change?); Endocrine: FSH−LH−Testosterone Toxic exposure Fever heat Infections Drugs Pharmaceuticals	Motile sperm yield; survival of motility; linear velocity Significance of CASA? (mean values only) *In vitro* mucus−sperm interaction; not PCT Testicular biopsy: don't overlook female factor	Antibodies (reduction of fertilizing potential and/or motility) Extended morphology: acrosomal cap; acrosine HOS−supravital stain (nonmotile vital sperm) SPA−hemizona: correlation to IVF? Demonstrate fertility (or lack of it) CK-activity CK-M concentrations: predict sperm; fertilizing potential	Better utilization insemination: cervical; uterine; tubal IVF (not GIFT!): SUZI; micro manipulation Donor insemination

---

CASA, computer assisted semen analysis; HOS, hypoosmotic swelling test; PCT, postcoital test; SPA, sperm penetration assay.

we are increasingly focusing upon better utilization of the sperm that exist in subfertile ejaculates. Within this approach we seek: (1) the determination of the fertilization potential or the lack of fertilization potential with objective biochemical sperm markers; (2) correction of sperm function defects (e.g., *in vitro* potentiation of acrosomal reaction, motility, etc.); and (3) more efficient utilization of the existing sperm in various assisted reproductive technologies.

10 Upon assessment of various parameters of sperm function and fertilizing potential and depending upon the total motile sperm available, therapy should be initiated with the appropriate modality of assisted reproduction. With at least 3 million motile sperm in the specimen the choice is intrauterine or intratubal insemination, whereas with lower total motile sperm concentrations, *in vitro* fertilization should be chosen. The techniques of enhanced *in vitro* fertilization such as SUZI for nonpenetrating sperm or micromanipulation for immotile sperm are presently considered to be experimental procedures. Gamete intrafallopian transfer is always inappropriate in couples with male factor infertility because if pregnancy does not occur this approach fails to provide essential information about fertilization.

11 The specialist may not be able to assist the couple with male factor infertility to achieve pregnancy, but it is his/her paramount duty to insure that good

information is generated toward a timely and well-thought-out decision between adoption and donor insemination if the couple desire to raise a child.

ACKNOWLEDGMENTS

The contribution by Mrs Susan Augir in editing the manuscript is greatly appreciated.

REFERENCE

1 World Health Organization. *WHO Laboratory Manual for the Examination of Human Semen and Semen–Cervical Mucus Interaction*, 2nd edn. Cambridge: Cambridge University Press, 1987.

2 Makler A, Murrillo O, Huszar G, DeCherney AH. Improved techniques for collecting motile spermatozoa from human semen. I. A self-migratory method. *Int J Androl* 1984; 7: 71–78.

3 Zanavelo LJD, Jeyendran RS. Biochemical analysis of seminal plasma and spermatoza. In: Keel BA, Webster BW, eds. *Handbook of the Laboratory Diagnosis and Treatment of Infertility*. Boca Raton: CRC Press, 1990.

4 Huszar G, Vigue L, Corrales M. Sperm creatine kinase activity in fertile and infertile oligospermic men. *J Androl* 1990; 11: 40–46.

5 Huszar G, Vigue L. Spermatogenesis related change in the synthesis of the creatine kinase B-type and M-type isoforms in human spermatozoa. *Mol Reprod Dev* 1990; 25: 258–262.

6 Huszar G, Vique L, Morshadi M. Sperm creatine phospholignase M-isoform ratios and fertilizing potential of men: A blind study of 84 couples treated with *in vitro* fertilization. *Fertil Steril* 1992; 57: 882–888.

7 Silber S, Cohen R. Simultaneous treatment of the wife in infertile couples with oligospermia. *Fertil Steril* 1983; 40: 505–511.

8 Huszar G, DeCherney A. The role of intrauterine insemination in the treatment of infertile couples: the Yale experience. *Semin Reprod Endocrinol* 1987; 5: 11–21.

Abnormal sperm motility

PETER N. SCHLEGEL

INTRODUCTION

Evaluation of the infertile man should include a carefully performed history and physical examination, laboratory evaluation of endocrine function, and a complete semen analysis. History and physical examination alone will result in a presumptive diagnosis for the cause of infertility in over 90% of men in our practice. Endocrine function tests (serum luteinizing hormone (LH), follicle-stimulating hormone (FSH), testosterone and 17β-estradiol levels) are used to quantify the performance of the hypothalamic—pituitary—gonadal axis in men. Semen analysis results provide the best individual parameter to predict the likelihood of a man fathering a child.

The semen analysis should be repeated with separate specimens over a period of at least 2 months. We agree with many andrologists that a single *normal* semen analysis is adequate to evaluate fertility potential for most men. However, fertility is defined by the presence or absence of children in a relationship, not the likelihood of fathering a child in the future. So, despite having a low fertility potential, a man may still be considered fertile. Similarly, a man considered to have normal fertility potential may not father a child by chance or other confounding (including female) factors. Therefore, a semen analysis evaluation does not automatically categorize an individual as fertile or infertile, despite the semen parameters. Rather, an abnormal semen analysis provides the clinician with the indication that it may be necessary to intervene for an individual patient to improve his chances to contribute to a pregnancy.

Many additional laboratory methods for evaluating sperm function have been proposed, including hamster zona-free oocyte penetration assay, computerized sperm motion analysis, biochemical evaluations (adenosine triphosphate and acrosin content), hypoosmotic swelling test, flow cytometry, and the human hemizona attachment assay. However, these additional and sometimes expensive tests have not yet been proven to be of value in guiding the clinician in the management of the infertile man. The evaluation of sperm motility may be quantified by computer-assisted sperm analysis (CASA); however, routine clinical use of CASA is not currently of value in the evaluation of infertile men. The evaluation of men with a suspected immunologic cause of infertility may be aided by assays for antisperm antibodies. Our experience is that a carefully performed history and physical examination with endocrine testing and semen analysis provide adequate information to allow delineation of the likely etiology of male factor infertility and to direct initial therapy.

SPERM MOTILITY

Sperm motility is defined both by the percentage of sperm that are motile as well as the quality of forward progression of sperm [1]. Criteria for normal motility have ranged from 30 to 85% of sperm in the ejaculate. We have used 50% of motile sperm in the ejaculate as our lower value for a normal semen analysis with forward progression of 2 on a scale of 1—4 (Table 92.1). Early results from several *in vitro* fertilization (IVF) centers indicated that sperm motility (and sperm concentration) was a good indicator of the likelihood of fertilization for a semen specimen [2]. Subsequent evaluations have shown that although sperm motility is not as good a predictive criterion of fertility potential as strict criteria morphology determinations [3], impaired sperm motility in a semen analysis (asthenospermia) may provide a sensitive clue to the presence of varicocele, immunologic factors, infection, toxic agents, epididymal dysfunction, or structural sperm tail defects that may impair fertility.

Collection and processing of semen specimens
Unfortunately, sperm motility is easily affected by

Table 92.1 Grading of motility (forward progression)

Forward progression	Description
0	No motility
1	Poor motility
2	Fair motility
3	Good forward progression
4	Excellent forward progression

Table 92.2 Potential technical factors that may impair apparent sperm motility during semen analysis

Excessive delay between production and delivery of speciment to semen analysis laboratory

Excessive heating or cooling of specimen during transport to laboratory

Contamination of specimen with K-Y jelly or soap during masturbation

Use of condoms containing contraceptive agents

Use of a container toxic to sperm (or containing traces of toxic agents, i.e., prescription drug containers)

Excessive delay at laboratory in examining specimens

a number of factors related to the collection and analysis of a semen specimen (Table 92.2). Semen specimens for analysis should be collected after 2–3 days of abstinence in a sterile container that has been previously evaluated and found not to affect the motility of normal sperm. Complete specimen collection should be stressed to the patient, with avoidance of contamination by soap, K-Y jelly, or other agents used during masturbation. The specimen should preferably be produced in a room reserved for that purpose at the laboratory. If necessary, the specimen may be transported to the laboratory within 1 hour of ejaculation, with the specimen maintained as close to body temperature as possible (e.g., in the inner pocket of a coat). Some plasticizers may affect sperm motility, so the patient should be encouraged to use the standard container tested by the laboratory [4]. After analysis of a first specimen, the importance of following the specific guidelines needed for semen collection should be reemphasized to the patient.

Some men are unable to produce a semen specimen by masturbation because of psychologic or religious reasons. In these cases, the man should use a silastic condom specially designed for collection of semen during intercourse without adversely affecting sperm quality.

After potential confounding causes of falsely decreased sperm motility in a semen specimen have been eliminated, the finding of decreased motility should be evaluated in view of the other semen parameters [5] (Fig. 92.1). This allows for an important distinction between isolated impairment of sperm motility and a finding of impaired motility in conjunction with low sperm concentration and abnormal sperm morphology, the oligoasthenoteratozoospermia (OAT) syndrome.

Multiple defects on semen analysis
Most commonly, impaired sperm motility is seen in conjunction with other semen abnormalities. As previously discussed, treatable causes of testicular

dysfunction should be addressed. The prognosis for recoverability of function may be additionally assessed in these patients based on serum levels of FSH, as well as the size and consistency of the testes. A man with small (<10 ml), soft testes, an FSH greater than three times the upper limit of normal, and no correctable cause for infertility, has virtually no chance of contributing to a pregnancy and should be counseled regarding adoption and donor insemination. Potential treatments for other patients with a globally impaired semen analysis, including nonspecific medical therapy and sperm separation techniques, are discussed in the last section of this chapter.

Impaired motility and necrospermia
Patients found to have isolated defects in sperm motility should also be evaluated to determine whether the sperm are viable, or if they are predominantly dead (necrospermic). Necrospermic specimens may result if the semen is contaminated with urine, if overwhelming infection is present, and in some patients affected by toxins. The presence of infection is evaluated by determining the number of white blood cells (WBC) present. If elevated (>3 WBC/sperm or >10^6 WBC/ml), then semen culture should be performed and specific therapy given for any pathogens isolated. "Shotgun" antibiotic therapy of men is discouraged because of the potential detrimental fertility effects of some antibiotics in the absence of specific indications for therapy [6].

Contamination of semen with urine is uncommon and may be difficult to diagnose. It is occasionally found in some patients with diabetes. For these patients, neurologic dysfunction may cause poor bladder neck closure during ejaculation, resulting

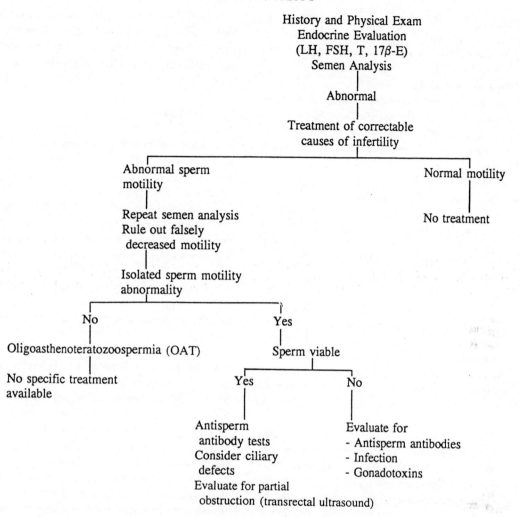

Fig. 92.1 Algorithm for management of men with abnormal sperm motility. (From [5].)

in retrograde ejaculation or an ejaculate partially containing urine. This condition may be associated with increased semen volume and decreased semen pH with otherwise unexplained poor sperm motility. These patients may be treated by alkalinizing the urine with Polycitra 20 ml four times a day starting the night before the specimen is produced. The man should empty his bladder just prior to masturbation and catheterization may be necessary if significant retrograde ejaculation occurs.

Most gonadotoxins will decrease spermatogenesis and decrease sperm counts as well as affecting sperm motility. However, some agents such as gossypol, the agent derived from cottonseed oil and used as an antifertility agent in China, may affect epididymal function without preventing sperm production, resulting in poor sperm motility.

Impaired motility and live sperm

Impaired sperm motility with live sperm may be associated with antisperm antibodies, infection, caused by defects in the sperm tail or abnormalities in sperm biochemistry. Abnormal sperm motility may also be associated with partial obstruction of the reproductive tract. Transrectal ultrasound may be useful to evaluate this possibility, most commonly found to be ejaculatory duct. The presence of sperm clumping (agglutination) in the semen specimen may be associated with immobilizing antisperm antibodies, or infection. For patients with impaired sperm motility, agglutination and elevated semen levels of antisperm antibodies, an immunologic cause of infertility should be suspected. These patients often have an improvement in sperm function that parallels a decrease in semen antisperm antibodies.

Isolated total lack of sperm motility, with viable sperm, strongly suggests the presence of sperm tail function abnormalities — the immotile cilia syndrome.

Antisperm antibodies

We use the immunobead test to evaluate for antisperm antibodies. Some sperm motility should be present in order to evaluate whether the beads are attached to sperm or merely overlying sperm in the immunobead test. Binding to greater than 10% of sperm by beads is considered a positive result, and if associated with infertility, is an indication for treatment. The advantages of the immunobead test include the ability to differentiate immunoglobulin (Ig) subtypes (IgM, IgG, IgA) present on sperm and to determine the location of antisperm antibodies on the sperm.

Optimal treatment for antisperm antibodies in men is controversial, because of the potential adverse effects of treatment with high-dose corticosteroids. Case reports of aseptic necrosis of the hip, as well as the known adverse effects of prednisone treatment on ulcer disease, have persuaded some clinicians to avoid corticosteroid treatment for infertile men. Alternative treatment involves referral of men with infertility associated with antisperm antibodies for IVF.

We have encountered no significant adverse effects of corticosteroid treatment for infertile men using low-dose intermittent therapy. Previous reports of adverse effects are associated with long-term high-dose corticosteroid treatment schedules. Men who are candidates for treatment are given 20 mg of prednisone daily for 1 week starting on the 21st day after the start of the wife's menstrual cycle. The maximum benefit of treatment is then achieved at the time of ovulation. Patients are followed with repeat semen analyses and immunobead tests every 3 months and the prednisone dose is titrated upward to a maximum of 60 mg/day for 7 days a month, until pregnancy, improvement in semen analysis, or reduction in antisperm antibody levels is noted. Although some investigators have suggested that corticosteroid therapy is indicated only under investigational review board approval, we feel that it is appropriate to treat these men with low-dose intermittent corticosteroids after providing detailed informed consent to the patient.

Infertile men with varicocele have a higher prevalence of antisperm antibodies than infertile men without varicocele. In our experience, microsurgical varicocelectomy is highly effective in eliminating these antibodies. Unilateral vasal, epididymal, or ejaculatory duct obstruction is also associated with high levels of antibodies against sperm surface antigens. When feasible, repair of obstruction may be indicated, since it should result in decreased antibody levels.

Sperm tail defects

A defect in ciliary function may be suspected if there is a history of bronchitis or sinusitis with impaired sperm motility. The best recognized clinical presentation involving these defects is Kartagener's syndrome. Kartagener's syndrome consists of situs inversus, chronic sinusitis, and bronchiectasis. These abnormalities are attributed to an absence in the dynein arms from the nine microtubular filament couplets in the axoneme complex of the sperm tail. The lack of dynein arms leads to the nonmotile condition of the sperm and appears to be associated with the immotility of cilia in the bronchial tree, as well as the rotational abnormalities that result in situs inversus.

Not all patients with the immotile cilia syndrome have all manifestations of Kartagener's syndrome. Some may have only minor defects of the spokes of dynein arms, absence of central microtubules, or a complete absence of the dynein arms, as occurs in Kartagener's syndrome. Therefore, the range of abnormalities in ciliary defects and associated clinical syndromes is wide. Ciliary dysfunction may present as tail-shaking or movement without purposeful action. Investigators of respiratory and other mucociliary clearance functions now commonly refer to these patients as having ciliary dyskinesia. This condition is thought to be rare, with a prevalence of less than one in 20 000 [7]. The association between chronic sinus or bronchial disease and nonmotile sperm should lead the clinician to suspect a ciliary defect. The diagnosis is made with ultrastructural studies of sperm by electron microscopy. Until recently, no treatment has been available to allow these patients to have children except artificial insemination or adoption. Advances in micromanipulation of eggs as part of IVF has allowed the subzonal insertion of nonmotile sperm and subsequent fertilization of those eggs, allowing implantation, pregnancies, and live births.

Young's syndrome (epididymal obstruction associated with chronic sinopulmonary infections) usually presents with azoospermia. The epididymal obstruction is associated with sludging of viscous fluid in the epididymal tubules. This syndrome is not associated with a primary defect in sperm tail function, but rather with altered sperm transport through the epididymis. Since the spermatozoa proximal to the obstruction are motile, these patients may be treated with vasoepididymostomy, usually to the caput region of the epididymis. Micropuncture aspiration of sperm from the epididymis in conjunction with IVF may also be effective for these men.

Sperm biochemical defects

Another alteration in sperm motility has been attributed to a defect in protein carboxyl-methylase (PCM) activity, an enzyme associated with chemotaxis in bacteria. Some researchers of protein carboxyl-methylase disagree with the purported action of this enzyme system as a mediator of mammalian sperm motility. It is possible that the level of biochemical enzymes, such as PCM, in semen may reflect the overall health of a population of sperm, rather than a specific cause of defective sperm motility. In some cases where no specific diagnosis can be reached, and an isolated lack of sperm motility is present, a defect in sperm biochemistry may be postulated. IVF is a possible therapeutic intervention for these patients. The male offspring obtained from IVF with sperm carrying a biochemical defect would probably be heterozygous for this defect, and should demonstrate no clinical stigmata of the defect, although this cannot be prospectively determined for certain.

EMPIRIC TREATMENT FOR IMPAIRED SPERM MOTILITY

Medical treatment

Several medical treatments have been proposed for the management of impaired sperm motility as well as oligospermia. These treatments include systemic administration of agents known to be associated with increased sperm motility *in vitro*, such as kallikrein and caffeine, as well as the phosphodiesterase inhibitor, pentoxifylline. These agents, as well as drugs with endocrinologic action such as clomiphene citrate, have not consistently demonstrated a significant increase in semen parameters or pregnancy rates [8]. Therefore, we do not currently advocate the non-specific medical treatment of patients with impaired sperm motility.

Topically administered caffeine, pentoxifylline, theophylline, carnitine and acetylcarnitine, arginine, cyclic adenosine monophosphate and kallikrein have all been shown in some cases to increase sperm motility. However, it is not well documented that the increase in motility is then translated into increased fertilization rates with these sperm. It is possible that some of these agents merely simulate the activation process of sperm that normally occurs within the female reproductive tract rather than changing the fertilizing potential of sperm. Others have cautioned against the topical use of methyl xanthines on sperm because methyl xanthines have a known teratogenic action in animals. This teratogenicity has not been demonstrated in humans. We do not advocate topical treatment of sperm to enhance sperm motility artificially until this intervention is shown to translate into improved fertilization and pregnancy rates.

Sperm motility selection techniques

Impaired sperm motility in a semen specimen (in the absence of a specific structural or biochemical defect) is reflective of poor fertilizing capacity. However, within the entire semen specimen there may be some spermatozoa with normal or near-normal fertilizing capability. The action of these sperm can be affected by dead or dying sperm and other contaminants within the seminal fluid. One mediator of the adverse action of dying sperm has been proposed to be reactive oxygen species. Reactive oxygen species have been shown to be highly toxic to spermatozoa. In the normal semen specimen, 70% of reactive oxygen species are released from leukocytes, with the remainder derived from spermatozoa. If many sperm are dead or dying, then release of reactive oxygen may be increased, affecting "normal" sperm. The concept behind sperm motility selection techniques is to separate the live (and motile) sperm from contaminants and dead sperm. Separation techniques utilize either the ability of motile sperm to swim away and isolate themselves from nonmotile sperm (swim-up or swim-down), differential sedimentation velocities of leukocytes, motile and nonmotile sperm (Percoll or iohexol gradient centrifugation), the predilection of dead and dying sperm to adhere to glass (glass-wool or glass bead column filtration), or the ability of motile sperm to avoid precipitation (sedimentation techniques). Sedimentation techniques may have the advantage of applicability to small-volume preparations of sperm, such as the microdroplets used by some IVF groups (J. Cohen, personal communication, 1991) [9]. All sperm selection techniques result in a variable quantitative loss of spermatozoa. Sperm washing (centrifugation with removal of supernatant) is usually performed prior to the above separation techniques and is necessary to remove prostaglandins, bacteria and other contaminants from semen prior to intrauterine insemination or IVF.

Intrauterine insemination and IVF

Both intrauterine insemination and IVF have been proposed as therapies for male factor infertility, including OAT. Prior to referral of a patient for these procedures, all correctable factors contributing to male infertility should be identified and addressed. Still, the overall results with intrauterine insemination and IVF for male factor infertility have not been very encouraging. We previously suggested intrauterine insemination for men with OAT, timed with the LH surge or in conjunction with ovulation stimulation. No more than three or four cycles of intrauterine insemination are recommended, as virtually all pregnancies are achieved before the fourth cycle in most series using this treatment.

We currently advocate referring men with impaired sperm motility or oligospermia (after optimizing the man's fertility potential) for IVF with assisted reproductive techniques. Subzonal insertion of sperm and partial zona dissection have been found by the Cornell IVF group significantly to increase fertilization rates for couples with male factor infertility. Unfortunately, failure of implantation is common for these embryos. This may be due in part to polyspermy, since the zona pellucida block to multiple fertilizations is bypassed with these techniques. The effect of assisted reproduction on pregnancy rates for male factor couples is yet to be fully delineated. It

is attractive to consider that a minimal number of selected spermatozoa derived from a patient with a poor semen analysis, previously thought to have no chance of fertility, may contribute to pregnancy with the use of assisted reproduction techniques.

REFERENCES

1 Amelar RD, Dubin L, Schoenfeld C. Sperm motility. *Fertil Steril* 1980; 34: 197–215.
2 Mahaderan MM, Trounsen A. The influence of seminal characteristics on the success rate of *in vitro* fertilization. *Fertil Steril* 1984; 42: 400.
3 Kruger TF, Acosta AA, Simmons KF, Swanson RJ, Matta JF, Oehninger S. Predictive value of abnormal sperm morphology in *in vitro* fertilization. *Fertil Steril* 1988; 49: 112–117.
4 Gagnon C ed. *Controls of Sperm Motility: Biological and Clinical Aspects*. Boca Raton: CRC Press, 1990.
5 Schlegel PN, Goldstein M. Abnormal sperm morphology and motility. In: Resnick MI, ed. *Current Therapy in Genitourinary Surgery*, 2nd ed. Philadelphia: BC Decker, 1991: 558–562.
6 Schlegel PN, Chang TSK, Marshall FF. Antibiotics: potential hazards to male fertility. *Fertil Steril* 1991; 55.
7 Boat TF, Carson JL. Ciliary dysmorphology and dysfunction — primary or acquired? *N Engl J Med* 1990; 323: 1700–1702.
8 Sigman M, Vance ML. Medical treatment of idiopathic infertility. *Urol Clin North Am* 1987; 14: 459–469.
9 Cohen J, Edwards R, Fehilly C *et al*. *In vitro* fertilization: a treatment for male infertility. *Fertil Steril* 1985; 43: 422–432.

Abnormal sperm morphology

CHARLES C. CODDINGTON

During evaluation of couples for fertility-related problems, analysis of semen should be performed, since at least 40% of the fertility problems can be related to the male [1]. Many different factors can alter or in some way impair male fertility. However, one of the most important parameters which can be measured related to fertility potential is sperm morphology, which is related to the shape of the acrosome or sperm head [2]. Morphology is particularly important, since it may affect the ability of the sperm to penetrate the cervical mucus, or the acrosome may be altered such that they cannot bind an oocyte or penetrate it properly.

Abnormal sperm morphology can be determined by at least two methods. One is the method described in the World Health Organization (WHO) manual [3] in which the sperm are evaluated with up to 200 counted in the hope that more than 50% have an oval form. This would be considered normal.

Another method utilizes exact measurements of the sperm [4]. Those which have an oval form, a smooth contour, and an acrosome comprising 40–70% of the distal part of the head, without any abnormalities from the neck, midpiece or tail, and with no cytoplasmic droplets of more than half of the sperm head, as described by Eliasson [5] and Menkveld and Kruger [6], would be considered normal. This type of specific measurement of sperm morphology has a lower limit of 14% normal forms. Confusion can occur if one is not clear which method is being utilized in the evaluating laboratory. However, the second method has been studied in conjunction with *in vitro* fertilization which led to a cutoff of 14% or greater normal forms, representing normal functional morphology range. Further studies suggest that there is a poor prognosis group below 4% normal morphology, as there were no pregnancies in this group [7]. In summary, poor morphology may mean a poor reproductive outcome.

In examining the initial screening results, one should try and explain what has occurred and if this result is consistent. Consideration should be given to repeating the semen analysis at least once and possibly twice. A thorough history and physical exam should be performed in an evaluation of abnormal sperm morphology. Historical aspects should focus on medications, including the possibility of drug abuse and other stressful activities (Table 93.1) [8]. Physical examination will help clarify abnormalities such as undescended testes, atrophic testes, or varicocele. All may lead to abnormal sperm parameters, including morphology. Furthermore, this examination may be helpful in determining acute infectious diseases which can affect the entire genital tract. Cultures for gonorrhea, *Chlamydia*, or *Ureaplasma* should be considered. Sperm penetration assays (SPAs) may not be as predictive when one is evaluating sperm with abnormal morphology because the SPA is performed on oocytes of hamsters which have had the zona pellucida removed. The absence of the zona may eliminate a functional barrier and thus sperm function may be reported as normal when in fact the sperm are not able to bind to the zona. Poor binding to the zona pellucida by sperm with abnormal morphology has been confirmed in the hemizona assay, a functional assay of sperm–zona interaction [9].

Table 93.1 Drugs which may affect spermiogenesis. (From [8])

Alcohol
Nitrofurantoin
Sulfa drugs
Sulfasalazine
Amebicides
Halogenated hydrocarbons
Marijuana
Cimetidine
Nicotine
Anabolic steroids

Lack of abstinence may play a significant role in lower morphology and other semen parameters as well. However, the effect of less frequent coitus in itself may have no impact. Since improvement may occur merely by changing coital frequency, one should consider this step before making an absolute diagnosis [6]. Hot seasons and heat-producing activity may also alter the true measurement of morphologically normal forms. Temperature of the testes may also be affected by clothes which compress these organs close to the body and thus raise the intratesticular temperature, as well as activities such as hot tub baths. These clothes and/or activities can be altered and the semen parameters can be repeated after 75 days to allow full benefit of the change in activity to occur, if any.

Occupational environment may also play a role, since exposure to various chemicals or compounds may increase the chance of occurrence or poor sperm morphology. As noted in one study, exposure to lead causes changes in all semen parameters [10]. Investigations of exposure to dibutyl phthalate in truck drivers may also have altered parameters of semen [11,12]. It is hard to alter environments or occupations, but it sometimes can be accomplished if the individual can see the benefits of doing so.

Severe physical stress such as illness may play a role in poor semen quality, including morphology. Even minor illnesses such as the common cold, influenza, or other apparent minor illness may cause an effect [6]. It is no surprise that more severe diseases such as severe viral infections, chicken pox, or pneumonia may alter sperm morphology [13]. These changes are hopefully short-lived and the evaluation of semen can be performed 3 months afterwards to determine what the semen parameters may be without the effect of the acute event. Mumps orchitis may cause irreversible changes in sperm morphology.

Treatment is not clearly defined for the difficult problem of abnormal morphology. Most importantly,

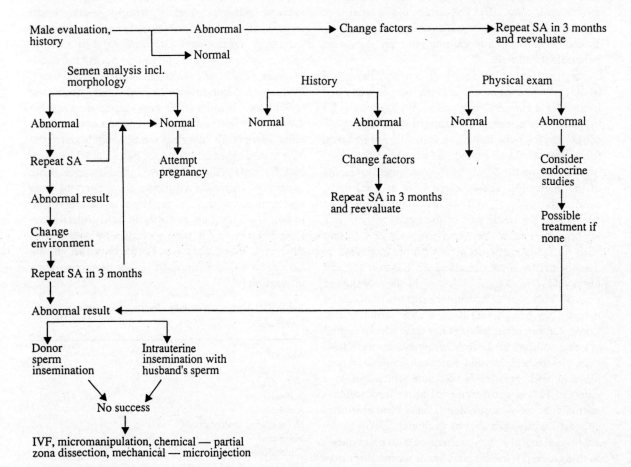

Fig. 93.1 Treatment for patients with abnormal sperm morphology.

environmental stress, clothes, drugs, or occupation should be altered to maximize the benefit of this change on semen parameters, including morphology. One should allow at least 75 days for the total effect to clear the system and even as much as 90 days in some cases before a repeat test is a true representation of semen quality. Once the confirmation is made, the alternatives described in Figure 93.1 are available. If one chooses not to be observed for the condition of abnormal sperm morphology, intrauterine insemination may be tried. The sperm may be prepared by standard washing techniques in Hams F10 with or without a swim-up [14]. This will improve the sperm morphology in the intrauterine insemination specimen, but timing is one of the most critical factors in success with this technique. Various methods of ovulation monitoring may be helpful. Use of donor sperm is another alternative which may be acceptable in the treatment of severe abnormal morphology. Assisted reproductive technology may aid couples in attaining their goals. Using increased sperm numbers in the *in vitro* fertilization incubation will have a result of increased fertilizations [14]. New techniques such as microinjection of sperm into the egg and dissection of the outer covering of the egg have had successful fertilizations, but to date very few have not been successful in producing a term pregnancy. However, utilizing these methods and others being developed, it is hoped a more improved outcome can be offered to individuals with poor sperm morphology.

REFERENCES

1 Glass R. Infertility. In: Yen SSC, Jaffe RB, eds. *Reproductive Endocrinology*, 3rd edn. Philadelphia: WB Saunders, 1991: 689−709.

2 Yanagimachi R. Mammalian fertilization. In: Knobil E, Neill J, eds. *The Physiology of Reproduction*. New York: Raven Press, 1988: 135−185.

3 World Health Organization. *Laboratory Manual for the Examination of Human Semen and Semen−Cervical Mucus Interaction*, 2nd edn. New York: Cambridge University Press, 1987.

4 Kruger TF, Menkveld R, Stander FSH *et al*. Sperm morphologic features as a prognostic factor in *in vitro* fertilization. *Fertil Steril* 1986; 46: 1118.

5 Eliasson R. Standards for investigation of human semen. *Andrologia* 1971; 3: 49.

6 Menkveld R, Kruger TF. Basic semen analysis in human spermatozoa. In: Acosta A, Swanson R, Ackerman S, Kruger T, Van Zyl J, Menkveld R, eds. *Assisted Reproduction*. Baltimore: Williams & Wilkins, 1990: 164−176.

7 Kruger TF, Acosta A, Menkveld R, Oehninger S. Basic semen analysis: clinical importance of morphology. In: Acosta A, Swanson R, Ackerman S, Kruger T, Van Zyl J, Menkveld R, eds. *Assisted Reproduction*. Baltimore: Williams & Wilkins, 1990: 176−181.

8 Male Infertility. ACOG Technical Bulletin. June 1990, No. 142: 1−8.

9 Burkman LT, Coddington CC, Franken DR, Kruger T, Rosenwaks Z, Hodgen G. The hemizona assay (HZA): development of a diagnostic test for the binding of human spermatozoa to the human hemizona pellucida to predict fertilization potential. *Fertil Steril* 1988; 49: 688−697.

10 Lancranjan I, Popescu HI, Gavonescu O, Kepsch I, Serbanescu M. Reproductive ability of workmen occupationally exposed to lead. *Arch Environ Health* 1975; 30: 396.

11 Whorton JD, Meyer CR. Sperm count results from 861 American chemical/agricultural workers from 14 different studies. *Fertil Steril* 1984; 42: 82.

12 Sas M, Szollosi J. Impaired spermiogenesis as a common finding among professional drivers. *Arch Androl* 1979; 3: 57.

13 MacLeod J. Effect of chicken pox and of pneumonia on semen quality. *Fertil Steril* 1951; 2: 523.

14 Kruger TF, Menkveld R, Scott R, Jeyendron R, Zanfeld L, Windt M. Spermatozoa motile fraction separation. In: Acosta A, Swanson R, Ackerman S, Kruger T, Van Zyl T, Mekveld R, eds. *Assisted Reproduction*. Baltimore: Williams & Wilkins, 1990: 181−185.

94

Sperm penetration assay

MICHAEL J. ZINAMAN

The sperm penetration assay (SPA), first described in 1976 [1], represents a valuable adjunctive aid for the clinician in determining male fertility potential. The test, using eggs obtained from hamsters mixed with human sperm, is also referred to as the hamster or humster test.

The need for the SPA to supplement the more routine semen analysis has been apparent since the 1950s' pioneering work of McLeod and Gold [2]. It was through their findings, and subsequently others, that the limitations of the semen analysis were clarified. Overlap of almost all semen parameters, between groups of fertile and infertile men, hampered the ability to manage the infertile couple. As our understanding of gamete biology has increased, so has the ability to put sperm "to the test," allowing us to increase our diagnostic and prognostic acumen.

This chapter will attempt to inform readers about the SPA sufficiently to allow them to use the test appropriately in the management of the infertile couple. The interpretation of an abnormal test can then be appreciated, enabling the clinician to better counsel the patient.

In the normal physiology of reproduction, human sperm need to exit seminal plasma, enter the cervical mucus en route to the fallopian tube, penetrate the cumulus mass of granulosa cells surrounding the oocyte, bind to the zona pellucida, undergo the acrosome reaction, penetrate the zona pellucida, and finally fuse the membrane with that of the oocyte [3]. This long journey requires two fundamental processes. The first is motility, (see Chapter 92) which is not the subject of this chapter, and the second are those membrane changes which are initiated upon entry into the cervical mucus and completed with fusion to the egg. These changes are referred to as capacitation.

As seen in Figure 94.1, the sperm head is composed of outer and inner membranes. When sperm leave seminal plasma these membranes, in a process of capacitation, begin to change. Capacitation basically refers to a poorly understood series of events that occur within the outer plasma and acrosomal membranes. The acrosome reaction, which is the culmination of capacitation, refers to the loss of these two outer membranes and the release of the acrosomal contents. These contents help to digest the oocyte's vestments and allow the sperm to penetrate the zona pellucida. The inner acrosomal membrane, which binds directly to the oocyte, is now exposed for fusion.

Much of this information has become available to us through research employing animal systems. While the use of heterologous gametes (gametes of

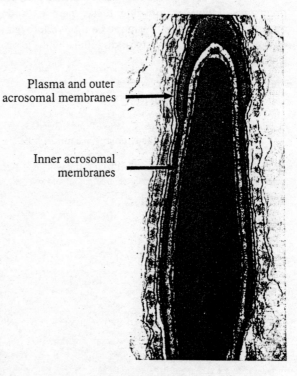

Plasma and outer acrosomal membranes

Inner acrosomal membranes

Fig. 94.1 Electron micrograph of sperm head.

different species) of an animal in a research setting is not new, it was not until 1976 that human sperm were shown to be able to penetrate a hamster oocyte whose zona pellucida had been previously removed.

As the SPA measures the ability of human sperm to fuse their inner acrosomal membranes with the membranes of zona-free hamster oocytes it was felt that it could become a useful test of sperm function. This idea led to a series of research publications evaluating its use as a clinical test. The functions that are ascertained are those of a sperm population's ability to complete the process of capacitation, including the acrosome reaction. In addition, the now exposed inner acrosomal membrane must fuse to the oocyte membrane, thereby gaining entry into the egg itself with release of its nuclear (chromosomal) material [4].

The performance of the SPA requires two basic sets of preparations involving eggs and sperm. Obtaining the zona-free eggs and capacitated sperm will be briefly described, along with some of the possible associated sources of laboratory variability.

Immature hamsters are superovulated and after sacrificing the animals the cumulus masses containing the oocytes are removed. The granulosa—cumulus mass of cells are digested away in the first enzymatic step, freeing the intact oocytes. The second enzymatic step removes the zona pellucida and is easily subject to error. Overdigestion can lead to partial loss of the oocyte membrane, allowing unimpeded penetration and defeating the test. Conversely, underdigestion of the zona pellucida can impede all penetration. Preparation of the sperm is equally critical. After being washed free of seminal plasma, sperm are incubated for a fixed period of time in a protein-containing (capacitating) media. A known number (usually several million motile) of sperm are then placed with some 25—30 zona-free hamster oocytes and the percentage of zona-free eggs penetrated by sperm are determined. Capacitation itself is a variable process dependent upon the sperm themselves, their handling, incubating conditions, and time. As the SPA is an attempt to assess the adequacy of this process, the latter three need to be tightly controlled and, most importantly, standardized for each laboratory.

These issues are to be stressed as the performance of the SPA is far more complex than almost any "routine" fertility test. The laboratory is of the utmost importance both for its methods as well as for its ability to have a sufficient inhouse database

to have analyzed the implications of its results. Therefore, commercial laboratories, lacking the ability to track patient outcome, should generally be avoided. The laboratory will almost always run known controls with the patient's specimens to bring to light any problems with its methods. The control values should be reported alongside those of the patient. The clinician is encouraged to speak with the laboratory director to familiarize him/herself with their procedures [5].

There are several situations which are encountered in the work-up of the infertile couple where the SPA can be of help. The first is when the semen analysis fails to reveal the presence of lesions in spermatogenesis and sperm maturation and other significant female-related infertility factors are absent. This is often referred to as unexplained infertility. The second situation could occur where the results of repeated semen analyses are subnormal, but not severely so. The overlap of parameters with those of fertile men then leaves the clinician in need of far more information to better determine the relative significance of the findings. In both of these settings the investigation has generally not yielded a sufficient basis to entirely explain the lack of conception.

There are other more specialized settings in which the SPA can also be useful. The findings of anti-sperm antibodies can also impair fertilization, especially when directed against the head of the sperm. The significance of such findings or changes related to treatment can be assessed with the SPA. In the realm of assisted reproduction, including *in vitro* fertilization (IVF) and gamete intrafallopian transfer (GIFT) and their variations, the SPA has been found to be a possible prognostic indicator of success. Several programs have found it useful to perform the SPA prior to the attempt of such invasive procedures and use the results in patient counseling. Additionally, some investigators have used the SPA to evaluate the effect of treatments (e.g., varicocelectomy, clomiphene citrate).

Clinical evaluation of the SPA is dependent upon the existing relationships between the results obtained and the fertility status of the male partner undergoing evaluation. Therefore, one can only relate the test results to what has been published in the literature and individual experience. This serves, once again, to point out the absolute necessity of having the test performed in a reliable laboratory with sufficient expertise and standardization to relate their results to others.

CHAPTER 94

When the results of an SPA are reported as normal (e.g., >10% penetration) this can be seen as reassuring. A result of 60%, though, is not to be interpreted as "more fertile" than, say, 30%. There is no relative fertility scale and the result is either normal or abnormal. The laboratory must report its ranges with each test result. While men with normal results generally have a shorter time to conception than those with abnormal results, the actual "passing grade" only serves to point out that the patient is potentially fertile. It by no means assures one that he is of normal fertility potential. On the other hand, normal results may serve to cause the clinician to reexamine the thoroughness of the female investigation and seek out other potential factors.

The case of an abnormal SPA result (e.g., 0% penetration) is more difficult. Like almost any other test, one should look for contributing factors to explain the poor result. Infections, recent illness, as well as adherance to guidelines for abstinence and collection procedures should be considered. Additionally, inquiries about technical problems in the laboratory should be made. If no mitigating or correctable factors are found a repeat SPA should be requested. A confirmatory poor result may well represent an indication of subfertility.

When an abnormal result is clearly at hand the prognosis is certainly poor and can be of value in the understanding of a patient's problem. A deficit in the ability of the sperm to undergo capacitation and fuse their membranes appropriately is suspected. Despite this, a variety of studies have shown that these men are still potentially fertile, albeit at a reduced rate. This should not be a surprise as the SPA by no means is an exact replica of *in vivo* conditions.

Unfortunately, there is little information in the literature to guide the clinician in this setting. A review of the patient's record is clearly indicated. If no other factors are felt to be significant enough to account for the problem and the male examination does not demonstrate any other problems (e.g., varicocele), the couple can be referred to an IVF program. In this manner the couple can determine whether the defect can be overcome allowing ultimate conception. Other treatment regimens can be attempted, such as induction of ovulation with menopausal gonadotropins in conjunction with intrauterine insemination, but they are to be considered empiric. There is not good evidence to suggest that they can overcome the problem.

The SPA represents a relatively new addition to the arsenal of fertility testing. For male fertility potential it is not at all meant to replace or usurp the role of the semen analysis. Its role in the evaluation of the infertile couple today is generally for those cases of unexplained infertility and where repeated semen analyses are neither good nor bad. As the test can be expensive, costing from $200 to $400 in many centers, it is appropriate for its usage to be limited to these types of cases. The interpretation of the results, as always, depends on the clinical setting and the results of other tests. Where doubt exists, consultation with a specialist can often be helpful.

REFERENCES

1 Yanagimachi R, Yanagimachi H, Rogers BJ. The use of zona-free animal ova as a test system for the assessment of the fertilizing capacity of human spermatozoa. *Biol Reprod* 1976; 15: 471.

2 MacLeod J, Gold RZ. The male factor in fertility and infertility, II. Spermatozoon counts in 1000 cases of known fertility and in 100 cases of infertile marriage. *J Urol* 1951; 66: 436.

3 Suarez S, Pollard J. Capacitation, the acrosome reaction, and motility in mammalian sperm. In: *Controls of Sperm Motility: Biological and Clinical Aspects*. Ann Arbor: CRC Press, 1990: 77.

4 Gould J, Overstreet J, Yanagimachi H et al. What functions of the sperm cell are measured by in vitro fertilization of zona-free hamster eggs? *Fertil Steril* 1983; 40: 44.

5 Rogers BJ. The sperm penetration assay: its usefulness reevaluated. *Fertil Steril* 1985; 43: 821.

Diagnosis and treatment of varicocele in the infertile male

RANDALL B. MEACHAM

The impact of varicocele on male fertility was recognized in the 1880s when the British surgeon Banfield reported improved fertility in a patient following bilateral varicuole repair [1]. A great deal has been written over the past 40 years regarding the diagnosis and treatment of this condition in men suffering from subfertility. Some 30–40% of men evaluated for subfertility will be found to have varicoceles. In many of these men, despite the fact that they have decreased semen quality, a varicocele will be the only treatable lesion identified. Decisions regarding the proper treatment of varicocele as well as the coordination of such treatment with the management of the female partner can therefore assume great significance in the care of the infertile couple. A basic understanding of the pathophysiology and treatment of this lesion is important for physicians involved in the treatment of both male and female infertility.

ANATOMY

A varicocele is a pathologic dilation of the pampiniform plexus of veins that drain the testis. The left testis generally drains into the left renal vein via the left gonadal vein. The right gonadal vein, however, normally drains directly into the vena cava (Fig. 95.1). Both gonadal veins normally have competent valves that prevent free reflux of blood back toward the testis. It is thought that in men suffering from varicoceles, these valves are incompetent and the resultant backflow causes dilation of the plexus of veins located immediately above the testis. This collection of dilated veins is identifiable on palpation, and in cases of large varicoceles, can be visualized through the scrotal wall when the patient is in the standing position. The majority of varicoceles are unilateral and located on the left side. Isolated left-sided lesions have been reported to account for 78–93% of varicoceles [2]. Unilateral right-sided

varicoceles have been noted in 1–7% of patients with this lesion, and bilateral varicoceles have been reported in 2–20% of cases.

The predominance of left-sided varicoceles is felt to be due to the asymmetry in the venous drainage of

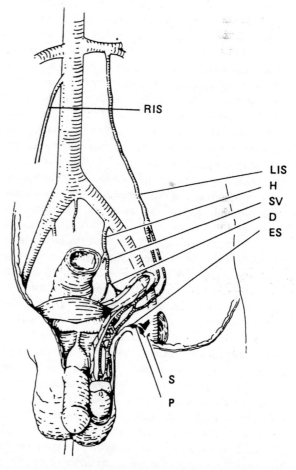

Fig. 95.1 Venous drainage of the testicle. LIS, left internal spermatic; RIS, right internal spermatic; ES, external spermatic; D, deferential; H, hypogastric; SV, superior vesical; S, saphenous; P, pudendal. (From [3].)

the two testicles, as described above. The left gonadal vein drains into the left renal vein and is 8–10 cm longer than the right gonadal vein. This longer length generates greater hydrostatic pressure within the left gonadal vein when the patient is in the upright position and contributes to the preponderance of left-sided lesions [3]. Anatomic studies have further indicated that the left gonadal vein has an absence of valves more often than does the right [3]. This finding also may help to explain the increased incidence of left-sided varicoceles.

DIAGNOSIS

Varicoceles may be associated with ipsilateral testicular pain. In such cases, the pain often is described as a dull, aching sensation located in the area of the testicle and made worse by prolonged periods of standing. Frequently, however, varicoceles are asymptomatic and are discovered only when the patient is evaluated for male factor infertility. The incidence of varicoceles in the general male population has been reported to be approximately 15% [2]. Reports describing the incidence of varicoceles among men evaluated in infertility clinics, however, indicate that the incidence of varicoceles in the subfertile population is 19–41% [4]. These data suggest that in many men the presence of a varicocele does not appear to significantly impair testicular function. The fact that the prevalence of varicocele is so much greater in the subfertile population, however, strongly supports an association between this lesion and male infertility.

The diagnosis of varicocele is generally based upon a careful physical examination. With the patient in a standing position, the scrotum is gently palpated. If present, a varicocele will be palpable within the spermatic cord just above the testis. Having the patient perform a Valsalva maneuver will increase intraabdominal pressure and make the varicocele more prominent. Varicoceles often are described according to their size. Grade 3 varicoceles are visible through the scrotal skin. Grade 2 lesions are palpable without Valsalva, and grade 1 varicoceles can only be palpated while the patient performs the Valsava maneuver. A variety of techniques have been explored to aid in the diagnosis of varicoceles. Such methods include Doppler examination, scrotal thermography, spermatic venography, radionuclide scanning, high-resolution scrotal ultrasonography and color flow Doppler ultrasonography. Although in selected cases these techniques may aid in the evaluation of men with suspected varicoceles, physical examination remains the most accepted method of diagnosing this lesion.

PATHOPHYSIOLOGY

Although the association between varicoceles and male subfertility is widely recognized, there are many theories regarding the pathophysiology of this lesion. The primary etiologic factor in testicular damage secondary to varicocele appears to be abnormal retrograde blood flow within the gonadal veins. Precisely how this damage is mediated remains a topic of research. Various authors have proposed a role for such entities as reflux of toxic renal or adrenal metabolites, altered hormonal metabolism, and testicular hyperthermia [5]. The concept that a varicocele raises testicular temperature and therefore impairs spermatogenesis is the most widely accepted explanation for the impact of varicocele on testicular function. A great deal of work remains, however, to elucidate the mechanisms of the varicocele effect.

Histologic evaluation of testis biopsies performed on patients with varicoceles has demonstrated abnormalities such as thinning and sloughing of the germinal epithelium as well as abnormalities of sperm maturation [4]. These abnormalities have been reported to diminish following varicocele repair [6]. Varicoceles often are associated with significant testicular atrophy [7]. Such atrophy generally involves the ipsilateral testis, but may at times be noted in the contralateral testis as well. Although varicocele repair may prevent further atrophy in such cases, in adults there rarely is significant testicular regrowth. Experience with adolescents undergoing varicocele repair, however, indicates that regrowth may occur among this group of patients following correction of the varicocele.

As discussed previously, varicoceles have long been associated with testicular dysfunction, especially impaired semen quality. In 1965, MacLeod described the so-called stress pattern of increased abnormal sperm forms, decreased sperm motility, and decreased sperm concentration, which he identified in a large group of patients with varicoceles [8]. Patients with varicoceles may manifest these semen characteristics but will not necessarily have all three abnormalities. Isolated defects in sperm motility or concentration are not uncommon. It is important to note that patients without varicoceles also may have these defects in semen quality. Semen analysis cannot, therefore, be used to diagnose a varicocele. Semen analysis is useful, however, for identifying those patients with varicoceles who might potentially benefit from repair as well as for following patients postoperatively to monitor clinical improvement.

RESULTS OF TREATMENT

Numerous communications describing the effect of varicocele on male fertility have been published [4]. The majority of these reports have demonstrated an improvement in semen quality postoperatively. A collected series from the literature, compiled by Lipshultz and Jarrow, described 2989 subfertile males treated by varicocele repair [5]. Among this group, 67% achieved improvement in their semen quality postoperatively and 39% subsequently achieved a pregnancy. This collected series includes patients with severely impaired semen quality (sperm counts less than 10 million/ml). Selected series that exclude patients with such profound preoperative defects in semen quality show even better results. Descriptions of the results of varicocele repair are often difficult to interpret since there generally is not a control group followed to assess critically the effectiveness of therapy. Data have been published, however, wherein pregnancy rates among patients treated by varicocele repair were compared to pregnancy rates among patients diagnosed as having varicoceles who elected not to undergo corrective therapy [5]. These studies indicated a marked increase in pregnancy rates among the group treated by varicocele repair compared to the group that declined such treatment.

Although achievement of an increased pregnancy rate is the ultimate measure of success in any form of infertility treatment, pregnancy data from reports describing the success of varicocele repair often are difficult to assess since little information is given regarding the fertility evaluation of the patients' partners. To study further the impact of varicocele repair on male fertility, attempts have been made to look at the effect of this procedure on sperm function in vitro. Seiber and coworkers reported on 34 subfertile males who underwent hamster egg penetration assay evaluations before and after varicocele repair. Although sperm density, percentage motility and forward progression did not increase significantly following surgery, there was significant improvement in the results of the postoperative sperm penetration assays [9]. The group reporting these data has found good correlation between the results of hamster egg penetration assays and successful fertilization during in vitro fertilization procedures. These findings suggest that varicocele repair may improve sperm function even in the absence of an improvement in bulk semen parameters.

The concept that varicocele repair may produce an increase in sperm function is supported by a report by Ashkenazi and colleagues who performed in vitro fertilization cycles before and after varicocele repair in couples in whom the male had a varicocele associated with decreased semen quality. They found that both fertilization and pregnancy rates improved significantly following correction of the varicocele [10]. Rogers et al., however, reported a study wherein patients with varicoceles underwent evaluation by sperm penetration assay performed before and after varicocele repair but failed to note a significant improvement in postoperative penetration assay results [11].

TECHNIQUE OF VARICOCELE REPAIR

Varicocele repair may be performed using either an open surgical technique or percutaneous venous embolization. Using the open approach, a small transverse incision is made either over the inguinal canal or just medial to the anterior superior iliac spine. The inguinal approach offers the advantages of very low morbidity as well as being relatively easy to perform. In this technique, the incision is carried down to the level of the external oblique fascia. The fascia is opened along the direction of its fibers, exposing the contents of the inguinal canal. The spermatic cord is then carefully mobilized and its fascial investments teased apart. The dilated spermatic vessels can then be visualized within the cord and are carefully identified and ligated. Care must be taken to avoid interruption of the lymphatic vessels running within the cord in order to prevent postoperative formation of a scrotal hydrocele. Caution must also be exercised to avoid damaging the arterial supply of the testicle. This procedure can be accomplished under local, regional, or general anesthesia and can be performed on an outpatient basis.

An alternative to open surgical repair of varicoceles is the use of percutaneous venous catheterization with occlusion of the ectactic spermatic vessels. Using this technique, an angiographic catheter is introduced via the femoral or jugular vein. The catheter is then advanced into the spermatic vein and the dilated vessels and collaterals are occluded using coils, balloons, or sclerosing agents. Although this approach can be effective in many cases, its success is clearly dependent upon the skill and experience of the radiologist performing the procedure. Due to venous anatomy, left-sided varicoceles are generally easier to treat via embolization than are right-sided varicoceles.

Although much work remains to be done elucidating the mechanisms by which varicoceles affect testicular function, there is a clear association between this lesion and impaired male fertility. Available data suggest that varicocele repair will result in an improvement in semen quality in many males who demonstrate decreased semen parameters. Repair of this lesion is safe and relatively free of morbidity. Varicocele correction, therefore, is indicated in subfertile males with impaired semen quality who have no other identifiable cause for male factor infertility.

REFERENCES

1 Zorgnotti AW. The Spermatozoa Count — a short history. *Urology* 1975; 5: 672.
2 Saypol DC. Varicocele. *J Androl* 1981; 2: 61.
3 Saypol DC, Lipshultz LI, Howards SS. Varicocele. In: Howards SS, Lipshultz LI, eds. *Infertility in the Male*. New York: Churchill Livingstone, 1983.
4 Nagler HM, Zippe CD. Varicocele: current concepts and treatment. In: Lipshultz LI, Howards SS, eds. *Infertility in the male*, 2nd ed. St Louis: Mosby Year Book.
5 Lipshultz LI, Jarrow JP. Varicocele and male subfertility. In: Sciarra JJ, ed. *Gynecology and Obstetrics*, Vol. 5. Philadelphia: JB Lippincott, 1989: 1–12.
6 Johnson SG, Agger P. Quantitative evaluation of testicular biopsies before and after operation for varicocele. *Fertil Steril* 1978; 29: 58.
7 Lipshultz LI, Corriere JN Jr. Progressive testicular atrophy in the varicocele patient. *J Urol* 1977; 177: 175.
8 MacLeod J. Seminal cytology in the presence of varicocele. *Fertil Steril* 1969; 20: 545.
9 Seiber A, Coburn M, Lipshultz LI. Effect of varicocele repair on sperm function. Presented at the eighty fifth annual meeting of The American Urological Association, abstract No. 767, 1990.
10 Ashkenazi J, Dicker M, Feldberg G *et al.* The impact of spermatic vein ligation on the male factor in *in vitro* fertilization-embryo transfer and its relation to testosterone levels before and after operation. *Fertil Steril* 1989; 51: 471.
11 Rogers BJ, Mygatt GG, Soderdahl DW *et al.* Monitoring of suspected infertile men with varicocele by the sperm penetration assay. *Fertil Steril* 1985; 44: 800.

Antisperm antibodies

WILLIAM D. SCHLAFF

The problem of antisperm antibodies is a confounding one for many clinicians. In many cases, the etiology of the antisperm antibodies is as unclear as the diagnosis. Even if one could establish agreement on the diagnosis, there continues to be a great deal of discord in the treatment of antisperm antibodies. Probably the only clear aspect of a discussion of antisperm antibodies is the agreement that such antibodies can have a major deleterious effect on sperm motility, fertilization, and fertility. An outline of the approach to antisperm antibodies is shown in Figure 96.1.

ANATOMY AND PHYSIOLOGY

During spermatogenesis, spermatogonia are confined to the germinal epithelium of the testis. The sperm are located between somewhat convoluted Sertoli cells which, in turn, are situated atop the basal lamina. The more immature germ cells are located at the periphery of the tubule and, during the course of spermatogenesis and spermiogenesis, they move generally toward the lumen. Ultimately, the mature spermatozoa with the nuclear material condensed in the head are shed into the lumen ultimately to become part of the ejaculate. During the process of spermatogenesis, many changes of conformation occur, and new protein antigens on the sperm surface develop. Therefore, proteins which may be antigenic on the immature spermatozoa may not be present on the mature spermatozoa as they are shed into the luminal compartment.

The immature sperm in the outer part of the germinal epithelium are relatively accessible to the immune system. Though there is no direct vascular connection between the interstitial area and the seminiferous tubule, it is clear that a variety of substances have easy access across the basal lamina. However, the intercellular gap junctions between Sertoli cells (as one moves towards the lumen) are among the tightest in the body. Therefore, germ cells within the adluminal compartment are relatively or completely sequestered from the testicular blood supply. Thus, the antigenic sites on maturing or mature spermatozoa are to a great extent unavailable for immunologic recognition, hence they are perceived as foreign.

Injury, surgery, or any trauma by which sperm cells are rendered available for immune recognition are likely to contribute to the development of sperm antibodies. The most common group of men known to have a high prevalence of antibodies are those who have undergone vasectomy. Antibody status is not modified by vasectomy reversal, and this may have a profound impact on fertility following sterilization reversal in men. Antibody formation has been identified after trauma, and there is some concern that antibodies may be initiated by testicular biopsy. Data to support this latter contention are largely lacking.

Sperm antibodies in women are relatively uncommon. This may reflect the presence of immune modulators either in seminal plasma or within the female genital tract that reduce the immunologic stimulus of these foreign proteins in the female tract.

CLINICAL PRESENTATION

Sperm antibodies have been identified on sperm heads, midpieces, and tails. Antibodies attached to each of these areas of the sperm cell may have different, though significant, manifestations and effects [1]. Sperm antibodies adherent to the tail may greatly decrease the ability of sperm to move normally. One should therefore have concern over the presence of sperm antibodies in men with normal sperm volumes and concentrations but reduced motility. This is particularly true in men who have undergone sterilization reversal. Tail-directed sperm antibodies may well decrease sperm movement

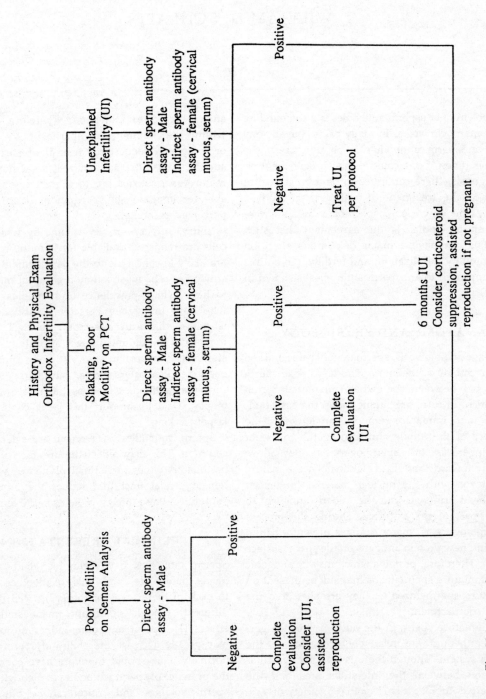

Fig. 96.1 Approach to antisperm antibodies.

ANTISPERM ANTIBODIES

within cervical mucus as well. Those antibodies that are head-directed may also have an impact on intracervical sperm progression, though this appears to be less of a problem. However, presence of head-directed sperm antibodies have been shown to decrease the likelihood of fertilization. Therefore, in couples with unexplained infertility, an evaluation of sperm antibodies should certainly be considered.

DIAGNOSTIC TESTING

A host of sperm antibody tests have been described and developed over the years. Initial tests of sperm agglutination (Kibrick) or immobilization (Isojima) had some correlation with clinical outcome, but this association was frequently unclear. More recently, an immunobead assay has been widely used and has several attractive aspects [2]. In this test, nonhuman-derived antihuman immunoglobulin is conjugated to a polyacrylamide bead and used to identify sites of antibody binding to sperm cells. This heterologous antibody will attach to any human immunoglobulin to which it is exposed. Therefore, when the beads are mixed with sperm on whose membrane an antisperm antibody is attached, the antihuman immunoglobulin will bind to the antibody, and microscopic examination will show a polyacrylamide bead apparently attached to the membrane at the point of the sperm antibody. This is called a direct immunobead test and can identify subclasses of immunoglobulins (i.e., IgG, IgA), depending on what immunobeads are used. An indirect test can also be performed by incubating various body fluids, including serum, cervical mucus, and seminal plasma with immunobeads and subsequently with normal sperm cells which do not have antibodies. When the polyacrylamide beads are seen to attach, one can infer that these fluids contain antisperm antibodies. This test provides both a quantitative assessment of sperm antibody presence by virtue of the number of beads binding, and a qualitative assessment of the primary locations of antibody binding. These observations may help the clinician to consider the likelihood of the antibodies interfering with motility, fertilization, or both. Generally, a test is considered positive if greater than 20% of motile (hence, presumed viable) sperm are found to have sperm antibodies attached to the head or to the tail. Antibody attachment to the tail tip is considered far less specific and may well be clinically irrelevant. Whenever these antibody tests are used, one should be sure that both negative and

positive controls are included to insure that results are accurate.

Other sperm antibody tests have also been described in recent years. These include primarily radioimmunoassays and enzyme-linked immunosorbent assays (ELISA) [3,4]. These tests also use a "tag" to identify presence of sperm antibodies, conceptually similar to the polyacrylamide bead. In the first case, a radioisotope is used as a tag rather than a microscopically visible bead, and in the second a substrate which undergoes colorimetric change in an ELISA reader is used. Flow cytometry tests have also been described in recent years. The clinician who chooses to use one of these tests should take the time to become fully aware of what is being measured. Specifically, tests are frequently reported as positive based on a certain number of deviations from the mean which may have no clinical correlation. That is to say, numeric relevance is not necessarily equal to biologic relevance. In some cases, those individuals with results that are mathematically positive may be found to have absolutely no decrease in fertility, while those who have mathematically negative results may have profound decreases in fertility. In summary, one should not make a clinical decision based on any sperm antibody assay unless it is clear that a normal result is suggestive of the absence of sperm antibodies interfering with fertility and an abnormal result confirms the presence of such an obstructive process.

TREATMENT

Treatment for sperm antibodies is frequently as confounding as is the diagnosis. It is fair to say at present that no standard treatment has been established. A number of studies using corticosteroid immunosuppression have been published and have frequently showed decreased sperm antibody load with treatment. However, the data regarding pregnancy outcome with corticosteroid suppression are conflicting. Alexander and her colleagues showed that a 7-day treatment with prednisone both decreased the load of immobilizing and agglutinating antibodies and increased pregnancy rates [5]. However, Haas and Manganiello failed to show a similar benefit using a radioimmunoassay to measure sperm antibodies [6]. Smarr et al. also failed to show a significant benefit of corticosteroid treatment in a prospective trial of patients with sperm antibodies [7]. However, they did note that treated patients who had a significant reduction of cytotoxic antibody titers with prednisone therapy had a much higher pregnancy rate (40–60%) compared to treated patients who had no reduction in titer (0–23%). This would suggest that prednisone treatment could be of benefit to those with reducible titers though, regrettably, there is not as yet any prospective study to allow us to predict who will respond in this positive way to steroid treatment. Other authors have suggested that intrauterine insemination with washed sperm should be used, and has been shown in some anecdotal studies to be of benefit [8]. Studies have clearly shown that washing does not remove the antibodies from sperm, nor has ejaculation into a buffered solution proved helpful. At present there are no controlled studies showing that intrauterine insemination is helpful in treatment of sperm antibodies despite its widespread use.

Ultimately, assisted reproductive technology in the form of *in vitro* fertilization may prove useful. Clarke and his colleagues showed that fertilization and pregnancy can occur even in the presence of relatively high titers of either IgG or IgA and antibodies [9]. However, when very high titers of IgA and IgG sperm antibodies were both present, the fertilization and pregnancy rates were significantly lower. Donor insemination may be the most effective therapy in the case of male antisperm antibodies, but would not be expected to be helpful should the female have antibodies.

Even in the virtual absence of any clear data, the clinician must ultimately choose some type of treatment. One must reemphasize the importance of being sure that the assay being utilized has biologic significance, and that all other factors of the infertility evaluation are normal. If the sole abnormality appears to be sperm antibodies, we recommend intrauterine insemination after either a Percoll or Sephadex washing. We also discuss corticosteroid suppression of the partner with antibodies. While most side-effects are transient and reversible, the specter of irreversible side-effects — most importantly avascular necrosis of the hip — must be clearly and specifically discussed with all patients. When patients agree to be treated with steroids, we use prednisone at a dose of 40 mg.

If the husband has sperm antibodies we treat him from days 4 to 14 of his partner's cycle, while we treat women with sperm antibodies from days 5 to 16. We must emphasize that this is purely an empiric treatment which is supported by some existing data, but should not be considered to be definitively established as the ideal treatment. We feel very strongly that this type of therapy should not be initiated without a careful history and physical examination of the partner taking corticosteroids, nor do we feel that it should be continued for a prolonged trial. If the couple has not conceived after 6 months of this approach, we do not recommend any further treatment with corticosteroids. At that point, we discuss assisted reproductive technologies or donor insemination if appropriate.

REFERENCES

1 Bronson R, Cooper G, Rosenfeld D. Sperm antibodies: their role in infertility. *Fertil Steril* 1984; 42: 171.
2 Bronson RA, Cooper GW, Rosenfeld DL. Sperm specific isoantibodies and autoantibodies inhibit the binding of human sperm to the human zona pellucida. *Fertil Steril* 1982; 38: 724.
3 Haas GG, Weiss-Wik R, Wolf DP. Identification of antisperm antibodies on sperm of infertile men. *Fertil Steril* 1982; 38: 54.
4 Witkin SS. Enzyme linked immunosorbent assay (ELISA) for detection of antibodies to spermatozoa. *Res Reprod* 1983; 15: 1.
5 Alexander NJ, Sampson JH, Fulgham DL. Pregnancy rates in patients treated for antisperm antibodies with prednisone. *Int J Fertil* 1983; 28: 63.
6 Haas GG, Manganiello P. A double-blind, placebo-controlled study of the rise of methylprednisolone in infertile men with sperm-associated immunoglobulins. *Fertil Steril* 1987; 47: 295.
7 Smarr SC, Wing R, Hammond MG. Effect of therapy on infertile couples with antisperm antibodies. *Am J Obstet Gynecol* 1988; 158: 969.
8 Confino E, Friberg J, Dudkiewicz AB, Gleicher N. Intrauterine inseminations with washed human spermatozoa. *Fertil Steril* 1986; 46: 55.
9 Clarke GN, Lopata A, McBain JC: Effect of sperm antibodies in males on human in vitro fertilization. *Am J Reprod Immunol Microbiol* 1985; 8: 62.

Artificial insemination: husband

MARY G. HAMMOND

Artificial insemination with husband's semen (AIH) has been widely applied in the management of infertility. A variety of clear indications exist for the utilization of this technique. In addition the procedure is also being used empirically to treat a number of disorders, in particular unexplained infertility. Few controlled studies have been reported supporting the efficacy of this treatment modality and it should be offered with reservation in settings in which no supportive data exist.

Indications for AIH include:

1 Intracervical insemination with stored husband semen obtained prior to chemotherapy or radiation therapy.

2 Intracervical insemination in situations in which intercourse or intravaginal deposition of semen is not possible, i.e., impotence, hypospadias.

3 Intrauterine insemination in cases of severe cervical factor.

4 Intrauterine insemination with sperm obtained from the bladder in cases of retrograde ejaculation.

5 Low semen volume (1 ml or less).

AIH has also been used empirically in the treatment of: (1) oligospermia; (2) asthenospermia; (3) unexplained infertility; (4) mild endometriosis; and (5) antisperm antibodies.

SELECTION OF COUPLES FOR AIH

Evaluation of the female partner

Because of the cost of inseminations and the time required, we feel that the female evaluation should be thorough. In cases in which intracervical insemination is planned, this evaluation would include assessment of tubal patency by hysterosalpingogram, documentation of normal ovulation by basal body temperature (BBT) and midluteal serum progesterone and assessment of the quality of midcycle cervical mucus.

When intrauterine insemination is anticipated, demonstration of tubal patency by hysterosalpingogram is indicated and laparoscopy should be done before the diagnosis of unexplained infertility is made. There is considerable debate in our group as to the advantage of medical therapy of mild endometriosis prior to intrauterine insemination therapy, but laser or cautery ablation of accessible lesions is always performed at the time of diagnosis.

Evaluation of the male partner

Serial semen analyses should be performed in the male so that an index of normal sperm numbers, motility, and abnormal forms is available. We prefer to have at least 10 million motile sperm per ejaculate and would not accept patients with less than 1 million motile sperm. We have found no benefit in storing or freezing sperm from serial ejaculates and combining them to increase numbers.

In males with increased round cell or white blood cell numbers we frequently treat with 14–30 days of Septra in an attempt to eradicate prostatitis.

TIMING OF INSEMINATION

Cycles of intracervical insemination should be monitored by BBT, cervical mucus checks, and ovulation predictor kits. If adequate stores of semen are available two inseminations per cycle are done.

If intrauterine insemination is anticipated we feel that more critical control of the time of ovulation is necessary and we prefer to superovulate the patient with either clomiphene or human menopausal gonadotropin (hMG). Our present protocol in normally ovulating women is to administer clomiphene 100 mg on days 3–7 and begin ultrasound evaluation on day 11 or 12. If medium-sized follicles are present, we begin daily home-testing of urinary luteinizing hormone (LH). If an LH surge is detected by day 16, insemination is scheduled for 48 hours later.

If the LH surge is delayed or not detected, more frequent ultrasounds are used and human chorionic gonadotropin (hCG) is administered in subsequent cycles. A single insemination is performed. This treatment is continued for four cycles. If patients fail to develop adequate follicle numbers (3–4) then rest cycles are initiated and clomiphene doses are increased.

After four cycles or if stimulation is inadequate, patients are transferred to an hMG protocol. They are treated with hMG 2 ampules daily, beginning on days 3–5 of the cycle. Monitoring with estrogen and ultrasound is begun on day 7 or 8. hCG is administered when the lead follicle is 16 mm and the estrogen is greater than 1000 pg/ml. Insemination is performed 40 hours later.

SEMEN PREPARATION FOR INSEMINATION

AIH can be performed intrauterine or intracervically. For most indications in which semen quality and quantity are normal and good-quality cervical mucus is present, intracervical insemination is preferred. This eliminates the necessity for facilities to process semen and also eliminates the need for precise timing of ovulation or ovarian hyperstimulation.

For intracervical insemination, semen is obtained by masturbation into a sterile container and inseminated directly after liquefaction.

Stored frozen samples of husband's sperm are thawed by the stringent instructions of the laboratory where the freezing was done and a formal analysis is done to determine viability. Many samples will be of poor quality and several vials may be required per insemination. We feel that 30 million motile sperm per insemination is optimal, although this much semen may not be available.

We no longer use whole semen for intrauterine insemination. A variety of methods are available for semen treatment. These range from simple washing with commercial media in a clinical centrifuge to elaborate gradient centrifugation and overlayering techniques.

For intrauterine insemination in most circumstances we use the following protocol:
1 Semen is collected under sterile conditions by masturbation into a sterile culture cup.
2 Semen is allowed to liquefy and a standard semen analysis is performed. Semen is then transferred into a disposable polystryene 15 ml sterile centrifuge tube

(Falcon 2099) using sterile Pasteur pipettes and the container rinsed with two to three times the semen volume with warm (37°C) prepared media (a 12 ml bottle of Irvine Scientific sperm-washing medium (#9983, Santa Ana, CA) containing 1.5 ml of heat-inactivated, sterile-filtered maternal or fetal cord serum screened for human immunodeficiency virus (HIV), hepatitis, VDRL, and antisperm antibodies. The mixture is inverted 10–15 times and divided evenly into two or more sterile centrifuge tubes.
3 Centrifuge for 10 min at 1200 rpm (350 g). Check supernatant for motile sperm. If present, increase centrifuge time. Discard supernatant and resuspend pellets in 1–2 ml of media and recentrifuge for 5 min. The supernatant is removed, pellets are combined, and resuspended in 0.25–0.5 ml of media.
4 Incubate specimen in 37°C incubator or water bath until ready for insemination.

This method eliminates seminal fluid which contains prostaglandins, which may cause uterine contractions, and may speed capacitation of the sperm. It also allows for concentration of the specimen. In some situations it is desirable to remove sediment as well as white blood cells. This can be accomplished by the standard swim-up used in in vitro fertilization. Unfortunately, most of the overlaying techniques used in this method yield only about 10% of the available motile sperm.

One method with better sperm yields is discontinuous Percoll gradient centrifugation. Sperm recovery near 60% has been reported with this method.

A number of techniques have been reported for collection of sperm in men, usually diabetics, with retrograde ejaculation. Males are identified by the presence of sperm in urine following ejaculation. Suitable numbers of sperm (>1 million) are required. The urine is alkalinized by ingestion of sodium bicarbonate and the bladder is emptied. The man then masturbates and urinates again. The specimen is centrifuged and redistributed in either his normal seminal plasma or in Ham's F10 media and inseminated. Counts and motility are recorded.

INSEMINATION

For intracervical insemination of husband sperm, semen is obtained by masturbation into a clean container and a semen analysis is performed. We place about 0.2 ml into the endocervical canal and the rest into a Mylex cervical cup. The patient remains supine for 15 min and then returns to normal activity. The cup is removed in about 6 hours or at bedtime. We feel the chances of conception may be improved by the use of a cervical cup which protects the semen from vaginal secretions and allows the patient greater mobility.

Intrauterine insemination is carried out in the lithotomy position. The cervix is visualized with a Graves' speculum and wiped clear of secretions. A Tomcat catheter which has been flushed three times with wash media is introduced through the cervix and into the uterine cavity. Care should be taken not to touch the top of the uterus as contractions will occur, which may expel the sperm. If difficulty is encountered in traversing the endocervical canal, then a suture or a tenaculum is placed on the anterior cervical lip and traction is used to straighten the uterus. The total volume of washed sperm is injected, the catheter is held in place for 1 min and then it is withdrawn. The patient rests supine for 15 min and then goes home.

Newer procedures are under investigation. One involves direct intraperitoneal insemination of sperm. Sperm are prepared by the swim-up technique which eliminates debris and gives a high percentage of normal, motile sperm. Standard ovarian stimulation regimes are utilized. Insemination is performed immediately after follicle rupture has occurred. The processed specimen is injected under ultrasound guidance into the pool of cul-de-sac fluid from follicle rupture. A 22.5-gauge spinal needle is used.

COMPLICATIONS

A number of potential complications exist for intrauterine insemination. The first is endometritis or salpingitis from agents introduced at the time of insemination. Many centers submit all sperm donors and recipients to a battery of microbiologic screening tests, including VDRL, HIV, gonorrhea, hepatitis and *Chlamydia*. We have not done that in our program as we feel that cohabiting couples are exposed to similar risks with intercourse. These would, however, be considerations in high-risk populations, as much for protection of laboratory personnel as for the patients. More likely the patients will be exposed to *Escherichia coli*, enterococcus, or other bowel flora which could represent problems. We have not as yet noted a clinical infection in our program.

A concern regarding the intrauterine instillation of sperm is the formation of antisperm antibodies in the recipient. In a recent study, two of 41 patients developed antibodies during therapy [10]. This was not felt to be significant by the authors, but does demonstrate that this is a real rather than theoretic complication of the treatment.

SUCCESS RATES

One of the major problems in evaluating reported pregnancy rates with AIH is the large number of clinical diagnoses treated. Many studies have small numbers of patients and do not analyze results by diagnoses. The second problem is that control cycles are rarely used and data are almost never analyzed by life-table analysis, nor is a per cycle pregnancy rate given. Tables 97.1–97.4 illustrate the results of a variety of studies. Each used different stimulation protocols and different methods of data analysis.

For the most part physicians must draw their own conclusions as to the cost : benefit ratio to their own patients of pursuing this treatment modality. We have offered it to patients with poor or absent cervical mucus, low semen volume, mild endometriosis and ejaculatory problems with no reservation as long as other conventional therapies have failed. We feel the results in unexplained infertility have not been demonstrated by controlled studies to exceed rates of nonintervention. There have been very poor success rates in male factor infertility. Patients are therefore advised that the therapy is empiric and may not significantly increase their chances of conception.

COUNSELING

For many couples AIH will represent the final treatment plan. *In vitro* fertilization may be too expensive or invasive for them and the physician must be prepared to counsel patients adequately about their options, including the need to terminate therapy and consider other alternatives to conception such as artificial insemination by donor, adoption, or childfree living. To continue to offer a treatment with low success rates to couples to keep their hopes alive may not be in the patients' best interests and may even be destructive to their relationship and continued growth.

REFERENCES

1 Hovatta O, Kurunmaki H, Tiitinen A, Lahteenmaki P, Koskimies AI. Direct intraperitoneal or intrauterine

Table 97.1 Results of recent intrauterine insemination (IUI) studies

Authors	Cycle no. (patient no.)	Diagnosis	Ovarian stimulation	Insemination	Control (intercourse)	Pregnancy cycle	Overall pregnancy rate
Hovatta et al. [1]	174 (63)	All	CC + hMG	Intraperitoneal	1.1%	8.6%	24%
	152 (61)	All	CC + hMG	IUI	0.6%	12.5%	31%
Hull et al. [2]	85 (27)	All	None	IUI	None	3.5%	11%
Margalloth et al. [3]	285 (67)	Antisperm antibodies	None	IUI	None	3%	13%
	86 (20)	Antisperm antibodies	CC	IUI	None	7%	30%
	102 (28)	Antisperm antibodies	hMG	IUI	None	11%	39%
Martinez et al. [4]	35 NA	All	CC	IUI	3.2	14.3%	NA
	32 NA	All	None	IUI		9.4%	
Dodson et al. [5]	148 (85)	All	hMG	IUI	None	16%	35%
	15 NA	Tubal	hMG	IUI	None	7%	
	93 NA	Endometriosis	hMG	IUI	None	17%	
Lalich et al. [6]	586 (138)	All	Multiple protocols	IUI	None	5%	27%
	NA (11)	Immune	Multiple protocols	IUI	None	NA	50%
Chaffkin [11]	357 (135)	All	hMG	IUI	6.3% (hMG)	19.6%	50%

CC, clomiphene citrate; hMG, human menopausal gonadotropin; NA, not applicable.

Table 97.2 Treatment of cervical factor: results of recent intrauterine insemination (IUI) studies

Authors	Cycle no. (patient no.)	Diagnosis	Ovarian stimulation	Insemination	Control (intercourse)	Pregnancy cycle	Overall pregnancy rate
Sunde et al. [7]	119 NA	Cervical	CC or hMG	IUI	None	10.8%	NA
Hull et al. [2]	65 (19)	Cervical	None	IUI		4.6%	16%
Dodson et al. [5]	7 NA	Cervical	hMG	IUI	None	29%	NA
Lalich et al. [6]	NA (62)	Cervical	Multiple protocols	IUI	None	NA	28%
Chaffkin [11]	91 NA	Cervical	hMG	IUI	7.6% (hMG)	26.3%	NA

CC, clomiphene citrate; hMG, human menopausal gonadotropin; NA, not applicable.

insemination and superovulation in infertility treatment; a randomized study. *Fertil Steril* 1990; 54: 339–341.

2 Hull ME, Magyar DM, Vasquez JM, Hayes MF, Moghissi KS. Experience with intrauterine insemination for cervical factor and oligospermia. *Am J Obstet Gynecol* 1986; 154: 1333–1338.

3 Margalloth EH, Sauter E, Bronson RA, Rosenfeld DL, Scholl GM, Cooper GW. Intrauterine insemination as treatment for antisperm antibodies in the female. *Fertil Steril* 1988; 50: 441–446.

4 Martinez AR, Bernardus RE, Voorhorst FJ, Vermeiden JPW, Schoemaker J. Intrauterine insemination does and clomiphene citrate does not improve fecundity in couples with infertility due to male or idiopathic factors: a prospective, randomized, controlled study. *Fertil Steril* 1990; 53: 847–853.

5 Dodson WC, Whitesides DB, Hughes CL Jr, Easley HA III, Haney AF. Superovulation with intrauterine insemination in the treatment of infertility: a possible alternative to gamete intrafallopian transfer and in vitro

Table 97.3 Treatment of idiopathic infertility results of recent artificial insemination by husband (AIH) studies

Authors	Cycle no. (patient no.)	Ovarian stimulation	Insemination type	Control (intercourse)	Pregnancy cycle	Overall pregnancy rate
Sunde et al. [7]	116 NA	CC or hMG	IUI	None	12.9%	NA
Dodson et al. [5]	31 NA	hMG	IUI	None	19%	NA
Lalich et al. [6]	NA (10)	Multiple protocols	IUI	None	NA	60%
Chaffkin [11]	46 NA	hMG	IUI	5.5% (hMG)	32.6%	NA

CC, clomiphene citrate; hMG, human menopausal gonadotropin; IUI, intrauterine insemination; NA, not applicable.

Table 97.4 Treatment of male factor: results of recent artificial insemination by husband (AIH) studies

Authors	Cycle no. (patient no.)	Ovarian stimulation	Insemination type	Control (intercourse)	Pregnancy cycle	Overall pregnancy rate
Sunde et al. [7]	726 NA	CC or hMG	IUI	None	7.4%	NA
Hughes et al. [8]	31 NA	None	Intracervical	1/21	0%	NA
	32 NA	None	IUI	3/14	0%	
Hull et al. [2]	20 (8)	None	IUI	None	0%	0%
Kerin et al. [9]	133 (severe)	None	IUI	4.5	8.8%	NA
	80 (moderate)	None	IUI	0	8.7%	
Ho (1989)	114 (47)	None	IUI	0.8	0%	0%
Lalich et al. [6]	NA (55)	Multiple protocols	IUI	None	NA	17%
Chaffkin [11]	111 NA	hMG	IUI	4.4% (hMG)	15.3%	NA

CC, clomiphene citrate; hMG, human menopausal gonadotropin; IUI, intrauterine insemination; NA, not applicable.

fertilization. *Fertil Steril* 1987; 48: 441–445.

6 Lalich RA, Marut EL, Prins GS, Scommegna A. Life table analysis of intrauterine insemination pregnancy rates. *Am J Obstet Gynecol* 1988; 158: 980–984.

7 Sunde A, Kahn JA, Holne K. Intrauterine insemination: a European collaborative report. *Hum Reprod* 1988; 3: 69–73.

8 Hughes EG, Collins JP, Garner PR. Homologous artificial insemination for oligoasthenospermia: a randomized controlled study comparing intracervical and intrauterine techniques. *Fertil Steril* 1987; 48: 278–281.

9 Kerin J, Quinn P. Washed intrauterine insemination in the treatment of oligospermic infertility. *Semin Reprod Endocrinol* 1987; 5: 23–33.

10 Moretti-Rojas, I, Rojas FJ, Leisure M et al. Intrauterine inseminations with washed human spermatozoa does not induce formation of antisperm antibodies. *Fertil Steril* 1990; 53: 180–182.

11 Chaffkin LM, Nulsen JC, Luciano AA, Metzger DA. A comparative analysis of the ciano cycle fecundity notes associated with combined human menopausal gonadotrophin (hMG) and intrauterine insemination (IUI) versus either hMG or IUI alone. *Fertil Steril* 1991; 55: 252–257.

FURTHER READING

Allen NC, Herbert CM, Maxson CM, Rogers BJ, Diamond MP, Wentz AC. Intrauterine insemination: a critical review. *Fertil Steril* 1985; 44: 569–580.

Berger T, Marrs RP, Moyer DL. Comparison of techniques for selection of motile spermatozoa. *Fertil Steril* 1985; 43: 268–273.

Urry RL, Middleton RG, McGavin S. A simple and effective technique for increasing pregnancy rates in couples with retrograde ejaculation. *Fertil Steril* 1986; 46: 1124–1127.

Artificial insemination: donor

WILLIAM D. SCHLAFF

Therapeutic donor insemination (TDI) has been practiced fairly commonly since the nineteenth century. It is one of the oldest and most successful therapies in infertility treatment. According to a recent survey published by the Office of Technology Assessment of the US Congress, over 170 000 women underwent TDI, and approximately 30 000 babies were born in this country as a result in 1987 alone [1]. This is over 10 times the number of successful pregnancies produced by all other forms of assisted reproduction combined. Yet, despite the widespread practice and success of TDI, there are numerous controversies regarding clinical strategies, techniques, and ethical concepts. These will be reviewed in this chapter.

INDICATIONS

The indication for therapeutic donor insemination is absence of sperm sufficient in quantity and/or quality to be likely to produce a pregnancy. Therefore, patients who could appropriately consider TDI are those whose husbands or partners have compromised production or fertilizing capacity of sperm, as well as those who do not have partners. While the medical issues for these two groups are virtually the same, social, ethical, and legal issues may be different and will be addressed in a later section of this chapter.

Women who seek TDI for male factor infertility should first be interviewed in depth with their partner regarding the nature of the diagnosis and alternative treatments. It is sometimes surprising how frequently patients seek TDI with only a cursory understanding of the indications of the male partner's diagnosis. The medical records of the male should be thoroughly reviewed to help the couple understand his diagnosis and the prognosis for pregnancy without TDI. These records should include at least three semen analyses to allow one to assess the severity of the male factor. In the absence of this information, it would be premature to initiate TDI. In such a case, the male should be referred for a complete evaluation including semen analysis, hormonal evaluation when appropriate, and physical examination to establish his reproductive potential.

Inherent in a couple's decision to undergo TDI is the decision to reject other alternatives using the partner's sperm. This is a moot point when the partner has no sperm nor any potential to produce them, such as in a male who has undergone bilateral orchiectomy for cancer. Other men may have no sperm in the ejaculate, but their situation could be amenable to medical therapy. Examples include men who have had a previous vasectomy or who have retrograde ejaculation secondary to retroperitoneal node dissection for cancer. In this situation, thorough counseling of the couple should be provided to inform them of the treatment alternatives, including the likelihood of success with therapy. Finally, many men will have severe oligospermia rather than azoospermia. Prior to initiating TDI in such a case, the physician is obliged to review the prognosis for establishing a pregnancy with the partner's sperm using all available techniques including assisted reproduction. It is only after such a discussion that the couple can elect to forego such therapy and pursue TDI in a fully informed manner.

SCREENING THE PATIENT

Once the decision has been made to proceed to TDI, a thorough history should be taken. Specific attention should be directed to previous obstetric performance and the presence of any risk factors which might interfere with normal fertility. Additionally, a family history of reproductive failure or heritable disease should be sought. Should the patient be at particular risk for suboptimal outcome by virtue of family or ethnic history (e.g., Tay–Sachs or sickle cell disease), she should be prospectively screened if accurate tests are available. Following the history, a physical and pelvic examination should be performed. Special attention should be directed at identifying any finding that might be associated with reduced fertility potential. At the time of the pelvic examination, cultures for gonorrhea and *Chlamydia* should be obtained, and a Pap smear should be performed if it is timely.

All patients who will be undergoing TDI should be screened with a VDRL test, rubella, and cytomegalovirus (CMV) titers, hepatitis antigen status, and blood type. It is recommended that the partner's blood type should also be obtained in an attempt to identify an appropriate donor whose blood type is compatible with a natural liaison of the couple. Human immunodeficiency virus (HIV) antibody status of the patient should be obtained after formal informed consent. New tests are becoming available including screening for the cystic fibrosis gene and polymerase chain reaction tests to identify the HIV virus in individual specimens. However, they are neither standard nor widely available at present.

It is not recommended routinely to screen all patients with invasive infertility testing such as hysterosalpingography or laparoscopy in the absence of risk factors (history of pelvic infection, previous prolonged unprotected intercourse without pregnancy, etc.) or concerning physical findings. Patients with a history of menstrual irregularity should undergo a diagnostic evaluation to elucidate the nature of the hormonal abnormality, but routine hormonal assessment is not indicated in women who appear to be normally ovulatory.

SELECTING A DONOR

Since early 1988 when the American Fertility Society, American Association of Tissue Banks, and, at least indirectly, the Food and Drug Administration agreed that the practice of TDI with fresh semen was no longer to be considered safe due to the risk of acquired immune deficiency syndrome (AIDS), standard practice of TDI has required insemination with frozen, quarantined sperm samples. Therefore, unless the practitioner is able to establish his or her own semen bank, reliance on commercial banks has increased. It is incumbent on the practitioner to know the screening program of any bank from which specimens are obtained as it is ultimately the practitioner's responsibility to provide safe, appropriately screened specimens. It is a good idea to contact the medical director of the semen bank from which specimens are ordered to inquire specifically about screening methods. At the very least, a thorough medical, sexual, genetic, and family history should be obtained from the donor. A physical examination should also be performed and updated periodically (every 4–6 months). Failure to meet standards set by the American Fertility Society should mandate disqualification as a donor [2]. The donors should be screened for HIV status, hepatitis antigen and antibody, CMV, gonorrhea, and *Chlamydia*. Blood type should be available. Karyotyping is not standard, though it is obtained by some programs. Semen specimens should be examined and found to meet normal standards [2]. Once the donor has satisfactorily completed this thorough screening process, specimens may be obtained and frozen using appropriate cryoprotective media. They should be maintained in liquid nitrogen for a minimum of 6 months during which time the donor must be rescreened for HIV and CMV (if originally negative) status. Only after testing has shown that the donor continues to be HIV-negative at least for a period of 6 months following the cryopreservation of the sample should the specimen be released for insemination. Specimens obtained from donors who become CMV-positive should be used only in CMV-positive women.

The process of donor selection is more taxing from a social than from a medical standpoint. Medical consideration demands that the CMV-negative patient be inseminated only with specimens from CMV-negative donors, and that Rh-negative women receive specimens only from Rh-negative donors whenever possible. Selecting a donor whose blood type is compatible with a natural child of the couple is also desirable. There are a number of social considerations, generally relating to the amount of information provided to couples. For example, there are different opinions regarding sharing of donor lists from commercial sperm banks with patients. These lists will commonly include ethnic background, educational level, body type, and hobbies. There are no data to establish whether this information should or should not be shared with the patient, or whether she should be able to make an active choice as to the donor she prefers. Therefore, the decision as to how to approach this process should be left to the individual practitioner.

PATIENT MONITORING AND INSEMINATION

As with many aspects of infertility practice, there is continued controversy in the area of patient monitoring for TDI and particularly insemination practices. While many new techniques and diagnostic adjuncts have been developed over recent years, the basal body temperature (BBT) chart continues to prove itself as a helpful technique for timing inseminations. TDI procedures can be performed successfully at the nadir or with the rise of the temperature. However, it is not clear that even the BBT chart is any more useful than counting backwards 14 days from the expected menses in women with regular periods and choosing that day for insemination. Urinary luteinizing hormone (LH) testing has also been extensively used, though again, no study has clearly shown this technique to provide better results than a BBT chart alone. More intensive (and expensive) monitoring, including ultrasound of the ovarian follicle along with serum hormonal assessment, should be reserved only for those women whose cycle irregularity renders more simple monitoring inaccurate or undependable. The use of clomiphene citrate or any other ovulation-inducing agent should be reserved for those women with identifiable ovulation abnormalities. The routine use of such agents for TDI in normally ovulatory women should be strongly discouraged.

Prior to the decision to utilize cryopreserved semen exclusively, intracervical insemination (ICI) was the standard approach to TDI. The procedure was performed by injecting the specimen into the cervical canal, by placing the semen into a small plastic cervical cup and then on to the cervix, or a combination of both. Fecundity rates (pregnancy rates per month of exposure) using this technique were generally about 15%, with an average time to conception of 4 months. With the exclusive use of cryopreserved sperm, the decision to use the intracervical as opposed to intrauterine route (IUI) has become more controversial. Most experts would concur that the cryopreservation–thawing cycle reduces the fecundity rate of insemination. One study found a pregnancy rate of 18% per cycle using fresh semen and only 6% per cycle with frozen specimens in a prospective study using the patient as her own control [3]. This observation emphasizes the importance of doing all one can to maximize the effectiveness of frozen specimens. A more recent study using exclusively frozen sperm showed a pregnancy rate of 10% using IUI and a rate of 4% with ICI in a similar prospective trial of TDI techniques using the patient as her own control [4]. While it would be attractive to conclude that IUI is thus shown to be superior, the relatively low fecundity in both groups leaves room for some skepticism regarding this conclusion, particularly in light of the increased expense of IUI compared to ICI.

Controversy also exists as to the optimal number of inseminations per cycle. We use urinary LH monitoring to detect the onset of the LH surge, and perform an insemination that day and the following day. In a prospective trial this approach has been shown to result in a fecundity rate of 21% compared to only 6% when insemination was performed only once per cycle on the day following detection of the LH surge [5]. We initially choose to perform inseminations intracervically using a combined approach. We thaw a 1 ml vial of cryopreserved sperm at room temperature, transfer it to a small glass test tube, and add 1 ml of culture medium at 37°C to it. Using a tuberculin syringe, we inject 0.2 ml intracervically and inseminate the rest via an oligospermia cup (Milex Corp., Arvada, CO). The cup has a string attached, and the patient is instructed to pull off the cup after 4 hours. Occasionally, she will need to insert a finger into the vagina to break the suction produced by the cup to allow its removal. If the patient has not conceived after 3–4 months of ICI, or if she has persistently poor cervical mucus during treatment by ICI, we elect to recommend IUI even with the associated increased expense.

A variety of preparation techniques of frozen donor specimens for IUI has been described without widespread agreement as to the ideal choice. Removal of as much cryoprotectant as possible is desirable. Therefore, fairly rapid dilution with warm culture medium to a volume of 10 ml is frequently the first step. Centrifugation at 200–300 g for 5 min will pellet the sperm and allow removal of much of the unwanted component in the supernatant. At this point, some centers will resuspend the pellet in another 5–10 ml of medium, recentrifuge, and suspend the final pellet in 0.3–0.5 ml of medium for IUI. Others choose to perform a swim-up by overlaying about 0.5–1.0 ml of media over the sperm pellet and allowing the most active sperm to swim into the supernatant over a period of 45–60 min in an incubator at 37°C. The supernatant is then aspirated for insemination. Unlike ICI, where the minimal number of motile sperm generally recommended is

20 million per insemination, there is no generally accepted lower limit for IUI, with pregnancies having occurred with 1 million motile sperm or less.

LEGAL ASPECTS

The legal status of the baby, donor, and practitioner should be thoroughly reviewed prior to initiating TDI. The obligations of the patient, her partner, and the physician must also be thoroughly discussed. After a detailed informed consent has been obtained, a permit should be signed by the patient, her partner, and a witness specifying the understanding with the physician. A copy should be given to the patient, and a copy maintained in the physician's records. Inherent in any informed consent is understanding and compliance with the state laws which might pertain. Many states have laws addressing TDI (34 at the last count) but the vast majority of such laws describe only legal rights and responsibilities of the couple and donor and do not specify any medical standards. Such laws generally specify that the husband and wife are the legal parents of any offspring of TDI (without adoption) once they have signed the permit, and that the donor has neither rights nor responsibilities to the child. However, other modifications on this theme may exist in some states. It would be very wise for all physicians to review their pertinent state statutes with a legal authority prior to initiating TDI.

A special situation exists in the case of donor insemination of single women, whether part of a couple or not. Only one state (Oregon) clarifies the parental responsibilities in cases of unmarried women. While one might infer that an unmarried woman who wishes TDI and signs the permit accepts all responsibilities of parenthood, it would be far wiser to require a detailed informed consent document specifying the patient's acceptance of this responsibility and releasing the practitioner, donor, or anyone else from parental responsibility. Aside from the legal concerns over parental rights and responsibilities, the patient should be thoroughly counseled regarding other risks. Sexually transmitted disease and significant emotional trauma are rare complications of TDI. Birth defects and adverse pregnancy outcome occur at a rate comparable to age-matched controls. Whether the practitioner prefers to include these risks as part of a formal permit or not is less important than the clear documentation that these potential adverse events have been discussed.

SOCIAL IMPLICATIONS

The most commonly asked question of the practitioner is, "What do I tell the child and my family?" Unfortunately, the answer to this, as well as many other social/sociologic questions is unclear. There are virtually no prospective data to provide a solid basis on which to counsel patients. Therefore, the answer to most such questions is to advise the couple to discuss their ideas and feelings thoroughly and reach a conclusion with which they can feel comfortable and live with indefinitely. Many couples will profit by at least short-term counseling regarding this and other topics, and counseling should be discussed with every couple considering TDI. Generally, a social worker or psychologist is better accepted by couples than a psychiatrist, but the latter should be consulted if there is concern over serious mental maladjustment or mental illness.

The long-term outcome (up to 12 years) of 427 women who conceived 606 pregnancies was recently described [6]. While not a prospective study, the authors found that 5.8% of the children had learning disabilities in school and 10.5% were considered gifted — neither of which appeared to be different from the expected. The majority of the couples (72%) told their obstetrician that they conceived through TDI, though only half told any family member or friends. Many couples (47%) did not or probably did not (14%) plan to tell their child about TDI. Strikingly, the divorce rate among these couples was only 7.2%, far below the national average. While these data are only observational and lack any compelling scientific weight, they are nevertheless very helpful in getting some early ideas as to the long-term social impact of a TDI baby.

CONCLUSIONS

TDI is an effective, safe, and overwhelmingly positive treatment for many infertile couples. It is the most successful of all available treatments for male factor infertility. TDI should only be initiated after a thorough review of the indications, comprehensive discussion of the nature of donor screening and selection, and sensitive consideration of the emotional, social, and legal implications of the process.

CHAPTER 98

REFERENCES

1 US Congress, Office of Technology Assessment. *Artificial Insemination: Practice in the United States: Summary of a 1987 Survey — Background Paper* (OTA-BP-BA-48). Washington: US Government Printing Office, 1988: 3.

2 New guidelines for the use of semen donor insemination: 1990. The American Fertility Society. *Fertil Steril* 1990; 53 (suppl 1): 1S.

3 Richter MA, Haning RV, Shapiro SS. Artificial donor insemination: fresh vs. frozen semen; the patient as her own control. *Fertil Steril* 1984; 41: 277.

4 Byrd W, Bradshaw K, Carr B, Edman C, Odom J, Ackerman G. A prospective randomized study of pregnancy rates following intrauterine and intracervical insemination using frozen donor sperm. *Fertil Steril* 1990; 53: 521–527.

5 Centola GM, Mattox JM, Raubertas RF. Pregnancy rates after double versus single insemination with frozen donor semen. *Fertil Steril* 1990; 54: 1089.

6 Amuzu B, Laxova R, Shapiro SS. Pregnancy outcome, health of children, and family adjustment after donor insemination. *Obstet Gynecol* 1990; 75: 899–905.

Part X
Climacteric

Menopause and hormone replacement therapy

WULF H. UTIAN

The current median age of menopause is 50 years, though approximately 8% of women undergo premature menopause before the age of 40 years. During the time of the climacteric, the phase in the aging of women that marks the transition from the reproductive to the non-reproductive stage of life, there may be abrupt cessation of menses or several months may pass between menstrual periods. The sometimes unpredictable perimenopausal menstrual pattern makes identifying the onset of menopause difficult for some women. This chapter will focus on practical problems associated with diagnosis and management of the menopause.

PHYSIOLOGY OF MENOPAUSE

As a woman ages and ovarian function begins to fall, the number of follicles in the ovaries decreases. A deficiency of follicular inhibin and estrogen leads to decreased negative feedback which results in an increase in levels of follicle-stimulating hormone (FSH) and luteinizing hormone (LH). Feedback sensitivity on the hypothalamus and anterior pituitary glands may also decrease [1]. The predominant estrogen of the reproductive years, estradiol, gradually declines during the climacteric period and gives way to estrone, a weaker estrogen produced in adipose tissue from androgen precursors. This gradual decline of total circulating estrogen may be associated with an alteration in menstruation which is frequently characterized by irregular cycles, a lighter menstrual flow, oligomenorrhea, and finally a total absence of menstruation.

The tissue or organs directly affected by this relative estrogen deficiency are those with specific estrogen receptors, such as the ovaries, endometrium, vaginal epithelium, hypothalamus, urinary tract, and skin. Other tissues in which estrogen receptors have not been consistently identified, such as bone, are nevertheless affected by a lack of estrogen. The resultant symptoms or problems that may occur when these various tissues and organs become estrogen-deficient are summarized in Table 99.1 [2].

Urogenital atrophy manifests as a loss of soft tissue elasticity and a decrease in muscle tone and secretions. Usually the uterus shrinks and the vagina undergoes progressive thinning and shortening, with a loss of the rugal pattern. These vaginal changes are a common cause of pruritis in postmenopausal women and they may be responsible for complaints of dyspareunia. Vaginal atrophy also puts the woman at increased risk of vaginal trauma and infection. The increased risk of infection is probably due, in part, to the slight increase in vaginal pH associated with changes in the bacterial flora. Similar changes also occur in the urethra and the trigone area of the bladder. Urethral atrophy may lead to the urethral syndrome, in which women have a recurrent abacterial urethritis characterized by symptoms of dysuria, frequency and urgency of urination, nocturia, and postvoid dribbling. Other visible changes include diminution of breast size and thinning of the skin, the latter a result of collagen loss.

Neuroendocrine problems are also relatively common in perimenopausal and postmenopausal women. Hot flashes, which can begin several years before the actual menopause, occur in 75–85% of climacteric women. One postulated mechanism is that the temperature-regulating set point of the hypothalamus may be reset downward. Most women describe a sudden onset of warmth and vasodilation, often visible as a red flush that is most apparent over the face and chest. The flush usually lasts from 30 seconds to 5 min and may occur every few minutes or only once or twice a week. Other vasomotor symptoms include nausea, dizziness, weakness, headaches, palpitations, diaphoresis, and night sweats. Women who experience hot flashes may also complain of sleep disturbances.

Many other psychologic changes supposedly

Table 99.1 Potential problems of the untreated climacteric. (Modified from [2])

Target organ	Possible symptom or problem
Vulva	Atrophy, dystrophy, pruritis vulvae
Vagina	Dyspareunia, blood-stained discharge, vaginitis
Bladder and urethra	Cystourethritis, ectropion, frequency and/or urgency, stress incontinence
Uterus and pelvic floor	Uterovaginal prolapse
Skin and mucous membranes	Atrophy, dryness, or pruritis; easily traumatized; loss of resilience and pliability; dry hair or loss of hair; minor hirsutism of face; dry mouth
Vocal cords	Voice changes (reduction in upper register)
Cardiovascular system	Atherosclerosis, angina, and coronary heart disease
Skeleton	Osteoporosis with related fractures, backache
Breasts	Reduced size, softer consistency, drooping
Neuroendocrine system	Hot flashes, psychologic disturbances

associated with menopause have been reported and studied. Such changes, including depression, mood swings, anxiety, and emotional lability, are probably due to the interactive effects of endocrine changes, sociocultural effects, and psychologic factors in each individual. The complaints are usually multiple, vague, and nonspecific. They may be related to vasomotor symptoms and a lack of sleep. The severity of psychologic complaints during the menopausal years is usually mild, not continuous, and tends to fluctuate [2]. Symptoms related to sexual dissatisfaction are common and are not only due to atrophy of genital tissues. The woman may be troubled by decreased libido, prolonged excitement phase, and decreased incidence of and satisfaction with orgasm.

Systemic risk factors of hypoestrogenism are also extremely important. The risk of cardiovascular disease is higher in men compared with age-matched women before the age of 40–45 years. During the perimenopausal period, the risk of cardiovascular disease in women begins to increase to a rate similar to that in men. The decrease in estrogen production is thought to be one factor responsible for this acceleration of risk. Numerous epidemiologic studies have shown a reduction of coronary artery morbidity and mortality in women who are provided with estrogen replacement therapy compared to controls. This apparent benefit of estrogen replacement may be manifest due to the effect of estrogen on the lipoprotein profile (increased high density lipoproteins, decreased low density lipoproteins) as well as a direct beneficial effect on the arterial wall.

A second major area of concern is osteoporosis. Women may lose 5–10% of their bone mineral density in the first year of hypoestrogenism, and their risk of fractures rises in a parallel fashion. By the age of 80 years, about 25% of all women have sustained one or more fractures of the proximal femur, vertebrae, or distal radius, any of which may be associated with high morbidity and mortality rates. The management of such fractures constitutes a major social and financial cost. Studies have clearly shown that estrogen replacement therapy stabilizes bone mineral status no matter when treatment is initiated in the postmenopausal years. This results in a decrease in fractures in estrogen-replaced women (up to a factor of 6 in some studies) and reduced morbidity and mortality.

DIAGNOSIS OF THE CLIMACTERIC

The diagnosis of the climacteric is straightforward when an older patient presents with prolonged amenorrhea (6–12 months) associated with symptoms of hypoestrogenism such as hot flashes. However, it is often difficult to confirm that a patient has entered the climacteric transition if she has not yet become menopausal, particularly when she is younger. Symptoms that should promote a high index of suspicion include alterations in menstrual pattern, specifically irregularity and reduced frequency of periods, decreased menstrual flow, or evidence of anovulation which may then be associated with hypermenorrhea. Hot flashes are also highly suggestive when present. Unfortunately, there are no satisfactory practical laboratory tests of confirmatory value. Plasma gonadotropins may be increased, but are helpful in diagnosis only when elevated. Normal gonadotropins do not preclude the climacteric transition. Dynamic tests of hormonal function are rarely of diagnostic help. Absence of withdrawal bleeding in response to a progestogen challenge (for example, medroxyprogesterone acetate 10 mg tablets orally for 7 days) is confirmatory of low estrogen production and can be helpful. Measuring serum estradiol can also be performed, with levels less than 35 pg/ml considered to be consistent with menopause. A maturation index can also be obtained from the vaginal side wall and will have few if any superficial cells in the absence of estrogen. Diagnostic difficulty often arises when a younger woman, perhaps in her 30s or early 40s, presents with secondary amenorrhea. Indeed, this is one of the most frequent symptoms for referral to a gynecologic endocrine unit. There are many possible causes for secondary amenorrhea which are addressed in chapter 8. A treatment oriented diagnostic protocol for secondary amenorrhea is presented in Figure 99.1.

A special problem arises in the older woman on oral contraceptives who asks if she is menopausal or if she can discontinue the pill without fear of pregnancy. One can usually reassure the patient regarding pregnancy on the basis of age alone, but sometimes further diagnostic testing can be helpful. A diagnosis of menopause can be made by discontinuing the pill and measuring estradiol and FSH levels 4 weeks later. A periovulatory surge of LH and FSH occurs normally and can be confused with menopausal levels of gonadotropins in some cases. These two situations can often be distinguished by the fact that periovulatory LH is usually higher than FSH, while the opposite is true in the menopause. If the results are unclear, it is wise to wait 2 weeks for a menstrual period to occur (or not) and repeat the LH and FSH levels to differentiate the two situations.

BENEFIT : RISK RATIO IN ESTROGEN THERAPY

Benefits of therapy can be directly related to both reducing symptoms as well as prolonging good health. Well-performed studies have shown that estrogen replacement will reduce vasomotor flushes, improve sleep patterns and sexual function, and decrease symptoms related to atrophy of the genitourinary tract. Perhaps more importantly in the long run, osteoporosis is significantly reduced in women receiving estrogen therapy and cardiovascular disease may be as well.

Patients frequently express concern over cancer as a potential risk. Data have shown that the excess risk of endometrial cancer associated with estrogen alone can be eliminated in women being replaced with an estrogen–progestin combination. There are conflicting data regarding estrogen use and the risk of breast cancer. A number of analyses have been published recently and, in sum, suggest (though do not demonstrate conclusively) that estrogen may slightly increase the risk of diagnosing breast cancer by about 10–30% [4]. Women who have been treated with estrogen for a prolonged period of time (greater than 10 years) seem to be at greatest risk. It is not clear whether estrogen can be implicated as causative, or whether this increased rate of breast cancer diagnosis can be attributed to a higher frequency of breast examinations or mammograms in women being treated with estrogen. Other data suggest that, even in the presence of a possible increase in the diagnosis of breast cancer, the death rate from breast cancer is, if anything, lower in estrogen-replaced women. The use of progestin with estrogen in women who have had a hysterectomy is another extremely controversial area. Though progestins have been shown to be mitogenic to breast tissue in culture, there are as yet no data which convincingly show that this is also true in women. Therefore, the physician and patient should have a thorough discussion of this prior to initiating therapy and select acceptable alternatives.

INDICATIONS AND EVALUATION FOR ESTROGEN REPLACEMENT

Prior to prescribing estrogen, the patient must be fully evaluated as to the general state of health by currently accepted methods including full history and physical examination (Table 99.2). Menopause should be confirmed, preferably by a minimum of 3 month's amenorrhea and the presence of specific estrogen deficiency symptoms, and by laboratory assessment when indicated. The patient should be fully informed regarding the nature of hormone replacement therapy, and should be made aware

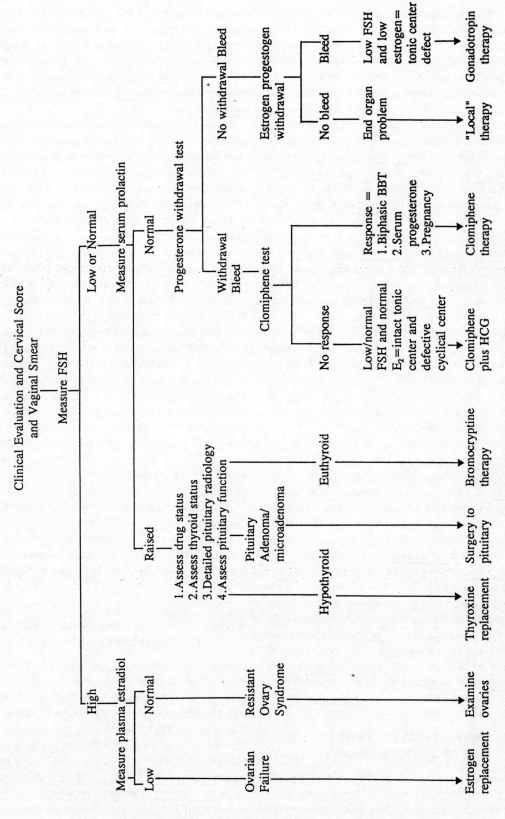

Fig. 99.1 Protocol for cost-effective treatment-oriented diagnosis of secondary amenorrhea. (Modified from [3].)

Table 99.2 List of important factors in the initial work-up before prescribing long-term hormone therapy. (Based on [2])

History	Presenting symptoms or complaints
Family history	Heart disease Cancer of the breast, uterus, cervix or ovary Diabetes Osteoporosis
Personal history	Menopausal age/menstrual pattern Vaginal bleeding (especially undiagnosed bleeding) Particulars of pregnancies Gynecologic operations Breasts Heart disease Thromboembolic disorders Liver disease Diabetes Allergy and contraindications to drugs Family relationships and personal problems

Current disorders	Menopausal
	  Hot flushes
	  Bouts of perspiration
	  Backache
	  Insomnia
	Psychosociocultural
	  Nervousness, irritability, headache, depression, etc.
	Other factors
	  Stress incontinence, urgency, or prolapse
	  Vaginal irritation
	  Aches in bone or joints
	Sexual relations
	  Frequency
	  Satisfaction
	  Pain
	  Change in interest or desire

General physical examination — note especially	Blood pressure Height and weight Breasts (mammography if necessary) Condition of skin, scalp hair, face
Pelvic examination	
Laboratory examination	Urinalysis — sugar and protein Hematocrit/hemoglobin Pap smear Hormone index on vaginal smear Mammography Hemoccult Bone density (as indicated)

of the various strategies of therapy along with the common side-effects [5]. She should also understand the importance of regular check-ups to be scheduled initially every 6 months to assess general health, clinical response, side-effects, and adequacy of dosage. Follow-up visits should include breast and pelvic examinations and blood pressure checks at the very least (Table 99.3).

Table 99.3 Recommended biannual follow-up procedures for women on long-term hormone therapy. (Based on [2])

History	Specifically any adverse effects

Physical	Especially
	  Blood pressure
	  Height and weight
	  Breast palpation
	  Pelvic examination

Laboratory tests	Cervical and vaginal smear* Fasting and 2-hour glucose[†] Hemoglobin/hematocrit[†] Fasting plasma cholesterol and lipid analysis[†] Urinalysis Endometrial biopsy[†] Mammography[†] Bone density[†] Stool blood[†]

* These procedures should be repeated once a year.
[†] Only to be undertaken when indicated.

There seem to be as many strategies for prescribing estrogen as there are estrogen preparations. Unfortunately, no perfect approach has been found or agreed on. Estrogen can be given continuously or intermittently, with progestin or without. The cyclic approach to estrogen administration, that is days 1–25 of the month, has long been used successfully. More recently, there has been a greater acceptance of a continuous, daily administration approach. Treatment with a progestin is indicated in all women who have maintained their uterus. At present there is a general consensus that progestins are unnecessary in women who have had a hysterectomy. Cyclic administration of progestin, generally days 13–25 or days 1–12, is almost always sufficient to prevent endometrial hyperplasia, but can result in menstrual-type bleeding, especially in women on cyclic estrogen. Medroxyprogesterone acetate 5–10 mg is frequently the preparation chosen. If one elects to give a progestin continuously, spotting is common in the first few months, but occurs in only about 10% of cycles thereafter. If medroxyprogesterone acetate is used, the dose is generally 2.5–5 mg daily. The safety and effectiveness of the long-standing cyclic approach are better established than the continuous approach. The choice should be made after a thorough discussion of the expectations and understanding of the patient.

Choice of preparation is far less critical than the decision to start estrogen in the first place and to be sure the patient remains compliant with the program. Frequently, patients have an idea of which estrogen

and which route they would prefer, and their input should be solicited. While complete comparative data are not available, it seems likely that virtually all preparations will be biologically effective in reducing the symptoms and risks of hypoestrogenism. Therefore, the choice rests with the physician and patient. It may be helpful to remember that conjugated estrogens (among other formulations) do not contain appreciable estrogen that is commonly measurable in the clinical laboratory. If confronted with a particularly difficult patient, one may wish to use a preparation containing estradiol which can be easily measured in the laboratory.

The incidence of estrogen-induced side-effects is usually low, provided the drugs are correctly selected and prescribed. The type and severity of adverse effects will be influenced by individual patient idiosyncracy, general health, selection of drug and dose, and the mode of administration. Nausea occurs in up to 20% of patients during the first 2–3 months of therapy. Treatment may require reduction in estrogen dose but is usually successfully achieved by reassurance, advice to take tablets with the evening meal, and prescription of antiemetic preparations. Alternatively, conversion to nonoral administration, usually the transdermal skin patch, may be helpful. Retention of excessive amounts of fluid may manifest as breast tenderness and/or weight gain. Reassurance, once again, is usually of value. The use of diuretics is not recommended. Occasionally, the dosage of estrogen or progestin will need reduction, or a change of preparation may be required.

Regular withdrawal bleeding with the cyclic progestin approach is common and should not cause a problem if the patient is prospectively alerted to the likelihood of this occurring. Any other pattern of abnormal bleeding, be it unpredictable, prolonged, or excessive, requires histologic evaluation of the endometrium. Once a histologic diagnosis has been made and cancer excluded, there are two ways to treat abnormal bleeding in association with hormonal therapy. The first is to cease therapy and observe. The second, and preferable approach, is to adjust the type and dose of hormone being administered.

A pretreatment endometrial sampling is not recommended or required unless the patient has manifested an abnormal bleeding pattern or is at high risk for endometrial atypia by virtue of a history of prolonged oligoovulation or, perhaps, of obesity. An annual endometrial biopsy is not recommended for the patient on cyclic progestin unless bleeding occurs at irregular or unexpected times. When indicated, there are various methods for obtaining endometrial specimens for cytologic or histologic diagnosis of the endometrial state.

Dilatation and curettage remains the most effective method for obtaining endometrial tissue for cytologic and histologic evaluation and has an overall accuracy of 95% or better. Unfortunately, this is not a practical screen for widespread use, and other methods have been developed. Endometrial biopsy can be effectively performed with a number of specifically designed instruments such as the Meigs or the Duncan endometrial biopsy curettes. However, endometrial biopsy can be difficult and painful in the postmenopausal woman. Furthermore, only a limited amount of tissue is obtained on most occasions, which makes the detection of localized lesions less reliable. Vacuum aspiration of endometrial tissue (Vabra aspirator) is effective in obtaining adequate endometrial specimens for histologic diagnosis from asymptomatic patients receiving estrogen. The method may yield inadequate tissue when endometrial atrophy is present, but a positive diagnosis can be made in up to 97% of cases with the Vabra aspirator. The Isaacs cell sampler and the Pipelle are other examples of safe, quick, comfortable, and reliable techniques giving adequate samples in 80–90% of patients.

CONTRAINDICATIONS

There is great disagreement as to absolute contraindications to estrogen therapy. Previously accepted standards are constantly undergoing reevaluation and renewed scrutiny [5]. There are probably very few absolute contraindications that are universally accepted. These would include undiagnosed or abnormal uterine bleeding, estrogen receptor-positive cancer, and active thromboembolic disease. There is great controversy regarding previously accepted contraindications such as a history of venous thrombosis, hypertension, or a family member with a history of breast cancer. Patients with some other previously accepted contraindications such as coronary artery disease are now considered appropriate for estrogen therapy. The physician must keep abreast of the data and be willing to discuss this frequently difficult risk: benefit dilemma with the patient prior to prescribing estrogen therapy.

A COMPREHENSIVE APPROACH

It is often gratifying to note the extent to which a comprehensive approach to the perimenopausal woman can greatly enhance her quality of life beyond that which estrogen alone can accomplish. Health advice, including establishment of a sound diet and physical fitness program, is highly desirable [4]. Counseling can also be extremely helpful, particularly in the area of marital problems or psychosexual adjustment. Finally, ongoing education is most helpful in having the woman thoroughly understand her treatment and will result in the best possible compliance with her program.

REFERENCES

1 Utian WH. Biosynthesis and physiologic effects of estrogen and pathophysiologic effects of estrogen deficiency: a review. *Am J Obstet Gynecol* 1989; 161: 1828.
2 Utian WH. *Menopause in Modern Perspective*. New York: Appleton Century Crofts, 1980.
3 Jacobs HS, Hull MG, Murray MA, Francis S. Therapy oriented diagnosis of secondary amenorrhea. *Horm Res* 1975; 6: 268.
4 Du Pont WD, Page DL. Menopausal estrogen replacement therapy and breast cancer. *Arch Int Med* 1991; 151: 67–72.
5 Utian WH, Jacobowitz R. *Managing Your Menopause*. New York: Fireside/Simon & Schuster, 1992.
6 Sitruk-Ware R, Utian WH. *The Menopause and Hormonal Replacement Therapy — Facts and Controversies*. New York: Marcel Dekker, 1991.

Osteoporosis

GIRAUD V. FOSTER

INTRODUCTION

Patients with osteoporosis frequently have multiple causes for their condition. The physician's duty is to know these causes, identify those individuals most likely to develop fractures, quantify bone mineral, and educate patients about the options that are available to them for treatment. This chapter reviews these topics.

CAUSES OF OSTEOPOROSIS

Factors that contribute to the development of osteoporosis are summarized in Table 100.1. Much attention has been paid to the two principal types: type 1, or menopausal osteoporosis, which occurs within 15–20 years of ovarian failure and is produced by accelerated bone resorption, particularly of metaphyseal bone in the vertebrae and the distal radii; and type II osteoporosis, which is a continuing process beginning about the age of 30 that affects both cortical and trabecular bone, causing fractures of the hip, especially during the eighth decade. In most female patients, not only do both types coexist but other causes may contribute as well. It is the role of the physician to identify all conditions present which accelerate the rate of bone loss or decrease the rate of bone formation.

Bone is most rapidly lost when the rate of bone formation is decreased consequent to immobilization, restricted activity, or prolonged bedrest. For example, radiologically detectable bone loss occurs within weeks in a 10-year-old child whose arm is casted for a Colles fracture; the same child, if put on full bedrest, develops a negative calcium balance within 1–10 days.

It is therefore mandatory to maintain as much activity as possible in order to prevent this rapid loss of bone, particularly in the elderly whose skeletons may be already compromised.

More difficult is the identification of factors that contribute to accelerated bone loss as a consequence of enhanced resorption. Hematologic and blood chemistry studies are needed to exclude dysfunctions of bone marrow, endocrine abnormalities, and acidosis. The history must determine if menopause has occurred early, estrogen secretion is deficient, bone marrow problems are present, medicines are enhancing bone loss, gastrointestinal problems are inhibiting calcium absorption, and if there is a familial history of bone fractures or renal disease (Fig. 100.1). The calcium in the diet must be estimated by inquiring about the amount of milk and cheese ingested, remembering that the daily need for elemental calcium is approximately 1 g/day and a quart of a milk supplies 800 mg or 80% of this need. Vitamin D levels are usually adequate if patients have had frequent exposure to sunlight or an average of at least one serving of fish or two eggs a week.

One should look for conditions that predispose to acidosis, whether respiratory, metabolic, or dietary. Smoking should be stopped since it impairs loss of carbon dioxide; diabetic or dietary ketosis should be avoided; and high-phosphate diets, like those rich in red meat, should be restricted. Acidosis is rarely reflected in laboratory findings, since buffering salts from the bone are mobilized to neutralize hydrogen ions at the expense of bone mass.

If there is a history of fractures, one should inquire about the conditions under which they occurred. Patients who have had multiple fractures or fractures occurring under nontraumatic circumstances are more likely to have osteoporosis which, by definition, is that condition in which there is insufficient normal bone to support the body to a degree that fractures occur.

Table 100.1 Factors that contribute to the development of osteoporosis

---

Hormonal causes
Luteal-phase defect
Oligomenorrhea
Early menopause
Hyperthyroidism
Hypercorticoidism
Diabetes mellitus
Hyperparathyroidism
Acromegaly
Addison's disease
Hypogonadism
Anorexia nervosa

Lack of exercise
Immobilization
Prolonged bedrest
Restricted activity

Medications
Antacids: Amphogel, Gelusil, Maalox, Mylanta, Riopan
Anticonvulsants: Dilantin, phenobarbital
Anticoagulants: Heparin
Antituberculosis medications: Isoniazid
Diuretics: Furosemide
Glucocorticoids: Cortisone, prednisone
Cyrotoxic drugs: Actinomycin D, mithramycin

Dietary deficiencies
Insufficient calcium
Low vitamin D intake
Excessive phosphate in diet

Increased bone mineral mobilization
Respiratory acidosis
Smoking
Metabolic acidosis
Liver disease
Chronic renal failure

Constitutional factors
Small skeletal frame
Family history for osteoporosis
Aging

Deficient calcium absorption
Alcohol
Hypercalciuria
Sprue-like conditions
Caffeine
Diets high in fiber, oxalates, or phytates
Gastrointestinal surgery with removal of segments of bowel

Table 100.1 (*cont.*)

Hematologic diseases
Systemic mastocytosis
Thalassemia
Leukemia
Lymphoma
Myelomatosis

Idiopathic osteoporosis

IDENTIFYING INDIVIDUALS AT RISK OF DEVELOPING OSTEOPOROSIS

In today's litigious society, patients should be advised if they are likely to develop osteoporosis. Those at risk are principally of two types; thin, Caucasian women under 1.65 m (5'6") and individuals of either sex who have several of the risk factors listed in Table 100.1.

A major problem is who should be treated. Obviously patients with depleted skeletons who have sustained fractures require treatment. On the other hand, for those who have less than normal bone and multiple risk factors, the physician must decide between immediate treatment or observation over a period of time to determine whether or not bone is being lost at a rate that will eventually lead to fractures. Unfortunately, there are no guidelines to help the physician make this decision. The decision is usually made empirically on the basis of the current condition of the skeleton and the willingness of the patient to be treated.

QUANTIFICATION OF BONE MINERAL

Four methods are currently available for measuring bone mineral density: single-photon absorptiometry, dual-beam photon absorptiometry, dual-energy X-ray absorptiometry, and quantitative computed tomography. Single-beam photon absorptiometry uses radiation from a nuclear source. The beam of radiation is usually passed across the distal radius or second metacarpal. The method estimates primarily cortical bone in the appendicular skeleton. Since the commonest fractures are of the vertebrae and the most costly and life-threatening are those of the hip, this technique is not of great diagnostic value for predicting fractures of the axial skeleton in these areas that consist principally of metaphyseal bone. Furthermore, since single-beam photon

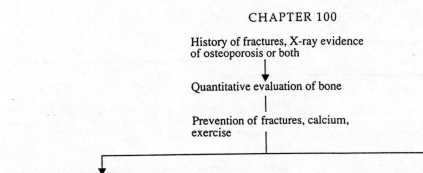

History of fractures, X-ray evidence
of osteoporosis or both

Quantitative evaluation of bone

Prevention of fractures, calcium,
exercise

If menopausal and no contraindications
to estrogen, treat with estrogen

If not menopausal, if contraindications to estrogen,
or if the patient selects it, coherence therapy

Fig. 100.1 Approach to osteoporosis.

absorptiometry measures fat in bone as well as bone mineral, the technique is not without error. Dual-beam photon absorptiometry has, until recently, been the most popular technique. It uses a rectilinear scanner and gadolinium as the nuclear source. Gadolinium emits radiation at two energy levels: one is used to measure fat and the other total bone density. By subtracting that density due to fat from total density, density due to bone mineral only is estimated. Scans of the total body, spine, and femur have precision errors of 1, 2, and 3%, respectively. The disadvantages of the method are its relatively poor reproducibility and the time it takes. A reading requires 30–45 min. As a result there is increasing use of dual-energy X-ray absorptiometry. The latter employs a high radiation flux which improves spatial resolution and precision while reducing scanning time to 5 or 10 min. Fortunately for those institutions that are changing from one system to another, the degree of correlation between the two is high. Because of its relative advantages, dual-energy X-ray absorptiometry is likely to replace dual-beam photon absorptiometry during the coming decade.

The latter two methods measure principally metaphyseal bone in vertebrae and hips. An alternate way of measuring metaphyseal bone is by quantitative computed tomography (CT). While CT scanning is accurate, because the slice read is thin, precision is often poor except in institutions with long-term experience.

Since metaphyseal bone is the most metabolically active bone, it is the bone most rapidly lost when the rate of bone resorption is high. Therefore for assessing vertebrae and femoral necks, techniques that measure metaphyseal bone are preferable. Most are computerized to compare results to both mean values observed in normal young individuals and normal individuals of similar age, sex, and body

weight and estimate the likelihood of the patient fracturing in the near future.

TREATMENT AND PREVENTION OF FRACTURES

Because of the attention the press devotes to osteoporosis, it behooves the physician to educate the patient by giving sufficient information that patient and doctor together can decide upon a satisfactory course of treatment. If the decision is made by the physician alone, all too frequently the patient will later hear of another form of therapy and change doctors in the hope of receiving more current therapy. Thanks to the improved methods of quantifying bone mineral, it has been demonstrated that each of the five treatments increases bone mineral at a similar rate of about 4–6% per year. Patients should be told in the office about these five treatments: calcium, estrogen, coherence therapy with biphosphonates, calcitonin, and fluorides. The merits and demerits of each of these should be discussed and one chosen on the basis of the patient's interaction with the doctor. The patient should then be written a letter of explanation upon which they can deliberate. If there are any misunderstandings, the physician can be called for further clarification and the strategy changed if need be. The advantages of this form of management are that the patient is: (1) more likely to be compliant if he or she has participated in the decision making process; (2) much less likely to change to another treatment; and (3) comforted that the physician has anticipated obvious questions.

The following is a suggested text for the physician to record on a word processor and use as it is or alter it for writing to patients about the treatment of osteoporosis.

Prevention of fractures

Prevention is probably more important than medication. There are six things that you should do:

1 Have "boating soles" put on all your shoes. These are made of rubber with multiple small parallel cracks which prevent slipping even on wet surfaces.

2 Remove scatter rugs and any other obstacles in your home that increase your chances of falling.

3 Avoid all heavy lifting. If you do have to pick up something, kneel down and pick it up with your back straight.

4 Do not open windows in the conventional way. If you need to open a window, approach it with your back to it and raise it using your cupped fingers.

5 Prevent unnecessary falls outside. If steps are icy in the wintertime, have a railing installed.

6 Practice correct posture. Sit and stand straight if you do not already do so.

Exercise

Exercise is helpful in two ways: by increasing your cardiac output, it improves circulation to your skeleton, and by strengthening your muscles it stimulates bone cells to build new bone.

Rapid walking or low-impact aerobic exercises are excellent. Be certain that in all activities the back remains straight or hyperextended and that you avoid forward-bending exercises. For patients who have sustained severe fractures, the assistance of a physical therapist is usually mandatory. Start your exercise program slowly, beginning with only 2 or 3 min a day and gradually working up to 15 or 20. If discomfort develops, reduce your program appropriately.

Fractures

Fractures of the vertebrae are common. Many occur without pain. Most, however, are associated with at least some discomfort and some are very painful. If fractures are frequent or severe, eventually a stooped posture develops. Good posture and exercise will help prevent these changes. However, fractures may still occasionally occur. For discomfort ibuprofen 800 mg three times a day always after meals and 5 mg Valium (diazepam), also three times a day, are helpful. The latter relaxes the muscles: it is also addictive, so it should not be taken for more than 2 weeks at a time.

If vertebral fractures cause severe pain, a removable light-weight body cast is helpful to provide support to the spine while allowing you to remain ambu-latory. With immobilization, the skeleton is very rapidly lost so keeping active is very important.

Medications

There are five treatments that are presently popular: calcium, estrogen, coherence therapy, calcitonin, and sodium fluoride. You should know about all of them.

Calcium

Who needs to take calcium supplements, how much calcium is needed to prevent osteoporosis, and what preparations should and should not be used are three important questions.

The answer to the first question is anyone needs calcium who has an insufficient dietary intake of calcium or impaired absorption of calcium. In practice it is usually difficult to identify who these individuals are. A good guess, however, is that probably about 25% of patients with osteoporosis have insufficient calcium intake in their diets. Most physicians therefore prescribe calcium for everyone.

The answer to the second question is that somewhere between 1.0 and 1.5 g of elemental calcium a day is needed to prevent osteoporosis. This is an inexact figure, because many factors affect absorption, like the amount of exposure to sunlight, the amount of vitamin D in the diet, the acidity of the stomach, the form in which calcium is taken, and medicines and foods that affect absorption. For example, milk increases absorption, probably as the result of fermentation of soluble calcium lactate, but at the same time delays transit time in the gastrointestinal tract, while diets rich in phosphates and fiber prevent intestinal absorption of calcium.

The third question is what calcium preparations are best. Calcium carbonate is usually given because it is the least expensive. Furthermore, since it contains 40% elemental calcium, only three 500 mg tablets supply half the daily requirement for calcium. However, calcium carbonate may be poorly absorbed by the elderly. Dissolution of calcium carbonate needs acid in the stomach and many patients in their seventh and eighth decades make little acid. Usually if there is not enough acid the undissolved tablets are seen in the stool.

In addition to stomach acid, compression of calcium carbonate during pill manufacture also reduces solubility. Insoluble preparations can be recognized by their inability to dissolve in a cup of vinegar when stirred for 2 min. If solubility is a problem, this can be solved by changing to another preparation, be it calcium carbonate or more soluble calcium citrate.

You should know the following additional facts about calcium replacement:

1 Calcium supplements do not prevent osteoporosis in most patients, despite the fact that theoretically they inhibit the secretion of parathyroid hormone, which has the potential to dissolve bones.

2 Dolomite, a carbonate of calcium and magnesium, should not be taken since some preparations contain lead.

3 Calcium carbonate is best taken after the main meal since food stimulates secretion of stomach acid that helps dissolve it.

4 Alcohol and some antacids, antibiotics, anticoagulants, and diuretics inhibit calcium absorption.

5 Calcium citrate is not usually initially prescribed because it is more expensive than calcium carbonate and more tablets must be taken — a factor that often leads to poor compliance.

Estrogen

Estrogen replacement in postmenopausal women and women who secrete insufficient estrogen inhibits bone loss by reducing the rate of bone resorption. This beneficial effect is additive to that produced by calcium supplementation. A daily dose of 0.625 mg usually prevents bone loss. The principal danger of estrogen replacement is hyperplasia of the lining of the uterus, which, if undetected, can lead to cancer. Hyperplasia is prevented if the conjugated equine estrogen preparation is prescribed for only 21 days of each month and is followed by a daily dose of progestogen for 8 days to insure monthly bleeding that occurs when the endometrial lining is sloughed.

You should know the following about estrogen:

1 To be effective estrogen must be given for life since stopping estrogen results in renewed and accelerated bone loss.

2 Estrogen has little effect in preventing osteoporosis in women over the age of 70.

3 Postmenopausal women frequently find menstruating again unacceptable and discontinue treatment.

4 A biopsy of the lining of the uterus must be carried out every 2 years to be certain that hyperplasia of the uterus has not developed.

5 Estrogen should not be given if there is a history of uterine or breast cancer, lipid problems, gallbladder disease, clotting disorders, or heavy smoking.

6 Estrogen can produce side-effects such as premenstrual symptoms, migraine headaches, hypertension, yeast infections, enlargement of breast lumps, and either an increase or decrease in weight.

7 Estrogen may cause an increase in the incidence of breast cancer in women who take it for more than 15 years but at the same time it probably reduces the likelihood of developing coronary artery disease.

8 Estrogen usually decreases other symptoms related to the menopause such as hot flashes, vaginal dryness, and sometimes even urinary incontinence.

Coherence therapy

Bone breakdown and build-up are processes that are continually taking place in bone remodeling units whose activity is not synchronous. If one synchronizes these units by first making them all active and then inhibits bone breakdown without altering the rate of bone build-up, the net effect is that they all act to increase bone. This treatment is called coherence therapy by some and ADRP, for activation-depression-free-repeat, by others. Several different ways of giving the medicines in coherence therapy have been used and most of the findings are encouraging. The method that appears the most promising uses 2 or 3 g of potassium neutral phosphate given orally for 3 days followed by 14 days of 400 mg a day of Didronel (disodium etidronate) and a 74-day rest period, during which 800 iu of vitamin D and 1.5 g of calcium as calcium carbonate are given daily. Every 91 days, this regime is repeated.

Since Didronel is not broken down in the body to metabolites, side reactions are rare but can include gastric irritation and skin rash. Potassium neutral phosphate, on the other hand, can cause diarrhea in some individuals. Recent studies suggest that the difference between giving and not giving neutral phosphate is not great, so that in older patients a good case can be made for deleting this part of the protocol.

Calcitonin

Calcitonin prevents bone breakdown. Since calcium ions are constantly going into bone and leaving bone, any medication that prevents their leaving bone results in an accumulation of bone mineral. Calcitonin is effective in doing just that. Its principal disadvantages are that it has to be given by injection and is expensive.

Sodium fluoride

Sodium fluoride also helps to build up bone. Unfortunately no commercial preparation is presently available that provides 20 mg. Therefore tablets of sodium fluoride must be specially prepared. To be effective 60–80 mg a day must be taken.

Sodium fluoride is not without its problems. The incidence of side-effects is high: 30% of patients develop gastric irritation and another 20% pain in their leg bones. In addition, about a quarter of patients are unresponsive to the medication. Finally, while bone density is increased by sodium fluoride, the strength of bone may actually be decreased in some patients, resulting in even more fractures. For these reasons, sodium fluoride is rarely prescribed for osteoporosis.

FURTHER READING

Dequeker J, Geusens P. Treatment of established osteoporosis and rehabilitation: current practice and possibilities. *Maturitas* 1990; 12: 1–36.

Johnston CC Jr. Treatment of osteoporotic patients. *Public Health Report* 1989; 104 (suppl): 75–77.

Nagant-de-Deuxchaisnes -C. Therapy for skeletal disorders. *Curr Opin Rheumatöl* 1989; 1: 98–111.

Riggs BL. A new option for treating osteoporosis. *N Engl J Med* 1990; 323: 124–125.

Seymour DG, Day JJ, Pathy MS. Review: sodium fluoride: too late and too toxic for the elderly osteoporotic patient? *Age-Ageing* 1990; 19: 222–228.

Storm T, Thamsborg G, Steiniche T, Genant HK, Srensen OH. Effect of intermittent cyclical etidronate therapy on bone mass and fracture rate in women with post-menopausal osteoporosis. *N Engl J Med* 1990; 322: 1265–1271.

Watts NB, Harris ST, Genant HK *et al*. Intermittent cyclical etidronate treatment of postmenopausal osteoporosis. *N Engl J Med* 1990; 323: 73–79.

Hot flashes

KENNETH A. STEINGOLD

INTRODUCTION

The hot flash is the most common symptom of the climacteric period with an estimated 20—45% of women seeking medical attention for this problem. Although these vasomotor complaints are often overshadowed by more serious medical concerns such as osteoporosis, the lifestyle of these women with severe hot flashes is truly affected by these problematic symptoms. The purpose of this chapter is to provide a brief overview of the hot flash process, including pathophysiology, differential diagnosis, and treatment.

DESCRIPTION OF HOT FLASHES

It is estimated that 75% of women undergoing spontaneous menopause experience hot flashes. In women with surgically induced menopause, the percentage of women with hot flashes may be higher — between 90 and 100% — although there is some controversy as to whether this abrupt withdrawal of estrogen production leads to an increase in symptomatology. Certainly there are some patients who require treatment for hot flashes prior to hospital discharge, but in general it appears there is a gradual increase in the frequency of hot flashes over time following the surgical procedure. In one study of 100 oophorectomized women, 50 women had symptoms while still in the hospital, while 84 women had vasomotor complaints within 6 weeks of the procedure. The length of time for the persistence of these complaints decreases with age. One year following the menopause, 80% of women continue to have hot flashes. However after 5 years, 25—50% of women persist in these complaints, and at 9 years, approximately 29% continue with hot flashes. It is encouraging that these symptoms may dissipate with time, but it is clear that a substantial number of women do continue to require treatment for these bothersome complaints.

The classical description of the hot flash is that of a periodic, episodic event. Usually the patient experiences a sudden onset of head and neck flushing which passes in waves to other parts of the body. With this subjective sensation of heat throughout the body and the subsequent recognition by the thermoregulatory centers, the body attempts to dissipate this heat with perspiration, predominantly in the head, neck, chest, and back. The patient also experiences the behavioral changes associated with this heat by actively trying to cool off, whether it be by fanning or removing articles of clothing and blankets. The terms flash and flush are often used interchangeably by most authors, although flushing refers to the reddening of the skin which usually but not always occurs with these vasomotor symptoms. Associated symptomatology is often noted, including headaches and palpitations. The most problematic association is the occurrence of insomnia. Flashing occurs with equal frequency between day and night; however when flashes do occur in the nighttime, the patient experiences night sweats and waking episodes. Sleep electroencephalogram studies have confirmed this decrease in sleep activity at night in patients with frequent hot flashes. This sleep disturbance carries over to impairment of daily activities on subsequent days.

PATHOPHYSIOLOGY

A clear understanding of the pathophysiology of hot flashes is still forthcoming. It was not until the last two decades that significant research was undertaken, since these symptoms were presumed to be psychogenic or emotional sequelae of the menopausal years. With greater understanding of thermoregulation, progress has been made in uncovering physiologic mechanisms and appropriate therapies. Objective studies have been performed on women experiencing frequent hot flashes by measuring various parameters, and the sequence of events has been constructed to delineate the physiologic changes.

The general sequence of events begins with peripheral cutaneous vasodilatation, followed by the subjective sensation of the flash, then an increase in peripheral skin temperature, a decrease in skin resistance, and finally as heat is lost, a decrease in core temperature. The initial event, cutaneous vasodilatation, is presumably in response to an alteration in the thermoregulatory center sensing a change in temperature. The body adapts with vasodilatation which usually occurs 1 min before the subjective sensation and lasts for approximately 8 min. Skin temperature rises approximately 90 seconds after the beginning of the subjective sensation and reaches a peak by around 9 min. The average skin temperature increases 4°C, although it may be substantially higher. Afterwards, in a response to perspiration, skin resistance decreases — maximum within 4 min. Occasionally palpitations and an increased heart rate are noted, probably secondary to increased sympathetic nervous system activity.

The cause of this disorder in thermoregulation is still not known. Clearly, the major associated event is a decrease in circulating estrogen levels, as evidenced by the menopausal status of the woman. However, 18% of women between the ages of 45 and 54 do experience hot flashes, but it is likely that the perimenopausal transition of these women reflects a decrease in total estrogen production during this particular phase of ovarian life. It also appears that the postmenopausal women with the lowest total estrogen levels (estradiol and estrone) have the more severe occurrence of hot flashes.

How hypoestrogenemia translates into vasomotor symptoms is unclear. The neuroendocrine link between estrogen-related events and the thermoregulatory mechanisms has not been elucidated. There is clearly an association between luteinizing hormone (LH) pulses and the occurrence of the individual hot flash, thus leading to speculation that the LH pulse was the initiator of the flash. However, patients who have had hypophysectomies performed and thus no endogenous LH and follicle-stimulating hormone (FSH) secretion still continue to have hot flashes. The next logical neurohormone to be implicated was gonadotropin-releasing hormone (GnRH); however, patients with isolated gonadotropin deficiency, and hence no endogenous GnRH secretion, after prior exposure to estrogen do experience hot flashes. Therefore GnRH and LH are not necessary for the occurrence of these events.

The modulating factor must reside in a suprahypothalamic area. Neurotransmitters such as norepinephrine, dopamine, endogenous opiates, and neurotensin have all been implicated as pathogenetic modulators. The decrease in estrogen may cause activation of the appropriate neurotransmitter pathway which affects thermoregulatory function and secondarily affects GnRH and LH secretion. It is the interconnection of these pathways that leads to these vasomotor events. Work continues in this interesting area trying to uncover the neuroendocrine basis for hot flashes.

DIFFERENTIAL DIAGNOSIS

The diagnosis of menopausal hot flashes is usually straightforward. An outline of the approach to the patient with hot flashes is shown in Figure 101.1. The combination of the characteristic episodic flash in a hypoestrogenic woman makes these symptoms a most likely menopausal vasomotor phenomenon. The perimenopausal patient can also experience hot flashes as she moves through the transitional phase from regular menses to amenorrhea. Also, women with premature ovarian failure can have significant hot flashes just like their older counterparts: age is much less important than the estrogen status.

The differential diagnosis arises in the patient experiencing flashes who is clearly not hypoestrogenemic. This is one subset of patients necessitating a search for alternate diagnoses. The second group of patients requiring evaluation are those who fail standard treatments. As discussed below, estrogen replacement therapy is highly effective in alleviating hot flashes. If one has persistent hot flashes despite adequate therapy, other medical conditions may be present.

The differential diagnosis list is straightforward and the diagnosis is usually evident based on routine historical data. Indeed, it is extremely unlikely for a menopausal women having hot flashes to have anything other than simple menopausal syndrome. The following is a list of other causes of flushing reactions:

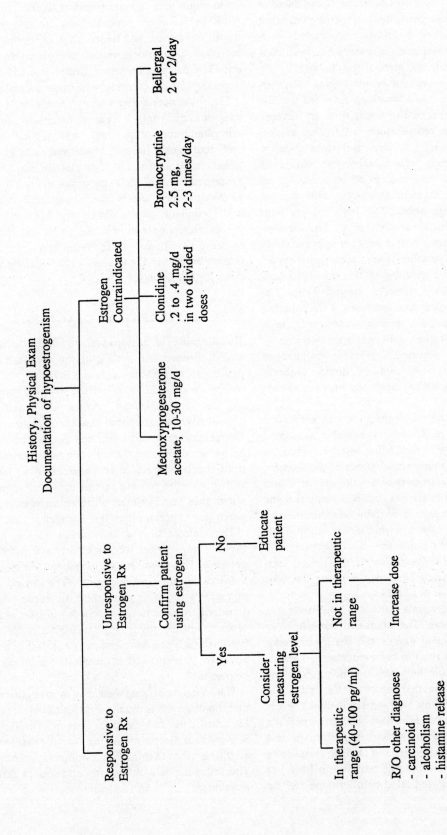

Fig. 101.1 Approach to the patient with hot flashes.

1 The most interesting entity associated with flashing is the carcinoid syndrome. In this syndrome, the patient experiences episodes of flushing reactions in association with a tumor of enterochromaffin-cell origin. These tumors can be found in the gut, a number of endocrine organs, and the lung, but most commonly in the terminal ileum. These flushes can be provoked by epinephrine, isoproterenol, alcohol, and food. The postprandial flushing in these individuals may be related to pentagastrin release. The diagnosis of carcinoid syndrome is based on elevated 5-hydroxyindole acetic acid levels followed by a search for the primary tumor.

2 There are a host of alcohol-induced flushing reactions. In these individuals, the alcohol may be acting as a vasodilator. In addition, some patients have impaired metabolism of ethanol and have predisposition to flushing.

3 There are also a number of drug interactions with alcohol that may induce flushes. Most notably disulfiram, metronidazole, and chlorpropramide can metabolically react with alcohol to produce these phenomena. Even in the absence of chlorpropramide, diabetic patients are prone to flushing.

4 There are also flushing reactions with other neoplasias besides carcinoid. Disorders associated with histamine release, such as basophilic chronic granulocytic leukemia and mastocytosis cause reactions due to the release of vasoactive peptides. Pancreatic tumors and insulinomas are also in the differential, with reactions from secreted peptides or prostaglandin release. In addition, medullary carcinoma of the thyroid can cause flushing, possibly from release of calcitonin.

5 Finally, idiopathic flushing and paroxysmal hypothalamic discharge are diagnoses of exclusion.

TREATMENT

The mainstay of therapy for hot flashes is estrogen replacement. The decision to undergo hormone replacement therapy with estrogen is complex and beyond the scope of this chapter. Obviously, one must weigh the benefits, which include prevention of osteoporosis and possibly a cardioprotective effect, with the known risks of long-term estrogen. However, estrogen remains almost completely effective in the alleviation of vasomotor symptoms. Previous teaching suggests that the smallest effective dose of estrogen be utilized; however, when other wanted actions of estrogen are taken into account, higher dosages are necessary. In general, for the prevention of bone loss, 0.625 mg of conjugated estrogens or its equivalent is the minimum necessary dose. This dose is also highly effective for the treatment of hot flashes. A dose of 10 µg of ethinylestradiol (which is more equivalent to 1.25 mg conjugated estrogen) is also commonly used. Oral micronized estradiol is also available in a standard dose of 1–2 mg daily. For patients unable to tolerate or with contraindications to oral estrogen, transdermal estradiol replacement has also been shown to be highly effective for the treatment of hot flashes; it is currently manufactured at 0.05 or 0.1 mg patches applied twice a week.

The dose of estrogen needs to be titrated according to symptoms, and occasionally the dosage needs to be increased in particularly susceptible individuals. If the patient does not experience symptomatic relief with oral or transdermal replacement, she should be switched to the alternate delivery route (oral to or from transdermal). In addition, injectable forms of estrogen are available. These may be pure estrogen (estradiol cypionate or valerate) or combinations of estrogen and testosterone. One advantage of the parenteral injection is that certain unwanted oral side-effects are avoided. Also, higher dosages are achieved, especially peak blood concentrations. In the patient who is significantly unresponsive to the oral or transdermal estrogen, utilizing an increased dose of intramuscular estrogen may help clarify if indeed these flashes are estrogen-responsive. If the injectable form does not prove to be effective, then the search should begin for alternative diagnoses.

In the patient with a contraindication to estrogen therapy, alternate forms of treatment are available. The second most effective treatment is the use of a progestational agent. In the patient with estrogen-sensitive tumors or an intolerance to estrogen therapy, progestins are logical alternatives. The progestational agent may be given via the oral or intramuscular route. Medroxyprogesterone acetate can be utilized in a dose between 10 and 30 mg orally per day. The average dose of 20 mg causes minimal side-effects, although rarely progestational spotting will be noted. This progestin may also be given intramuscularly in a depot form, 150 mg monthly. The advantage of this injection is that adequate levels can be achieved rapidly, but the disadvantage is the unpredictable nature of this medication with irregular bleeding sometimes noted, even in these postmenopausal women. Alternatively, megestrol, 20–80 mg a day, is as effective. Another advantage of the progestins is they provide a positive calcium balance and are protective to bone.

In patients who cannot tolerate or have a contraindication to progestin therapy, nonhormonal medications have been studied. This group of women includes patients with previously treated breast cancer where all hormonal therapy tends to be withheld. In studies of the pathophysiology of hot flashes, various neurotransmitter pathways have been implicated, thus providing a basis for the nonhormonal treatments. Clonidine, an α-adrenergic agent, has been used with success in some objectively studied patients. The response to this medication is variable, but, in general, studies appear to be in agreement on the efficacy of this antihypertensive agent. The dose ranges between 0.2 and 0.4 mg in two divided doses. Patients need to be observed for hypotensive episodes, especially with the initial dosing. The success of clonidine has provided evidence of increased α-adrenergic activity as a possible mechanism for these thermoregulatory disturbances. Another antihypertensive, α-methyldopa, has also been evaluated. The dose administered is 250 mg t.i.d., although success with this agent is less impressive than with clonidine.

The dopaminergic pathway has also been modulated with both dopamine agonists as well as antidopaminergic agents studied. Interestingly, both agonists and antagonists of dopamine have been shown to be effective in the subjective relief of hot flashes. Bromocriptine has shown some promise in a dose of 2.5 mg two to three times a day. An antidopaminergic agent, veralipride, has recently been shown to provide 60–80% of patients with relief. Further studies with these agents will delineate the role of dopaminergic pathways in the treatment of hot flashes, but these agents may be used in the refractory patients. Finally, Bellergal is another nonhormonal agent that has been used for a number of years for the relief of vasomotor-associated symptoms. This medication is a combination agent consisting of ergotamine, belladonna alkaloids, and phenobarbital. This provides inhibition of adrenergic and cholinergic impulses in addition to the sedative effect of the barbiturate. Placebo-controlled studies in the past have provided evidence for relief of nervousness, hot flashes, insomnia, dizziness, and irritability associated with menopausal syndrome. Therefore, this drug should not be forgotten if other medications have failed.

It is also clear that activities in the daily life can modulate the hot flashes, with heat being a major predisposing factor. Hot weather makes symptoms worse, as does a hot environment within the house. It is important for patients to be aware of this and try to modify environmental stimuli.

In conclusion, hot flashes remain the most common problem associated with the menopausal patient, causing impairment of sleep, interruption of normal daily activities, with episodic symptoms that are both discomforting and embarrassing. Many women seek treatment for this condition since it is such a bothersome complaint. Adequate therapies are available, both hormonal and nonhormonal, and treatment can be tailored for the patient who has a contraindication to hormonal replacement therapy. In the resistant patient, a search is necessary for alternative diagnoses, although most of these conditions are rare and may be obvious from the general medical history of the patient. Otherwise, the treatment of hot flashes is very satisfying both to the patient and physician and should provide long-term relief.

FURTHER READING

Meldrum DR. The pathophysiology of postmenopausal symptoms. *Semin Reprod Endocrinol* 1983; 1: 11.

Steingold KA, Laufer L, Chetkowski R *et al*. Treatment of hot flashes with transdermal estradiol administration. *J Clin Endocrinol Metab* 1985; 61: 627.

Tataryn IV, Lomax P, Bajorek JG *et al*. Postmenopausal hot flashes: a disorder of thermoregulation. *Maturitas* 1980; 2: 101.

Tulandi T, Lal S. Menopausal hot flash. *Obstet Gynecol Surv* 1985; 40: 553.

Wilkin JK. Flushing reactions: consequences and mechanisms. *Ann Intern Med* 1981; 95: 468.

Hormone replacement in cancer patients

ELY BRAND

Approximately half of all cancer patients become long-term survivors. As the quality of life improves for these patients, the long-term consequences of estrogen deficiency become increasingly important. In this chapter, we discuss guidelines for estrogen replacement therapy (ERT) in cancer patients. An outline of ERT in endometrial cancer patients is shown in Figure 102.1 In general three principles guide this discussion. First, in a cancer-free patient ERT cannot cause recurrence. Secondly, in cancer cells which lack estrogen receptors, estrogen usually does not have a mitogenic effect. Thirdly, while ERT has not been proven detrimental to any group of cancer patients, virtually no prospective studies exist in patients with potentially hormone-sensitive tumors. Therefore, the recommendations presented represent the bias of the author and are not based on well-established clinical data.

BREAST CANCER

A total of 150 000 cases of breast cancer are diagnosed in the USA annually, affecting one in 10 women over the course of their lifetime. The patient with breast cancer may ask, "Did my use of the birth control pill or estrogen replacement cause this cancer?"

Oral contraceptives (OCs) and breast cancer

Several large studies have failed to provide a link between using OCs and later development of breast cancer. Patients who develop breast cancer after OC use may actually have a slightly better prognosis, possibly due to earlier detection. On the other hand, first child-birth after age 35 almost doubles the risk of breast cancer. While some studies of OCs found increased breast cancer risk in users, the 1984 case control study performed by the US Centers for Disease Control found no increased risk [1]. However, long duration of use, as well as use by teen-agers, may be major contributors to the attributable

risk. One retrospective analysis concluded that "progesterone dominant" formulas given to teenage women for 6 or more years quadrupled the breast cancer risk [2]. While the methodology in that work was seriously questioned, recent studies also find increased risk associated with increasing duration of use. Keep in mind that the average age of OC users is much younger than the average age of breast cancer patients, so large prospective studies will require many years before firm conclusions emerge.

ERT and breast cancer

There are few convincing data that ERT increases the risk of breast cancer. The relative risk of breast cancer in most studies of ERT is between 0.8 and 3.4, with a plethora of research demonstrating no increased risk in conjugated estrogen users. While the effects of ERT on relative risk may be higher in women with natural menopause than in those with surgical menopause, confounding variables plague the research. For instance, ERT patients are followed closely and may obtain more frequent examinations and mammograms, thus increasing the detection rate. Secondly, patients at risk for breast cancer may be dissuaded from ERT. Several studies of breast cancer patients who received ERT prior to diagnosis have found decreased mortality (up to 40%) compared to the cohort who did not receive ERT [3].

Most studies do not evaluate the effect of concomitant progestin therapy, which may reduce the risk of breast cancer [4]. The majority of breast cancer cell lines are inhibited by progestins *in vivo*, which block the mitogenic effects of estrogens. *In vitro*, breast epithelial cells divide more in the luteal phase in the presence of progestins than in the follicular phase. Nonetheless, anovulatory women who have a relative deficiency of progesterone have up to five times the risk of breast cancer. The incidence rises sharply after menopause when progestins are no longer produced. In one of the few randomized,

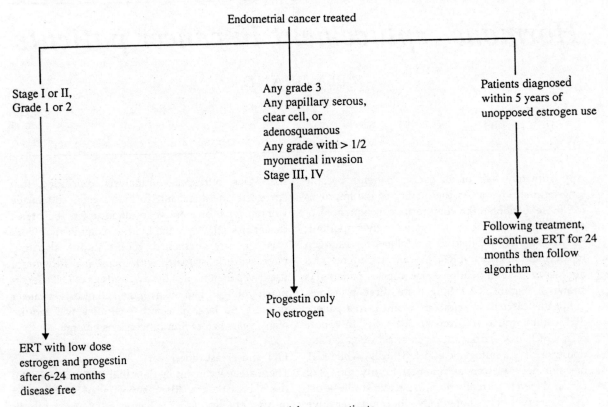

Fig. 102.1 Suggested estrogen therapy (ERT) in endometrial cancer patients.

blind, placebo-controlled and prospective studies (168 women), after 10 years, breast cancer developed in 5% of the women on placebo and none on combination therapy [5].

In a large study of 23 000 women in Sweden the use of conjugated estrogens was not associated with increased risk. Ethinylestradiol, more commonly used in Europe than conjugated estrogens, did appear to increase breast cancer risk about twofold [6]. In the largest study to date — over 280 000 women — there was a 1.5% increase in relative risk after 20 years or more of ERT [3]. Thus, the risk of breast cancer in women on ERT is controversial and uncertain.

ERT in breast cancer patients

Even if ERT slightly increases a woman's risk of developing breast cancer, it does not follow that ERT would stimulate recurrence in patients clinically free of disease. One prospective study has been conducted using oral contraceptives as hormone replacement therapy with tumor regression in 22% of 65 cases and no adverse effects. In a follow-up study, no evidence of increased recurrence was seen in the continuous low-dose estrogen—progestin group [7]. Since there are inadequate data to address the safety of ERT in breast cancer patients, the safest course is to use progestins in these patients for treatment of vasomotor flashes and to retard bone loss. The new antiresorptive agents (e.g., etidronate), which retard bone loss, should also be considered.

The natural history of breast cancer results in recurrences as late as 30 years after diagnosis. Over 25% of recurrences occur after 10 years. These patients harbor occult breast cancer cells that divide very slowly, or not at all, until unknown triggers promote recurrence. Since estrogen can be mitogenic in breast cancer cells in culture, one could theoretically hasten recurrence in patients treated with ERT. The Halstedian hypothesis that breast cancer spreads from the primary site to regional lymphatics in an orderly fashion before systemic spread has not held up. Many oncologists consider breast cancer to be a systemic disease from its inception. Even a 1 cm breast cancer contains 1 billion cells and has been present for many years. Supporting the systemic hypothesis are recent data that adjuvant chemotherapy or tamoxifen in node-negative patients reduces recurrences. Clearly, if no cancer cells remain, estrogens should be safe. But can we ever be sure that no cancer cells remain? Probably not.

Endocrine ablation by medical or surgical adrenalectomy, hypophysectomy, or oophorectomy has resulted in clinical remission in advanced cases. Therefore, the use of unopposed estrogen is generally contraindicated in breast cancer patients, of whom two-thirds are ER-positive. However, diethylstilbestrol has also been used as an anticancer agent in breast cancer with some remissions, in high doses.

Further studies may show that the combination of continuous estrogen and progestin *may* be safe in stage 1 node-negative breast cancer after a disease-free interval of at least 5 years. However, only 80% of these patients will be disease-free at 5 years. In stage 2 node-negative breast cancer (2–5 cm primary) only 65% are disease-free at 5 years. With such high recurrence rates in early breast cancer, the physician who prescribes ERT places him- or herself and the patient in a precarious position. In node-positive cases, well over half relapse within 5 years, and ERT cannot be recommended without further study. Any breast cancer patient who develops a recurrence while on ERT presents an ethical and medicolegal dilemma which cannot be resolved until prospective studies are complete. In addition the lifetime risk of developing a second primary breast cancer is about 1% per year.

The use of estrogen receptor status as a guide to ERT is alluring. However, several caveats are in order. First, some estrogen receptor-negative tumors (5–10%) respond to hormonal therapy. Secondly, tumor heterogeneity suggests that estrogen receptor-negative tumors can contain low levels of estrogen receptor-positive cells. For instance, tumors that contain 1–5 fm/mg of receptors are defined as estrogen receptor-negative. Furthermore, there may be technical problems in performing the assay or estrogen receptor-positive clones may be present in portions of the tumor not assayed. Thirdly, low levels of estrogen receptors may be increased by estrogen-promoting synthesis of its own receptor. Finally, keep in mind that disease-free intervals are shorter in estrogen receptor-negative tumors, which are usually poorly differentiated, and that breast cancers which develop in women on ERT tend to have lower estrogen receptor levels than cancers in women not treated with ERT.

Benign breast disease

Women with benign breast disease should not be denied the benefits of ERT. Conjugated estrogens in low doses (0.625 mg) do not increase the incidence of fibrocystic breast disease or fibroadenoma and may lower breast cancer risk in women with atypical hyperplasia [8]. Studies have yielded conflicting results as to whether patients with benign breast disease — already at higher risk — have an elevated attributable risk due to ERT. Regardless of whether ERT causes breast cancer, the interpretation of mammograms is more difficult in these patients due to estrogen effects on the ductal parenchyma, effects which can be minimized by the addition of progestins. Dose and duration of ERT may play a role, and may be important in long-term studies that enlist cases from the 1950s and 1960s when higher doses of estrogen were routinely used.

The following points about ERT and breast cancer should be noted:

1 Do not administer ERT to breast cancer patients if:
  (a) estrogen receptor-positive tumors are present;
  (b) there are positive lymph nodes or metastases;
  (c) the patient is within 5 years of diagnosis;
  (d) the patient is taking tamoxifen.

2 Patients at low risk of recurrence include:
  (a) stage I patients after 5 years;
  (b) any patient who is disease-free after 10 years;
  (c) Patients with small (5 mm) intraductal carcinomas after 5 years. (With lobular carcinoma *in situ* the long-term risk of developing invasive cancer is significant.)

3 Patients should be advised that ERT may shorten the disease-free interval in breast cancer and the physician should document informed consent if ERT is used. The Food and Drug Administration requires estrogen package inserts to state that estrogens are "contraindicated" for "hormone sensitive cancers."

4 Mammograms in patients on ERT may show increased benign ductal proliferation, which can make interpretation more difficult.

ENDOMETRIAL CANCER

ERT with unopposed estrogens increases the risk of endometrial cancer several-fold. The average relative risk is two to eight times the baseline risk of one in 50 women. Of women who use unopposed estrogen for more that 10 years, 5% will develop endometrial cancer. These cancers are *not* more benign than spontaneously arising endometrial cancers of the same stage and grade, although most will be stage I, grade 1. The risk of death from ERT-related endometrial cancer is estimated at less than one in 4000 estrogen users. The addition of progestins to estrogen replacement reduces the risk of endometrial cancer to control levels, or lower. Progestins suppress cell mitoses, decrease estrogen receptor levels, increase estrogen metabolism, and promote differentiation of the endometrium to a secretory state. Recently, alarming reports of endometrial cancer in breast cancer patients receiving tamoxifen have been cited, presumably due to agonistic action on endometrial estrogen receptors [9]. Breast cancer patients are at higher risk of endometrial cancer and should be followed closely if placed on ERT at all.

Patients who undergo hysterectomy and oophorectomy and/or irradiation for endometrial cancer should have a risk profile for osteoporosis before considering estrogen replacement. Tumor estrogen and progesterone receptor status are favorable prognostic factors, independent of stage and grade, and should be considered. Many patients with endometrial cancer are obese, non-smokers, and continue to produce high enough levels of estrone, from peripheral fatty conversion of androstenedione, so that they have little risk of osteoporosis. Patients who develop vasomotor symptoms can be effectively treated with 10 mg of medroxyprogesterone acetate or 40 mg of megesterol acetate daily. Vaginal dryness and dyspareunia can often be improved with vaginal lubricants.

The use of progestins as a means of prophylaxis against cancer recurrence is of no benefit. Progestins should not be prescribed for recurrence prevention since they may alter the lipoprotein profile in an adverse way.

Two retrospective nonrandomized studies have demonstrated no increased recurrences in endometrial cancer patients at low risk who were given ERT at the discretion of their physician [10,11]. Stage I, grade 1 and 2 patients without myometrial invasion (International Federation of Gynecologists and Obstetricians (FIGO) stage IA) have less than a 5% risk of recurrence. These patients can be treated with low doses of estrogen and progestin after an arbitrary disease-free interval (6−24 months), after which the recurrence risk drops further. However, in these studies the patients chosen for ERT were selected by the authors and a randomized trial should be undertaken to confirm this preliminary recommendation. Patients who are not surgically staged and in whom

there is myometrial invasion past the inner third should not currently receive ERT (Fig. 102.1). The position of the American College of Obstetricians and Gynecologists is that estrogen replacement could be used in selected patients with favorable prognostic indicators [12].

OVARIAN CANCER

The prognosis of patients with ovarian cancer remains poor for those with advanced disease. Some 75% of ovarian cancers present with advanced disease. Since only 20% of stage III ovarian cancer patients survive for 5 years, ERT to prevent osteoporosis or atherosclerosis is not a concern in the majority of patients. However, as patients survive longer, and for patients with stage I and II disease (80% survival), ERT becomes increasingly important.

Approximately half of ovarian epithelial tumors contain estrogen and progestin receptors. However, the response rate to megesterol acetate and/or tamoxifen in ovarian cancers is between 10 and 20%, inferring some risk with estrogen stimulation. Responses have been documented in estrogen receptor-negative tumors and estrogen/progestin receptors themselves are not a prognostic indicator in ovarian cancer. Since 80% of recurrences occur in the first 2 years, waiting 2 years reduces the risk to an acceptable degree. The following recommendations seem prudent in the absence of any scientific studies:
— Stage I and II: ERT after 2 years.
— Stage III: ERT after 5 years in estrogen receptor-negative patients.
— Estrogen receptor-positive tumors: no ERT except in selected patients who are disease-free at 5 years.

ERT AFTER PELVIC IRRADIATION

Loss of ovarian function occurs after as little as 4 Gy radiation. However, even after full pelvic irradiation (50 Gy) some endometrial activity in response to estrogens can persist, though these patients are amenorrheic. Adenocarcinoma of the endometrium has been reported after pelvic radiotherapy for cervical cancer. While some authors suggest that ERT in these patients should include concomitant progestins, these relatively young women face years of potential therapy and the reduced benefit of combined therapy against cardiovascular disease should also be considered.

About 10−15% of patients with uterine sarcomas

will have had prior pelvic irradiation, and these tumors often contain estrogen receptors. However, most uterine sarcomas recur in the first 2 years. Therefore, ERT is contraindicated in patients with uterine sarcoma for 2—5 years. In patients with cellular leiomyomas and leiomyoblastomas there is no evidence of increased risk with estrogen therapy. However, these tumors may recur 5—10 years later, may recur during pregnancy, and can respond to progestins. Therefore, ERT must be considered risky in these women until further information accrues.

MALIGNANT MELANOMA

There may be a slightly increased risk of melanoma in women on OCs. About one-third of melanomas contain estrogen receptors. There was a slightly higher risk of melanoma in one study of over 20 000 women on ERT (relative risk 1.5). However, premenopausal women seem to have a slightly better prognosis than postmenopausal women or men, with the same stage and depth of tumor, suggesting a possible ameliorating effect of sex steroids. As in endometrial and breast cancer, progestin receptor-positive tumors are associated with longer survivals. Both diethylstilbestrol and tamoxifen have shown low-level activity against melanomas. Therefore, there are conflicting data about the risk of hormone therapy in melanoma patients. Until further data are available, no scientific recommendation about the safety of ERT in these patients can be made.

OTHER CANCERS

A variety of cancers, not thought to be hormonally sensitive, contain estrogen and progestin receptors, including brain tumors, colorectal cancers, sarcomas, and cervical carcinomas. Whether estrogen replacement in these patients is safe may not be known for some time. In general, ERT has not demonstrated adverse outcomes in *any* cancer patients, and should not be withheld from patients with gastrointestinal tumors, squamous cancers, or lymphomas and leukemias when there are clinical indications for therapy. OCs or estrogens are frequently useful in patients who develop uterine bleeding associated with coagulation or platelet disorders from cancer or chemotherapy.

ENDOMETRIOSIS

Malignancy arising in endometriosis is a rare event. However, several cases have developed in women given unopposed estrogens shortly after surgery for endometriosis [13]. We recommend an estrogen-free interval of several months before starting ERT if there might be residual endometriosis. No cases of malignancy arising in endometriosis have been reported in patients given a progestin in addition to ERT.

REFERENCES

1 Centers for Disease Control and Steroid Hormone Study. Oral contraceptive use and breast cancer risk. *N Engl J Med* 1987; 316: 405—409.
2 Pike MC, Henderson BE, Krailo MD, Duke A, Roy S. Breast cancer in young women and use of oral contraceptives: possible modifying effect of formulation and age at use. *Lancet* 1983; ii: 926—930.
3 Brinton LA, Hoover R, Fraumeni JF. Menopausal oestrogens and breast cancer risk: an expanded case control study. *Br J Cancer* 1986; 54: 825—832.
4 Gambrell RD. Estrogen-progestogen replacement and cancer risk. *Hosp Pract* 1990; 25: 81—100.
5 Nachtigall LE, Nachtigall RH, Nachtigall RD, Beckman EM. Estrogen replacement therapy. II. A prospective study in the relationship to carcinoma and cardiovascular and metabolic problems. *Obstet Gynecol* 1983; 62: 435—443.
6 Bergkvist L, Adami H-O, Persson I, Hoover R, Schairer C. The risk of breast cancer after estrogen and estrogen-progestin replacement. *N Engl J Med* 1989; 321: 293—297.
7 Stoll BA. Hormone replacement therapy in women treated for breast cancer. *Eur J Clin Oncol* 1989; 25: 1909—1913.
8 Dupont WD, Page DL, Rogers LW, Parl FF. Influence of exogenous estrogens, proliferative breast disease, and other variables on breast cancer risk. *Cancer* 1989; 63: 948—957.
9 Gusberg SB. Tamoxifen for breast cancer: associated endometrial cancer. *Cancer* 1990; 65: 63—64.
10 Lee RB, Burke TW, Park RC. Estrogen replacement therapy following treatment for stage I endometrial carcinoma. *Gynecol Oncol* 1990; 36: 189—191.
11 Creasman WT, Henderson D, Hinshaw W, Clarke-Pearson DL. Estrogen replacement therapy in the patient treated for endometrial cancer. *Obstet Gynecol* 1986; 67: 326—330.
12 American College of Obstetricians and Gynecologists. Estrogen Replacement Therapy and Endometrial Cancer. Washington, DC: ACOG Committee Opinion 80, 1990: 990.
13 Reimnitz C, Brand E, Hacker NF. Malignancy arising in endometriosis associated with unopposed estrogen replacement. *Obstet Gynecol* 1988; 71: 444—447.

Index